Principles and Methods
of Sterilization
in Health Sciences

Principles and Methods of Sterilization in Health Sciences

By

JOHN J. PERKINS, M.S., LL.D., F.R.S.H.

Vice President
American Sterilizer Company
Erie, Pennsylvania

Second Edition, Sixth Printing

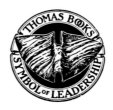

C H A R L E S C T H O M A S • P U B L I S H E R

Springfield   •   Illinois   •   U.S.A.

Published and Distributed Throughout the World by

CHARLES C THOMAS ● PUBLISHER

Bannerstone House

301-327 East Lawrence Avenue, Springfield, Illinois, U.S.A.

© *1956 and 1969, by* CHARLES C THOMAS ● PUBLISHER

ISBN 0-398-01478-7

Library of Congress Catalog Card Number: 68-20794

First Edition, First Printing, 1956
First Edition, Second Printing, 1960
First Edition, Third Printing, 1963
First Edition, Fourth Printing, 1965
Second Edition, First Printing, 1969
Second Edition, Second Printing, 1970
Second Edition, Third Printing, 1973
Second Edition, Fourth Printing, 1976
Second Edition, Fifth Printing, 1978
Second Edition, Sixth Printing, 1980

With THOMAS BOOKS *careful attention is given to all details of
manufacturing and design. It is the Publisher's desire to present books that
are satisfactory as to their physical qualities and artistic possibilities and
appropriate for their particular use.* THOMAS BOOKS *will be true to those
laws of quality that assure a good name and good will.*

Printed in the United States of America

R-1

EXCERPT:—

The mode of life of modern men is profoundly influenced by hygiene and medicine and the principles resulting from the discoveries of Pasteur. The promulgation of the Pasteurian doctrines has been an event of the highest importance to humanity. Their application rapidly led to the suppression of the great infectious diseases which periodically ravaged the civilized world, and of those endemic in each country.

—ALEXIS CARREL: *Man The Unknown*

PREFACE TO THE SECOND EDITION

TEN YEARS have elapsed since the appearance of the first edition of this book. During that time many advances have occurred in the field of sterilization, with particular emphasis upon medical-surgical applications. These developments rendered much of what had been written obsolete, and made necessary an extensive revision of the text including the graphics and illustrations. Nearly every chapter has undergone considerable change, and new knowledge relating to automation, mechanical equipment, methods, techniques, and procedures has been added.

Several sections have been reworked completely, particularly those dealing with the thermal destruction of microorganisms, processing of instruments, the central service department, and ethylene oxide gas sterilization. The impact of prepackaged, presterilized disposables on the modern hospital has been the cause for deletion or restricted treatment of certain material such as processing of surgeon's gloves, syringes and needles, and infant formulas.

Although the text and illustrations have been altered extensively, the structure of the book remains unchanged. Moreover, the general objective remains the same: to offer a coherent reference guide for sterilization practices in hospitals, clinics, laboratories, allied institutions and services. The tremendous strides being made in the field of medicine and in the hospital care of patients make it increasingly evident that decontamination, sterilization, disinfection, and environmental sanitation are subjects upon which lives depend. An adequate understanding of the many problems of sterilization, disinfection, and the aseptic barrier is a necessity for those who must shoulder the responsibility for the preparation and use of sterile supplies in our hospitals. The author has intentionally omitted any discussion on radiation sterilization for the simple reason that it is considered impractical to attempt to cover the subject in any depth in one chapter of the book. Also, equipment required for the use of high-energy ionizing radiations, whether in the form of a linear accelerator machine or a cobalt-60 source, is costly and currently impractical for installation in hospitals. An excellent source of information on radiation is the U.S. Atomic Energy Commission and Atomic Energy of Canada, Ltd.

A further word of explanation seems desirable for the large number of bibliographic references attached to the majority of the chapters. It is believed that for the serious student, the text may not be sufficient, and he should, therefore, have the opportunity of examining original papers and thoughtful reviews that give a more detailed picture.

JOHN J. PERKINS

Erie, Pennsylvania

vii

PREFACE TO THE FIRST EDITION

THIS BOOK is an attempt to integrate basic principles upon which conventional sterilizing processes depend with practical methods for the preparation and sterilization of materials and supplies. It was written primarily to serve as a reference guide for sterilization practices in hospitals, clinics, laboratories, allied institutions and services. It is in this institutional environment that we find a host of professional and nonprofessional workers daily depending upon the science of sterilization and surgical asepsis as the chief means of protecting the patient against the ravages of infectious disease. The need for helpful information on the subject is acute, particularly among operating room supervisors and central service supervisors—the key persons largely responsible for sterilization techniques in hospitals.

The goal of the author has been to systematize the study, giving all of the important principles and methods of which he is aware, at the same time keeping the work within the limits of a textbook rather than an extensive reference volume. Many important references on the subjects of sterilization and disinfection have been freely consulted. Without the long list of reference material this book should not have been written. Any subject as extensive as that of sterilization which, conservatively, covers the past seventy-five years, is not the work of a few, but many people. Scientific minds pave the way and open the door to progress, but actual advancement does not take form until industry through the designing engineer is able to build the necessary equipment. Even then, the maximum benefits of progress in sterilization are not realized by the patient until hospital personnel are thoroughly trained to apply the principles and to intelligently operate the equipment.

The question may logically arise as to whether nurses or nursing students, as a group, are sufficiently prepared to profit by the study of scientific journals and technical publications. It is the author's opinion that if nurses are to be charged with the responsibility for sterilization in hospitals they must be encouraged to read and search for pertinent reference material. Certainly it is desirable to stimulate an open-minded, questioning attitude on the part of all nurses for the subject of sterilization. The operating room supervisor and the central service supervisor particularly should realize that sterilization is an expanding subject with the constant addition of new knowledge, the discarding of old theories or their reinterpretation in the light of new experimental evidence.

For any errors, omissions or misstatements found in this book, the author must assume full responsibility. The long hours spent in the preparation of the manuscript have been a work of love rather than labor. It is hoped that it will be found useful in some measurable degree by those for whom it is intended.

ACKNOWLEDGMENTS

THE AUTHOR wishes to acknowledge his indebtedness to the American Sterilizer Company, for the generous grant of time expended in preparing the manuscript, and for permission to use the large number of photographs and diagrams from which many of the illustrations have been made. An expression of gratitude is also due the American Sterilizer Company for permission to use certain copyrighted material from the Textbook on Sterilization by the late W. B. Underwood.

Sincere thanks and appreciation are extended to the friends and colleagues of the author who have rendered valuable assistance, in particular: to Miss Edna Prickett, of the American Hospital Association, for review and criticism of the sections dealing with surgical sterilization; to Miss Marian Fox, of the American Hospital Association, and Miss Margaret Giffin, formerly of the National League of Nursing, for the opportunity to observe the everyday problems of the operating room supervisor and the central service supervisor through the medium of Institutes; to the Research Staff of the American Sterilizer Company for skillful assistance in the accumulation of material and the reading of proof.

Grateful acknowledgment is also made to the many authors whose works have been quoted in this book. Thanks are extended to the various publishers who have generously granted permission for the reproduction of illustrations and quotations from their publications. In these cases, specific acknowledgment has been made in the appropriate places throughout the text.

In the preparation of this revision, the author has profited greatly from the kind suggestions and generous technical advice received from many friends and colleagues both in the United States and abroad. It is a pleasure to record my appreciation of the help and assistance rendered by the Research and Development staff of the American Sterilizer Company; also for permission to excerpt copyrighted material from the *Journal of Hospital Research*. Grateful appreciation is extended to the following for their substantial contributions to the text and for resource information and data:

Ultrasonics—

G. G. Brown,
Senior Engineering Consultant,
American Sterilizer Company.

Ethylene Oxide—

> R. S. Lloyd, M.S.,
> Research Assistant,
> American Sterilizer Company.

Pyrogens—

> S. A. Marcus, Ph.D.,
> Department of Microbiology,
> University of Utah.

Surgical Scrubs—

> P. B. Price, M.D.,
> Emeritus Professor of Surgery,
> University of Utah.

Surgical Environment—

> Miss E. A. Prickett, B.S., R. N.,
> American Hospital Association.

Chemical Disinfection—

> E. H. Spaulding, Ph.D.,
> Department of Microbiology,
> Temple University Medical Center.

Central Service Department—

> Mrs. M. D. Young, B.S., R. N.,
> Nurse Consultant,
> American Sterilizer Company.

Special thanks are due John R. Raup for general assistance in the preparation of the manuscript, the procurement of illustrations, and the reading of proofs. Acknowledgment is also due Mrs. E. H. Garwood for her splendid assistance in the preparation of graphs, charts, and other illustrative material. Finally, the author wishes to thank his secretary, Mrs. Goldie Kreider, for devoted assistance in organizing material and for typing the many manuscript revisions.

J.J.P.

CONTENTS

Principles and Methods

of Sterilization

in Health Sciences

Chapter 1

HISTORICAL INTRODUCTION

IT HAS OFTEN been said that nothing is more difficult than the beginning. This remark seems particularly appropriate as the opening phrase to the Historical Introduction on the subject of sterilization. To be sure, one cannot claim that related material is lacking as a preparatory measure, because the literature contains a wealth of information dealing either directly or indirectly with the subject. However, any attempt to trace the origin of various practices which form the basis of our modern concept of sterilization leads eventually to the conclusion that gradual development of the art has been so closely allied with the development of microbiology that it is difficult to discuss the former without bringing into the picture more than the desirable amount of the latter. Just as the science of microbiology is said to have originated from the various attempts to solve the origin of life and the origin of death, so has the advancement of our knowledge of sterilization kept pace with each important contribution to these age-old problems of nature. To the historian, it is also evident that the many investigations and researches which have led us to our present state of knowledge on this subject, as well as that of microbiology, were actually stimulated by certain controversies and ideas originating hundreds of years before the beginning of the Christian era.

OUR ANCIENT HERITAGE

From the dawn of recorded history man appears to have practiced in one form or another the process of purification or disinfection, the latter a precursor of sterilization. The use of antiseptics such as pitch or tar, resins and aromatics was widely employed by the Egyptians in embalming bodies even before they had a written language. From the work of Herodotus[1] (484-424 B.C.), there are indications that the Egyptians were acquainted with the antiseptic value of dryness resulting from the use of certain chemicals such as niter and common salt. The fumes of burning chemicals were also used by the ancients for deodorizing and disinfecting purposes. Of early importance was sulfur, apparently the first of the useful chemicals to be mentioned. In the Odyssey[2] the following passage may be found:

> *To the nurse Eurycleia then said he:*
> *"Bring cleansing sulfur, aged dame, to me*
> *And fire, that I may purify the hall."*

The purification of premises and the destruction of noxious and infectious material by fire also seem to have originated among the Egyptians. The cremation of bodies of animals and of persons, especially in the case of war, was often resorted to by the ancients as a means of their disposal, as well as a way of destroying putrefactive odors.

Moses was the first to prescribe a system of purification by fire, and we learn from the books of Leviticus and Deuteronomy that he also developed the first system for the purification of infected premises. The stern mandates given by Moses (about 1450 B.C.) on the disposal of wastes, camp sanitation, treatment and prevention of leprosy, the touching of unclean objects or eating of unclean foods, formed the basis of the first sanitary code as established by the ancient Hebrews. It is noteworthy that they forbade tattooing (Lev. 19:28) with its attendant risk of needle-transmitted hepatitis, and it is probable that they suspected the role of flies in the transmission of disease.[3] From the precepts as laid down in the Mosaic law are based the various systems of purification of the succeeding ages.

History has recorded that the thinkers of antiquity never seem to have doubted that under favorable conditions life, both animal and vegetable, might arise spontaneously. Certain of the early Greek philosophers held the theory that animals were formed from moisture. Empedocles (450 B.C.), an early advocate of fumigation as a means of combatting epidemics, attributed to spontaneous generation all of the living beings which he found inhabiting the earth. Aristotle (384 B.C.) also asserted that "sometimes animals are formed in putrefying soil, sometimes in plants, and sometimes in the fluids of other animals." He also formulated a principle that "every dry substance which becomes moist, and every moist body which becomes dried, produces living creatures, provided it is fit to nourish them." During this era it is worthy of note that Hippocrates (460-370 B.C.), the greatest of all physicians, who was responsible for the dissociation of philosophy from medicine, recognized the importance of boiled water for irrigating wounds, the cleansing of the hands and nails of the operator, and the use of medicated dressings for wounds.

An early exponent of the germ theory of disease was Marcus Terentius Varro (117-26 B.C.), one of Caesar's more competent physicians. His *Rerum Rusticarum* contains these words: "Small creatures, invisible to the eye, fill the atmosphere, and breathed through the nose cause dangerous diseases."[4]

THE MIDDLE AGES

In the period from 900 to 1500 A.D., progress from the standpoint of noteworthy contributions having a direct bearing on the development of the art of sterilization was virtually at a standstill. For medicine this period is also regarded as an age of decadence and stagnation. Filth, pestilence, and plague ravaged all Europe in the Middle Ages. Attempts were made to combat the pestilence in hospitals, lazarettos, and infected houses by means of cleansing solutions, aeration, the smoke of burning straw, fumes of vinegar, and, not the least, by the fumes of sulfur, antimony, and arsenic. The Middle Ages witnessed the rise of the monastic infirmaries under the influence of the early Church. It is believed that the modern doctor-staffed hospitals had their true origin in these monastic infirmaries comprising patient wards, apothecary shops, and other facilities.

In 1546, Fracastorius, the world's first epidemiologist, published his famous work *De Contagione*, which dealt with airborne pestilence. He presumed the existence of imperceptible "seeds of disease which multiply rapidly." Moreover, he declared that diseases were spread in three ways: by direct contact, by handling things that infected persons had handled previously, and by transmission from a distance.[5]

THE DISCOVERY OF BACTERIA

The existence of bacteria was considered possible by many people long before their discovery. However, actual proof of their existence had to await the development and construction of a compound microscope suitable for the observation and study of forms of microbial life. For this achievement, credit must be given to Antonj van Leeuwenhoek, a Dutch linen draper, for marked perfection of lenses of short focal distance with which he was able to see for the first time some of the larger forms of bacteria. In 1683, he observed and described a great variety of microbial forms in various body fluids, intestinal discharges from animals, water, and beer with a high degree of accuracy and painstaking detail. He also made important contributions to microscopic anatomy and is regarded by certain authorities as the real discoverer of the blood corpuscles.[6] Leeuwenhoek's observations and development of the microscope provided the foundation of bacteriology and reopened the question concerning the causation of fermentation and disease.

THE DOCTRINE OF SPONTANEOUS GENERATION

Following the discovery of bacteria, the age-old question of spontaneous generation of living things again became a subject for discussion. Some few individuals did combat the theory, but the belief was general that bacteria did originate spontaneously and this belief persisted until Louis Pasteur finally settled the question with convincing experimental data in 1862. One of the early opponents of the theory was L. Spallanzani,[7,8] who in 1765 demonstrated that boiling an infusion of decomposable matter for 2 minutes did not suffice to destroy all the microbes; but when the infusion was placed in a hermetically sealed flask and boiled for an hour, no generation of microbes or fermentation occurred, so long as the flask remained sealed. Although Spallanzani proved to his own satisfaction that vegetative power does not exist in inanimate material, it was still maintained by some, notably John Needham

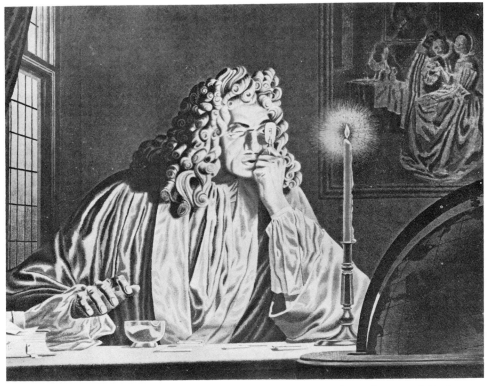

FIGURE 1-1. Antonj van Leeuwenhoek. (Courtesy Lambert Pharmacal Co.)

(1713-1781) and George Buffon (1707-1788), that the boiling process had weakened or destroyed the "vegetative force," thereby preventing spontaneous generation from taking place.

The attack on spontaneous generation was continued in 1836 by Franz Schulze,[9] who failed to find evidence of living organisms in boiled infusions to which air had been admitted only after passage through sulfuric acid. Similar experiments were conducted by Theodor Schwann,[10] in 1837, except that the air admitted to the infusions was first heated to a high temperature, but the results were the same—no evidence of fermentation or bacterial growth. In connection with the work of Schwann, it is interesting to note that he considered the process of fermentation could be arrested or inhibited by an agent capable of destroying fungi, such as heat or potassium arsenate. Because of this belief, Schwann is regarded by certain authorities as the founder of the science of disinfection.[11]

In 1854, H. Schroeder and T. von Dusch[12] made additional contributions in favor of the opposing forces to the theory of spontaneous generation. These workers employed a new technique of admitting air into flasks of boiled infusions by filtering the air through a layer or plug of cotton wool. This was

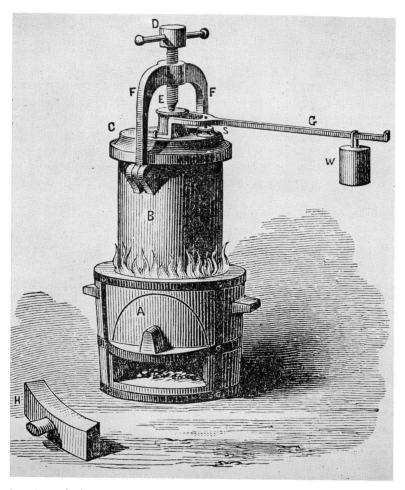

FIGURE 1-2. Papin's "Digester." Invented by Denys Papin in 1680—a collaborator of Robert Boyle in study of pneumatics. The "digester" consisted of a vessel, B, capable of being tightly closed by screw, D, and lid, C, in which food could be cooked in water raised by furnace, A, to temperature of any desired safe pressure of steam. Pressure was determined and limited by weight, W, on safety valve lever, G. Papin is given credit for having first made use of safety valve to control pressure of steam. (Courtesy Cornell Univ. Press.)

done to combat the argument against any possible change in the properties of the air which could have occurred in the experiments of Schulze and Schwann, and which might give rise to a condition unfavorable to the support of life. Although the results showed that sterile solutions were obtained by this method, it was later demonstrated that the same procedure was unsuccessful in preventing fermentation of milk, meat, or egg yolk unless these materials were subjected to prolonged boiling at 100°C, heated in an oil bath to 130°C or heated in Papin's "digester" under a pressure of 15 to 75 pounds (see Fig. 1-2).

By the year 1859 the problem of spontaneous generation was still in a state of uncertainty. The primary issue at stake was decisive proof of the presence of microbes in the atmosphere. The controversy was further aggravated by the appearance of a publication entitled *Heterogenie*, by F. A. Pouchet.[13] Apparently the author had repeated the experiments of Schulze and Schwann and his results were diametrically opposed to the findings of the earlier investigators. Pouchet also ridiculed the assumption of organisms being present in the atmosphere—a view in direct conflict with the current reasoning of Pasteur that microorganisms responsible for fermentation came from outside the fermenting material.

LOUIS PASTEUR

For an account of Pasteur's contributions to the development of the art of sterilization, it is necessary to begin with the year of 1860. Here we find Pasteur, having previously completed his brilliant researches on the microbic cause of fermentation, now ready to begin his epoch-making studies on the problem of spontaneous generation. He began his attack with a microscopic investigation of atmospheric air, and with the aid of the most ingenious devices he demonstrated that the air in different localities differed in its content of microorganisms. His paper published in 1862,[14] "On the Organized Corpuscles Existing in the Atmosphere," was destined, according to some scientific minds of that day, to remain forever as a classic. With a severity typical

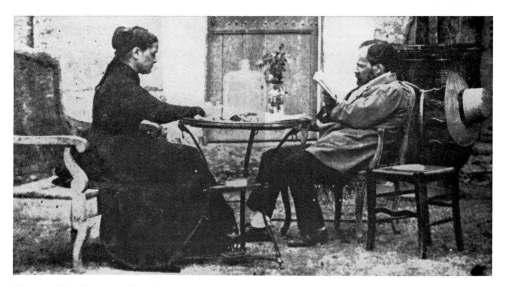

FIGURE 1-3. Pasteur dictating notes on silkworm disease to his wife (1868). (Courtesy The Upjohn Co.)

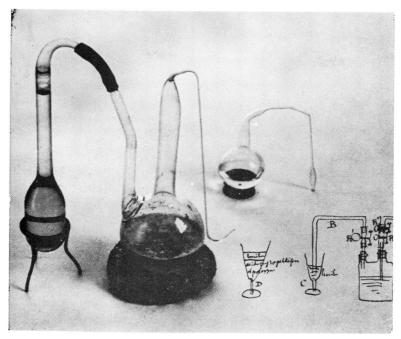

FIGURE 1-4. Pasteur's double flask for demonstrating anaerobic fermentation, and notes on the subject. In background, flask of barley water prepared and pasteurized by Pasteur in 1860. It was protected from dust, but not from air, by its long neck. It is still sterile and unfermented. (Courtesy The Upjohn Co.)

of the thoroughly disciplined experimenter, Pasteur repeated and confirmed the experiments of Schwann, Schroeder, and von Dusch. He showed that after passing air through a filter or plug of cotton wool the filter contained organized particles similar in appearance to mold spores, and if these particles were then introduced into sterilized nutritive fluids, they would induce fermentation. Finally, Pasteur showed that fermentation in boiled infusions could be prevented if the neck of the flask was drawn out and bent in a simulated U tube form, so that microorganisms and dust particles present in the air could enter the open end of the U tube, but then due to the absence of air currents the microorganisms were unable to ascend the other arm of the tube to reach the contents of the flask. With this type of flask, he also showed that fermentation could be immediately induced by tilting the apparatus so as to permit the infusion to contact the organisms deposited in the bent arm of the U tube. In brief, this experiment constituted the greatest blow yet delivered against the doctrine of spontaneous generation.

The importance attached to this phase of Pasteur's work can best be summarized by saying that, where previous investigators had concerned themselves with experiments to demonstrate the absence of fermentation in sterilized infusions in contact with germ-free air, he not only did this, but also proved that the microorganisms present in the air were unquestionably responsible for the changes which occurred in his sterilized infusions. In the words of W. W. Ford:[15]

> The great practical result of this phase of Pasteur's work is not so much that he finally settled the controversy regarding spontaneous generation, but that his observations on the pollution of the atmosphere by bacteria paved the way for Lister's antiseptic surgery which has revolutionized surgical practice throughout the world.

One of the last defenders of spontaneous generation was the English physician Bastian. In 1876, he attacked the previous work of Pasteur in which it had been stated that urine, sterilized by boiling, did not undergo fermentation or show evidence of bacterial growth upon incubation. Bastian claimed that such sterility was attainable only under certain conditions, and if the urine were made alkaline in the beginning, bacterial growth would frequently take place. This led Pasteur to reconsider certain phases of his past work, and together with his collaborators, Joubert and Chamberland, he repeated and confirmed Bastian's experiments. As the result, it was demonstrated that liquids with an acid reaction could be rendered *apparently sterile* by boiling, because certain organisms not destroyed by the process were unable later to develop in the notably acid media; but if the liquids were made slightly alkaline beforehand, the surviving bacteria would grow and multiply freely.

This controversy with Bastian finally led to the establishment of the fact that certain microbes exist in nature which are capable of resisting prolonged boiling at 100°C; for example, the spores of *B. subtilis,* discovered by Cohn in 1876.[16] Where formerly Pasteur had been content to boil his liquids, he was now forced to heat them to a temperature of from 108° to 120°C in order to insure sterility. The custom of raising liquids to a temperature of 120°C in order to sterilize them dates from that conflict with Bastian.[17]

In addition, other articles common to sterile technique, such as glassware, vessels, and tubes, were required to be put through a flame at a temperature of from 150° to 200°C. Vallery-Radot[18] has given Pasteur's definition of what he meant by putting glass receptacles, tubes, and cotton through a flame:

> In order to get rid of the microscopic germs which the dusts of air and of the water used for the washing of vessels deposit on every object, the best means is to place the vessels (their openings closed with pads of cotton wool) during half an hour in a gas stove, heating the air in which the articles stand to a temperature of about 150° to 200°C. The vessels, tubes, *et cetera* are then ready for use. The cotton wool is enclosed in tubes or in blotting paper.

To meet the requirement of more effective methods of sterilization at

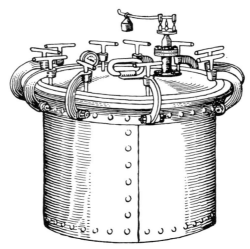

FIGURE 1-5. Chamberland's Autoclave. The first pressure steam sterilizer (autoclave) was built in 1880 by Charles Chamberland, a pupil and collaborator of Louis Pasteur. It was patterned after Papin's steam "digester" and resembled a modern pressure cooker. Chamberland also invented the porcelain bacterial filter.

temperatures higher than boiling demanded of Pasteur the invention of new apparatus. During this period (1876-1880) of marked advances in bacteriological technique, Pasteur's pupil and collaborator, Charles Chamberland,[19] developed the first pressure steam sterilizer, or autoclave, with which it was possible to attain temperatures of 120°C and higher (Fig. 1-5). This sterilizer was patterned after the steam "digester" invented by the French physicist, Denys Papin, in 1680 (Fig. 1-2). It resembled the modern pressure cooker, with the cover held in place by means of toggle bolts. It was equipped with a safety valve and a small pet cock in the cover which could be opened for expulsion of air as pressure developed from heating. It contained a small quantity of water and the materials to be sterilized were suspended above on a rack. Although this sterilizer, which became known as Chamberland's Autoclave, an indispensable apparatus for hospitals and laboratories, was criticized later by the German school and other investigators because the higher and more uncertain temperatures developed were harmful to heat-sensitive forms of media, it did, nevertheless, usually sterilize in one performance, and it must be considered as the "father" of our modern precision sterilizers.

Pasteur's researches were not restricted to fermentation or to the settlement of the spontaneous generation theory. Of even greater importance were his accomplishments culminating in the establishment and laboratory verification of the true germ theory of disease. This, however, is a story so well known and so competently recorded in the literature that it would be an injustice to attempt to recount the events in the limited space available. Perhaps it will suffice to say that, in the author's opinion, the literature records no greater contribution to the development of applied sterilization than the statement made by Louis Pasteur in his celebrated lecture on the germ theory, delivered on April 30, 1878, before the Academie de Médecine:[20]

> If I had the honour of being a surgeon, convinced as I am of the dangers caused by the germs of microbes scattered on the surface of every object, particularly in the hospitals, not only would I use absolutely clean instruments, but, after cleansing my hands with the greatest care and putting them quickly through a flame (an easy thing to do with a little practice), I would only make use of charpie, bandages, and sponges which had previously been raised to a heat of 130°C to 150°C; I would only employ water which had been heated to a temperature of 110°C to 120°C. All that is easy in practice, and, in that way, I should still have to fear the germs suspended in the atmosphere surrounding the bed of the patient; but observation shows us every day that the number of these germs is almost insignificant compared to that of those which lie scattered on the surface of objects, or in the clearest ordinary water.

MICROBE AND MICROBIOLOGY

In 1878, Charles Sedillot, a French surgeon, introduced the term *microbe* during the course of a discussion in the Paris Academy of Medicine.[21] His intention was to initiate a term suitable for describing any living organism so small as to be visible only under a microscope. In the scientific community the term *microbe* has not been popular—having given way to *microorganism* with a more sophisticated appeal. Pasteur also considered that the term *bacteriology* was much too limited, and he suggested that the newly developing science should be called *microbiology*.

IGNAZ SEMMELWEIS

One of the early crusaders for the development of the aseptic barrier was a Hungarian obstetrician, Ignaz Semmelweis. Although he knew little about the causative germs of disease, it is important to recognize that he preached asepsis from an empirical point of view and unquestionably saved the lives of many women from the ravages of puerperal fever.

In 1847, at the maternity hospital in Vienna, Semmelweis instituted a strict rule that all students should wash their hands in a chloride of lime solution and scrub their fingernails with a brush before entering the ward and carrying out internal examinations on women. By this simple measure the mortality rate on his wards was reduced from 18 per cent in 1847 to 1.27 per cent of the 3,556 patients delivered in 1848.[22,23] The remarkable success of Semmelweis in preventing infection in parturient women unfortunately estranged him from his colleagues in both Vienna and Budapest. To boldly assert, as he did, that the dirty hands of doctors were transmitting disease to women patients was an affront to professional pride and his position became untenable. In 1861, Semmelweis published *The Cause and Prevention of Puerperal Fever*, but he was unsuccessful in convincing his critics of the necessity of washing hands before contacting parturient patients.

THE DISCOVERY OF THE HEAT RESISTANCE OF BACTERIA

Any history of sterilization would be considered incomplete unless something more than passing recognition were given to the discovery of the heat resistant phases of bacteria. For this enduring contribution we are indebted to the English physicist, John Tyndall. In 1876,[24] he made his entry into this field with a series of researches devoted to the phenomena of fermentation and putrefaction. Prior to this time, Tyndall had concerned himself with the problem of atmospheric germs and dust, and by means of a concentrated beam of light he developed a most searching test for suspended matter both in air and in water. He firmly believed that microorganisms present in the air were associated with dust particles. With the aid of an ingenious wooden chamber fitted with a glass front and side windows through which was passed a beam of light, he demonstrated that dust-free air which did not scatter the beam of light would not initiate growth in tubes of boiled infusions exposed to it.

Further studies made by Tyndall revealed that infusions prepared from old dried hay were far more difficult to sterilize by boiling than those prepared from fresh hay.[25] This observation led him to investigate extensively the heat resistance of bacteria. From numerous exacting experiments, he finally concluded that at certain times in the life history of organisms they developed heat resistant phases in which they were most difficult to kill even by prolonged boiling. This heat-resistant (spore) stage of bacteria was also recognized by Pasteur and independently discovered by the German botanist, Ferdinand Cohn, in 1876.[16] Typical of Tyndall's conclusions on this subject is the following quotation taken from one of his detached essays:[26]

> As regards their power of resisting heat, the infusorial germs of our atmosphere might be classified under the following and intermediate heads: Killed in 5 minutes; not killed in 5 minutes but killed in 15; not killed in 15 minutes but killed in 30; not killed in 30 minutes but killed in an hour; not killed in an hour but killed in 2 hours; not killed in 2 but killed in 3 hours; not killed in 3 but killed in 4 hours. I have had several cases of survival after 4 and 5 hours' boiling, some survival after 6, and 1 after 8 hours' boiling. Thus far has experiment actually reached; but there is no valid warrant for fixing upon even 8 hours as the extreme limit of vital resistance. Probably more extended researches (though mine have been very extensive) would reveal germs more obstinate still. It is also certain that we might begin earlier and find germs which are destroyed by a temperature far below that of boiling water. In the presence of such facts, to speak of

a death-point of bacteria and their germs would be unmeaning—but of this more anon.

It is also apparent from Tyndall's publications that he was quite aware of the role played by moisture in the growth and destruction of bacteria. His early analysis of the importance of prompt interchange of moisture (wetting action) from the surrounding liquid to the bacterial cell for destruction is strikingly similar to present day theory advanced in explanation of bacterial destruction by means of moist heat. In one of his papers published in 1877, there appears the following remark:[27]

> It is not difficult to see that the surface of a seed or germ may be so affected by desiccation and other causes as practically to prevent contact between it and the surrounding liquid. The body of a germ, moreover, may be so indurated by time and dryness as to resist powerfully the insinuation of water between its constituent molecules. It would be difficult to cause such a germ to imbibe the moisture necessary to produce the swelling and softening which precede its destruction in a liquid of high temperature.

Tyndall is probably best known and generally recognized as the originator of the method of *fractional sterilization* by discontinuous (intermittent) heating. This method was originally developed as a practical means of sterilizing infusions containing heat-resistant forms of bacteria. The process involved heating the infusions to the boiling point on five consecutive occasions with appropriate intervals of holding at room temperature (10, 12, or 24 hours) in between each period of heating. The purpose of the intervals of holding between the heating periods was to allow sufficient time for the resistant bacterial spores to change or germinate into the more susceptible vegetative stage. Tyndall[28] has described the process as follows:

> An infusion infected with the most powerfully resistant germs, but otherwise protected against the floating matters of the air, is gradually raised to its boiling point. Such germs as have reached the soft and plastic state immediately preceding their development into bacteria are thus destroyed. The infusion is then put aside in a warm room for 10 or 12 hours. If for 24, we might have the liquid charged with well-developed bacteria. To anticipate this, at the end of 10 or 12 hours we raise the infusion a second time to the boiling temperature, which, as before, destroys all germs then approaching their point of final development. The infusion is again put aside for 10 or 12 hours, and the process of heating is repeated. We thus kill the germs *in the order of their resistance,* and finally kill the last of them. No infusion can withstand this process if it be repeated a sufficient number of times.

Fractional sterilization, which later became known as tyndallization, was actually the forerunner of developments leading up to the nonpressure steamer type sterilizer (Fig. 1-7) devised by Robert Koch and his associates in 1880-1881. The process of tyndallization constituted an important advance in the development of practical sterilizing methods. Its usefulness and popularity can best be judged by the fact that to this day the procedure is followed in many laboratories for the sterilization of heat-sensitive media by steaming for 30 minutes on 3 consecutive days. From his experimental findings in the sterilization of organic infusions, Tyndall concluded that in the life history of certain bacteria there may exist two distinct phases: one, thermolabile; the other, incredibly thermostable. In retrospect, it seems unfortunate that his name is not more closely associated with Pasteur and Lister as well as the early history of bacteriology, putrefaction, and wound infection.

JOSEPH LISTER AND ANTISEPTIC SURGERY

Lord Joseph Lister has been recognized the world over as the Father of Antiseptic Surgery. His work is too well known to justify any extensive presentation of his achievements here. Without doubt he was the first surgeon to employ a chemical disinfectant for the maintenance of an antiseptic atmosphere designed to prevent the entrance of bacteria into surgical wounds. Lister's antiseptic system was prescribed long before the germ theory had been accepted. In fact, it was toward the end of 1864 that he first became interested in Pasteur's work on the causes of fermentation and putrefaction. After carefully repeating and confirming many of Pasteur's experiments, Lister conceived the theory that airborne bacteria are responsible for suppuration and putrefaction in operative wounds. This led him to the formulation of certain principles which ultimately comprised the basis of the antiseptic system.[29,30]

> Germs must be prevented from entering the wound during or after operation.
> If germs are present in the wound, they must be prevented from spreading after operation.
> Germs on the outside or surrounding the wound should be destroyed.
> All instruments, dressings, and everything else in contact with the operation, including the hands of surgeon and assistants, should be rendered antiseptic.

In order to carry out the principles of the antiseptic system, Lister was obliged to develop suitable methods and materials. In his search of chemical compounds as a possible means of destroying bacteria, his attention was directed to a newspaper account describing the use of carbolic acid for the destruction of sewage in the town of Carlisle, near Glasgow. He immediately recognized this antiseptic as peculiarly adapted to his experiments. His first application of the antiseptic principles occurred in March 1865, Glasgow Royal Infirmary, in a case of compound fracture. The air about the wound was subjected to a fine spray of carbolic acid solution. Also, the hands, instruments, and ligatures were washed and soaked in the same solution. Although this first test of the antiseptic system proved unsuccessful, Lister attributed it

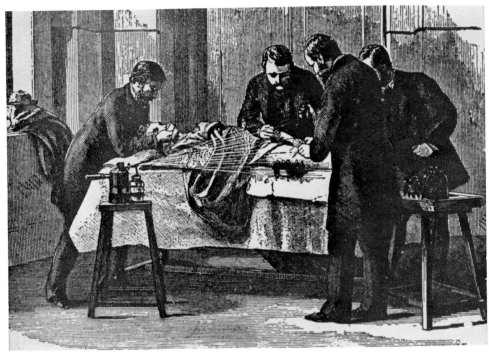

FIGURE 1-6. Lister operating with carbolic spray. (Courtesy W. B. Saunders Co.)

to improper management. Then followed a long series of experiments with repeated attempts at improvement of dressings and techniques that would permit more effective application of the antiseptic principles. Finally, in 1867 his first papers, "On the Antiseptic Principle in the Practice of Surgery," appeared in *Lancet*.[29,31] Here it was recorded that with the application of the antiseptic treatment his mortality in cases of compound fracture was reduced from 45 per cent to 9 per cent—a remarkable stride toward the elimination of postoperative sepsis.

It is to Lister that full credit must be given for an organized system of antiseptic surgery—the basis upon which our modern aseptic surgery has been founded. He is responsible for introducing the sterilization of instruments, dressings, glassware, and other supplies used in the operating room. Although equipment and methods employed in modern surgery differ greatly from those used by Lister, it should not be forgotten that the original listerian principles remain as inviolable today as when they were first proclaimed. To emphasize the necessity of becoming bacteriology-minded, Lister offered the following advice:[32,33]

> In order, gentlemen, that you may get satisfactory results from this sort of treatment, you must be able to see with your mental eye the septic fer-

ments as distinctly as we see flies or other insects with the corporeal eye. If you can really see them in this distinct way with your intellectual eye, you can be properly on your guard against them; if you do not see them you will be constantly liable to relax in your precautions.

It is of interest to note that Lister did not introduce the term antiseptic. Robinson[34] has stated that "perhaps the first who used it was the wholly unknown Place, who wrote in his *Hypothetical Notion of the Plague* (1712): 'As this phenomenon shows the motion of the pestilential poison to be putrefactive, it makes the use of (antiseptics) a reasonable way to oppose it, and whatever resists and is preservative against putrefaction, admits not of the generation of insects.' In the next generation, Sir John Pringle, father of military sanitation, published his important *Experiments upon Aseptic and Antiseptic Substances* (1750). By this time the word was evidently familiar to the public, for it occurs in the *Gentlemen's Magazine* (1751): 'Myrrh in a watery solution is twelve times more antiseptic than sea salt.' Yet over a hundred years later, Lister had to begin at the beginning."

It is a rather remarkable fact that Lister's extensively practical results were secured, in the destruction of bacteria in his surgical work, with no definite knowledge of pathogenic bacteria. To be sure, Pasteur and others had suggested the relationship between bacteria and infection, but no one had proved that relationship. A great part of Lister's presentation occurred in the eighteen-sixties; while it was not until 1876 that Robert Koch was able for the first time to cultivate artificially, outside the body, a pathogenic organism (anthrax) and to produce the disease in animals with his cultures. Shortly thereafter Pasteur was able to confirm all of Koch's observations, and in 1878, in association with Joubert and Chamberland, he threw his great influence in favor of the thesis that all infectious disease is caused by the growth of microorganisms within the body.

CONTRIBUTIONS FROM THE GERMAN SCHOOL

The researches of Koch and his associates in 1881 on the disinfecting properties of steam and hot air mark the beginning of the science of disinfection and sterilization. In collaboration with Wolffhügel,[35] Koch demonstrated that there was a marked difference in the effect of dry heat on bacteria as contrasted with that of moist heat. These investigators determined that dry heat at a temperature of 100°C would destroy vegetative bacteria in 1½ hours, but the more resistant spores (anthrax) required a temperature of 140°C for 3 hours in order to insure their destruction. In conjunction with Gaffky and Loeffler,[36] Koch also investigated the germicidal action of moist heat. This study showed that the spores of anthrax were destroyed in boiling water at 100°C in 1 to 12 minutes. It is certain that Koch was not impressed with dry heat as an efficient method of sterilization because in one of his experiments he demonstrated clearly the greater powers of penetration of moist

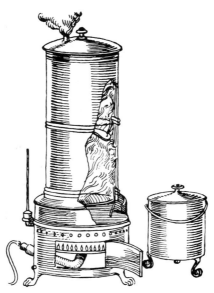

FIGURE 1-7. Nonpressure steamer type sterilizer devised by Robert Koch and his associates in 1880-1881. It was utilized broadly by Germans for intermittent or fractional sterilization of media.

heat. This particular experiment has been summarized by Zinsser[37] as follows:

> Small packages of garden soil were surrounded by varying thicknesses of linen with thermometers so placed that the temperature under a definite number of layers could be determined. Exposure to hot air and to steam were then made for comparison, and the results were as tabulated:

| Temperature | Time of Application Hours | Temperatures Reached Within Thickness of Linen | | | Results |
		20 Thickness	*40 Thickness*	*100 Thickness*	
Hot Air 130°–140°C	4	86°C	72°C	Below 70°C	Incomplete Sterilization
Steam 90°–105.3°C	3	101°C	101°C	101.5°C	Complete Sterilization

The German school seems to have preferred the nonpressure steamer type sterilizer for the sterilization of media by the fractional or intermittent process. This may have been due, in part, to the difficulties experienced with the early models of autoclaves of the Chamberland type developed by Pasteur and his group. In any event, it is known that Koch and his associates devised the first nonpressure flowing steam sterilizer in 1881, and studied its bactericidal value (Fig. 1-7). In brief, it consisted of a metal cylinder in which water was heated through the bottom by a gas flame, the resulting steam enveloping shelves above the water on which materials were placed. It should not be

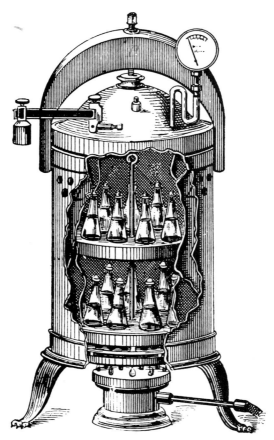

FIGURE 1-8. Early modification of Pasteur-Chamberland type of laboratory autoclave, probably of German make. It had improved type of cover lock and was equipped with pressure gauge but no thermometer. There was no apparent means for expelling air from chamber. Steam was generated from water contained in bottom of chamber and heated by gas flame.

construed, however, that interest on the part of the German school was confined solely to the development and usage of the nonpressure sterilizer. On the contrary, Koch and other workers showed that steam under pressure is a more efficient sterilizing agent than steam at atmospheric pressure. Also, one may gather from the literature of the first sterilizer manufacturers that the original autoclave of the Pasteur-Chamberland type underwent early modification at the hands of the Germans, and later became known as the Koch (Upright) Autoclave (Fig. 1-8).

Koch also developed methods and equipment for the disinfection of clothing. In this application he likewise found moist heat to be superior to dry heat because of its greater penetrating power. His studies revealed that upon exposing a roll of flannel contaminated with spores to dry heat at 140 to

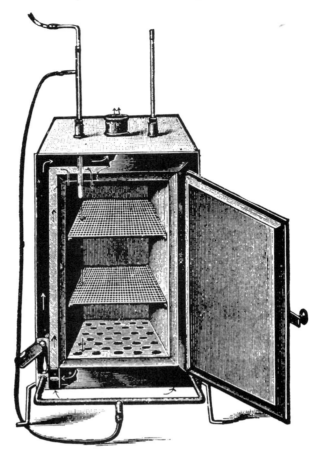

Figure 1-9. One of the early types of hot air sterilizers used in bacteriological laboratories in the 1890's. It was patterned after design developed by the German school, double walled, gas heated, in which an attempt was made to circulate heated air by gravity convection. Relatively it served its purpose to much greater advantage than steam sterilizers of that day because actual temperature of heated air was measured by thermometer.

150°C for 4 hours, the temperature inside the roll was only 83°C, and the contained spores germinated freely. When the flannel was exposed to moist heat at 120°C for 1½ hours, the temperature inside the roll was 117°C, and all the spores were destroyed. The apparatus shown in Figure 1-11 is typical of a flowing steam disinfector for clothing constructed according to Koch's specifications by the firm of W. Budenberg, Dortmund, for the King's Government at Arnsberg in 1888.

Although Ernst von Bergmann (1836-1907) is sometimes credited with having introduced steam sterilization into surgery, it has been pointed out by Walter,[38] in his discussion on the development of the concept of asepsis, that

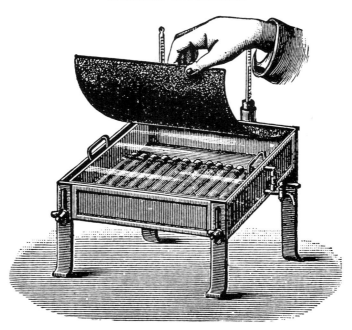

FIGURE 1-10. Koch's Inspissator. Water bath type of apparatus developed for coagulation and sterilization of blood serum media. Temperature was maintained at 60°C (140°F) or higher for one hour on each of 5 or 6 consecutive days.

Schimmelbusch, one of von Bergmann's assistants, first used the steam sterilizer for the sterilization of surgical dressings in 1885. Apparently Schimmelbusch devoted much of his time and efforts to the establishment of a highly formalized pattern of operating room asepsis. He also recommended the addition of alkali (1% sodium carbonate) to boiling water for the sterilization of instruments in order to prevent corrosion and to increase its bactericidal value. On this same subject, it is interesting to note that Hugo Davidsohn, another of Koch's assistants, first demonstrated in 1888[39] the practicality of boiling water as a means of sterilizing surgical instruments.

Following the discoveries and advances made by Robert Koch in the etiology of wound infections and in bacteriologic technic, other workers made significant contributions to the science of disinfection and sterilization. Von Esmarch,[40] for example, emphasized the great practical importance of using saturated steam containing the maximum amount of water vapor in all methods of steam sterilization. Max Rubner[41] also proved that the bactericidal effect of steam is diminished in proportion to the amount of air present in the sterilizer. From the literature it is evident that during the period of 1885 to 1900 the Germans made many notable contributions to the principles governing steam sterilization and chemical disinfection. Widespread application of these principles, including their adaptation to sterilizing equipment, did not,

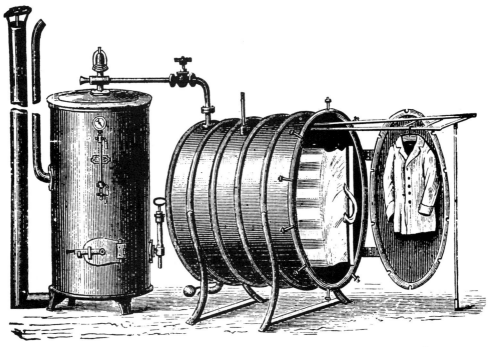

FIGURE 1-11. The Budenberg Steam Disinfector, built in 1888 by W. Budenberg, Dortmund, Germany, according to specifications of Koch and his associates. The assembly consisted of small boiler for generation of low pressure steam to which was connected an oval-shaped disinfecting chamber. It was used for disinfection of clothing and mattresses by means of flowing steam.

however, take place until some thirty years later with the introduction of the modern temperature-controlled sterilizer—a product of American manufacturers.

AERIAL OR GASEOUS DISINFECTION

From the discovery of formaldehyde gas by Von Hoffman in 1867 until about 1888, the only gaseous agents used for disinfection of dwellings, clothing, *et cetera* were sulfurous acid, chlorine, hydrocyanic acid, oxygen, ozone, and nitric acid fumes. In the year of 1888, Blum and Loew[42] demonstrated the disinfecting properties of formaldehyde. Later, Buchner discovered that a 10% solution of the gas would destroy anthrax spores. This period may be said to be the beginning of formaldehyde disinfection, but it remained for Walter, Miquel,[42] and others to point out the real bactericidal properties and to partially determine its range of usefulness as a disinfecting agent.

In Germany, the Breslau method of formaldehyde disinfection was widely employed.[43] The formaldehyde gas was generated by evaporation of a dilute formalin solution and in such a manner that polymerization did not occur.

Flügge,[44] in 1898, detailed the requisites of a practical gaseous disinfectant as follows:

1. It should be producible in a fixed and controllable concentration with ease and certainty, and such concentration should be sufficient to destroy the disease germs with certainty and within a definite time.
2. A practically useful disinfectant must penetrate objects exposed to it to a certain extent; mere destruction of the superficially located disease germs is not enough.
3. The disinfectant must not damage the articles exposed to it, and it must not leave any odor behind which would interfere with the use of the room or anything in it after the process is completed.
4. The price of the disinfectant must be relatively small.

The term *aerial disinfection* was employed to mean the use of the air as a vehicle for diffusing a gaseous germicide to all exposed surfaces of a room and its contents. In this connection it is interesting to note that Rosenau[45] in his standard work *Disinfection and Disinfectants* (1902) stated:

A gas is the ideal weapon for destroying such an invisible foe as the infection of the communicable diseases, but the ideal gas for this purpose is still to be discovered. By reaching all portions of a room or confined space, it lessens the risk of overlooking any surface upon which the infective agent may be lodged. Germicidal solutions are difficult to apply to all the surfaces of an ordinary room, and it is furthermore difficult to hold the solution in contact with the ceiling, walls, and other surfaces a sufficient length of time in order to obtain the certain action of the substance. There is practically only one gas suitable for general application—*viz.* formaldehyde. This substance comes nearer to being an ideal disinfectant than any of the gases so far exploited. It is not poisonous, does not injure fabrics, colors, metals, or objects of art and value.

EARLY AMERICAN DEVELOPMENTS IN STERILIZATION

During the period of brilliant researches and discoveries in bacteriology in Europe, workers in this country were also engaged in furthering progress in the same field. By 1890, the new science of bacteriology had become well known in the United States. It is believed that Thomas J. Burrill (1839-1916) first introduced the study of bacteriology into this country at the University of Illinois sometime in the seventies.[46] Perhaps the earliest contributor to the subject of disinfection and sterilization was George M. Sternberg, who in 1878 conducted experiments on the evaluation of certain commercial disinfectants including chlorine. He also studied the thermal death point of pathogenic bacteria[47] and determined that nonspore-bearing organisms were killed in 10 minutes' exposure to a temperature of 62° to 70°C (143.6°-158°F) and spore bearers were destroyed in 5 minutes exposure to moist heat at 100°C (212°F).

Much of the bacteriological apparatus and sterilizing equipment used by the early American bacteriologists was brought to this country from Europe. Precise records of the early sterilizers produced in the United States seem not to exist, but certain it is that sometime prior to 1895 the industry of sterilizer manufacture had its origin. The best records available to the author have been taken from a publication entitled:

Pressure Sterilization
THE NECESSITY TO THE BEST RESULTS IN
ASEPTIC SURGERY

SPRAGUE-SCHUYLER COMPANY
Works: Rochester, N.Y., Main Office: 136 Liberty St., New York City
(Dated 1895)

Pertinent information may be gathered from the introduction to this brochure with respect to the first comprehensive installations of sterilizers in hospitals in this country:

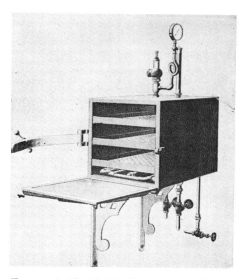 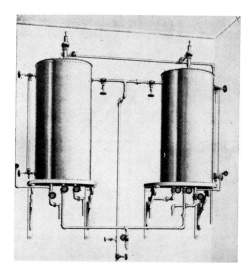

FIGURE 1-12. (*left*) This rectangular dressing sterilizer was part of group installed at City Hospital, Rochester, N.Y., in 1890. It was described by the producers, Sprague-Schuyler Co., as "The first complete plant for pressure sterilization of surgical appliances in the history of the art." The sterilizer was heated by direct steam from institution's service lines. Chamber had dimensions of 15″ × 15″ × 20″ long and was made of cast bronze, highly polished. Fittings included a thermometer, pressure gauge and safety relief valve.

FIGURE 1-13. (right) Pair of steam-heated pressure water sterilizers, 25 gallons capacity, part of group mentioned in Fig. 1-12, installed at City Hospital, Rochester, N.Y., in 1890. Water filters were not provided and there were no thermometers or pressure gauges. Evidently the control necessitated blowing of safety valves to indicate adequate pressure. Certainly these were among the first pressure water sterilizers used in this country.

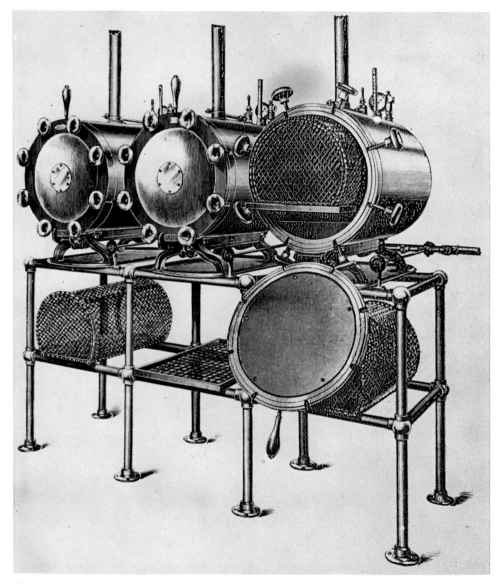

FIGURE 1-14. Group of three dressing sterilizers installed in 1892 in W. J. Syms Surgical Theatre, Roosevelt Hospital, New York City, produced by Sprague-Schuyler Co. They were heated by steam direct from service lines and equipped with pressure gauges and thermometers located in extreme tops of chambers.

The first complete plant for pressure sterilization of surgical appliances in the history of the art was installed in the Whitbeck Memorial Surgical Pavilion, connected with the Rochester City Hospital, Rochester, New York, in the year 1890, by A. V. M. Sprague, and is now in daily use, and appreciated as an invaluable auxiliary to their work. We illustrate the sterilizers for surgical dressings, for water, and the irrigation outfit employed (see Figs. 1-12 and 1-13. In the year 1892 we installed in the W. J. Syms Surgical Theatre, Roosevelt Hospital, New York City, an object lesson for the world in the way of a perfect plant for sterilization under pressure. Embraced in this outfit are two tanks for the sterilization of water, each having a capacity of 100 gallons; six of our No. 3 horizontal dressing sterilizers; two special instrument sterilizers; besides the innumerable small items by aid of which the operations are carried on, and the articles processed safely and conveniently (refer to Figs. 1-14, 1-15, and 1-16).

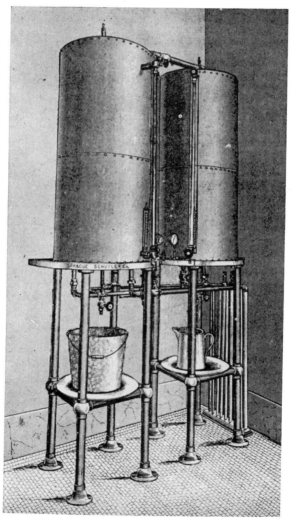

FIGURE 1-15. These water sterilizers were also installed in the W. J. Syms Surgical Theatre, Roosevelt Hospital, New York City, in 1892. Tanks were equipped with thermometers and pressure gauges but no water or air filters.

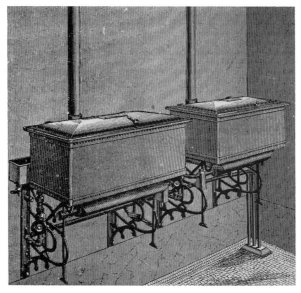

FIGURE 1-16. Pair of instrument sterilizers (boilers) on wall brackets, heated by gas. Installed in Roosevelt Hospital, New York City, in 1892 by Sprague-Schuyler Co. Covers were elevated by hand and chambers were vented for disposal of excess steam.

Historically, it is known that the major parts of the Sprague-Schuyler Company sterilizers were built by the Shipman Engine Company of Rochester, hence the reference to "Works: Rochester, N. Y." This latter firm, together with the Sprague sterilizer patents, was taken over early in the 1900's by J. E. and G. F. Hall, the founders of the American Sterilizer Company, Erie, Pennsylvania. These men originally began their activities under the name of Hall Bros. in 1894. It is also known that the Sprague-Schuyler Company and another pioneer producer in this field, the Kny-Scheerer Company of New York (1888), were responsible for the introduction of the steam-tight radial-locking-arm door on pressure sterilizers—a door which could be opened or closed simply by the manipulation of a single handwheel. Figure 1-17 illustrates this feature.

Another early contributor to the sterilizer industry was the Wilmot Castle Company,[48] which began operations in 1883 by producing the Arnold steam cooker, which was later transformed into the Arnold (flowing steam) sterilizer (Fig. 1-18). This device and modifications thereof have continued throughout the years as a popular means of sterilization of heat-sensitive forms of media in laboratories. The Arnold sterilizer largely replaced the non-pressure steamer devised by Koch and his associates.

A significant advance in the development of sterilization in this country came about through the introduction of the Kinyoun-Francis steam and formaldehyde disinfecting chamber (Fig. 1-22). The fundamental principles

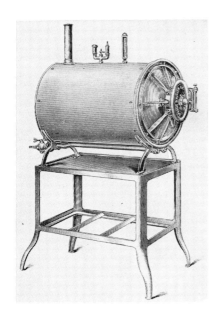

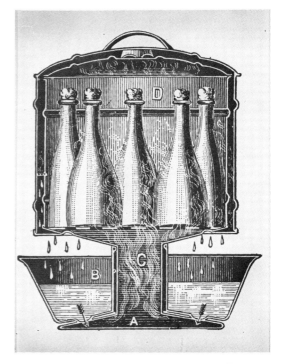

FIGURE 1-17. (*left*) Early type of horizontal pressure sterilizer, known as Kny-Sprague Steam Sterilizer. This type was steam jacketed and water from which steam was generated was contained in jacket to which heat was applied directly. No precise system of air elimination was provided. A pressure gauge was furnished but no thermometer. The door was one of the first equipped with radial arms for locking.

FIGURE 1-18. (*right*) Early form of Arnold flowing steam sterilizer, modified from original steam cooker invented by W. E. Arnold in 1883. This constituted an improvement on Koch's nonpressure steamer. Water placed in the reservoir B, flowed into shallow receptacle A, formed by the double bottom. Upon applying flame to the bottom, steam was generated in area C, and circulated through main chamber D. Steam escaped through lid at top of chamber and condensed under outer hood and ran back into reservoir.

and design of this equipment were conceived and developed by J. J. Kinyoun, Past Assistant Surgeon of the U. S. Public Health and Marine Hospital Service, working in conjunction with W. H. Francis, one of the founders of the Kensington Engine Works Co., Philadelphia. In 1888, on the recommendation of Kinyoun,[49] the Louisiana Quarantine Board constructed the first steam chamber in the United States for the application of steam under a pressure of 1 to 2 atmospheres, to be used for the disinfection of garments, mattresses, bedding. Prior to this time the only bulk disinfecting apparatus available was of the Dumond, or French model, type, constructed for operation at a maxi-

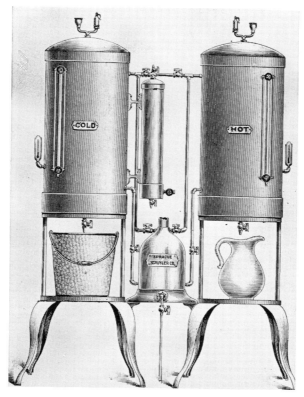

FIGURE 1-19. Typical water sterilizers produced in 1895. Here for the first time we find evidence of attempt to filter air drawn in, as water was drawn out. Small cup located on top of each tank, fitted with check valve, prevented escape of steam under pressure and also opened to let air in, as water was withdrawn. These cups were supposedly filled with fresh cotton daily for air filtration. Actually, they were more hazardous than helpful. Tanks were equipped with thermometers, water filter containing granulated quartz rock and animal charcoal as filtering medium, and combination gas heater. Sterilization was accomplished by maintaining water at 116°C (240°F) for 15 minutes.

mum steam pressure of 7 pounds, equivalent to 111°C. The Dumond disinfector, as shown in Figure 1-21, consisted of a cylinder (4½ feet in diameter by 7 feet in length), equipped with a door at either end. It was also equipped with heating coils or radiators on top and bottom of chamber to maintain temperature of the desired degree without condensation of the steam in the chamber. Steam was admitted to the chamber by means of a perforated pipe extending the whole length of the cylinder.

Kinyoun devoted considerable time to remedying defects of the early steam disinfectors. The pattern which he eventually recommended consisted of an oblong cylinder, jacketed, with an outer and inner shell instead of heating

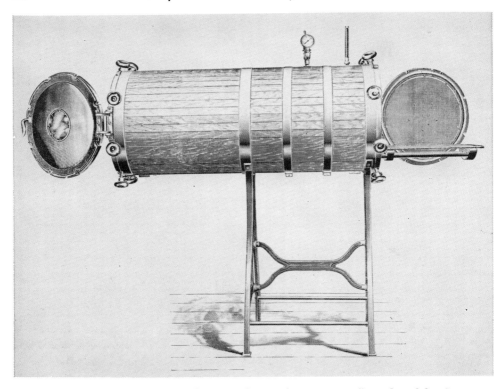

FIGURE 1-20. A "Combined Sterilizing and Disinfecting Oven," produced by Sprague-Schuyler Co. in 1895. Apparatus was steam jacketed and outer walls were insulated with hardwood strips. Doors were provided at each end of oven, the design being to receive contaminated articles at one end and remove them, following disinfection, at other end. It was arranged for recessing—a feature which apparently had its origin with the German school.

coils, and the entrance of steam at the top of the chamber rather than the bottom. By this system it was claimed that the currents of steam in the chamber could be easily controlled. A partial vacuum was also recommended for the rapid removal of air from the chamber prior to the introduction of steam.

In his experiments with formaldehyde as a disinfecting agent, Kinyoun[50] found that a greater penetration of formaldehyde could be obtained if the process was conducted in a steam disinfector provided with special apparatus such as shown in Figure 1-22. The main feature of the process consisted of the partial displacement of the air in the chamber by means of a vacuum apparatus and then admitting formaldehyde gas into the chamber so as to replace the exhausted air. Steam was admitted to the jacket only of the disinfector in order to heat the articles and to maintain the chamber at a temperature of about 90°C (194°F).

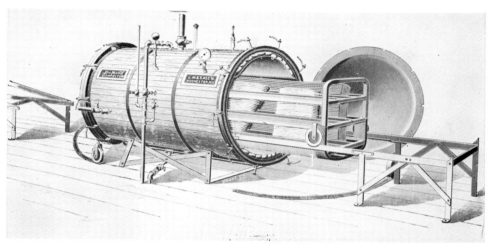

FIGURE 1-21. The Dumond Disinfector—a development of the French school. This apparatus, widely used in Europe, was designed for pressure steam disinfection of mattresses, pillows, fabrics, *et cetera*. It consisted of cylinder 4½ feet in diameter by 7 feet long, with door at either end. Radiators (heating coils) along top and bottom of chamber reduced condensation of steam and permitted rapid drying of goods following exposure to steam. The great advantage claimed for this apparatus was to the effect that one man could disinfect as many as one hundred mattresses in a day—a remarkable feat difficult to accomplish even with present-day equipment.

Directions for Operating Kinyoun-Francis Disinfector:

By opening Valve 1, steam was admitted to the pressure-reducing Valve 2, and reduced to the recommended operating pressure for the chamber, namely, 10 pounds. By opening Valve 3, steam was admitted to the jacket surrounding the chamber. When the jacket was thoroughly heated, the contaminated goods were loaded onto a car which was then pushed into the chamber. The door was closed and made steamtight. When the temperature had risen, the exhaust was opened until the gauge showed about 15 inches vacuum. The valves "CC" to the inner chamber were then opened, and, when the pressure had risen partially, they were closed and the exhauster again opened until 15 inches vacuum was shown by the gauge. At this point the exhauster valve was closed and the steam valves again opened until the thermometer indicated the proper temperature of the inner chamber, usually 115°C (239°F). This condition was maintained during the required exposure period. Finally, the steam was shut off and the exhausters opened to draw off all vapor. After a short time, the door was opened and the car removed.

When using formaldehyde gas as the disinfectant, steam was first admitted into the jacket until a temperature of at least 80°C (176°F) was obtained within the chamber. The articles to be disinfected were placed in the rack, or car, which was then rolled into the chamber, the door closed,

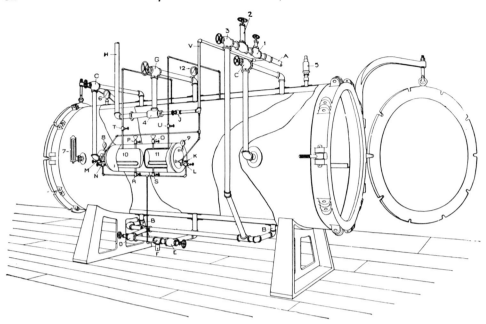

FIGURE 1-22. Kinyoun-Francis Steam and Formaldehyde Disinfecting Chamber. This apparatus, constituting marked improvement over earlier forms of pressure steam sterilizing equipment, could be used for application of steam under pressure at 1 to 2 atmospheres or for formaldehyde disinfection, combined with dry heat in vacuum chamber. It was widely used for the disinfection of clothing, bedding, *et cetera* in quarantine stations, municipal disinfecting plants, and hospitals. Kinyoun-Francis disinfectors ushered in era of bulk (large cylindrical and rectangular) sterilizer design and application.

1 Admits steam from Boiler to Reducing Valve.
2 Reduces steam to pressure used in Chamber.
3 Admits reduced steam to jacket at bottom.
4 Vacuum Apparatus.
5 Safety Valve.
6 Steam Pressure Gauge.
7 Thermometer.
8 Formaldehyde Pressure Gauge.
9 Ammonia Pressure Gauge.
10 Copper Formaldehyde Retort.
11 Steel Ammonia Retort.
12 Vacuum Gauge.

A Steam Pipe from Boiler.
B B Steam Pipes to Jacket.
C C Admit steam from Jacket to Chamber.
D Drip Valve from Jacket.
E Drip Valve from Chamber.
F Outboard Drip and Circulation
G Vacuum Valve.
H Exhaust Pipe of Vacuum Apparatus.
J High pressure steam to Vacuum Apparatus.
K High pressure steam to Ammonia Coil

L Drip from Ammonia Coil.
M High pressure steam to Formaldehyde Coil.
N Drip from Formaldehyde Coil.
O Filler for Ammonia Retort.
P Filler for Formaldehyde Retort.
R Drain from Formaldehyde Retort.
S Drain from Ammonia Retort.
T Admits Formaldehyde Gas to Chamber.
U Admits Ammonia Gas to Chamber.

and a vacuum of 15 to 20 inches obtained. By this time, steam having been allowed to course through the coil in the generator containing the formalin mixture, a gauge pressure of 40 to 60 pounds should have developed. (The formalin mixture consisted of formalin [100 parts], calcium chloride [20 parts], glycerin [10 parts]).

When the heat in the chamber approximated 90°C (194°F) the valve between the generator and the chamber was opened just enough to permit the escape of gas in sufficient quantity to cause the pressure to gradually decrease. At the end of 10 to 15 minutes most of the gas had been expelled and the valve was then closed. At this point, the vacuum gauge would usually read 7 to 8 inches, dependent upon the quantity of gas entering the chamber. At the end of 30 minutes, the vacuum was broken and air allowed to fill the chamber. This mixture of air plus formaldehyde gas was then exhausted, and the ammonia generator, previously supplied with aqua ammonia, was operated in the same manner as described for formalin. The introduction of the ammonia resulted in prompt neutralization of the residual formaldehyde gas. Finally, air was again admitted to the chamber and the door opened.

The efficiency of the formaldehyde disinfection process in a vacuum chamber was studied in detail by E. K. Sprague, Past Assistant Surgeon, U. S. Marine Hospital Service in 1899.[51] His report stated, in part:

> The writer would be distinctly understood as not recommending formaldehyde, even when combined with a high degree of heat, as a disinfecting agent upon which reliance can always be placed for the treatment of articles requiring much penetration, especially when the exposure is limited to ½ hour. A critical examination of nearly all the published experiments with this agent will reveal instances in which organisms that there was every reason to expect would be killed have survived, and vice versa. It is that occasional unaccountable uncertainty of action that calls forth the warning not to attempt disinfection with formaldehyde in a case in which there is any doubt as to the result.

The evolution and approach toward perfection of the pressure steam sterilizer has been, like all other apparatus of kindred nature, slow in development. Practically all of the pressure steam surgical dressing sterilizers employed in hospitals during the period from 1900 to 1915 were designed for operation by what was then known as the vacuum system of control. This system or method of operation, with few exceptions, consisted of the partial evacuation of air from the sterilizer chamber obtained by means of a steam ejector or vacuum attachment, and then subjecting the dressings or load in the chamber to steam at a pressure of 15 to 20 pounds for a period of from 20 to 30 minutes. The stated purpose of the initial vacuum (5 to 15 inches) was to aid in the displacement or removal of air from the chamber so as to insure a thorough penetration of the dressings or materials by the steam when it was next admitted to the chamber.

About the year 1915, there was introduced to hospitals in this country an entirely new conception of pressure-steam-sterilizer performance, in which the newly discovered gravity process of eliminating air from the chamber was substituted for the previously accepted standard of vacuum system of control. Much of the credit for the establishment of the gravity process of eliminating air from the chamber of the sterilizer, together with certain mechanical features of design, must be attributed to the efforts and accomplishments of the early investigator, W. B. Underwood, and his co-workers, who were responsible for notable advances in this field.[52] Whereas the advantage of gravity air clearance from the pressure steam sterilizer was recognized by other workers[53] prior to this time, it is generally conceded that the first sterilizers for operation on this newly developed principle appeared about the year 1915, thus constituting the first approach to modern methods of steam sterilization.

A typical pressure steam sterilizer of early design and construction for

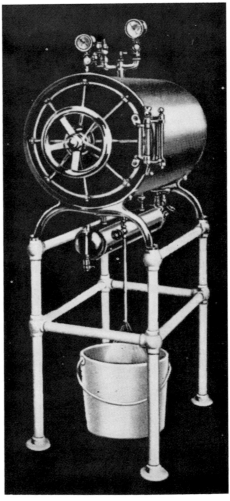

FIGURE 1-23. Typical pressure steam sterilizer of 1915, utilizing newly developed principle of gravity air discharge from chamber—first approach to modern temperature-controlled sterilizer.

gravity air discharge from the chamber is shown in Figure 1-23. The chamber was equipped with a drain outlet at the extreme bottom near the front end. This drain emptied into a pail on the floor, discharging into the open air so that the quality of the discharge could be observed by the operator. It was known, of course, that when steam is admitted to such a chamber with the bottom drain open, the lighter steam would literally float to the top of the chamber, and as the pressure was permitted to build up from the incoming steam it would force the air out at the bottom. The drain was left open until a full body of steam was observed to discharge into the pail, then the drain was closed in part so that only a slight discharge of steam occurred. When this process was followed with proper care, it left little to be desired from the standpoint of insuring the use of pure steam as the sterilizing medium.

Shortly after the introduction of the gravity system for air discharge as described above, a serious obstacle was encountered. The required performance of the sterilizer necessitated close attention on the part of the operator and in many cases, hospitals in particular, this close attention was not given. As the result, frequent failures in sterilization occurred. Fortunately, certain sterilizer manufacturers were prone to recognize the need for a more effective system of air discharge that would eliminate the hazard of faulty operation. Consequently, there appeared several modifications to the nonvacuum system described above, each contributing its share to the development of the modern (automatically controlled) pressure steam sterilizer. Because operators did not like the idea of the pail on the floor to catch the discharge from the chamber, the use of steam traps (thermostatic valves) to control the chamber discharge was introduced on sterilizers shortly after 1915. In 1919, Scanlan, Larson, and Clark[54] showed the value of the automatic air and condensate ejector and its influence on the efficiency of steam sterilization in an autoclave.

INTRODUCTION OF SANITARY CONNECTIONS TO STERILIZERS

Prior to 1928, it was general practice to connect all discharge outlets from sterilizers directly to the institution's waste lines. Also, most of the boiling type sterilizers for instruments and utensils, pasteurizers, bedpan washers, and water sterilizers had their water inlet connections directly joined to the respective reservoirs at a point actually below the normal level of the water. This meant that under adverse conditions, such as a sudden failure of the water pressure while the sterilizers were being filled, the polluted water in the sterilizers could, and often did, drain back into the supply line. Examples of these faulty connections, which today are recognized as violations of sanitary codes, are shown in Figures 1-24 through 1-30.

Water sterilizers were, perhaps, the worst offenders of all from the standpoint of recontamination (see page 281). When the tanks were permitted to

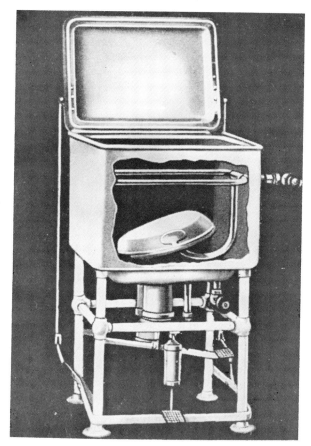

FIGURE 1-24. Early model of the so-called Typhoid Sterilizer for heat treatment of bedpans. Pan containing excreta was placed upright on an inner rack, the cover closed, and control lever turned to empty pan, leaving it suspended vertically. Then pan was flushed with cold water, steam valve opened and contents of chamber boiled, after which, waste valve was opened to discharge excreta into sewage disposal system. Today any similar apparatus would be promptly condemned as unsanitary because of possibility of pollution of water supply.

cool down following sterilization, a relatively high degree of vacuum was produced which then had to be relieved through (sanitary) intake of room air. This feature was accomplished through the medium of cotton air filters, as furnished on all water sterilizers for many years. The cotton filters were actually more hazardous than helpful because the cotton invariably became wet during the sterilizing process, and afterwards the intake of supposedly filtered air resulted in drawing back droplets of moisture highly laden with dust particles and bacteria. The older types of water sterilizers which were connected directly to the waste lines were particularly offensive. The waste valves, because of the accumulation of scale, were often leaky; and, conse-

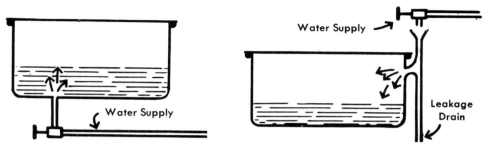

FIGURE 1-25. (*left*) With this type of connection the hospital's water supply could easily become polluted by backflow from the sterilizer.

FIGURE 1-26. (*right*) Correct method of connecting water supply to sterilizer. Open air-break prevents any backflow from sterilizer to water supply line.

quently, when the tanks were under vacuum, it was easily possible to draw back polluted water from the waste line into the sterile reservoirs. The water filters also became unspeakably foul from the accumulation of sediment; and, because one filter served both tanks, a leaky valve permitted the slow seepage of unsterile water into the sterile tanks.

In the late 1920's, public health authorities became "sterilizer conscious," with special emphasis upon the hazards of cross connections. The City Department of Health, Chicago, Illinois, showed that with such connections it was easily possible, through the medium of leaky valves, to conduct waste or sewage back into the sterilizers. Similarly it was shown that with many sterilizers the water supply connections could be polluted by backflow from the sterilizers. As a result of these investigations, all manufacturers of sterilizers were compelled to take drastic action to the end that protective features were

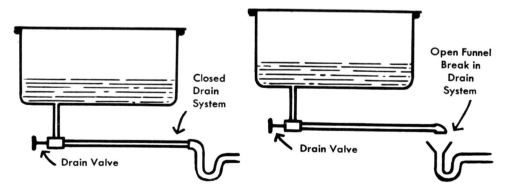

FIGURE 1-27. (*left*) With closed connection to drainage system, as shown here, sterilizer could be easily contaminated through backflow if waste valve were left open or if it did not close tightly.

FIGURE 1-28. (*right*) This is recognized as safe and practical method of connecting drain line of sterilizer to hospital's soil stack or waste system.

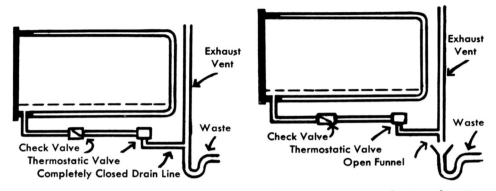

FIGURE 1-29. (*left*) Typical of many early installations, prior to introduction of sanitary connections, this chamber was drained through thermostatic valve direct to combination waste and vent. Obviously, a leaky check valve would permit contamination to be drawn into chamber, especially when latter was subjected to vacuum of 10 to 20 inches.

FIGURE 1-30. (*right*) Sterilizer shown in Figure 1-29 can be fully protected against pollution from waste by application of open funnel air-break.

provided for the elimination of the so-called cross connections through which, under all possible conditions, the sterilizers were freed from contamination influences arising from water and waste connections, and which also guarded against pollution of the water supply system from the sterilizers. Slowly but surely, progress had been made toward safer and more efficient sterilization.

THE MODERN ERA OF STERILIZATION

It is generally accepted that the year of 1933 marked the beginning of the modern era of scientific sterilization. At that time the American Sterilizer Company introduced the first pressure steam sterilizer (Fig. 1-31) in which the entire control of performance was centered in the measurement of temperature by a mercury thermometer located in the discharge outlet (chamber drain line) at the bottom of the chamber. Sterilizers manufactured and installed in hospitals prior to 1933 were operated with "pressure" as the sole indication of control, with no means for measuring the temperature developed by the steam or the degree of air elimination.

The introduction of temperature control marked the departure from unscientific guesswork methods of gauging sterilizer performance and ushered in a period of more precise sterilization which has remained largely unchanged up to the present time, with the exception of automatic control mechanisms. All sterilizers of recognized merit have long since been equipped with reliably accurate thermometers so located that under all conditions of performance, they register the true temperature of the steam applied to the load.

The reader may gather from the foregoing pages that the first three de-

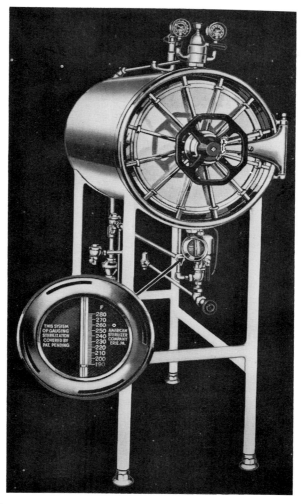

FIGURE 1-31. This sterilizer, introduced in 1933—some of these are still in service—was equipped with dialed top operating valve and entire control of performance was centered in measurement of temperature by mercury thermometer located in discharge outlet at bottom of chamber.

cades of the twentieth century witnessed important and far-reaching advances in the science and methodology of sterilization. Many of these developments have contributed greatly to the safety of the patient and to the convenience of the surgical and nursing personnel in our hospitals. From these advances there has finally emerged a clear understanding and disquisition of the scientific principles involved in sterilization, together with a means or system whereby sterilization of hospital supplies can now be accomplished with greater economy, an increased factor of safety, and a higher degree of precision than ever before.

IMPORTANT (PAST) CONTRIBUTORS TO THE DEVELOPMENT OF THE ART OF STERILIZATION

1680 PAPIN, DENYS: French physicist (1647-1714). Invented steam digester (pressure cooker) to which was later added first safety valve on record. He also discovered that the boiling points of liquids vary with the pressure.

1765 SPALLANZANI, LAZZARO: Italian naturalist (1729-1799). A leading opponent of the theory of spontaneous generation. Studied the effectiveness of heat in the destruction of bacteria and the sterilization of liquids. Proved to his own satisfaction that there is no vegetative power in inanimate material.

1807 DALTON, JOHN: English chemist (1766-1844). Investigated the properties of gases and formulated the Law of Partial Pressures. His greatest work was the establishment of the Atomic Theory.

1810 APPERT, NICOLAS: Parisian confectioner (?-1841). Credited with discovery of process of food preservation by canning. Introduced the use of sealed containers followed by heating in boiling water. Published first treatise on canning.

1832 HENRY, WILLIAM: English chemist (1775-1836). Investigated the disinfecting powers of increased temperatures and demonstrated that infected clothing could be rendered harmless by heat. He devised a jacketed dry heat (hot air) sterilizer.

1847 SEMMELWEIS, IGNAZ: Hungarian physician (1818-1865). Recognized as the true pioneer of antisepsis in obstetrics. He proved the contact transmissibility of puerperal (childbed) fever from physician, midwife, or nurse to the patient. One of the immortals of medicine.

1861 PASTEUR, LOUIS: French chemist-bacteriologist (1822-1895). Generally recognized as the "Father of Bacteriology." Noted for his brilliant researches on fermentation and the prevention of anthrax and rabies. He disproved the doctrine of spontaneous generation and proved that putrefaction is a fermentation caused by the growth of microbes. He also originated the process of pasteurization; postulated the role of bacteria in disease, and contributed greatly to the foundation of modern surgical asepsis.

1867 LISTER, JOSEPH: English surgeon (1827-1912). Founder of antiseptic surgery. He applied Pasteur's principles of fermentation to surgical practice and postulated the theory that "infection was due to passage of minute bodies capable of self multiplication from infector to infected." Lister's contributions led directly to the establishment of sterile technic in the operating room.

1877 TYNDALL, JOHN: English physicist (1820-1893). Discovered the heat-resistant phase (spore stage) of bacteria. He was the originator of the method known as fractional (intermittent) sterilization or tyndallization.

1880 CHAMBERLAND, CHARLES: French bacteriologist (1851-1908). Pupil and collaborator of Pasteur on the germ theory of disease. He built the first pressure steam sterilizer—known as "Chamberland's Autoclave."

1881 KOCH, ROBERT: German bacteriologist (1843-1910). Widely acclaimed as the "Father of Bacteriological Technic." He discovered the use of solid (liquefiable) culture media and investigated the etiology of infective diseases. He also discovered the cause of tuberculosis and advocated the use of bichloride of mercury as a germicide. Many important contributions to the field of sterilization and chemical disinfection originated in Koch's laboratory, with the able assistance of Wolffhügel, Gaffky, and Loeffler.

1885 SCHIMMELBUSCH, CURT: German surgeon (1860-1895). He developed and evaluated the various details of aseptic technic. Also credited as the first to use the steam sterilizer for sterilization of surgical dressings. He advocated addition of sodium carbonate to boiling water to enhance its germicidal value and prevent corrosion of instruments. Published *Aseptic Treatment of Wounds.*

1888 VON ESMARCH, ERVIN: (1855-1915). Investigated the sterilizing efficiency of unsaturated or superheated steam. Also recommended the use of bacteriologic tests as proof of sterilization.

1888 KINYOUN, J. J.: American bacteriologist (1860-1919). He made important contributions to design of steam pressure chambers and first recommended the vacuum process to augment steam penetration of objects. He also studied gaseous disinfectants, particularly formaldehyde, and was largely responsible for development of steam-formaldehyde disinfector used in quarantine stations, hospital and municipal services.

1933 UNDERWOOD, WEEDEN: American engineer (1880-1946). Responsible for notable advances in design and application of pressure steam sterilizers. His investigations influenced the development of the modern temperature-controlled sterilizer. He promoted the modern concept of sterile supply centralization for hospitals. Published *Textbook of Sterilization.*

1948 MELENEY, FRANK, L.: American surgeon (1889-1963). Widely acclaimed for his many contributions to surgical bacteriology. Established standards for functional control of and continuous supervision of sterile technic of operating rooms. Promoted improvements in design and reliability of sterilizers. Published *Treatise on Surgical Infections.*

REFERENCES

1. BRYAN, A. H., and BRYAN, C. G.: *Principles and Practice of Bacteriology,* 3rd ed. New York, Barnes & Noble, 1942, p. 2.
2. HOMER: *The Odyssey,* translated in verse by J. W. Mackail. London, Oxford, 1932, Book XXII, p. 474.
3. LEVIN, S.: Bacteriology in the Bible. *Practitioner, 192:*820-827, 1964.
4. BETTMANN, O. L.: *A Pictorial History of Medicine.* Springfield, Illinois, Thomas, 1956, p. 35.
5. TURNER, T. A., and COMPERE, E. L.: *Microbes That Cripple.* Elyria, Ohio, National Society for Crippled Children, 1944, p. 8.
6. FORD, W. W.: *Clio Medica, Bacteriology.* New York, Hoeber, 1939, p. 34.
7. SPALLANZANI, L.: Saggio di osservazioni microscopiche relative al sistema della generazione di Signore Needham e Buffon. Reprinted in Wolf, A.: *A History of Science, Technology and Philosophy in the 18th Century.* New York, Macmillan, 1939, p. 474.
8. HAMILTON, J. B.: The shadowed side of Spallanzani: *Yale J Biol Med,* 7:151-170, 1934.
9. SCHULZE, F.: Vorläufige Mittheilung der Resultate einer experimentellen Beobachtung über Generatio aequivoca. *Ann Physik Chemie,* 39:487-489, 1836.
10. SCHWANN, T.: *Ann Physik Chemie,* 41:184-192, 1837.
11. TANNER, F. W.: *Bacteriology,* 3rd ed. New York, Wiley, 1937, p. 9.
12. SCHROEDER, H., and VON DUSCH, T.: Ueber Filtration der Luft in Beziehung auf Fäulniss und Gahrung. *Ann Chemie Pharmacie,* 89:232-241, 1854.
13. POUCHET, F. A.: *Heterogenie ou traite de la generation spontanee, base sur des nouvelles experiences.* Paris, 1859.

14. PASTEUR, L.: Memoire sur les corpuscles organises qui existent dans l'atmosphere, examen de la doctrine des generations spontanees. *Ann chimie physique (Paris)* 64:5-110, 1862.
15. FORD, W. W.: *Textbook of Bacteriology.* Philadelphia, Saunders, 1927, p. 22.
16. FORD, W. W.: *Clio Medica, Bacteriology.* New York, Hoeber, 1939, p. 88.
17. VALLERY-RADOT, R.: *The Life of Pasteur,* Transl. by R. L. Devonshire. New York, Doubleday, 1926, p. 255.
18. *Ibid.*
19. METCHNIKOFF, E.: *The Founders of Modern Medicine (Pasteur, Koch, Lister).* New York, Walden Publications, 1939, p. 39.
20. VALLERY-RADOT, R.: *op. cit.,* p. 274.
21. BALDRY, P. E.: *The Battle Against Bacteria.* London, Cambridge U. P., 1965, p. 24.
22. BETTMANN, O. L.: *A Pictorial History of Medicine.* Springfield, Illinois, Thomas, 1956, p. 258.
23. SEMMELWEIS, I.: *Die Aetologie, der Begriff und die Prophylaxis des Kindbettfiebers.* Pest, C. A. Hartleben's Verlags-Expedition, 1861.
24. TYNDALL, J.: On the optical deportment of the atmosphere in relation to the phenomena of putrefaction and infection. *Phil Trans Roy Soc, 166:*27-74, 1876.
25. TYNDALL, J. Further researches on the deportment and vital persistence of putrefactive and infective organisms from a physical point of view. *Phil Trans Roy Soc, 167:*149-206, 1877.
26. TYNDALL, J. *Selected Works of John Tyndall, Fragments of Science,* Westminster ed. New York, Appleton, Vol. II, p. 320.
27. TYNDALL, J.: *Ibid.,* p. 323.
28. TYNDALL, J.: *Ibid.,* p. 321.
29. LISTER, JOSEPH: On the antiseptic principle in the practice of surgery. *Brit Med J, 2:*246-248, 1867. Also, *Lancet, 2:*353, 1867.
30. PELTIER, L. F.: A brief account of the evolution of antiseptic surgery. *Journal-Lancet,* Nov. 1950, pp. 442-444.
31. LISTER, JOSEPH: On a new method of treating compound fracture, abscess, etc., with observations on the conditions of suppuration. *Lancet, 1:*326, 357, 387, 507, 1867.
32. LISTER, JOSEPH: Demonstrations of antiseptic surgery before members of the British Medical Association. *Edinburgh Med J, 21:*193, 1875-6.
33. LISTER, JOSEPH: An address on the effect of the antiseptic treatment upon the general salubrity of surgical hospitals. *Brit. Med J, 2:*769-771, 1875.
34. ROBINSON, V.: Story of medicine. From Underwood, W. B. (Ed.): *Story of Sterilization. Surgical Supervisor, 6:*3-61, 1946.
35. KOCH, R., and WOLFFHÜGEL, G.: Untersuchungen über die Desinfection mit heisser Luft. *Mitt Kaiserl Gesund, 1:*301-321, 1881.
36. KOCH, R.; GAFFKY, G., and LOEFFLER, F.: Versuche über die Verwerthbarkeit heisser Wasserdämpfe zu Desinfektionszwecken. *Ibid.,* p. 322-340.
37. ZINSSER, HANS: *Textbook of Bacteriology,* 6th ed. New York, Appleton, 1927, p. 67.
38. WALTER, C. W.: *The Aseptic Treatment of Wounds.* New York, Macmillan, 1948, p. 18.
39. DAVIDSOHN, H.: Wie soll der Arzt seine Instrumente desinficirin? *Berl Klin Wchnschr, 25:* 697, 1888.
40. VON ESMARCH, E.: Die desinficirende Wirkung des strömenden überhitzen Dampfes. *Ztschr Hyg Infektionskr, 4:*197, 1888.
41. RUBNER, M.: Zur Theorie der Dampfdesinfektion. *Hygienische Rundschau, 8:*721, 1898. *Idem.:* Modern Steam Sterilization, Harvey Lectures, Harvey Soc. of New York, 1912-13, Philadelphia, Lippincott, p. 15-27.
42. BARNES, C. L.: *Contagious and Infectious Diseases.* Chicago, Trade Periodical, 1903, p. 122.
43. FORD, W. W.: *Textbook of Bacteriology,* Philadelphia, Saunders, 1927, p. 165.
44. FLÜGGE: On disinfection of dwellings. From Barnes, C. L. (Ed.): *Contagious and Infectious Diseases. Ztschr Hyg Infektionskr, 29,* 1898.
45. WILLIAMS, S. W.: Aerial or gaseous disinfection. *Amer Pharm Ass* (Chicago Branch), Nov. 16, 1915, p. 23.

46. WINSLOW, C. E. A.: Some leaders and landmarks in the history of microbiology. *Bact Rev., 14*:99-114, 1950.

47. STERNBERG, G. M.: Experiments to determine the germicide value of certain therapeutic agents. *Amer J Med Sci, 335* (April), 1883.

48. WILMOT CASTLE Co., Personal Communication, July, 1952.

49. *Report on the Louisiana Quarantine.* Abstract of Sanitary Reports, 1888.

50. KINYOUN, J. J.: *Public Health Rep,* Sept. 4, 1897.

51. SPRAGUE, E. K.: Formaldehyde disinfection in a vacuum chamber. *Public Health Rep, XIV* (Sept 22), 1899.

52. UNDERWOOD, W. B.: The story of sterilization. *Surgical Supervisor, 6*:3-61, 1946.

53. FROSCH, P., and CLARENBACH, A.: Ueber das Verhalten des Wasserdampfes im Desinfektionsapparate. *Ztschr Hyg Infektionskr, 9*:183, 1890.

54. SCANLAN, S. G.; LARSON, G. L., and CLARK, P. F.: High pressure dressing sterilizers or autoclaves. *Mod Hosp XII* (April), 1919.

Chapter 2

DESCRIPTIVE TERMINOLOGY

BIOLOGICAL

Bacterial anatomy: Has to do with the shape and elucidation of the surface structure of the cell. From the older study of bacterial cytology to the modern advances in microbiology, anatomy dates from the introduction of the electron microscope and the development of precise methods for slicing the bacterial cell into incredibly thin sections (see Fig. 4-9). The first commercial electron microscopes were manufactured in Germany in 1939.

D value: Refers to what is known as the decimal reduction time (DRT), or in other words, the time required to destroy 90 per cent of the cells. It is convenient to express the resistance of an organism in terms of the D_{10} value, which is the exposure time to the lethal agent required to reduce a given population to 10 per cent of the original number. Also, it means the time required for the survivor curve to traverse one log cycle.

Exponential killing (or survival): The kinetics of inactivation give a straight line when logarithms of survivors are plotted against time of exposure to, or dosage of, the inactivating agent. The slope of this line (D value) is the (fractional) *rate of inactivation* and it measures sensitivity of the bacterium relative to the dosage.

Forespore: The first indication of the onset of sporulation in living cells is the appearance within the cytoplasm of a smooth, transparent area known as the *forespore* (see Fig. 4-8). The forespore gradually assumes the characteristic, highly refractile appearance of the mature spore.

Germination: Infers a loss of heat resistance. In terms of a bacterial spore, it may be regarded as the change from a heat-resistant phase to a heat-labile entity which may not necessarily be a true vegetative cell.

Inactivation: To render anything inert by the application of heat or other means, as in the inactivation of viruses with the resulting disappearance of the infectivity factor.

Phage: A bacteriophage is a virus that infects bacteria. More specifically it refers to the ability of the phage to bring about lysis of growing bacterial cultures. A certain phage will attack a certain bacterium, and in this connection they may be used as labels.

Pyrogens: The term *pyrogen* means "fever producing." It is generally accepted that pyrogens are by-products of bacterial growth or metabolism

44

closely related to or identical with bacterial O antigen (the antigen which occurs in the bodies of bacteria) and commonly called endotoxin.

Temperature coefficient: The temperature coefficient, Q_{10}, is defined as the increase in the killing rate constant per $10°C$ rise in temperature. It follows that the larger the value of the coefficient, the greater the increase in killing rate upon increasing the temperature or concentration of a disinfectant. In practice, this means that when a coefficient is large, a slight change in the conditions may cause a great change in the efficiency of a disinfectant.

MEDICAL-SURGICAL

Aerosol: Refers to particles suspended in the air and capable of causing an airborne infection. In general, the particles exist in the micron size range, with diameters from 100 microns to 1 micron or less, consisting partially or wholly of microorganisms. At the lower size limit are those particles which transport single infectious microorganisms. The upper size limit is set by characteristics of the respiratory system and the hygroscopic nature of the particles. The term *aerosol* came into use during the latter part of World War I, and it was applied to the fine aerial suspensions of arsenical smokes.

Carrier: An infected person who harbors a specific infectious agent in the absence of discernible clinical disease and serves as a potential source of infection for man. The carrier state may occur with infections inapparent throughout their course (commonly known as healthy carriers) and also as a feature of incubation period, convalescence, and postconvalescence of a clinically recognizable disease (commonly known as incubatory and convalescent carriers). Under either circumstance the carrier state may be short or long (temporary or chronic carriers). The same applies to other vertebrate animals.[1]

Clean: Freedom of or removal of all matter in which microorganisms may find favorable conditions for continued life and growth. Similarly, cleaning means the removal of soil and microorganisms adherent to surfaces by a process such as scrubbing with hot water and detergent.

Communicable disease: An illness due to a specific infectious agent or its toxic products, which arises through transmission of that agent or its products from a reservoir to a susceptible host, either directly as from an infected person or animal, or indirectly through the agency of an intermediate plant or animal host, a vector, or the inanimate environment.[1]

Concurrent disinfection: The application of disinfection as soon as possible after the discharge of infectious material from the body of an infected person, or after the soiling of articles with such infectious discharges, all personal contact with such discharges or articles being prevented prior to such disinfection.[1]

Contact: A person or animal who has been in such association with an infected person or animal or with a contaminated environment as to have had opportunity to acquire the infection. Exposure may be direct and involve physical touching as in kissing, shaking hands, or in sexual intercourse. Persons thus exposed are variously characterized as direct, immediate, or intimate contact. Exposure may be indirect, with no established physical touching, through living in the same household, being in the same room, or through remote or close association at school, work, or play. Exposure may be long or short; single, continued, or repetitive; and casual or close. Such indirectly exposed persons are often denoted as either familial, school, or work contacts; or as close, casual, or remote contacts, in expression of varying degrees of risk of a developing infection.[1]

Contamination: The presence of an infectious agent on a body surface; also on or in clothes, bedding, toys, surgical instruments or dressings, or other inanimate articles or substances including water, milk, and food. Contamination is distinct from pollution which implies the presence of offensive but noninfectious matter in the environment.[1]

Decontamination: In the biological sense, a process or method whereby an object or material such as a surgical instrument or bed linens is freed of the contaminating agent(s) and rendered safe for human handling without further recourse to individual protective measures. In effect, the decontamination process is the equivalent of sterilization in that *all* agents of infection must be destroyed or irreversibly inactivated.

Disinfestation: Any physical or chemical process serving to destroy undesired small animal forms, particularly arthropods or rodents, present upon the person, the clothing, or in the environment of an individual, or on domestic animals. This includes delousing as applied to infestation with *Pediculus humanus,* the body louse.[1]

Endemic: The habitual presence of a disease within a given geographic area; may also refer to the usual prevalence of a given disease within such area. *Hyperendemic* expresses a persistent activity in excess of expected prevalence.[1]

Epidemic: The occurrence in a community or region of a group of illnesses of similar nature, clearly in excess of normal expectancy, and derived from a common or from a propagated source. The number of cases indicating presence of an epidemic will vary according to the infectious agent, size and type of population exposed, previous experience or lack of exposure to the disease, and time and place of occurrence; epidemicity is thus relative to usual frequency of the disease in the same area, among the specified population, at the same season of year. A single case of a communicable disease long absent from a population (as smallpox in Boston) or first invasion by a disease not previously recognized in that area (as American trypanosomiasis in Arizona) is to be considered as a potential epidemic meeting the requirements in respect to reporting of epidemics.[1]

Fumigation: Any process by which the killing of animal forms, especially arthropods and rodents, is accomplished by the employment of gaseous agents.[1]

Host: A man or other living animal, including birds and arthropods, affording under natural conditions subsistence or lodgment to an infectious agent. Some protozoa and helminths pass successive stages in alternate hosts of different species. Hosts in which the parasite attains maturity or passes its sexual stage are primary or definitive hosts; those in which the parasite is in a larval or asexual state are secondary or intermediate hosts.[1]

Incidence: A general term used to characterize the frequency of occurrence of a disease, an infection, or other event over a period of time and in relation to the population in which it occurs. Incidence is expressed more specifically as a rate, commonly the number of new cases during a prescribed time in the unit of population in which they occur; thus, cases of tuberculosis per 100,000 population per year.[1]

Infection: The entry and development or multiplication of an infectious agent in the body of man or animal. Infection is not synonymous with infectious disease; the result may be inapparent or manifest. The presence of living infectious agents on exterior surfaces of the body or upon articles of apparel or soiled articles is not infection but contamination of such surfaces and articles. The term *infection* should not be used to describe conditions of inanimate matter such as soil, water, sewage, milk, or food; the term *contamination* applies.[1]

Infectious agent: An organism, mainly microorganisms (bacterium, protozoan, spirochete, fungus, virus, rickettsia, bedsonia, or other) but including helminths, capable of producing infection or infectious disease.[1]

Infestation: By infestation of persons or animals is meant the lodgment, development, and reproduction of arthropods on the surface of the body or in the clothing. Infested articles or premises are such as harbor or give shelter to animal forms, especially arthropods and rodents.[1]

Isolation: The separation for the period of communicability of infected persons from other persons, in such places and under such conditions as will prevent the direct or indirect conveyance of the infectious agent from infected persons to persons who are susceptible or who may spread the agent to others. This applies also to animals. Strict isolation of the patient for the period of communicability is necessary in certain diseases, notably smallpox. Isolation of the patient has but little effect in limiting the spread of many diseases, for instance poliomyelitis.

When used in connection with such diseases as the common cold, influenza, chickenpox, mumps, and the pneumonias, isolation is not to be understood, under ordinary circumstances, as a necessary or practicable procedure for official requirement or enforcement, but a modified practice to be instituted under the direction of the attending physician, and its duration to be generally, if not exclusively, at his direction.[1]

Microbial persistence: This term is used to designate a phenomenon whereby microorganisms which are drug-susceptible when tested outside the body are, nevertheless, capable of surviving within the body despite intensive therapy with the appropriate antimicrobial drug.[2]

Reservoir of infectious agents: Reservoirs are man, animals, plants, soil, or inanimate organic matter in which an infectious agent lives and multiplies and depends primarily for survival, reproducing itself in such manner that it can be transmitted to a susceptible host. Man himself is the most frequent reservoir of infectious agents pathogenic for man.[1]

Source of infection: The thing, person, object, or substance from which an infectious agent passes immediately to a host. Transfer is often direct from reservoir to host, in which case the reservoir is also the source of infection (measles). The source may be at any point in the chain of transmission, as a vehicle, vector, intermediate animal host, or contaminated article; thus, contaminated water (typhoid fever), an infective mosquito (malaria), beef (tapeworm disease), or a toy (diphtheria). In each instance cited the reservoir is an infected person. Source of infection should be clearly distinguished from source of contamination, such as overflow of a septic tank contaminating a water supply, or an infected cook contaminating a salad.[1]

Terminal disinfection: This is no longer practiced after the patient has been removed by death or to a hospital, or has ceased to be a source of infection, or after isolation practices have been discontinued. Terminal cleaning suffices along with airing and sunning of rooms, furniture, and bedding. Necessary only for diseases spread by indirect contact; steam sterilization of bedding is desirable after smallpox.[1]

Transmission of infectious agents: Modes of transmission of infection are the mechanisms by which an infectious agent is transported from reservoir to susceptible human host. They are as follows:

1. *Contact:*

   a. Direct contact: Actual touching of the infected person or animal or other reservoir of infection, as in kissing, sexual intercourse, or other contiguous personal association. In the systemic mycoses, by skin contact with soil, compost or decaying vegetable matter where the agent leads a saprophytic existence.

   b. Indirect contact: Touching of contaminated objects such as toys, handkerchiefs, soiled clothing, bedding, surgical instruments and dressings, with subsequent hand to mouth transfer of infective material; less commonly, transfer to abraded or intact skin or mucous membrane.

   c. Droplet spread: The projection onto the conjunctivae and the face or into the nose or mouth, of the spray emanating from an infected person during sneezing, coughing, singing, or talking. Such droplets usually travel no more than 3 feet from the source. Transmission by droplet infection is considered a form of contact infection, since it involves reasonably close association between two or more persons.

2. *Vehicle:* Water, food, milk, biological products to include serum and plasma, or any substance serving as an intermediate means by which an infectious agent is transported from a reservoir and introduced into a susceptible host through ingestion, through inoculation, or by deposit on skin or mucous membrane.

3. *Vector:* Arthropods or other invertebrates which transmit infection by inoculation into or through the skin or mucous membrane by biting, or by deposit of infective materials on the skin or on food or other objects. The vector may be infected itself (in some instances becoming infective only after appropriate extrinsic incubation) or act as a mechanical carrier of the agent.

4. *Airborne:* The dissemination and inhalation of microbial aerosols, or their deposition on skin, mucous surfaces or wounds. Microbial aerosols are suspensions in air of particles, ordinarily with diameters from 100 microns to 1 micron or less, consisting partially or wholly of microorganisms. Particles in the lower ranges of that size may remain suspended in air for long periods of time. Microbial aerosols arise from the following:

   a. Droplet nuclei: The small residues which result from evaporation of droplets. Droplet nuclei also may be created purposely by a variety of atomizing devices, or accidentally in abattoirs, rendering plants, autopsy rooms, or by many laboratory procedures.

   b. Dust: The particles of widely varying size which may arise from contaminated floors, clothes, bedding, or other articles; from soil, especially mycotic spores or cells leading a saprophytic existence there; or from contaminated animal hair, cotton, or similar products. The larger particles remain suspended in the air for relatively short periods of time; the finer particles may be indistinguishable from droplet nuclei.[1]

PHYSICAL-CHEMICAL

Absolute temperature: In addition to the Fahrenheit and Celsius scales, the absolute temperature scale is commonly used in physics and engineering. On this scale the lowest fixed point is $-273°C$. This point is known as absolute zero. It is the temperature at which all molecular movement would cease. To convert from the absolute temperature indicated in degrees K (Kelvin) to the Celsius scale, it is necessary to subtract $273°C$ from the absolute reading. For example:

$$C = K - 273$$
$$K = C + 273$$

Alkylation: The replacement of a hydrogen atom in a molecule by an alkyl group is called alkylation. A compound which can effect this replacement of a hydrogen atom or addition is known as an alkylating agent.

Angstrom unit: The Angstrom unit (A) is used to express the wave length of light. One Angstrom unit is equal to (10^{-7} mm) one ten-millionth of a millimeter or 1/250,000,000 of an inch. Wave length may also be measured in microns (μ) and millimicrons (mμ).

10 Angstrom units $= 1/1,000,000$ millimeter or 1 millimicron (mμ).
1000 millimicrons $= 1$ micron (μ).
1000 microns $= 1$ millimeter (mm) or 1/25 inch.

Cavitation: Gas-filled, vapor-filled, or empty cavities ranging in size from submicroscopic to very large may be produced in a liquid by methods such as chemical, thermal, or mechanical actions, and they may have a short or prolonged life. The production of these cavities and the effect that they induce on the medium in which they are produced is known as cavitation.[3]

Celsius versus centigrade temperature scale: The temperature scale used by scientists in America has been called centigrade, while in many countries it was called Celsius for its inventor. Anders Celsius, a Swedish astronomer, is credited with having invented a thermometer, in 1742, whose scale had 100 degrees between the ice and steam points. In 1948, the Ninth General Conference on Weights and Measures, representing thirty-three nations that subscribed to the Treaty of the Meter, adopted the name Celsius. This name, however, did not come into general use by scientists in America, partly because they were unaware of the official action of the conference and partly because some preferred the old name.

At the Eleventh General Conference in 1960 the scale was defined in a way that makes the adjective *centigrade* inexact. The name Celsius is correct and its use by American scientists and technicians would help make the nomenclature of temperature uniform in all countries. The National Bureau of Standards now uses the name Celsius in all of its scientific publications.[4]

Chelating or sequestering agents: Certain compounds such as ethylenediaminetetracetic acid (EDTA) have the property of forming complexes with polyvalent metallic ions, e.g., calcium, magnesium, iron, which, when present as their salts in hard water, interfere with soaps by causing precipitation, or with the germicidal action of quaternary ammonium compounds.

Conductivity: This is a measure of the ability of a solution to conduct an electric current. It changes with the concentration of ions and the velocities of the ions in an electric field. Ionically pure water has a high resistivity (resistance) and a low conductivity. The conductivity is measured by an electronic instrument incorporating a Wheatstone bridge—an electrical balance measurement made by comparing a known resistance with an unknown.

Deflocculation: The process of dispersing aggregates of small particles so that they will go into suspension in the cleaning liquid.

Degassing: The removal of an excess quantity of dissolved gas from a liquid. The action of ultrasonic energy on a liquid is an excellent method for degassing.

Energy of activation: The energy of activation represents the energy that molecules must acquire in order to be capable of undergoing reaction. During the course of a reaction the reactant molecules become activated by collisions with one another.

First-order reactions: A reaction is said to be of the first order if the number of molecules reacting at any given time is proportional to the number of molecules present at that time. First-order reactions are those in which a single molecule, without collision, can produce the products of the reaction.

Fusion: When the temperature of a solid is gradually raised, a stage is reached at which the substance passes into the liquid state. For each crystalline substance, there is, generally, a specific temperature at which it changes from the solid to the liquid state. This temperature is called the fusing point. Certain sterilization indicators or controls react in this manner when subjected to sterilizing temperatures.

Heat of vaporization: Every liquid has a particular boiling point which is constant at a specific pressure. If the pressure is increased the boiling point increases; if the pressure is decreased the boiling point is decreased. The number of calories needed to change one gram of a liquid at a specific temperature to a gas at the same temperature is called the heat of vaporization of that substance. The heat of vaporization of water is 539.5 calories per gram at 100°C.

Heat unit: The unit of heat measure employed in this country is the *British thermal unit,* more commonly written and referred to as the BTU. It represents the quantitative energy required to be added to one pound of water at a temperature of its greatest density, i.e. 39°F, to raise its temperature one degree on the Fahrenheit scale. Expressed more simply, the BTU means the quantity of heat required to raise the temperature of 1 pound of water 1 degree Fahrenheit.

Passivation: The process of forming a passive film on stainless steel by the use of nitric acid. This treatment of stainless steel renders it less susceptible to corrosion.

Practical sterility: This term is used in the milk industry to describe a situation wherein not all bacterial spores are killed, but the survivors are unable to grow and cause spoilage under most practical conditions. Oftentimes, this is the case with evaporated milk. The reasons for the inability of the surviving spores to germinate are not completely understood.

Pressure: This term may be defined as the force per unit of area. The use of the "atmosphere" or "cm of mercury" to express pressure is relative. To say that the pressure of a gas is as great as so many atmospheres, or equal to that of a column of mercury of a certain height does not convey the actual pressure, unless the force exerted by a standard atmosphere or by a column of mercury 1 cm high is known. The absolute unit is the *dyne*. A dyne is that force which will give a mass of 1 gram an acceleration of 1 centimeter per second per second (1 cm/sec^2). Normal atmospheric pressure = 1,000,000 dynes/cm^2.

Radiation: By classical definition, radiation means the flow of energy from one point to another across empty space. With the advent of the atomic age, the term radiation has been used in its narrowest definition for those electromagnetic waves of higher energy, such as x-rays and gamma rays, and limiting the class of particles to those of atomic size and smaller.

Stress corrosion: The rate of uniform or general corrosion may be affected by the presence of stress. A metal under tensile stress is more susceptible to corrosion, particularly in the presence of an acid solution.

Ultrasonic: This term is used to describe a vibrating wave of a frequency above that of the upper frequency limit of the human ear; it generally embraces all frequencies above 16 kilocycles per second.[3]

Vapor permeability: The property of a film or sheet which permits the passage of vapors. This property must be measured under carefully specified conditions of total pressure, partial pressures of the vapor on the two sides of the film, temperature, and relative humidity. Since paper has a specific affinity for water vapor, the vapor permeability should not be confused with air permeability or porosity.

Vapor pressure: At a given temperature a definite quantity of a liquid will evaporate in a given space, and the pressure it exerts in this space is a function of the temperature only. If the space is increased, more liquid, if present, will evaporate, and if the space is reduced some of the vapor will condense. In this case the vapor (or space) is said to be saturated, and the corresponding pressure is the maximum vapor pressure for this temperature.

MECHANICAL

Cross connection: A cross connection may be defined as any physical arrangement in a plumbing system whereby a public or semipublic water supply is connected directly or indirectly to any other water supply system, sewer, drain, conduit, storage reservoir, or other device which contains contaminated water, sewage, or other waste capable of imparting contamination to the public supply as a result of backflow or siphonage. One of the common defects in sanitary plumbing systems responsible for contamination of water and fixtures is a cross connection.

Entrainment: The collecting or transporting of solid particles or a second fluid by the flow of the primary fluid or vapor at high velocity is known as entrainment.

Entropy: The concept of entropy is complex. It represents a thermodynamic quantity. In simple terms it can be considered as a measure of the total energy of a system (or of a chemical reaction) unavailable for doing useful work. It can be more generally defined as the property which measures that portion of the heat added which cannot be converted into work no matter how nearly perfect the operation may be. The increase in entropy of any system is equal to the heat which it absorbs, divided by the absolute temperature at which the heat is absorbed. Entropy is commonly represented by the symbol S. The use of the Greek letter delta (Δ) in combination with S is for the purpose of emphasizing that such a symbol represents an increase or a change.

Probability: True probability is the limit of the ratio of favorable outcomes to the total number of trials as the total number of trials approaches infinity. An estimate of probability can be obtained by performing a number of tests or trials. The results constitute an exact measure of the likelihood of how close the estimate is to the true value. Statistical methods have been developed which enable us to calculate, from the obtained estimate and from the number of trials, confidence limits for the true probability and the confidence in per cent that the true probability lies within these limits. Success in sterilization is dependent upon the laws of probability and reliability.

Reliability: This is a yardstick of capability to perform within required limits when in operation. It normally involves a parameter which measures time. The reliability of a component is its conditional probability of performing its function within specified performance limits at a given age for the period of time intended and under the operating stress conditions encountered.

Sanitary ventilation: Any combination of ventilation and other means of destroying infectious particles in the air is known as sanitary ventilation. The removal of airborne organisms, whether by ventilation or by ultraviolet irradiation disinfection, follows an exponential die-away curve. Epidemiologic evidence indicates that at least one air change per minute, or an equivalent reduction in air borne organisms by disinfection, is needed. One air change means the introduction of a volume of air equal to the volume of the room; it does not mean necessarily the replacement of all the air in the room by fresh air.[5]

Thermocouple: A thermocouple is two lengths of wire, each made of a different homogeneous metal. The wires are welded together at one end (measuring junction) and connected to a measuring instrument at the other end (reference junction) to form an electric circuit. When one end is hotter than the other, an electromotive force (EMF) develops that starts a current flowing through the wires. This EMF can be used to measure temperature changes by connecting a potentiometer into the thermocouple circuit.

MATERIALS

Disposables: The term *disposable* as used in the medical field applies to a product which is used only once and then discarded, or to an article which is used on only one patient and then discarded. Disposables should not be confused with items normally consumed in use, such as bandages, gases, soap, and sutures.[6]

Glassine paper: A smooth, dense, transparent, or semitransparent paper manufactured primarily from chemical wood pulps which have been beaten to secure a high degree of hydration of the stock. This paper is greaseproof and when waxed or lacquered it is practically impervious to air and vapors. Steam-sterilizable glassine permits passage of water vapor and air.

Kraft paper: This paper is made entirely from wood pulp produced by an alkaline process. It is a coarse paper particularly noted for its strength. It is used primarily as a wrapper or packaging material. The natural, unbleached color is brown, but by use of semibleached or fully bleached sulfate pulp, it can be produced in lighter shades of brown, and white. Kraft paper is commonly made in weights ranging from 25 to 60 pounds.

Plastics: Plastics are a class of synthetic organic materials (resins) which are solid in finished form but, at some stage in their processing, are fluid enough to be shaped by application of heat and pressure. In the finished form, plastics consist of long-chain molecules known as polymers. There are two basic types of plastics:

1. Thermoplastic resins. They may be softened and resoftened repeatedly without undergoing change in chemical composition. The maximum continuous service temperature for thermoplastics ranges from 140°F for polystyrene, 175°F for polyethylene, to 250°F for nylon.
2. Thermosetting resins. They undergo a chemical change with application of heat and pressure and cannot be resoftened. Examples of this class are silicones, phenolics, and epoxies. In general they are resistant to temperatures ranging from 300° to 500°F.[7]

Tensile strength: The resistance offered by a material to its being pulled apart is recognized as tenacity. Tensile strength is the tenacity of an object per unit area of its cross section. It is measured in pounds per square inch. The tensile strength of textiles is of particular importance to hospitals. Also, the choice of a suture material depends largely upon the tensile strength of the tissues to be sutured and the strength of the suture material.

Ultrapure water: A water having a specific resistance of 10,000,000 ohm-cm or greater and containing less than 20 parts per billion of electrolyte. Theoretically pure water has a specific resistance of 18,000,000 ohm-cm at 18°C and no electrolyte.

Vegetable parchment: This is a paper made by passing a waterleaf sheet prepared from rag or pure chemical wood pulp through a bath of sulfuric acid, after which the sheet is washed and dried. Parchment is odorless and tasteless, greaseproof or grease resistant, and it has a high wet strength which is maintained over a long period of time. It is resistant to many solutions, either hot or cold.

REFERENCES

1. Gordon, J. F. (Ed.): *Control of Communicable Diseases in Man,* 10th ed. New York, Am. Public Health, 1965.
2. McDermott, W.: Microbial persistence. *Yale J Biol Med, 30:*257-291, 1958.
3. Crawford, A. E.: *Ultrasonic Engineering.* London, Butterworths Scientific Publications, 1955, p. 26.
4. Stimson, H. F.: Celsius versus Centigrade: The nomenclature of the temperature scale of science, *Science, 136:*254-255, 1962.
5. Riley, R. L., and O'Grady, F.: *Airborne Infection.* New York, Macmillan, 1961, p. 168.
6. American Medical Association: *Report of Commission on Cost of Medical Care,* Vol. III, 1964.
7. Clauser, H. R. (Ed.): *Encyclopedia of Engineering Materials and Processes.* New York, Reinhold, 1963, p. 484.

Chapter 3

GROWTH AND DEATH OF MICROORGANISMS

CHARACTERISTICS OF GROWTH

IT IS COMMONLY accepted that in a biological sense the process of growth represents an orderly increase in all of the components of an organism. This signifies that the living cell is a dynamic system with a specific pattern of organization, imposed by its genetic structure, and which is perpetuated through the assimilation of energy-yielding nutrients and the ability to reproduce.

In studying growth phenomena, the rate at which the organism is dividing, i.e. how many generations are occurring within a period of time is of greater interest than simply determining the actual number of living organisms from hour to hour. Bacterial species are characterized by exceptionally high growth rates and this factor is recognized as of the utmost importance in the scheme of biological survival. Since the growth rate is directly related to the rate of metabolism, it can be said that the larger the organism, the more slowly it grows.

In any cell the process of reproduction requires the presence of a large number of different enzymes and proteins. In addition, other molecules must be present, such as nucleic acids, lipids, and carbohydrates. That all organisms share a common chemical composition is well established. Foremost in importance in this composition is the invariable presence of three kinds of complex organic macromolecules: deoxyribonucleic acid (DNA), ribonucleic acid (RNA), and proteins. The DNA is the cellular substance which serves as the repository of information identifying the organism in terms of specific properties. It is largely confined to the nucleus of the cell. RNA appears to be deeply involved in the complex patterns of protein synthesis and most of this substance is located in the cytoplasm of the cell. The proteins, in turn, function as the catalysts or enzymes responsible for all of the varied operations of the cell.

The size of the smallest of microbial cells is governed by molecular limitations basic to the maintenance of cellular function. A definition of "cell size" is difficult to comprehend until one can visualize that an organism occupying only 10^{-12} ml and consisting of only 2.5×10^{-13} gm of dry matter contains hundreds, perhaps thousands, of different kinds of nucleic acid and protein molecules organized in space and time in such a manner that

TABLE 3-1

SIZE OF UNICELLULAR PROTISTS AND OF VIRUSES

(From Stanier, Doudoroff, and Adelberg[1])

| | | *Volume of Unit—Cubic Microns* | | |
Major Group	*Subgroups*	*Normal Range*	*Extreme Limits*	*Limits for Major Group*
Higher Protists	Unicellular algae	5,000–15,000	5–100,000	
	Protozoa	10,000–50,000	20–150,000,000	5–150,000,000
	Yeasts	20–50	20–50	
	Eubacteria	1–5	0.1–5,000	
Lower Protists	Spirochetes	0.1–2	0.05–1,000	
	Myxobacteria	1–5	0.5–20	0.01–5,000
	Blue-green algae	5–50	0.1–5,000	
	Rickettsiae	0.01–0.03	0.01–0.03	
	Pox group	0.01		
Viruses				
	Rabies virus	0.0015	Fixed per group	0.00001–0.01
	Flu virus	0.0005		
	Polio virus	0.00001		

their functioning results in perpetuation of the species. Because of the great variation in shape of cells, it has been proposed that size should be defined in terms of cellular volume for the various structural units, representative of the higher and lower forms of microbial life, as shown in Table 3-1.

In practice, it is customary to express the growth rate in terms of the number of generations per hour. A generation is defined as the doubling of the cell number or, in other words, the time required for a culture to double in concentration or mass is referred to as the mean generation time or, as commonly stated, the *doubling time*. Since unicellular organisms multiply by geometric progression in a given period of time, the total population increases as the power (exponent) of 2. For example, one bacterium produces 2; 2 produce 4; 4 produce 8; 8 make 16. . . . On the assumption that no cells die during the process, this relationship may be expressed in the following way:

$$2^0 \rightarrow 2^1 \rightarrow 2^2 \rightarrow 2^3 \rightarrow 2^4 \rightarrow - - - \rightarrow 2^n$$

The exponents represent the number of generations.

If the logarithms of the numbers of organisms in a culture growing exponentially are plotted against units of time, a straight-line relationship is obtained as shown in Figure 3-1. When the graphic representation of exponential growth is plotted on a semilogarithmic scale, the slope of the line marks the growth rate of the culture. The steeper the slope ascends, the greater is the rate of cell multiplication. Also, the shallower the slope or the more closely it approaches the horizontal axis of the plot, the lower is the rate of growth. When the numbers of cells present at any two times are known from

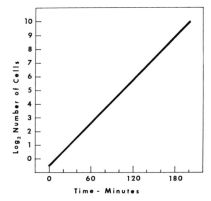

FIGURE 3-1. Typical exponential growth of organisms. The logarithms of the numbers of cells are plotted against units of time.

an exponentially growing culture, the generation time may be calculated directly by means of the following equation:

$$\text{g (number of generations)} = \frac{\log N_1 - \log N_0}{\log 2}$$

where

N_0 is the number of cells at time zero and

N_1 is the number of cells at a later time.

If, for example, the initial culture contained 100 cells and following exponential growth the number increased to 100,000,000, the number of generations would be

$$\frac{\log (10^8) - \log (10^2)}{\log 2} = \frac{8 - 2}{0.3} \text{ or 20 generations.}$$

If this increase in population occurred over a period of 10 hours, the growth rate would be 20/10, or 2 generations per hour.

THE GROWTH CURVE

Studies made on many different species of microorganisms have shown that the full reproductive power of the cells cannot be maintained over long periods of time. Microbial populations become self-limited through depletion of essential nutrilites, or when an unfavorable ionic equilibrium (pH) develops and/or by the accumulation of toxic substances in the environment.

The history of any culture is marked by a series of relatively distinct and consecutive phases of growth which, if plotted as in Figure 3-2, will show a

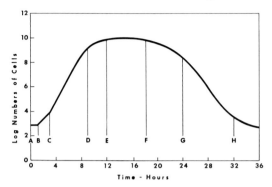

FIGURE 3-2. The growth and death cycle in a culture of bacteria. The logarithms of the numbers of viable cells are plotted against time.

typical growth curve. This curve may be divided into various sections or phases as shown in Table 3-2 and represented by the letters A through H on the graph.

INITIAL LAG PHASE

Following inoculation of a liquid medium with viable microbial cells, there occurs a stationary period, lasting for 2 or 3 hours, during which the number of cells shows no increase over the original number present in the inoculum. This is known as the *lag phase*. It represents a period of adjustment and adaptation of the cells to their new environment. The course and length of this initial stationary period depend upon the nature of the cells, the culture medium, and the temperature. The lag phase extends over that portion of the growth curve designated A to B in Figure 3-2.

EXPONENTIAL PHASE

The logarithmic or exponential period of growth is characterized by a maximum and constant rate of cell multiplication in the specific environment. Here, certain factors govern the rate of growth, such as the microbial spe-

TABLE 3-2

TYPICAL GROWTH CURVE

Section of Curve	Descriptive Phase Buchanan[2] and Clifton[3]	Monod[4]	Growth Rate
A–B	Initial stationary	Lag	Zero
B–C	Positive acceleration	Acceleration	Increasing
C–D	Logarithmic	Exponential	Constant
D–E	Negative acceleration	Retardation	Decreasing
E–F	Maximum stationary	Stationary	Zero
F–G	Accelerated death	Decline	Negative (death
G–H	Logarithmic death		
H–	Negative acceleration of death		

cies, nature and concentration of nutrients in the medium, pH, and the temperature of incubation. In ordinary liquid cultures the exponential phase of growth does not last more than 2 to 4 hours, but it can be prolonged by aeration so as to provide an adequate oxygen supply to the medium. When aeration is employed it does not necessarily increase the multiplication rate, but rather maintains it constant for a longer time and thereby affects the yield, resulting in a larger crop of cells. Usually when the cell concentration becomes greater than about 1×10^7 or 10,000,000 per ml, the growth rate will decrease unless oxygen is added through the process of agitation or by bubbling a current of air through the medium.

During this phase the numbers of organisms increase exponentially with time, and when the logarithms of numbers of cells are plotted against time a straight-line relationship results. This feature is shown by section C to D on the growth curve in Figure 3-2. Throughout the exponential growth all cells produced are viable. Generation times vary according to hereditary differences in microbial species. Under optimum conditions, *Escherichia coli* divide every 20 minutes approximately. The staphylococci and streptococci exhibit a similar generation time, but the tubercle bacillus requires 5 or more hours for division. Other species show intermediate rates of multiplication.

MAXIMUM STATIONARY PHASE

The logarithmic increase phase is followed by the so-called stationary phase, during which the maximum number of viable organisms remains constant. This comprises section E to F on the growth curve. During this period the rate of death and the rate of formation of new cells balance each other. The exhaustion of the food supply resulting in starvation, possible overcrowding, and accumulation of toxic products from metabolism are factors contributing to the cessation of growth and the appearance of the maximum stationary phase. A deficient oxygen supply is recognized as one important limiting factor in this phase. In units of time, a culture may remain in this condition for hours, perhaps days, before death of the cells becomes demonstrable. In the event that the organism is capable of producing resistant spores, the stationary phase may be extended indefinitely.

DEATH PHASE

With a progressive increase in the rate of dying, the culture enters the death phase or the phase of decline as shown by section F through H on the growth curve. As soon as a constant death rate is established, the culture proceeds to die exponentially and the number of survivors becomes smaller and smaller until finally sterility occurs and the growth cycle is complete. It must be noted, however, that deviations from the exponential order of death are not uncommon. For example, after the majority of cells have died, the death rate may show a marked decrease to the extent that a small number of cells continue to survive for many months. The continued growth of this small population of survivors has been attributed to the availability of nutrients released from cells which die and slowly decompose or lyse. Some workers believe[5,6] that "cannibalism" may be one mechanism that operates in maintaining a viable culture over long and possibly indefinite periods. This condition is also referred to as cryptic growth[7] and regrowth.[8]

THE MEANING OF DEATH

Microbial death is a statistical phenomenon. As applied to the individual cell, death represents an irreversible cessation of those vital processes which are essential for growth and reproduction. The death of microorganisms can be measured only by determining the diminution in the number of viable cells in a population. For this reason, the viable count or the number of survivors remaining after contact with a destructive influence is the only valid means by which death can be (pronounced) made known.

CRITERIA OF DEATH

The diagnosis of death in a population of unicellular organisms is not a simple process. The one practical criterion of death is failure of the organism to reproduce when planted in a suitable medium or when subjected to an optimum environment. The choice of culture medium and the conditions of incubation are critical factors in testing for viability or "kill." An injured organism may grow in one type of medium but not in another, or it may exhibit an abnormally long lag period. For example, heat-shocked tubercle bacilli have been found to remain dormant for several months in the body of a guinea pig before causing infection. Following exposure to x-rays, ultraviolet light, or to certain toxic chemicals, the organisms may lose their ability to reproduce, yet continue to function in an otherwise normal manner for a long time. These conditions demand that the medium selected for testing of survival be specified carefully, including properties that aid in repair of cell damage acquired through exposure to sublethal agents, and the incubation time allowed for growth to occur.

Considering further the criteria of death, it must be recognized that a microbial cell is "dead" only insofar as test conditions are held inviolable and permit the factual determination of viability or nonviability. A point worthy of the greatest respect is the adaptability of the microbial cell, its powers of repair and recovery, and the impact of these biologic characteristics upon man's ability to develop safe, practical methods for sterilization, disinfection, and sanitization. In the words of King,[9]

> The death of a cell may be caused by a multitude of injurious agents. The fate of the cell is dependent on its inherent reserve, its state of differentiation, its capacity to adapt to the degree of injury it suffers. If the reserve

capacities and synthetic potentialities of the cell are not badly interrupted, the autoregulatory mechanism will tend to repair and replace the damaged areas. If the injury is so severe as to preclude this compensatory response, structural and chemical disorganization quickly ensues; the fate of the cell is thereby determined and the process proceeds remorselessly, relentlessly to its inexorable conclusion.

REFERENCES

1. STANIER, R. Y.; DOUDOROFF, M., and ADELBERG, E. A.: *The Microbial World,* 2nd ed. Englewood Cliffs, N. J., Prentice-Hall, 1963, p. 140.
2. BUCHANAN, R. E., and FULMER, E. I.: *Physiology and Biochemistry of Bacteria.* Baltimore, Williams & Wilkins, 1928.
3. CLIFTON, C. E.: *Introduction to Bacterial Physiology.* New York, McGraw 1957, p. 291.
4. MONOD, J.: The growth of bacterial cultures. *Ann Rev Microbiol, 3:*371-394, 1949.
5. STEINHAUS, E. A., and BIRKLAND, J. M.: Studies on the life and death of bacteria. *J Bact,* 38:249-261, 1939.
6. HARRISON, A. P., JR.: The response of *Bacterium lactis-aerogenes,* when held at growth temperature in the absence of nutrient: an analysis of survival curves. *Proc Roy Soc [Biol], 152:*418-428, 1960.
7. RYAN, F. J.: Spontaneous mutation in nondividing bacteria. *Genetics, 40:*726-731, 1955.
8. STRANGE, R. E.; DARK, F. A., and NESS, A. G.: The survival of stationary phase *Aerobacter aerogenes* stored in aqueous suspensions. *J Gen Microbiol, 25:*61-76, 1961.
9. KING, D. W.: Effect of injury on the cell. *Fed Proc, 21:*1143-1146, 1962.

Chapter 4

THERMAL DESTRUCTION OF MICROORGANISMS

SINCE the total temperature range for the development or growth of living organisms extends from about 23°F (—5°C) to 176°F (80°C), it follows that exposure to temperatures above this range will result usually in rapid death of the organisms, with the exception of the heat-resistant spores. It is believed that the upper limit of this temperature range is determined in large measure by the thermal lability of the chemical constituents of living matter, namely, the proteins and nucleic acids. These substances are rapidly destroyed (denatured) at temperatures ranging between 122°F (50°C) and 194°F (90°C).

The mechanism responsible for the death of microorganisms when subjected to heat is not clearly understood. The traditional theory is that death of bacteria at elevated temperatures is closely linked to the alteration of proteins involving some irreversible protoplasmic change within the bacterial cell. It is held by certain investigators[1,2] that death is associated with the heat inactivation of vital enzymes or some enzyme-protein system in the cell. That other mechanisms may be operative when bacteria are destroyed by high temperatures was advanced as early as 1908 by Chick.[3,4,5] The original quantitative measurements made by Chick have contributed greatly to the evolution of a useful tool known as the "logarithmic order of death of bacteria."

More recent studies [6,7,8] have led to the concept that the mode of action of heat on bacteria closely parallels the heat coagulation of proteins. In support of this view, Amaha and Sakaguchi[9] believe that the cause of death of bacterial spores subjected to moist heat can be attributed to the denaturation of an essential protein molecule in the spore cell. Assuming this view to be correct, it is reasonable to conclude that the effect of moisture on the coagulation temperature of proteins must bear some relationship to the temperatures at which bacteria are destroyed. This point was investigated many years ago by Lewith,[10] who found that proteins are coagulated by heat at lower temperatures when they contain an abundance of water, as shown on page 286. Also, when moisture is present, bacteria are destroyed at considerably lower temperatures and in much shorter periods of time than when moisture is absent. This phenomenon can be explained on the basis that all chemical reactions, including the coagulation of proteins, are catalyzed by the presence of water.

If the frequency of statements in the literature is a valid criterion, it would be fair to say that today the concept is widely accepted that bacterial death by moist heat is caused by the denaturation and coagulation of a critical proteinaceous site within the genetic structure of the cell[11] (see Figs. 4-1, 4-2, 4-3); whereas death by dry heat is primarily an oxidation process.[12] This theory is supported by experimental observations showing that the high temperature coefficients, Q_{10} values, of bacterial death are also characteristic of protein coagulation;[13] by the increase in death rate as the result of changes in the hydrogen-ion concentration (pH) of the medium;[14,15] and by the fact that bacterial spores show a much greater resistance to dry than to moist heat.[16] The question of the mechanism of death is, indeed, a difficult one. As so aptly expressed by Ball and Olson,[17] . . . "if we knew precisely what causes a cell to die, we would be in a much better position to predict, evaluate, and improve our sterilizing technics."

DENATURATION

It is believed that the proteins of the bacterial cell, most of which are enzymatic, exist in a finely dispersed colloidal state. When subjected to antimicrobial agents such as moist heat, alcohols, or phenol, the proteins coagulate (precipitate) and become nonfunctional as, for example, in the conversion of raw egg white into rigid egg white by heat. This transformation involves an important characteristic reaction of proteins known as denaturation.[18] It implies any change in the physical or chemical properties of the

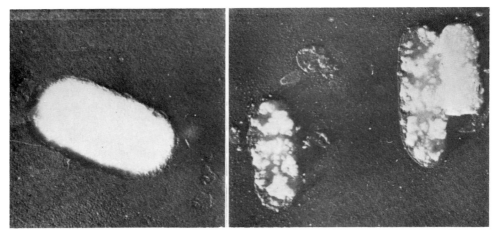

Figure 4-1. Typical colon bacillus from a one-hour broth culture. ×28,000. This shows the apparent uniformity of the cellular protoplasm. (From Heden and Wyckoff.[126])

Figure 4-2. Typical colon bacilli after being heated for 10 minutes in saline at 50°C. ×16,000. Heating the organisms in saline at temperatures above 50°C granulates their protoplasm in an irreversible fashion.

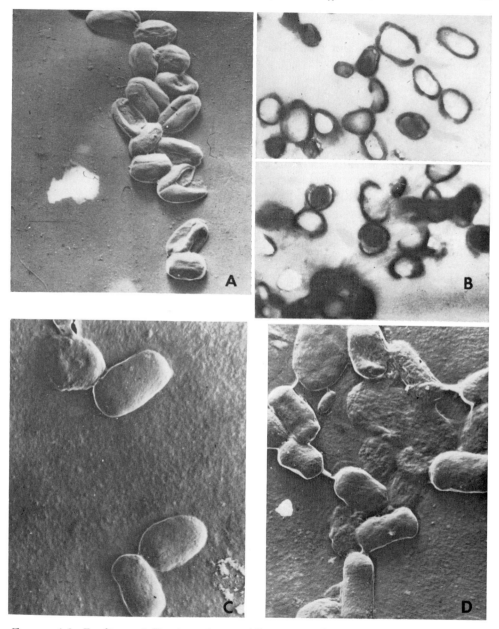

FIGURE 4-3. Replicas of *B. stearothermophilus* spores (×22,000). The structures in sections A and B are typical of unheated spores. The effect of heating at 100°C for 30 minutes is shown in C. This treatment caused swelling of the spores with evidence of cracking or splitting at one end. Section D is typical of spores heated at 115°C for 15 minutes. Here the spores have broken open at one end allowing some or all of the contents to extrude. (From Franklin and Bradley.[127] Courtesy A. H. Walters, Milton-Deosan Research Laboratory.)

protein, like solubility, and including any change in the structure of the protein molecule. If the exposure to heat is not unduly prolonged, the denaturation may be reversed by restoring the conditions under which the protein is stable. In effect, this means that one must distinguish between *reversible* and *irreversible* denaturation of proteins. After reversal of denaturation, few proteins have been shown to be identical in all respects with the original native protein.

In addition to heat, other agents capable of the denaturation of proteins are radiation, ultrasonic waves, freezing, pressure, and a variety of chemical agents, e.g., acids, alkalis, alcohol, urea, and detergents. Reactions involving denaturation are extremely complex and little understood. The significance of protein denaturation to sterilization is in the lethal action of heat on bacterial spores which was reported on very early by Chick and Martin.[5] They characterized protein denaturation as a monomolecular reaction with water.

ORDER OF DEATH

When a population of microorganisms is exposed to a sterilizing influence, the rate or velocity at which the individual organisms die is directly proportional to the concentration or number per unit volume at any given time. Generally, the order of death, as may be determined experimentally, follows a uniform and consistent course and it is commonly described as being logarithmic. This implies further that when a microbial population is in contact with a sterilizing medium the number of living cells decreases gradually, in such a manner that the logarithms of the numbers of the surviving cells at any one time, when plotted against this time, fall on a descending straight line (Fig. 4-4). Although there is some evidence to support a nonlogarithmic order of death,[19,20,21] it must be conceded from the overwhelming amount of data in the literature, dating from the earliest quantitative measurements by Chick[4] to the present time, that the death of vegetative cells as well as the death of spores is essentially logarithmic.

Knowledge of the logarithmic order is highly important because it permits the microbiologist to compute the death rate constant, designated K. This term expresses by a single number the rate of death which bears a direct relationship to the efficiency of the sterilizing agent. The constancy of the death rate signifies that the number of bacteria that are killed each minute or per time unit is a constant percentage of the number of living bacteria at the beginning of each new minute. It is customary to compute the death rate constant, K, from the formula:

$$K = \frac{1}{t} \log_{10} \frac{N_o}{N_t}$$

in which t = time in minutes or exposure period, N_o = initial number of

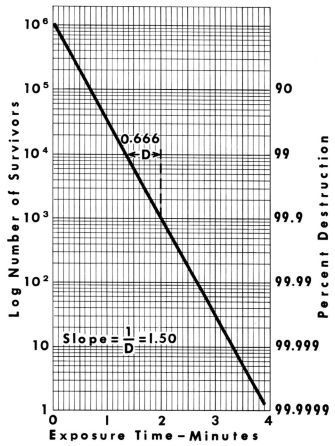

FIGURE 4-4. Survivor Curve. Numbers of survivors are plotted against times of exposure at constant temperature. The D value equals 0.666 minutes.

organisms at beginning of time interval, and N_t = number of organisms surviving at the end of the time interval.

Example: From Figure 4-4 assume that $N_o = 1$ million or 10^6 organisms, $t = 2$ minutes, and $N_t = 1$ thousand or 10^3 organisms. Then,

$$K = \frac{1}{2} (10^6 - 10^3) = \frac{6 - 3}{2} = 1.50$$

The determination of death rates makes it possible to compare the heat resistance of different organisms at the same temperature, or the heat resistance of one particular organism at different temperatures. They also enable one to describe quantitatively the effect of environmental factors, such as pH, upon sterilization. It is important to note that the logarithmic order of death implies that the same percentage of living bacteria die each minute.

Theoretically this means that complete sterilization is never attained. For example, the figures given in Table 4-1 are illustrative of a theoretical case, based upon the assumption that when a suspension of 1 million bacteria per milliliter is subjected to a sterilizing influence, 90 per cent of the organisms are killed each minute of exposure.

TABLE 4-1

A THEORETICAL EXAMPLE OF THE ORDER OF DEATH OF A BACTERIAL POPULATION

Minute	Bacteria Living at Beginning of New Minute	Bacteria Killed in One Minute	Bacteria Surviving at End of Minute	Logarithm of Survivors
First	1,000,000	90% = 900,000	100,000	5
Second	100,000	= 90,000	10,000	4
Third	10,000	= 9,000	1,000	3
Fourth	1,000	= 900	100	2
Fifth	100	= 90	10	1
Sixth	10	= 9	1	0
Seventh	1	= 0.9	0.1	−1
Eighth	0.1	= 0.09	0.01	−2
Ninth	0.01	= 0.009	0.001	−3
Tenth	0.001	= 0.0009	0.0001	−4
Eleventh	0.0001	= 0.00009	0.00001	−5
Twelfth	0.00001	= 0.000009	0.000001	−6

The figures near the end of the survivor column—0.1 or 0.01 bacteria per ml —mean that only 1 bacterium remains alive in 10 ml or in 100 ml of the suspension. At the end of 12 minutes' exposure, 1 bacterium would still survive theoretically in 1,000,000 ml, equivalent to 1000 liters or approximately 250 gallons of the suspension.

As a practical measure, the above example shows the necessity of allowing a proportionately greater period of exposure for the sterilization of a liquid containing a high concentration of bacteria than for a liquid containing only a few organisms. This condition holds true for heat sterilization, chemical disinfection, or pasteurization. However, application of this principle is oftentimes overlooked in establishing minimum exposure periods for the sterilization of materials or products.

Various explanations have been proposed to account for the logarithmic order of death of microorganisms. One of the most plausible is that advanced by Rahn[22] in which he reasoned that the death process resembles a unimolecular or first-order bimolecular reaction. With this as a basis, the logarithmic order of death is mathematically possible only when the death is due to the destruction (denaturation) of a single molecule in the cell. The logarithmic order is entirely impossible if more than one molecule must be inactivated to produce death of the cell. Whatever the true cause of death may be, it is apparent that, after a half century or more of investigation, the process remains inadequately defined.

SURVIVOR CURVES

The rate of death may also be expressed as the D value or decimal reduction time. This principle introduced by Katzin *et al.*,[23] is based upon the application of the unimolecular reaction rate constant to microbial death under uniform conditions. By definition, the D value is the time required at any temperature to destroy 90 per cent of the organisms. From Figure 4-4 it may be noted that the D value also represents the time required for the survivor curve to traverse one log cycle. Where the rate of kill is exponential, the D value becomes the reciprocal of the death rate constant K, and both D and K represent the slope of the survivor curve. It is convenient to express the relationship of these terms as:

$$D = \frac{2.303}{K}$$

Since D values may be determined for any temperature, a subscript is normally used to designate the temperature employed, such as D_{250} or D_{150}.

Decimal reduction times are important in the food processing industry, especially in the evaluation of methods for the preservation of foods by heat processing and in research studies on the microbiology of canned foods. Stumbo[24] and Schmidt[25] have contributed markedly to advances in this field. For those who may wish to gain a deeper insight into the significance of D values and thermal resistance of microorganisms, their publications should be consulted. The thermophilic organism *B. stearothermophilus* produces spores characterized by D_{250} values in excess of 4.00 minutes. The obligate anaerobes of which Types A and B *botulinum* are typical give D_{250} values of the order of 0.10 to 0.20, and the resistant spores of the putrefactive anaerobe (P.A. 3679) are characterized by D_{250} values in the range of 0.50 to 1.50. Most spores of obligate aerobic bacilli show D_{250} values of the order of a fraction of a minute, and the resistant nonsporebearing bacteria, yeasts, and molds are characterized by D_{150} values of 1.00.[24]

It is not unusual to observe a marked decrease in the death rate of survivor curves after exposure to a constant lethal temperature. These deviations from the straight line relationship and the significance of the variation in shape of time-survivor curves have been the subject of many investigations.[8] It is acknowledged that several factors influence and can be responsible for the development of nonlinear curves. The following factors should not be overlooked.

Nature of subculture medium.

Mixed flora—two strains of one species which cannot be distinguished by conventional means.

Heat required for activation of spores.

Nature of suspending medium in which spores are stored.

Age of spores.

Temperature of heating. At higher temperatures the lag due to heat activation requirement may be short and undetectable by the usual techniques.

THERMAL DEATH POINT AND THERMAL DEATH TIME

Some years ago the concept arose among bacteriologists that if a suspension of bacteria were gradually heated, a point would be reached on the ascending scale of temperature at which all of the cells in the suspension would be killed instantaneously. This gave rise to use of the expression "thermal death point" (the lowest temperature at which an aqueous suspension of bacteria is killed in 10 minutes), formerly the standard of comparison of heat tolerance of organisms of different species.[26] Use of this term has been criticized by various investigators,[27,28,29] and quite rightly, on the grounds that it is misleading because it implies that a certain temperature is immediately lethal to a microbial population, without regard to the exposure period, the number of organisms, the environment surrounding the organisms, or their physiological state.

In view of the evidence that death of microorganisms under the influence of heat follows an orderly process, due to the irreversible coagulation of cellular protein, it must be admitted that there is no one temperature at which all of the cells in a suspension would be killed instantaneously. The process occurs chiefly as a function of time within a certain range of temperature. *If the temperature is increased, the time may be decreased, or if the temperature is lowered, the time must be lengthened.* In other words, the killing of microorganisms by heat is a function of the time-temperature relationship employed. A given number of survivors cannot be said to result solely from a certain exposure, but can occur from any one of many combinations of exposure time and intensity of the sterilizing agent. Generally speaking, a process conducted at a high temperature for a short time is preferable to that performed at a lower temperature for a longer time. For these reasons, the expression "thermal death point" has in recent years given way to a more practical measurement known as thermal death time (TDT) or thermal death time temperature. These terms refer to a determination of the shortest period of time necessary to kill all of a known population of microorganisms in a specific suspension at a given temperature.

When making thermal death time determinations, it is first necessary to prepare a standardized suspension of the test organism in a suitable medium. This is usually done in a sterile phosphate buffer solution at pH 7.0. The number of organisms per milliliter of the suspension may be determined by dilution of samples and standard plate counts or counted microscopically. Quantities of the test suspension (usually 1 to 2 ml) containing 5×10^7 (50 million) organisms per milliliter are aseptically transferred into sterile TDT tubes (9 mm OD, 1 mm thickness and 150 mm in length) of Pyrex® glass.

The tubes are then sealed with the aid of oxygen flame and immersed completely in a preheated oil bath maintained constant at the desired heating temperature. At the end of each time interval of heating (5 minutes or less), four or more tubes are removed from the bath and plunged into ice water. The tips of the sealed tubes are then broken aseptically and the test suspension inoculated into sterile recovery culture media. The cultures are then incubated at the optimum temperature for thirty days, following which, colony counts are made to determine the number of survivors.

The nature of the medium in which the organisms are suspended has an important bearing on the thermal death time. Toxic substances, if present, become increasingly germicidal with slight increases in temperature. Also, products of metabolism show increased toxicity at higher temperatures. A pronounced acid or alkaline pH decreases the thermal death time; whereas the presence of oils or fats retards heat penetration and increases the time. At best, it is difficult to obtain consistent determinations of thermal death time values. Regardless of the precautions taken, certain inaccuracies may occur which are not easily controllable, such as variations in heat tolerance of organisms of the same species, number of cells, and nature of suspending medium. Comparable results can only be expected when conditions are standardized as to history and age of culture, number of cells or spores, pH of suspension, uniformity of suspension, size of test tubes, thermal conductivity and thickness of glass in test tubes. Table 4-2 gives the comparative resistance of vegetative cells and spores of certain aerobic sporeforming bacilli, expressed in terms of thermal death times.

TABLE 4-2

THE RESISTANCE OF VEGETATIVE CELLS AND SPORES OF AEROBIC SPOREFORMING BACILLI
(*From Williams and Zimmerman*[125])

Organism	Vegetative Cells Thermal Death Time In Minutes at 53°C		Spores Thermal Death Time in Minutes at 99.5°C	
	Lived	*Died*	*Lived*	*Died*
Bacillus brevis	2	4	14	16
Bacillus cereus	2	4	4	6
Bacillus subtilis, SI	2	4	4	6
Bacillus subtilis, UT	10	12	10	12
Bacillus globigii	4	6	6	8
Bacillus mycoides, 420	4	6	10	12
Bacillus mycoides, SIII	4	6	6	8
Bacillus megatherium	4	6	4	6
Bacillus fusiformis	4	6	12	14
Bacillus mesentericus	20	22	10	12

THERMAL DEATH TIME CURVE

In brief, the thermal death time curve shows the relative resistance of organisms to different lethal temperatures. This curve can be constructed by

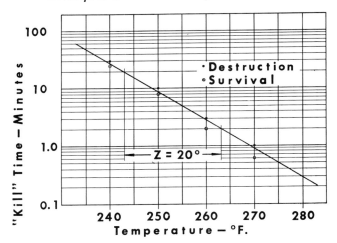

FIGURE 4-5. Thermal Death Time Curve with survival and destruction times plotted against temperature of moist heat. z = 20°F (11.2°C). The curve passes through 9 minutes at 250°F. *B. stearothermophilus* at 100,000 population of dried spores.

plotting the thermal death times (TDT's), determined experimentally, on a logarithmic scale and the corresponding temperatures on a linear scale. Such a curve is shown in Figure 4-5. It is important to note that any TDT value is meaningless unless the original number of organisms is known, because different populations result in different curves. Bingel[12] has stated that TDT determinations require a minimum number of organisms, 10^6 to 10^7 or 500 to 1000 mg of spore (garden) soil, respectively.

The slope of the curve in Figure 4-5, symbolized by z, is defined as the number of degrees F required for the curve to traverse one log cycle. This is the equivalent of the number of degrees the temperature must be raised or lowered from a given reference temperature to effect a tenfold increase or decrease in destruction time. Further inspection of the curve shows that the value of z is a measure of how the TDT varies with the temperature. It follows then, that if the z value is large, the temperature has a lesser effect on the TDT than when z is a small number. Most resistant bacterial spores exhibit z values within the range of 18 to 27°F (10 to 15°C). In Table 4-4 the average figures are 19.8°F (11.0°C). In the plotting of TDT data certain conditions should be observed. These conditions, as stipulated by Townsend, Esty, and Baselt,[30] are as follows:

A survival point is considered as positive data and the curve must be above (higher in temperature or longer in time) every survival point.

Destruction points are indicative but not positive owing to the phenomenon of "skips" (survival of organisms at a time beyond that at which sterility is indicated). In general, a thermal death curve should lie beneath as many destruction points as possible and still be above all survival points.

The slope of the thermal death time curve should be parallel to the general trend of the survival and destruction points.

The temperature coefficient, Q_{10}, equivalent to the z value, also indicates the slope of the straight line obtained by plotting logarithms of death times against temperatures. The value F, which gives one point on the curve (equal to 9 minutes at 250°F in Fig. 4-5), and z, or its corresponding Q_{10} value, are sufficient to characterize the thermal resistance of the spores of a particular species at any temperature. The symbol Q_{10} is used to designate the temperature coefficient over a range of 10°C. It means the ratio of the death rate constant at a particular temperature to the death rate constant at a temperature 10°C lower. If the constants at any two temperatures, t_1, and a temperature 10°C higher, t_2, are known, then Q_{10} may be calculated from the equation:

$$\log Q_{10} = \frac{10}{t_2 - t_1} \log \frac{K_2}{K_1}$$

The relationship of z to Q_{10} may be expressed as:

$$z \ (in \ °F) = \frac{18}{\log Q}$$

$$z \ (in \ °C) = \frac{10}{\log Q}$$

Rahn[22] has calculated that the temperature coefficient per 10°C increase is between 8 and 10 for most bacterial spores over the range of 212° to 275°F (100° to 135°C). Vegetative cells give somewhat higher values in the range of 122° to 176°F (50 to 80°C).

Thermal death time studies are highly important in the field of applied bacteriology as, for example, in the canning industry, where information is required on the resistances of food-spoilage bacteria as a basis for developing adequate heating processes for canned foods. It should be remembered that thermal death times are not precise values. Also, Q_{10} values are often falsely assumed constant over a broad temperature range. Actually, they diminish as the temperature is raised. All death time data have a certain range of possible error, the magnitude of which depends upon the spacing of the time intervals. The number of survivors is never zero, but becomes very small, e.g. 1 in 100 liters or 1 in 1000 liters.

RESISTANCE OF MICROORGANISMS TO HEAT

The resistance of microorganisms to external destructive agents such as heat, chemicals, and ionizing radiations forms the basis for all methods of sterilization and disinfection. It must be explained, however, that today our knowledge of "why and how" certain species are more resistant than others to destructive influences is very limited. This situation calls for the greatest respect of the fact that the microbial cell is composed of a highly complex system which controls its ability to survive in an undesirable environment. According to Wyss,[31] "when stresses are brought to bear upon the system three possibilities are revealed: 1) the system breaks down and the organism dies or fails to leave progeny for the continuation of its line; 2) the system develops means of resisting, and 3) the system changes by accommodating itself temporarily or permanently to the presence of the undesirable influence."

VEGETATIVE FORMS

The resistance of microorganisms to heat covers a broad range of temperature. The extremes extend from approximately 122°F (50°C) for a few minutes' exposure to moist heat for the highly susceptible forms, to 572°F (300°C) for 30 minutes' exposure to dry heat for the most resistant bacterial spores.

Yeasts

Probably the yeasts and the yeast-like fungi are typical of the most readily killed forms of microbial life. In contact with moist heat at 122° to 140°F (50° to 60°C) vegetative yeast cells are usually killed in 5 minutes. However, in the spore stage these organisms require a temperature of 158° to 176°F (70° to 80°C) for killing in the same period of time. Beamer and Tanner[32] found that *Saccharomyces ellipsoideus in* dextrose bouillon (about 5 million cells/ml, pH 8.0) were killed at 140°F (60°C) in 15 minutes, and in grape must with 8 million cells/ml, pH 2.6, at the same temperature in 20 minutes.

Molds

The vegetative forms of molds or fungi are usually destroyed in 30 minutes' exposure to moist heat at 144°F (62°C); whereas certain spores may require a temperature of 176°F (80°C) for killing in the same period of time. Most of the organisms classified as the *Actinomycetes* group are killed by moist heat at 140°F (60°C) in 15 minutes. According to Goyal,[33] these organisms, including the spores, are killed by a time-temperature relationship of 30 minutes at 140°F (60°C) to more than one hour at 162°F (72°C). In contact with dry heat, mold spores require a temperature of 230° to 240°F (110° to 116°C) for 90 minutes to insure their destruction.

Streptococci

In general, vegetative bacterial cells in high populations are killed by exposure to moist heat at 149°F (65°C) for 10 minutes or 176°F (80°C) for 5 minutes. Certain organisms may offer an exception to this rule. For example, *Streptococcus faecalis* is reputed to withstand a temperature of 140°F (60°C) for 30 minutes.[34] Also, it has been shown that S. *faecalis* var. *liquefaciens* survives 30 minutes at 145°F (63°C) or 10 minutes at 149°F (65°C), unless the initial number of cells is of the order of 50,000 per ml or less. In comparison, *Streptococcus lactis* in skim milk medium at 2,450,000 per ml was completely destroyed in 5 minutes at 140°F (60°C).[35] Ott, El-Bisi, and Esselen[36] determined the thermal destruction rates of *Streptococcus faecalis* in a group of precooked frozen products. Their data showed that at 150°F (65.5°C) a time of 18 minutes was required to achieve a 99.99999 per cent destruction.

Staphylococci

The staphylococci are among the most resistant of the non-sporebearing species of bacteria. *Staphylococcus pyogenes* var. *aureus* is not destroyed with certainty by exposure to a temperature of 140°F (60°C) for 30 minutes, but it is destroyed at 149°F (65°C) within that time.[37] Most coagulase-positive strains of staphylococci are killed within 30 minutes at 140°F (60°C) to 149°F (65°C). Thermal death time studies by Angelotti, Foter, and Lewis[38] indicate that heating perishable foods to 150°F (65.5°C) for at least 12 minutes reduces 10 million or less staphylococci or salmonellae per gram to nondetectable levels.

The practical importance of the relatively high heat resistance of staphylococci lies in their ability to survive occasionally in pasteurized food and on utensils that have been inadequately disinfected. Staphylococci show exceptional ability to survive in pus as demonstrated by Bormann,[39] who kept sealed tubes at room temperature and obtained abundant growth after two to three years. It has been claimed that the survival time of staphylococci and E. *coli* subjected to heat can be doubled or tripled by the addition of heat-killed cells of the same species.[40]

Walker and Harmon[41] studied the thermal resistance of *Staphylococcus aureus,* four coagulase-positive strains, in milk, whey, and phosphate buffer. The logarithmic order of death prevailed until about 99.99 to 99.999 per cent of the organisms were destroyed, after which there was a decline in the rate of destruction. The data further indicated that the D value increases at least threefold as the age of the cells increases from 12 to 60 hours or more. If a 99.999 per cent destruction of staphylococci is desired, then whole and skim milk should be heated at 140°F (60°C) for 12 and 21 minutes, respectively.

Salmonellae

Because of the continued occurrence of foodborne salmonellosis throughout the world, many studies have been conducted to determine conditions necessary for thermal destruction of *Salmonella* organisms in foods. When using *Salmonella senftenberg,* strain 775 W, Beloian and Schlosser[42] found that this organism requires 83 to 95 minutes' exposure at 140°F (60°C) for destruction when heated in liquid whole egg at pH 5.5. Also, the results indicate that if baked goods reach a temperature of 160°F (71°C) or higher, they can be considered safe from any *Salmonella* organisms if those organisms are present in the ingredients. Other studies[38] of a similar nature performed on perishable foods have shown that at 140°F (60°C) a holding time of 78 to 83 minutes would reduce 10 million salmonellae per gram to nondetectable levels.

Rickettsiae

The great mass of evidence in support of a temperature of 145°F (63°C) for 30 minutes, such as is employed in the pasteurization of milk, leaves little doubt that this time-temperature relationship is fatal to all pathogenic nonsporulating bacteria in that medium, with the occasional exception of the staphylococci. It is of special interest to note, however, that the causative agent of Q fever, *Coxiella burnetii,* was found by Ransom and Huebner[43] to survive temperatures as high as 145°F (63°C) when suspended in milk, sealed in vials, and submerged for 30 to 40 minutes in water baths. In more recent observations,[44,44a] it has been reported that the present minimum standard of pasteurization by the vat method of 143°F for 30 minutes is inadequate, but the temperature of 145°F for 30 minutes will eliminate the organism. The pasteurization of milk according to present standards of high-temperature short-time equipment of 161°F (72°C) for 15 seconds seems adequate to destroy *C. burnetii.* One of the most distressing thoughts is to have to admit that in certain states, raw, dirty, unpasteurized milk is still legally saleable—a black mark against progress in public health.

The heat resistance of diphtheroids and known species of *Corynebacterium* has been studied by Alford, Wiese, and Gunter.[45] They found these organisms capable of surviving 162°F (72.5°C) for 2.5 minutes in moist heat.

Zamenhof[46] showed that the dried vegetative cells of *E. coli* when heated in a vacuum to 275°F (135°C) for 16 minutes, were almost as resistant as the spores of *B. subtilis.* This unusual degree of resistance to high temperatures was attributed to efficient removal of water and oxygen from the cells with subsequent slowing down of the heat denaturation reactions.

Mycobacterium tuberculosis

The tubercle bacillus is one of the most difficult to destroy of all vegetative forms of bacteria. Although it offers approximately the same level of resistance to heat as other nonsporing bacteria, it has a much higher resistance to chemical agents because of the waxy envelope, the hydrophobic nature of the cell surface and the clumped growth characteristic. It will remain viable for many months in polluted water, foods, or in the dry state surrounded by organic matter. Smith[47] has stated that in books contaminated with the sputum of tuberculous patients the organisms remain viable from 2 weeks to 3½ months. In contact with dry heat, it is generally recognized that tubercle bacilli will withstand a temperature of 212°F (100°C) for 20 minutes but are destroyed in 45 minutes at this temperature.

According to Wilson,[37] the mammalian tubercle bacilli are completely destroyed by exposure to a temperature of 138°F (58.9°C) for 30 minutes, 140°F (60°C) for 20 minutes, 145°F (62.8°C) for 5 to 10 minutes, 150°F (65.6°C) for 2 to 5 minutes, or 160°F (71.1°C) for 12 seconds. Harrington and Karlson[48] tested 195 strains of *Mycobacteria* in milk by pasteurization and found no survivors in the strains of *M. tuberculosis, M. bovis, M. avium, M. fortuitum,* and BCG when exposed to 145°F (62.8°C) for 30 minutes or 161°F (71.7°C) for 15 seconds.

In determining the thermal death time curve for *M. tuberculosis* var. *bovis,* Kells and Lear[49] found a linear relationship in the temperature range of 147°F (64°C) to 156°F (69°C), with a corresponding z value of 8.6°F (4.8°C). This work further indicates that the present pasteurization standards provide a margin of safety of approximately 28½ minutes at 143°F and approximately 14 seconds at 161°F. Figure 4-6 shows an experimental thermal death time curve for *M. tuberculosis* var. *bovis* compared with the conventional standard pasteurization curve.

From studies on *M. tuberculosis* var. *bovis,* strain No. 9805, Bundeson *et al.*[50] showed that this organism failed to produce tuberculosis in guinea pigs after exposure to temperatures of 160°F to 180°F for periods of 15 to 30 seconds in chocolate drink, 12% milk and 12% ice cream mix. For effective pasteurization of ice cream mix it has been recommended that a temperature of 155°F (68°C) for 30 minutes be employed to insure destruction of *E. coli.* This has been confirmed by Speck,[51] who found that 175°F for 21.2 seconds was equivalent to the 155°F for 30 minutes.

The primary purpose of a pasteurization process is to provide assurance, with a reasonable factor of safety, that a food is free from pathogenic microorganisms. Milk standards as related to pasteurization have been to some extent the result of a compromise between conditions required for bacterial destruction and those which might impair certain properties of the milk. Following extensive research, the low temperature holding method of pasteurization has been raised from 143°F to 145°F for 30 minutes. The high-temperature short-time (HTST) standard of 161°F for 15 seconds continues to be recognized as adequate.

BACTERIAL SPORES

Spores are a normal resting stage in the life-cycle of certain groups of organisms, namely the Bacilli and Clostridia, and they constitute a phase of

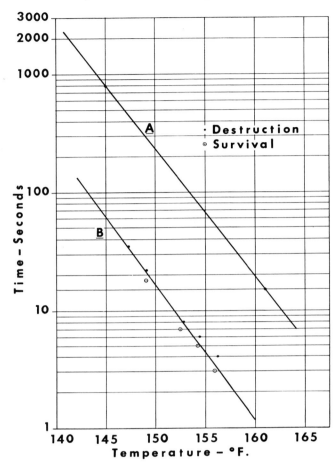

FIGURE 4-6. Thermal Resistance Curves. A represents present milk pasteurization standards. B, thermal death time curve for *M. tuberculosis*, var. *bovis*, with a viable cell population of 10^4/ml milk. z value = 8.6°F. (Adapted from data by Kells and Lear.[49])

bacterial life in which the processes of the living cell are carried on at a minimum rate. This does not mean that the bacterial spore possesses a metabolically inert system. It has been demonstrated[52] that intact resting spores contain a large number of active enzymes which make it possible to transform the dormant passive cell into an actively growing vegetative cell in a short period of time in contact with a favorable environment. Formerly it was believed that sporulation was stimulated by adverse conditions, such as extreme temperatures, aridity, or the accumulation of toxic products of metabolism. It now appears that many species of bacteria sporulate in a favorable environment.

Longevity

It is commonly recognized that bacterial spores are the most resistant of all living organisms in their capacity to withstand external destructive agents. Anthrax spores, for example, dried on silk threads have been found viable after sixty years. Also, it has been reported that *B. anthracis* survived for sixty years in dried soil kept at room temperature.[53] Other viable spore-formers have been recovered from canned and hermetically sealed meat after a lapse of 115 years.[54] Murray[55] found 34 strains of *C. tetani* in brain heart agar in test tubes, sealed in 1930, to be viable with typical growth and spore formation when examined in 1959. Miller and Simons[56] reported on the survival of bacteria after twenty-one years in the dried state. Their findings indicated that the gram-positive cocci and bacilli survive drying and storage *in vacuo* better than gram-negative organisms.

The maximum time that microorganisms can survive in the dormant state is of interest to biologists in general. Such information may serve as a guide to the preservation of cultures, to assist in explaining the mechanism of dormancy and in helping to answer the question of transmission of life through space. An interesting account of the survival records of spores was made by Sneath,[57] who determined the number of microorganisms present (viable counts) in the soil dried on the roots of plants from collections of the Royal Botanical Gardens and the British Museum. Some of the plants were more than three hundred years old, maintained in the dry state, and some had been treated with mercuric chloride, making unlikely the possibility of multiplication during this time period. Fungi and streptomyces were found in samples less than fifty years old, whereas only species of *Bacillus* were observed in older samples.

From Sneath's data it appears that 90 per cent of the organisms die every fifty years for a period and that later, due presumably to the presence of a more resistant fraction, 90 per cent die every one hundred years. On the assumption that the last figure is correct, one can estimate that a ton of dry soil would still contain a few viable spores after a lapse of one thousand years. From this study one may conclude further that life could probably be preserved for periods of more than a million years, if suitably protected and maintained at temperatures close to absolute zero.

Explanation of Spore Resistance

From studies on the structure of bacterial forms by means of the electron microscope, it appears that spores are dense concentrations of bacterial protoplasm (Figs. 4-7, 4-8). There are two regions in the interior of spores: a kernel of dense protoplasm, and a rind, or *cortex*, of less dense material. The inner region comprises the dormant bacillus as shown in Figure 4-8. Just how this small mass of protoplasm differs in its chemical and physical prop-

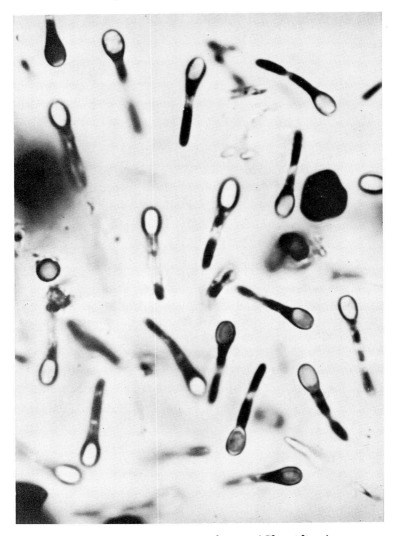

FIGURE 4-7. Bacterial spores. Anaerobic sporeformer (*Clostridium*) in course of sporulation. Stained wet mount ×2700. The rod-shaped cells are swollen at one end by the presence of oval, high refractile spores. (Courtesy of Dr. C. F. Robinow, University of Western Ontario.)

erties from the protoplasm of vegetative cells is not clearly understood. However, the thermal resistance of spores is generally attributed to a low water content or to a relatively low salt content. Certain investigators hold that most of the water present in spores is bound, not in the free state, intimately associated with the colloids of the cell, and as such it is less reactive and more resistant to physical and chemical agents.

Henry and Friedman[58] showed that spores of the *Bacillus* group have a

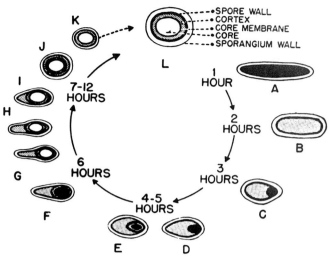

FIGURE 4-8. Diagrammatic summarization of observed stages in sporulation cycle of *Clostridium perfringens*. A, vegetative cell. B, cell enlargement, forespore not obvious. C, forespore is terminally located; sporangium ellipsoid in shape. D, enlargement of forespore. E, encystment of forespore. F, contraction of sporangium. G, forespore seen which resists staining effect. H, forespore becomes subterminal within sporangium. I, sporangium progressively contracts around forespore. J, final stages of sporangium contraction. K, morphologically mature spore. L, cytological aspect of mature spore. (From Smith and Ellner.[128])

bound water content of the order of 60 to 70 per cent, as compared with 3 to 21 per cent in the vegetative cells. Others[59,60] have expressed the view that the water content of spores is exceedingly low, comparable to that of dehydrated protein. In contrast, Black and Gerhardt[61] found the water content of dormant spores and vegetative cells of *Bacillus cereus* to be 64.8 and 73.0 per cent, respectively. This work on water distribution and permeability led them to propose that the core of the dormant spore exists as an insoluble and heat-stable gel. The presence of lipoid material in the spore may also contribute to its heat resistance.

One of the most outstanding characteristics of bacterial spores is their resistance to heat inactivation. The specific mechanism and biochemical properties responsible for this resistance have been the subject of considerable research with practical implications for those concerned with the medical-surgical field and the preservation of foods and other perishable materials. As far back as 1932, ultraviolet photomicrographs of sporulating bacteria revealed that the developing spore absorbs ultraviolet light more intensely than the surrounding vegetative cell.[62] Some twenty years later, Powell[63] identified the specific chemical substance responsible for this light absorption as dipicolinic acid (DPA). Since the identification of DPA from aerobic spores, this compound has been found in all spores examined to the extent of 5 to 15 per cent of the dry weight. It is believed to have an essential role in the property of thermoresistance,[64,65,66] but it is not the determinant of the differences in heat resistance between species. Even within a species, the DPA content can apparently become divorced from the heat-resistant state. Schmidt[25] has advanced the hypothesis "that dipicolinic acid or a polymer thereof may confer thermal stability upon spore protein molecules either by direct linkage or by further chelate linkages between dipicolinic acid, protein, and calcium or other heavy metals.

Dipicolinic acid is synthesized during sporulation and is completely lost, presumably as a calcium chelate, during the germination process. When a suspension of bacterial spores is subjected to thermal inactivation, there is a progressive loss of DPA, proteins, and other constituents from the cell.[65] The exact relationship between heat inactivation of spores and release of these cellular materials remains to be explained.

Spore resistance appears to vary widely from species to species and to a considerable extent within a species and within a given spore population. Williams and Harper[67] claim that luxuriance of growth and luxuriance of sporulation are not governing factors in determining heat resistance of spores. Incubation at the optimum temperature favors increased thermal resistance. In the case of obligate thermophilic spores an increase in incubation temperature, up to 60°C, may show a marked increase in resistance.[68] Most spores attain their maximum resistance several days after entering into the spore stage, whereas others such as *Cl. botulinum* and *Cl. tetani* appear to be more resistant when young.

In seeking an explanation of the mechanism of spore resistance, Curran[54] has mentioned that the nature of the nutrients in the spore-producing medium is significant. Media deficient in certain metallic ions, such as phosphate, calcium, magnesium, and iron yield spores of low thermal resistance. Potassium is essential for spore formation by *B. cereus,* and minute amounts of manganese are required by *B. subtilis.* Calcium has been recognized as playing a role in heat resistance and spores contain about ten times as much calcium as the vegetative forms. Spores produced in media deficient in calcium but rich in other ions appear to be heat-sensitive.[66]

The higher the concentration of spores in a medium, the greater is their resistance, and proportionately more heat or a longer time is required to effect sterilization. In high populations of 10^7 or 10^8 spores, a minute fraction may possess extreme heat resistance.[19] Descendants of spores surviving extreme heat treatments do not show increased heat tolerance. The reaction of the medium is another important factor affecting heat resistance. The pH of maximum heat tolerance of different species may vary from 6.0 to 8.0. Also, when spores are suspended in oily materials their heat resistance is markedly increased and the resistance of dry spores in strictly anhydrous fat approaches that of dry sterilization.

Germination

Within the past few years there has emerged a generalized picture of the processes occurring in the transformation of a dormant spore into a vegetative cell. At least three different kinds of sequential events are recognized in the transformation. These are referred to as activation, germination, and outgrowth. The first step in the breaking of dormancy known as activation or "heat shock" is a process which conditions the spore to germinate under the appropriate environment. The usual way to activate spores is by exposing them to heat. Curran and Evans[69] were the first workers to demonstrate systematically that sublethal heat of 143°F (62°C) to 203°F (95°C) could induce dormant spores to germinate. Germination may be regarded as the change from a heat-resistant phase to a heat-labile entity which may not be a true vegetative cell. If germination is not induced after heat activation, the spore reverts to its previous dormant state.[70,71]

In the process of outgrowth the synthesis of new macromolecules takes place, which results in the emergence of a new vegetative cell. Keynan and Halvorson[72] have mentioned the fact that activation is frequently a reversible process consistent, perhaps, with the notion that it involves a reversible denaturation of proteins. The sites in the spore activated in this manner are at present unknown (Fig. 4-9). Possibly an "unblocking" of an enzyme system or a change in permeability of some structure could account for the known effects of activation.

Powell,[73] who has studied extensively the biochemistry of spores, has summarized our general "working hypothesis" in these words: "The resting spore is a highly condensed waterproofed structure stabilized by the incorporation of calcium dipicolinate and possibly by the constitution of the spore coat. We think it likely that a hydration and depolymerization of this structure occurs during germination." These views do not differ essentially from the very early ideas of Lewith[10] in 1890.

Relative Resistances

Rahn[22] has presented a summary of the relative resistances of bacterial spores, mold spores, and of viruses, based on the resistance of a vegetative organism (*E. coli*) as unity. These data are given in Table 4-3. The contrast between bacterial spores and the other forms is immediately apparent, where in the case of moist heat as the sterilizing agent, the computed death rate of *E. coli* is 3,000,000 times as great as that of spores. It should be understood that the ratios given in Table 4-3 are not precise values. They reflect only the order of magnitude of the lethal reactions. Murrell and Warth[66] analyzed a number of *Bacillus* species with a wide range in heat resistance. They calculated decimal reduction times from survival curves and the D values at 212°F (100°C) were found to range from 0.83 min-

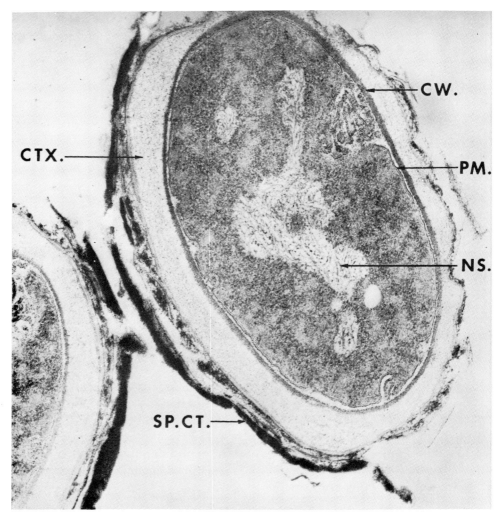

FIGURE 4-9. Section through a germinating spore of *Bacillus megaterium* with much of the cortex still left in place. The outer coat (SP. CT.) is not well preserved. The cortex (CTX.) has a loose, spongy structure and is in the process of being dissolved. Cell wall (CW.) is still thin but will soon become thicker. Plasma membrane (PM.) is dense and shows irregularities of outline characteristic of fully developed vegetative cells. Nuclear structure (NS.) is well defined. Cytoplasm appears coarse grained and typical of that of a growing bacterium. (Electron micrograph. Courtesy of Dr. C. F. Robinow, University of Western Ontario.)

utes to 714 minutes. The temperature coefficient or z value equaled 18°F (10°C). The magnitude of resistance can be further illustrated by the fact that certain spore cultures will withstand a temperature of 240°F (116°C) for over 3 hours, whereas the vegetative forms of most sporulating species

TABLE 4-3

RELATIVE RESISTANCES OF BACTERIAL SPORES, MOLD SPORES, AND OF VIRUSES
REFERRED TO THE RESISTANCE OF E. COLI AS UNITY

(From Rahn[22])

Sterilizing Agent	Escherichia Coli	Bacterial Spores	Mold Spores	Viruses and Bacteriophage
Phenol	1	100,000,000	1–2	30
Formaldehyde	1	250		2
Dry heat	1	1,000	2–10	±1
Moist heat	1	3,000,000	2–10	1–5
Ultraviolet	1	2–5	5–100	5–10

are killed in a few minutes at temperatures ranging from 131°F (55°C) to 149°F (65°C).

From the literature it is evident that authorities are not always in agreement concerning the thermal death requirements of microbial life. Various time-temperature ratios have been recommended for moist heat sterilization, some of which carry a proportionately greater factor of safety than others in assuring the destruction of the most resistant spores. Most of the data in the classical literature are of little value in establishing thermal death time curves because they lack essential information on populations of organisms used, rate of rise in temperature, points of survival and kill, or other such data. The data given in Table 4-5 are typical of recommended thermal death time temperatures necessary to kill all life.

The commonly quoted statement that "no living thing can survive 10 minutes *direct exposure* to saturated steam at 121°C (249.8°F)" would seem to be reasonably close to a minimum standard of time and temperature required for hospital sterilization. It is noteworthy, however, that Bigelow and Esty[75] reported the existence of thermophilic spores which required 23 minutes of direct exposure to saturated steam at 248°F (120°C) for their destruction. Also, Black and Tanner[76] found that certain aerobic thermophiles survived 212°F (100°C) for 24 hours, 239°F (115°C) for 1 hour, and 248°F (120°C) for 25 minutes. More recently, Williams and Robertson[68] were able to show that thermophilic spores of five obligate strains of *B. stearothermophilus* survived 25 to 44 minutes at 248°F (120°C).

For long it has been known that garden soil (spore-earth) is a highly thermoresistant medium. Tests made by Dobberstein[77] showed a striking degree of resistance in that samples of spore-earth, in aerobic and anaerobic cultures, exposed to tense steam at 273°F (134°C) for 4½ hours survived when incubated at 60°C. Similarly, Kurzweil[78] has mentioned a thermoresistant anaerobic organism from the soil spore species (*B. cellulosae dissolvens*) which survives 30 to 40 minutes in saturated steam at 248°F (120°C) and 2 to 3 minutes at 273°F (134°C). From the destruction times of bacterial spores subjected to moist heat as given in Table 4-4, it is known that most resistant spores can rarely withstand 5 minutes' exposure to satu-

TABLE 4-4

TYPICAL DESTRUCTION TIMES (IN MINUTES) OF BACTERIAL SPORES SUBJECTED TO MOIST HEAT

(Revised from Perkins[74])

Organism	212°F 100°C	221 105	225 107	230 110	239 115	248–250 120–121	257 125	266–270 130–132	273–275 134–135	z Value °F	z Value °C	Investigator
B. anthracis	2											Schneiter and Kolb[78]
B. anthracis	15											Stein and Rogers[80]
B. anthracis	10	10										Murray[81]
B. cereus	14.2D									18.0	10.0	Murrell and Warth[66]
B. coagulans	270D									18.0	10.0	Murrell and Warth[66]
B. larvae	160			41		8.6		1.9	1.2	30.0	16.8	Calesnick and White[82]
B. subtilis	17											Schneiter and Kolb[79]
B. subtilis					1.6D	0.35D	0.10D	0.017D		14.8	8.3	Pflug[16]
B. subtilis	10											Ecker[83]
B. subtilis	14	6								23.4	13.0	Williams[84]
Cl. botulinum	330	100		32	10	4				18.0	10.0	Esty and Meyer[85]
Cl. botulinum				30	10	4				19.8	11.0	Hoyt, Chaney, and Cavell[86]
Cl. botulinum	300	120		90	40	10						Tanner and McCrea[87]
Cl. botulinum	300	40				6				18.0	10.0	Weiss[88]
Cl. botulinum	360				10							Ball[89]
Cl. bifermentans	45	21								27.0	15.0	Esty and Meyer[85]
Cl. oedematiens				10	4	1				19.8	11.0	Hoyt, Chaney, and Cavell[86]
Cl. oedematiens				15								Ecker[83]
Cl. sporogenes	150	45		12						16.2	9.0	Esty and Meyer[85]
Cl. septicum			5									Ecker[83]
Cl. tetani	90	25								16.2	9.0	Esty and Meyer[85]
Cl tetani	25	10								21.6	12.0	Murray and Headlee[90]
Cl. welchii		5								23.4	13.0	Headlee[91]
Cl. welchii		5	5									Ecker[83]
Cl. welchii				10								Underwood[92]
Putrefactive anaerobe	780	170		41.6	15.6	5.6						McCulloch[93]
Putrefactive anaerobe				8.0D		0.37D		0.028D				Frank and Campbell[94]
Putrefactive anaerobe				110	30	9	4			20.0	11.2	Schmidt[75]
"Thermophiles"	834			100	40	12	4.6					Bigelow[95]
B. stearothermophilus	714D	405		120				2.2		18.0	10.0	Murrell and Warth[66]
Spore soil	660	420			15					18.0	10.0	Ecker[83]
Spore soil	1020		420		15	6			0.9	16.2	9.0	Konrich[96]
Average										19.8	11.0	

D value = Decimal Reduction Time. Minutes required to destroy 90 per cent of the cells when exposed to given temperature

z Value = Number of degrees F per tenfold change in thermal death time.

TABLE 4-5

TIME-TEMPERATURE RELATIONSHIP FOR MOIST HEAT STERILIZATION

(*Revised from Perkins*)[74]

Authority	Degrees Celsius	Degrees Fahrenheit	Time, Minutes
Novy	130.0	266	$\frac{1}{2}$
Hoyt, Chaney, and Cavell	121.0	250	1
Konrich	120.0	248	6
Muntsch	120.0	248	5
Jordan	120.0	248	5
Muir and Ritchie	120.0	248	$7\frac{1}{2}$
Gerard	115.5	240	10
Eyre	115.0	239	15
Beeson	115.0	239	20
Sternberg	115.0	239	25
Bingel	114.0	237	10
Novy	110.0	230	15
McFarland	110.0	230	15

rated steam at 250°F (121°C), while apparently none of the pathogenic organisms have been shown to be resistant to an exposure of even 3 minutes.

HEAT INACTIVATION OF VIRUSES

In terms of thermal resistance, the viruses are more closely related to the vegetative bacteria than the spore-bearing organisms. Whereas all appear to be inactivated by high temperatures, it is also evident that wide variations exist between different viruses. In the classical work of d'Herelle,[97] published in 1926, it was reported that several bacteriophages were inactivated by heating for 30 minutes at 167°F (75°C), whereas some survived and some did not after heating at 158°F (70°C). These observations eventually led to the general concept of a qualitatively defined inactivation temperature, characteristic of each phage and analogous to the thermal death point of bacteria.

Moist heat at 131° to 140°F (55 to 60°C) for 30 minutes is fatal for most viruses, but when dried and in contact with dry heat they may withstand considerably higher temperatures. The vaccinia virus, for example, in dry form withstands a dry heat temperature of 212°F (100°C) for 10 minutes.[98] Under moist conditions at 133°F (56°C) the infectivity of vaccinia virus particles is destroyed rapidly, but even when it is reduced by a factor of 10^6, the particles are capable of producing strong interference in tissue cells.[99]

The virus of poliomyelitis is moderately susceptible to heat. Early references[100,101] indicate that it is inactivated at or below 167°F (75°C) for 30 minutes. More recent information[102] indicates that the poliovirus, as found in fecal material, is destroyed in aqueous suspension when heated at 122° to 131°F (50° to 55°C) for 30 minutes, but in the presence of certain cations such as magnesium no loss of the virus occurs under these conditions. It is also known that milk, cream, and ice cream exert a protective effect in that the poliovirus is able to withstand temperatures about 9°F (5°C) higher when suspended in these materials than when present in water. Pasteurization of milk experimentally contaminated with the fecal virus destroys the agent.

According to the British Commission,[103] the virus of foot-and-mouth disease in defibrinated blood is rendered inactive in 20 minutes at 131°F (55°C), and in filtered, diluted vesicular fluid in 15 to 40 minutes. Other investigators[104] have shown that this virus is destroyed at 140° to 145°F (60° to 63°C) within 10 minutes. The virus associated with swine fever appears to be unusually resistant. In filtered blood it will withstand a temperature of 136°F (58°C) for 2 hours, but at 172°F (78°C) it is destroyed in 1 hour.[105]

The herpes virus has long been considered to be one of the most thermolabile viruses. Recently, Wallis and Melnick[106] showed that by manipulating its environment with respect to salt concentration, this virus could be stabilized at 122°F (50°C) for 15 minutes. Apparently the cytomegalovirus (salivary gland) possesses a most unusual property in that it can be inactivated more rapidly at 39°F (4°C) than at higher temperatures.[107] Rapp *et al.*[108] found the infectivity of measles virus in water to be rapidly destroyed at temperatures of 98.6°F (37°C) and above. More than 50 per cent of the infectivity was lost after 1 hour at 77°F (25°C). In a study involving six outbreaks of lethal infantile diarrhea in hospitals, Light and Hodes[109] determined that the infectious agent, a filtrable virus, was wholly inactivated by boiling for 5 minutes, but it resisted heating at 158°F (70°C) for 1 hour.

It has been well established that normal commercial pasteurization is not sufficient for bacteriophage destruction. Prouty,[110] for example, reported that a temperature of 158°F (70°C) and an exposure of 15 to 30 minutes were required for inactivation of lactic streptococcus bacteriophage. Likewise, other workers[111] have shown that various strains of bacteriophages exhibit differences in resistance to heat inactivation, the conditions required ranging from 167°F (75°C) for 12 minutes, down to 140°F (60°C) for 30 minutes.

Kinetics of Inactivation

The inactivation of viruses by heat is a complex phenomenon, and in a number of instances differences have been found in the thermodynamic parameters of the reaction when carried out at high and low temperatures.[99] It is generally accepted that the destruction process is exponential in nature with the rate of the reaction dependent on temperature. The reaction rate is customarily expressed as a function of the absolute temperature according to the Eyring theory of absolute reaction rates.[112] The Eyring equation which relates the reaction rate constant, k, to thermodynamic values is written as:

$$\ln k = \ln \frac{KT}{h} + \frac{\Delta S}{R} - \frac{\Delta H}{RT}$$

in which k is the observed velocity constant at absolute temperature T; K is Boltzmann's constant (1.380×10^{-16} ergs/degree); h is Planck's constant (6.625×10^{-27} erg sec); R is the gas constant equal to 1.986 calories per degree per mole; ln* is the base e of natural logarithms; ΔH is the energy of activation, and ΔS is the entropy of activation for the process. The energy of activation is determined by plotting the logarithm of the rate constant against the reciprocal of the absolute temperature ($1/T$). This is known as an Arrhenius plot. The activation energy is generally expressed as cal/mole, or as kcal/mole. Table 4-6 gives examples of activation energy

TABLE 4-6

HEAT INACTIVATION CONSTANTS OF VIRUSES

Virus	Activation Energy $\Delta H \pm$ cal.	Temp. Range °C	Reference
T 1 phage—*E. coli*	95,000	60–75	Pollard and Reaume[119]
Staph phage	137,000	above 65	Chang, Willner, and Tegarden[120]
Staph phage	14,000	below 65	Chang, Willner, and Tegarden[120]
Rous sarcoma	77,900	45–60	Dougherty[121]
Rous sarcoma	19,900	37–45	Dougherty[121]
Variola	28,000	40–55	Hahon and Kozikowski[122]
Polio-PV ribonucleic acid	31,000	40–75	Norman and Veomett[123]
TMV—tobacco mosaic virus	74,000	43–49	Wu and Rappaport[124]

values for several viruses. For a more thorough discussion on the thermal inactivation of viruses, the reader is referred to the work of Pollard[113] and Hiatt.[114]

Viral Hepatitis

For the past 20 years the causative agent of infectious hepatitis and/or homologous serum (jaundice) hepatitis has been the subject of many investigations. It is now generally recognized that "infectious hepatitis" (IH) differs from "serum hepatitis" (SH) in that it is caused by a different virus. The causative agents of viral hepatitis are now classified etiologically as Virus A and Virus B. The A virus demonstrated in feces and blood can withstand heating at 132.8°F (56°C) for 30 minutes, whereas the B virus found in blood only survives heating at 140°F (60°C) for 1 hour and remains active in a desiccated state at room temperature for 1 year.[115] Murray[116] reported that heating plasma containing Virus B for 4 hours at 140°F (60°C) was ineffective. On the other hand, Neefe[117] found that this virus in human albumin was inactivated by heating for 10 hours at 60°C.

Hepatitis A and B may be transmitted by parenteral inoculation, and instruments contaminated with blood are infective when they puncture the

* The factor 2.303 converts $\log_{10}$ to $\ln_e$; ln of a number = 2.303 $\times$ log of that number.

skin or mucous membranes. Experimentally, as little as 0.01 ml of blood from a patient with hepatitis A and 0.00004 ml of blood from a patient with hepatitis B have produced the disease in volunteers.[118] The commonly used methods of sterilization of syringes, needles, and lancets by brief exposure in boiling water or immersion in chemical disinfectants are recognized as inadequate for the destruction of these viruses, particularly in the presence of organic substances. The National Institutes of Health stipulate that apparatus and instruments capable of transmitting viral hepatitis from one person to another be heat-sterilized with minimum requirements as follows: "Heat sterilization shall be by autoclaving for 30 minutes at 121.5°C, by dry heat for 2 hours at 170°C, or by boiling in water for 30 minutes." Since the thermal resistance of these viruses is not well established but appears to approach that of bacterial spores, it would seem unwise to attempt sterilization or decontamination by any other means than the most reliable methods.

REFERENCES

1. Isaacs, M. L.: From F. P. Gay, (Ed.): *Agents of Disease and Host Resistance.* Springfield, Illinois, Thomas, 1935, p. 228.
2. Virtanen, A. I.: On the enzymes of bacteria and bacterial metabolism. *J Bact,* 28:447-460, 1934.
3. Chick, H.: An investigation of the laws of disinfection. *J Hyg (Camb),* 8:92-158, 1908.
4. Chick, H.: The process of disinfection by chemical agencies and hot water. *J Hyg (Camb),* 10:237-286, 1910.
5. Chick, H., and Martin, C. J.: On the "heat coagulation" of proteins. *J Physiol (London),* 40:404-430, 1910.
6. Rahn, O.: The size of bacteria as the cause of the logarithmic order of death. *J Gen Physiol,* 13:179-205, 1929.
7. Rahn, O.: *Physiology of Bacteria.* Philadelphia, Blakiston, 1932.
8. Rahn, O.: The problem of the logarithmic order of death in bacteria. *Biodynamics, 4:* 81-130, 1943.
9. Amaha, M., and Sakaguchi, K.: The mode and kinetics of death of the bacterial spores by moist heat. *J Gen Appl Microbiol (Tokyo)* 3:163-192, 1957.
10. Lewith, S.: Ueber die Ursache der Widerstandsfähigkeit der Sporen gegen hohe Temperaturen. Ein Beitrag zur Theorie der Desinfektion. *Arch Exper Path Pharmakol,* 26: 341-354, 1890.
11. El-Bisi, H.; Lechowich, R. V.; Amaha, M., and Ordal, Z. J.: Chemical events during death of bacterial endospores by moist heat. *J Food Sci,* 27:219-231, 1962.
12. Bingel, K. F.: Absterbekurven gröberer Temperatur-Zeitbereiche von vegetativen Keimen und Sporen unter Einwirkung feuchter oder trockener Hitze und ihre gegenseitigen Beziehungen. *Arch Hyg Bakt,* 142:26-48, 1958.
13. Rahn, O.: Disinfection. In O. Glasser (Ed.): *Medical Physics.* Chicago, Year Bk. 1961, vol. 1, p. 327.
14. Xezones, H., and Hutchings, I. J.: Thermal resistance of *Cl. botulinum* spores as affected by fundamental food constituents. *Food Tech,* 19:113-115, 1965.
15. Walker, H. W.: Influence of buffers and pH on the thermal destruction of spores of *Bacillus megaterium* and *B. polymyxa. J Food Sci,* 29:360-365, 1964.
16. Pflug, I. J.: Thermal resistance of microorganisms to dry heat: design of apparatus, operational problems and preliminary results. *Food Tech,* 14:483-487, 1960.
17. Ball, C. O., and Olson, F. W.: *Sterilization In Food Technology.* New York, McGraw, 1957, p. 159.
18. Kauzmann, W.: Denaturation of proteins and enzymes. In W. D. McElroy and B.

Glass, (Eds.) *The Mechanism of Enzyme Action.* Baltimore, Johns Hopkins, 1954, pp. 70-110

19. VAS, K., and PROSZT, G.: Observations on the heat destruction of spores of *Bacillus cereus. J Appl Bact, 21*:431-441, 1957.

20. HUMPHREY, A. E., and NICKERSON, J. T. R.: Testing thermal death data for significant nonlogarithmic behavior. *Appl Microbiol, 9*:282-286, 1961.

21. LICCIARDELLO, J. J., and NICKERSON, J. T. R.: Some observations on bacterial thermal death time curves. *Appl Microbiol, 11*:476-480, 1963.

22. RAHN, O.: Physical methods of sterilization of microorganisms. *Bact Rev, 9*:1-47, 1945.

23. KATZIN, L. I.; SANDHOLZER, L. A., and STRONG, M. E.: Application of the decimal reduction time principle to a study of the resistance of coliform bacteria to pasteurization. *J Bact, 45*:265-272, 1943.

24. STUMBO, C. R.: *Thermobacteriology in Food Processing.* New York, Academic, 1965.

25. SCHMIDT, C. F.: Thermal resistance of microorganisms. In G. F. Reddish (Ed.): *Antiseptics, Disinfectants, Fungicides, and Chemical and Physical Sterilization,* 2nd ed. Philadelphia, Lea & F., 1957, pp. 831-884.

26. MAGOON, C. A.: Studies upon bacterial spores. *J Bact, 11*:253-283, 1926.

27. TOPLEY, W. W. C., and WILSON, G. S.: *Topley and Wilson's Principles of Bacteriology and Immunity,* 3rd ed. Edited by G. S. Wilson and A. A. Miles. Baltimore, Williams & Wilkins, 1946, Vol. I, p. 115.

28. TANNER, F. W.: *Bacteriology,* 3rd ed. New York, Wiley, 1937, p. 158.

29. McCULLOCH, E. C.: *Disinfection and Sterilization,* 2nd ed. Philadelphia, Lea & F., 1945, p. 69.

30. TOWNSEND, C. T.; ESTY, J. R., and BASELT, F. C.: Heat resistance studies on spores of putrefactive anaerobes in relation to determination of safe processes for canned foods. *Food Research, 3*:323-346, 1938.

31. WYSS, O.: Bacterial resistance and dynamics of antibacterial activity. In G. F. Reddish (Ed.): *Antiseptics, Disinfectants, Fungicides and Sterilization,* 2nd ed. Philadelphia, Lea & F. 1957, p. 210.

32. BEAMER, P. R., and TANNER, F. W.: In A. Jorgensen (Ed.): *Microorganisms and Fermentation.* London, Charles Griffin, 1948, p. 262.

33. GOYAL, R. K.: From Topley and Wilson: *Principles of Bacteriology and Immunity,* 3rd ed. Baltimore, Williams & Wilkins, 1946, Vol. I, p. 378.

34. TOPLEY and WILSON: *op. cit.,* p. 601.

35. KRISHMA IYENGAR, M. K.; LAXMINARAYANA, H., and IYA, K. K.: Heat resistance of streptococci. *Indian J Dairy Sci, 10*:90-9, 1957.

36. OTT, T. M.; EL-BISI, H., and ESSELEN, W. B.: Thermal destruction of *Streptococcus faecalis* in prepared frozen foods. *J Food Sci, 26*:1-10, 1961.

37. WILSON, G. S.: *The Pasteurization of Milk.* London, Edward Arnold & Co., 1942, p. 148.

38. ANGELOTTI, R.; FOTER, M. J., and LEWIS, K. H.: Time-temperature effects on salmonellae and staphylococci in foods. *Appl Microbiol, 9*:308-315, 1961.

39. BORMANN, F.: Beitrag über die Haltbarkeit der Staphylococcus im Eiter. *Zbl Bakt,* I, Abt Orig, *146*:68-69, 1940.

40. LANGE, B.: Keimmenge und Desinfektionserfolg. Ein Beitrag zur Methodik von Desinfektionversuchen. *Z Hyg Infektionskr, 96*:92-117, 1922.

41. WALKER, G. C., and HARMON, L. G.: Thermal resistance of *Staphylococcus aureus* in milk, whey, and phosphate buffer. *Appl Microbiol, 14*:584-590, 1966.

42. BELOIAN, A., and SCHLOSSER, G. C.: Adequacy of cooking procedures for the destruction of salmonellae. *Amer J Public Health, 53*:782-791, 1963.

43. RANSOM, S. E., and HUEBNER, R. J.: Studies on the resistance of *Coxiella burnetii* to physical and chemical agents. *Amer J Hyg, 53*:110-119, 1951.

44. ENRIGHT, J. B.; SADLER, W. W., and THOMAS, R. C.: Observations on the thermal inactivation of the organism of Q fever in milk. *J Milk Food Tech, 19*:313-318, 1956.

44a. ENRIGHT, J. B.; SADLER, W. W., and THOMAS, R. C.: Pasteurization of milk containing the organism of Q fever. *Amer J Public Health, 47*:695-700, 1957.

45. ALFORD, J. A.; WIESE, E. E., and GUNTER, J. J.: Heat resistance in *Corynebacterium* and the relationship of this genus to *Microbacterium. J Bact, 69*:516-518, 1955.
46. ZAMENHOF, S.: Effects of heating dry bacteria and spores on their phenotype and genotype. *Proc Nat Acad Sci USA, 46*:101-105, 1960.
47. TOPLEY, W. W. C., and WILSON, G. S.: *op. cit.,* Vol. I, p. 419.
48. HARRINGTON, R., JR., and KARLSON, A. G.: Destruction of various kinds of *mycobacteria* in milk by pasteurization. *Appl Microbiol, 13*:494-495, 1965.
49. KELLS, H. R., and LEAR, S. A.: Thermal death time curve of *Mycobacterium tuberculosis* var. *bovis* in artificially infected milk. *Appl Microbiol, 8*:234-236, 1960.
50. BUNDESON, H. N.; DANFORTH, T. F.; WOOLLEY, H., and LEHNER, E. C.: Thermal destruction of *Mycobacterium tuberculosis* var. *bovis* in certain liquid dairy products. *Amer J Public Health, 43*:185-188, 1953.
51. SPECK, M. L.: Bactericidal aspects of high temperature pasteurization of ice cream mix. *J Milk Food Tech, 24*:378-381, 1961.
52. LAWRENCE, N. L.: Enzymes active in the intact spore. *Spores,* (Pub. 5). *Amer Inst Biol Sci,* 1957, 94-104.
53. WILSON, J. B., and RUSSELL, K. E.: Isolation of *Bacillus anthracis* from soil stored sixty years. *J Bact, 87*:237-238, 1964.
54. CURRAN, H. R.: Symposium on the biology of bacterial spores. V. Resistance in bacterial spores. *Bact Rev, 16*:111-117, 1952.
55. MURRAY, T. J.: Survival of *Clostridium tetani. J Bact, 78*:293-294, 1959.
56. MILLER, R. E., and SIMONS, L. A.: Survival of bacteria after twenty-one years in the dried state. *J Bact, 84*:1111-1114, 1962.
57. SNEATH, P. H. A.: Longevity of microorganisms. *Nature (London), 195*:643-646, 1962.
58. HENRY, B. S., and FRIEDMAN, C. A.: The water content of bacterial spores. *J. Bact, 33*: 323-329, 1937.
59. ROSS, K. F. A., and BILLING, E.: The water and solid content of living bacterial spores and vegetative cells as indicated by refractive index measurements. *J Gen Microbiol, 16*:418-425, 1957.
60. POWELL, J. F., and STRANGE, R. E.: Biochemical changes occurring during the germination of bacterial spores. *Biochem J, 54*:205-209, 1953.
61. BLACK, S. H., and GERHARDT, P.: Permeability of bacterial spores. IV. Water content, uptake and distribution. *J Bact, 83*:960-967, 1962.
62. WYCKOFF, R. G., and LOUW, TER A. L.: Some ultraviolet photomicrographs of *B. subtilis. J Exp Med, 54*:3, 1931.
63. POWELL, J. E.: Isolation of dipicolinic acid from spores of *B. megaterium. Biochem J, 54*:210-211, 1953.
64. WALKER, H. W.; MATCHES, J. R., and AYRES, J. C.: Chemical composition and heat resistance of some aerobic bacterial spores. *J Bact, 82*:960-966, 1961.
65. WALKER, H. W., and MATCHES, J. R.: Release of cellular constituents during heat inactivation of endospores of aerobic bacilli. *J Food Sci, 30*:1029-1036, 1966.
66. MURRELL, W. G., and WARTH, A. D.: Composition and heat resistance of bacterial spores. *Spores III. Amer Soc Microbiol,* 1965, pp. 1-24.
67. WILLIAMS, O. B., and HARPER, O. F., JR.: Studies on heat resistance. IV. Sporulation of *Bacillus cereus* in some synthetic media and the heat resistance of the spores produced. *J Bact, 61*:551-556, 1951.
68. WILLIAMS, O. B., and ROBERTSON, W. J.: Effect of temperature of incubation at which formed on heat resistance of aerobic thermophilic spores. *J Bact, 67*:377-378, 1954.
69. CURRAN, H. R., and EVANS, F. R.: Heat activation inducing germination in spores of thermotolerant and thermophilic aerobic bacteria. *J Bact, 49*:335-346, 1945.
70. POWELL, J. F.: Factors affecting the germination of thick suspensions of *B. subtilis* spores in L-alanine solution. *J Gen Microbiol, 4*:330, 1951.
71. KEYNAN, A., *et al.*: Activation of bacterial endospores. *J Bact, 88*:313-318, 1964.
72. KEYNAN, A., and HALVORSON, H.: Transformation of a dormant spore into a vegetative cell. *Spores III.* Symposium, Ann Arbor, Michigan, *Amer Soc Microbiol,* Oct. 1964, p. 176.

73. Powell, J. F.: Biochemical changes occurring during spore germination in *Bacillus* species. *J Appl Bact, 20*:349-358, 1957.

74. Perkins, J. J.: Bacteriological and surgical sterilization by heat. In G. F. Reddish (Ed.): *Antiseptics, Disinfectants, Fungicides, Chemical and Physical Sterilization.* Philadelphia, Lea & F., 1954, p. 657. Also 2nd ed., 1957, p. 782.

75. Bigelow, W. D., and Esty, J. R.: The thermal death point in relation to time of typical thermophilic organisms. *J Infect Dis, 27*:602-617, 1920.

76. Black, L. A., and Tanner, F. W.: A study of thermophilic bacteria from the intestinal tract. *Zbl Bakt [Naturwiss], 75*:360-375, 1928.

77. Dobberstein, H.: Sterilisations- und Kulturversuche mit hochthermoresistender Sporenerde. *Zbl Bakt [Naturwiss], I Orig, 168*:606-626, 1957.

78. Kurzweil, H.: Neue Methoden der bakteriologischen Testung von Dampfsterilisationsapparaten. *Schweiz Z Allge Path Bakt, 20*:505-510, 1957.

79. Schneiter, R., and Kolb, R. W.: Heat resistance studies with spores of *Bacillus anthracis* and related aerobic bacilli in hair and bristles. *Public Health Rep* (Supp 207): 1-24, 1948.

80. Stein, C. D., and Rogers, H.: Resistance of anthrax spores to heat. *Vet Med, 40*:406-410 1945.

81. Murray, T. J.: Thermal death point. II. Spores of *Bacillus anthracis. J Infect Dis, 48*: 457-467, 1931.

82. Calesnick, E. J., and White, J. W., Jr.: Thermal resistance of *Bacillus larvae* spores in honey. *Appl Microbiol, 64*:9-15, 1952.

83. Ecker, E. E.: Sterilization based on temperature attained and time ratio. *Mod Hosp, 48*:86-90, 1937.

84. Williams, O. B.: The heat resistance of bacterial spores. *J Infect Dis, 44*:421-465, 1929.

85. Esty, J. R., and Meyer, K. F.: Heat resistance of spores of *Bacillus botulinus* and allied anaerobes. *J Infect Dis, 31*:650-663, 1922.

86. Hoyt, A.; Chaney, A. L., and Cavell, K.: Steam sterilization and effects of air in the autoclave. *J Bact, 36*:639-652, 1938.

87. Tanner, F. W., and McCrea, F. D.: *Clostridium botulinum.* IV. Resistance of spores to moist heat. *J Bact, 8*:269-276, 1923.

88. Weiss, H.: The heat resistance of spores with special reference to the spores of *B botulinus. J Infect Dis, 28*:70-92, 1921.

89. Ball, C. O.: Short-time pasteurization of milk. *Ind Eng Chem, 35*:71-84, 1943.

90. Murray, T. J., and Headlee, M. R.: Thermal death point. I. Spores of *Clostridium tetani. J Infect Dis, 48*:436-456, 1931.

91. Headlee, M. R.: Thermal death point. III. Spores of *Clostridium welchii. J Infect Dis, 48*:468-483, 1931.

92. Underwood, W. B.: *A Textbook of Sterilization,* 2nd ed., Chicago, Lakeside, Donnelley, 1941, p. 3.

93. McCulloch, E. C.: *Disinfection and Sterilization,* 2nd ed. Philadelphia, Lea & F., 1945, p. 138.

94. Frank, H. A., and Campbell, L. L., Jr.: The nonlogarithmic rate of thermal destruction of spores of *Bacillus coagulans. Appl Microbiol, 5*:243-248, 1957.

95. Bigelow, W. D.: Logarithmic nature of thermal death time curves. *J Infect Dis, 29*: 528-536, 1921.

96. Konrich, F.: Die bakterielle Keimtötung durch Wärme. From A. Jorgensen, (Ed.): *Microorganisms and Fermentation.* London, C. Griffin, 1948, p. 113.

97. d'Herelle, F.: *The Bacteriophage and Its Behavior.* Baltimore, Williams & Wilkins, 1926.

98. Topley and Wilson: *op. cit.,* p. 962.

99. Galasso, G. J., and Sharp, D. G.: Effects of heat on the infecting, anti-body absorbing, and interfering powers of vaccinia virus. *J Bact, 89*:611-616, 1965.

100. Flexner, S., and Lewis, A. P.: The transmission of epidemic poliomyelitis to monkeys. *JAMA, 53*:1913, 1909.

101. Breed, R. S.; Murray, E. G. D., and Hitchens, A. P. (Eds.): *Bergey's Manual of Determinative Bacteriology,* 6th ed. Baltimore, Williams & Wilkins, 1948, p. 1258.

102. JAWETZ, E.; MELNICK, J. L., and ADELBERG, E. A.: *Review of Medical Microbiology* Los Altos, Calif., Lange, 1964, p. 339.
103. British Commission, Foot-and-Mouth Disease Research Committee, Ministry of Agriculture and Fisheries, London, 1927.
104. ZELLER, H.; WEDEMANN, W.; LANGE, L., and GILDEMEISTER, E.: From Wilson, G. S. (Ed.): *The Pasteurization of Milk,* London, Arnold, 1942, p. 148.
105. TOPLEY and WILSON: *op. cit.,* Vol. II, p. 1964.
106. WALLIS, C., and MELNICK, J. L.: Thermostabilization and thermosensitization of herpesvirus. *J Bact, 90:*1632-1637, 1965.
107. VONKA, V., and BENYESH-MELNICK, M.: Thermoinactivation of human cytomegalovirus. *J Bact, 91:*221-226, 1966.
108. RAPP, F.; BUTEL, J. S., and WALLIS, C.: Protection of measles virus by sulfate ions against thermal inactivation. *J Bact, 90:*132-135, 1965.
109. LIGHT, J. S., and HODES, F. L.: Studies on epidemic diarrhea of the newborn: Isolation of a filtrable agent causing diarrhea in calves. *Amer J Public Health, 33:*1451, 1943.
110. PROUTY, C. C.: The problems of bacteriophage in relation to cheese starters. *Canad Dairy Ice Cream J, 27:*46-48, 1948.
111. WILKOWSKE, H. H.; NELSON, F. E., and PARMELEE, C. E.: Heat inactivation of bacteriophage strains active against lactic streptococci. *Appl Microbiol, 2:*250-253, 1954.
112. EYRING, H.: The activated complex in chemical reactions. *J Chem Phys, 3:*107-115, 1935.
113. POLLARD, E. C.: *The Physics of Viruses.* New York, Academic, 1953.
114. HIATT, C. W.: Kinetics of the inactivation of viruses. *Bact Rev, 28:*150-163, 1964.
115. WORLD HEALTH ORGANIZATION. Expert Commission on Hepatitis, *Technical Report Series,* No. 62, Geneva, 1953.
116. MURRAY, R.: Razors and homologous serum hepatitis. *JAMA, 152:*656, 1953.
117. NEEFE, J. R.: Recent advances in knowledge of "virus hepatitis." *Med Clin N Amer, 30:*1407, 1946.
118. EICHENWALD, H. F., and MOSLEY, J. W.: *Viral Hepatitis,* U. S. Dept. Health, Education and Welfare, Publ. No. 435, 1959.
119. POLLARD, E., and REAUME, M.: Thermal inactivation of bacterial viruses. *Arch Biochem, 32:*278, 1951.
120. CHANG, S. L.; WILLNER, M., and TEGARDEN, L.: Kinetics in the thermodestruction of bacterial virus in water. *Amer J Hyg, 52:*194-201, 1950.
121. DOUGHERTY, R. M.: Heat inactivation of rous sarcoma virus. *Virology, 14:*371-372, 1961.
122. HAHON, N., and KOZIKOWSKI, E.: Thermal inactivation studies with variola virus. *J Bact, 81:*609-613, 1961.
123. NORMAN, A., and VEOMETT, R. C.: Heat inactivation of poliovirus ribonucleic acid. *Virology, 12:*136-139, 1960.
124. WU, J., and RAPPAPORT, I.: Kinetic studies of heat inactivation of tobacco mosaic virus infected centers and potentially infectible sites on *Nicotiana glutinosa. Bact Proc, 67:*161, 1961.
125. WILLIAMS, O. B., and ZIMMERMAN, C. H.: Studies on heat resistance. III. The resistance of vegetative cells and spores of the same organism. *J Bact, 61:*63-65, 1951.
126. HEDEN, C. G., and WYCKOFF, R. W. G.: The electron microscopy of heated bacteria. *J Bact, 58:*153-160, 1949.
127. FRANKLIN, J. G., and BRADLEY, D. E.: A further study of the spores of species of the genus *Bacillus* in the electron microscope using carbon replicas, and some preliminary observations on *Clostridium welchii. J Appl Bact, 20:*467-472, 1957.
128. SMITH, A. G., and ELLNER, P. D.: Cytological observations on the sporulation process of *Clostridium perfringens. J Bact, 73:*1-7, 1957.

Chapter 5

PRINCIPLES OF STEAM STERILIZATION

M OIST HEAT in the form of saturated steam under pressure is the most dependable medium known for the destruction of all forms of microbial life. The microbe-destroying power is composed of two factors, both of which are essential: moisture and heat. Atmospheric (flowing) steam has no value in surgical sterilization. Boiling water likewise is an inadequate microbicide and its use should be discouraged wherever pressure steam is available. Saturated steam possesses the following characteristics:

ADVANTAGES

· Rapid heating and rapid penetration of textiles or fabrics.
· Destruction of most resistant bacterial spores in brief interval of exposure.
· Easy control of quality and lethality for various materials and supplies.
· No toxic residue on materials following sterilization process.
· Most economical sterilizing agent.

LIMITATIONS

· Incomplete air elimination from sterilizer, depressing temperature and preventing sterilization. Air is a stubborn opponent to the diffusion and expansion of steam.
· Possible superheated steam with diminished microbicidal power, if sterilizer is used incorrectly.
· Unsuitable method for sterilization of anhydrous oils, greases, and powders.

In order to gain a clear conception of the functions of steam in sterilizing processes as well as an accurate working knowledge of the operation of sterilizers, it is essential to understand the physical and thermal properties underlying the production and control of steam. To the scientist or engineer it may appear superfluous to devote space and attention to the meaning and interpretation of such fundamental terms as heat, temperature, and pressure. However, it should be borne in mind that in the broad field of applied sterilization there are today many individuals responsible for the daily operation and care of sterilizers whose limited background of technical training and experience would hardly permit them to qualify as skilled sterilizer technicians. It is to this group primarily that the following details are directed:

HEAT AND TEMPERATURE

The usual conception of heat is that it comprises a basic form of energy produced by the vibratory motion or activity of the molecules of a body or substance. The hotter the substance or the more heat that is added to it, the more vigorous will be the activity of the molecules. Heat itself is not a substance, because when it is added to or absorbed by a body there is no increase in weight. In one sense, heat may be likened to water in that it will only flow downhill, or rather, pass from the higher (hotter) range of temperature to the lower or colder level. The transfer of heat, upon which sterilization depends, involves an energy exchange between the sterilizing agent and the external object or receiver of heat. The process of heat transfer from one body to another may be accomplished by either conduction, convection, or radiation.

If the transmission of heat from one part of a body to another or from one body to another in intimate contact occurs by molecular impact or agitation, the process is termed conduction heating. For example, if one end of a bar of metal is heated, the other end also becomes hot. The molecular agitation set up in the heated end of the bar is transmitted from molecule to molecule until the opposite end is reached. The sterilization of instruments by means of dry heat is also an example of conduction heating.

Convection heating takes place only in liquids and gases. It implies a transference of heat from one point to another by means of a circulation of the liquid or gas itself. When a flask of solution, for example, is heated over a burner, the heated portion or bottom layer expands and rises through the entire volume. The bottom layer is replaced by a colder portion which also becomes heated and rises in its turn. Thus convection currents are set up and the heat is distributed throughout the solution by actual motion within the liquid itself.

The process of heat transfer by radiation involves the passage of heat from one object to another without warming the space between the objects. In other words, the heat is passed by means of a wave motion similar to that of light. In the strict sense, radiant heating is not used for sterilization purposes, although dielectric or induction heating utilizing radio frequency energy is employed to some extent for sanitization purposes in industry.

In distinguishing between heat and temperature, it should be understood that the latter term is used to define the hotness of a mass or body, according to some arbitrarily selected scale such as Fahrenheit or Celsius. Temperature is not a measure of the quantity or amount of heat contained in a substance, but rather it gives an idea of the intensity or quality of heat present. For example, a glass of water at 140°F (60°C) is hotter, or at a higher temperature, than a pail of water at 60°F (15.6°C), but it does not contain as much heat because the quantity of heated substance is considerably less.

ATMOSPHERIC PRESSURE AND GAUGE PRESSURE

Since pressure is considered one of the fundamental properties of a working substance, it follows that atmospheric pressure, gauge pressure, and vacuum must have a direct bearing on the behavior of a gas, vapor, or liquid confined in a sterilizing chamber. Generally speaking, the average person is not inclined to recognize that he is living at the bottom of a great ocean of air which, by virtue of its weight, exerts upon the surface of the earth an enormous pressure of more than 300,000 million tons. The pressure of this great mass of air is commonly referred to as atmospheric or barometric pressure, which, simply explained, means the weight of the column of air above the point or place in question.

Atmospheric pressure is known to diminish with elevation above the earth's surface because with increasing altitude there is a lesser quantity of air to exert a downward pressure. Also, atmospheric pressure varies from day to day due to atmospheric conditions, temperature changes, winds, etc. For these reasons, it is necessary to adopt some standard to which all variations of pressure can be referred. The standard accepted for this purpose is the weight of a column of the atmosphere at sea level which has been determined to be 14.7 pounds per square inch at a standard temperature of 32°F or 0°C. It is also known that a column of atmosphere with pressure equivalent to 14.7 pounds per square inch will balance or support a column of mercury 29.92 inches (760 mm) high. Since measurements of atmospheric pressure are made by means of a barometer, it is customary to express the results in terms of the height (inches or millimeters) of a mercury column rather than in pounds or on a weight basis. At an altitude of 250 miles (400 km) the pressure averages only 3×10^{-8} mm Hg, compared to 760 mm Hg at sea level.

When a gas, vapor or liquid is confined in a container, the instrument commonly used for recording the pressure within the container is a pressure gauge. This device measures the difference between the pressure in the container and the external atmospheric pressure in pounds per square inch. The standard type of low pressure gauge used with steam sterilizers is shown in Figures 5-1 and 5-2. This is often referred to as a compound gauge because its construction permits a reading of both pressure in pounds per square inch and vacuum in inches of mercury. In the manufacture of pressure gauges the instruments are usually adjusted to indicate zero pressure at normal atmospheric sea level pressure which in reality is 14.7 pounds per

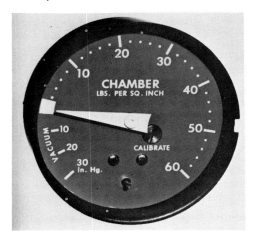

FIGURE 5-1. Low pressure gauge used on steam sterilizers. This permits reading of pressure in pounds per square inch and vacuum in inches of mercury.

square inch. Practically all steam and pressure gauges are initially set in this manner and the pressures indicated by the instruments are termed gauge pressures.

The basic elements of a Bourdon tube (sometimes referred to as Bourdon spring) gauge are shown in Figure 5-2. One end of a tube, usually formed

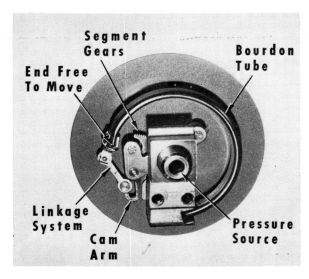

FIGURE 5-2. Interior construction details of pressure gauge used on steam sterilizers. It consists essentially of a coiled brass tube closed at one end. The open end of tube is connected to pipe through which steam under pressure is admitted. When pressure is applied, tube tends to straighten out, moving a pointer to which it is connected by means of a gear arrangement.

into a segment of a circle, is fastened to a socket which connects to the pressure source. The tube is flat on opposite sides and has an approximately elliptical cross section. When pressure is applied inside the tube, the walls deflect and tend to assume a round cross section. This sets up stresses which increase the coiling radius and the free end of the tube moves a small amount. This movement is translated into rotary motion of an indicating pointer by a linkage-and-gear arrangement. The Bourdon tubes are subject to fatigue failure. Principal factors influencing fatigue are frequency and magnitude of pressure cycling and a corrosive environment.

In scientific and experimental studies another pressure scale is employed. This scale is known as absolute pressure because zero on the scale indicates no pressure at all, or in other words, a perfect vacuum. To obtain a pressure reading relative to the true zero of pressure, the absolute zero, the pressure gauge reading must be added to the atmospheric pressure. This may be written as follows:

$$\text{Abs. pressure} = \text{gauge pressure} + 14.7 \text{ pounds.}$$

Also,

$$\text{Gauge pressure} = \text{abs. pressure} - 14.7 \text{ pounds.}$$

Vacuum gauges indicate the difference, expressed in inches of mercury, between atmospheric pressure and the pressure within the vessel or container to which the gauge is attached. For all practical purposes, 2.04 inches height of mercury may be considered equal to a pressure of one pound per square inch. Hence for any reading of the vacuum gauge in inches, G, the absolute pressure for any barometer reading in inches, B is

$$\frac{B - G}{2.04}$$

For example, if a vacuum gauge on a sterilizer reads 15 inches and at the same time the barometer reads 29.4 inches of mercury, what would be the absolute pressure in pounds per square inch in the sterilizer?

Using the above formula,

$$\frac{29.4 - 15}{2.04} = 7.0 \text{ lb. per sq. in. abs.}$$

Figure 5-3 shows the relationship existing among atmospheric, gauge, absolute, and partial vacuum pressures.

SATURATED STEAM

Moist heat in the form of saturated steam under pressure is the most dependable medium known for the destruction of all forms of microbial life. Today, in every modern hospital, there may be found a variety of sterilizers

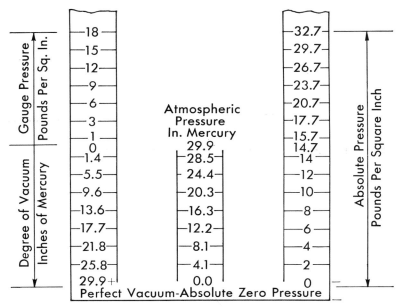

FIGURE 5-3. Numerical relationship between gauge, atmospheric, absolute, and partial vacuum pressures.

or autoclaves, each performing a vital service in protecting the patient and employee against infection, but all are dependent upon the application of certain fundamental principles allied with the use of steam as a sterilizing agent.

Steam is water vapor and, as such, it represents a physical state of water as truly as ice does; but, as a gas, it may be near or far away from its condensing or liquefying temperature. Saturated steam is water vapor in the condition in which it is generated from the water with which it is in contact. Saturated steam cannot undergo a reduction in temperature without a lowering of its pressure, nor can the temperature be increased except when accompanied by a corresponding increase in pressure. Thus, given the pressure of steam as it is ordinarily formed its temperature may be considered fixed; or, given its temperature, the pressure may be, of course, as readily deduced, pressure and temperature being convertible terms. Therefore one may speak of saturated steam at a certain temperature or at a certain pressure. The relationship of pressure and temperature in steam is shown in Figure 5-4. The phase boundary curve for saturated steam also represents the vapor pressure of water. The terms *boiling, vapor, steam, mixture, heat of vaporization,* and *superheat* are all relevant to the process of steam generation, and they help to define the physical states or properties of the working substance.

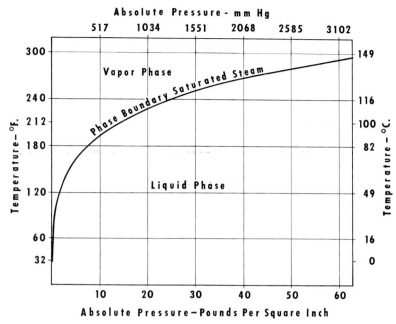

FIGURE 5-4. The relationship of pressure and temperature in steam.

MECHANISM OF STEAM GENERATION

Figure 5-5 illustrates an electrically heated steam generator. This apparatus consists of a pressure vessel, made of steel, partially filled with water, and provided with a pressure gauge, thermometer, safety valve, an adjustable steam outlet valve, water feed inlet, condensate return port, and a source of heat. The application of heat to the water in the vessel, if the steam outlet valve is open to the atmosphere, will increase the thermometer reading to 212°F (100°C), at which point it will remain constant while steam escapes to the atmosphere through the discharge valve. If the rate of heat input is increased or decreased, the rate of steam discharged will be changed correspondingly, but the temperature will remain constant at 212°F (100°C) if the pressure in the vessel remains constant and equal to standard atmospheric pressure or 14.7 pounds per square inch absolute (psia).

During the heating process, steam bubbles are formed on the surface of the heating element, they rise through the water, break at the liquid surface, and release their steam into the space above the liquid surface. The steam in the free space above the liquid is known as *saturated steam*. If the source of heat is cut off temporarily so that all of the steam bubbles rise to the water surface, the bubble-free water is designated *saturated water,* and this saturated water is at the same temperature as the saturated steam. Also, this temperature is referred to as the *saturation temperature*. When heat is ap-

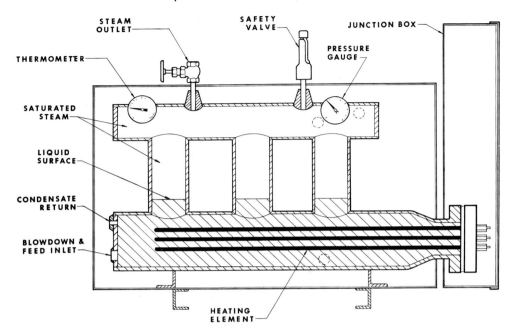

FIGURE 5-5. Diagram of an electrically heated steam generator.

plied to the water in the generator and the steam outlet valve is partially closed so as to restrict the escape of saturated steam to the atmosphere, the pressure in the vessel will rise and the temperature of the steam will show a corresponding increase. When this condition occurs it will be observed that at any specific pressure there is only one temperature of the saturated steam. This saturation temperature is plotted against steam pressure in Figure 5-4.

If the rate of heat supplied to the generator in Figure 5-5 is sufficiently low so that the liquid surface is only slightly disturbed by the bursting steam bubbles which are rising through the water, the steam that is generated will be free of entrained droplets of water and it is known as *dry saturated steam*. It is a misnomer to state that dry saturated steam contains no water, because all steam is a physical state of water. From a practical standpoint, saturated steam is always wet to at least some small degree as the result of some small quantity of unvaporized water held in suspension or mechanically entrained with the steam. Dry saturated steam is actually a theoretical line of demarcation between the wet saturated and superheated steam phases. By referring once again to the generator in Figure 5-5, if the rate of heat input is high, the liquid surface will be violently disturbed by the rapidly bursting steam bubbles and droplets of water will become entrained with the steam and discharged through the steam outlet valve.

Steam produced in this manner is called *wet steam*. It will be at the saturation temperature corresponding to the steam pressure because the saturated water and saturated steam are at the same temperature.

QUALITY OF STEAM

The quality of steam may be defined as the weight of dry steam present in one pound of the mixture of dry saturated steam and entrained water. Thus, if the quality of the steam is said to be 98 per cent, it means that the wet-steam mixture delivered from the boiler or generator, as in Figure 5-5, is composed of 2 parts by weight of saturated water, usually in the form of a fine mist, and 98 parts by weight of dry saturated steam. In other words, the dryness fraction is 0.98. Much of the contamination of steam is caused by dissolved solids or particles contained in the tiny droplets that may remain in the steam following primary separation in the boiler. Therefore, as boiler water concentration increases, steam contamination may be expected to increase. Also, gross impurities in steam may occur as the result of an abnormally high water level in the boiler, allowing the water to be carried over in gulps—commonly referred to as "priming." Excessive foam in the boiler may also contribute to the contamination of the steam. The percentage of free moisture, due to entrained water droplets, in the steam should be maintained at a very low level if the steam is to be used for the sterilization of fabrics or textiles. This requires that the dryness fraction of the steam should not fall below 97 per cent; otherwise surgical dressings and other muslin wrapped articles may become soaked with excess moisture during the initial phases of the sterilizing cycle and subsequently offer difficulty in terminal drying of the load. This point is commonly overlooked in analyzing the causes of wet dressings.

BOILER AMINES

During the past fifteen years, boiler water feed compounds have been developed to control corrosion in steam-condensing and condensate-return systems. When steam is generated in a pressure boiler system these compounds, because of their volatility, are carried over with the steam. The compounds used are generally referred to as filming amines and neutralizing amines. Filming amines are preferred in usage since they protect against oxygen corrosion as well as carbonic acid attack. The following compounds are typical of the various corrosion inhibitors:

     neutralizing amines—morpholine; cyclohexylamine.
     filming amines—octadecylamine; fatty acid
     cyclic amidines.

The presence of these compounds in steam distribution lines may present a problem because they are toxic substances and they must be dealt with accordingly. Instances where problems have occurred include the following:

Steam kettles of the direct steam injection type have contaminated food when amines were present in the steam supply.

Cases of dermatitis have developed as the result of persons bathing in hot water heated by injection of steam containing amines.

Hazards that should be considered when steam containing amines is used include the preparation of infant formulas, intravenous solutions, steam condensate as a substitute for distillate, laboratory chemical solutions, and various media for growth of microorganisms.[1]

Holmlund and Tärnvik[2] investigated the cytotoxic effect on HeLa cells of cyclohexylamine and decylamine, per se, and of the corrosion products from instruments autoclaved in steam or steam containing these compounds. Their results showed that cyclohexylamine is about ten times and decylamine about thirty times more cytotoxic than phenol. No cytotoxic effect, however, could be detected with corrosion products containing possible traces of amines or amine salts or both—nor with corrosion products alone— when these surface products were removed from the instruments by means of ultrasonic cleaning.

According to the Food and Drug Administration, USDA,[3]

octadecylamine is classed as a poisonous and deleterious substance; therefore, it may not be used in the steam lines of steam that may be incorporated into food products unless it can be established that it is required in the production of the food and a tolerance is established for the amount that would be safe for such use. There is no objection to the use of octadecylamine in steam lines where the steam may be used for autoclaving surgical instruments and gauze if the octadecylamine in the steam is not more than 2.4 parts per million.

SUPERHEATED STEAM

If saturated steam at any given temperature is subjected to a higher temperature, as, for instance, by passing it over heated surfaces or coils, it becomes *superheated steam*. The term "superheat" is used to denote the excess of the temperature over the saturation temperature corresponding to the pressure for the vapor state. The difference between the temperature of the superheated steam and the saturation temperature at the pressure of the steam is called the degrees of superheat. It is important to note, however, that superheating does not increase the pressure of the steam. It will occur only when heat is added to dry steam in the absence of water. By this process the steam is literally dried out (no longer saturated) and the peculiar advantages of the high moisture content, so necessary to sterilization, are dissipated. One common cause of superheating is the maintenance of a higher pressure and temperature in the steam jacket of a sterilizer than in the chamber. This condition raises the temperature of the steam in the chamber to a level above the actual boiling point or condensation temperature of the saturated steam. Mild degrees of superheat in the range of 2° to 5°F (1° to 3°C) may occur in steam distribution or supply lines coming from a central boiler source and connected to sterilizers in hospitals.

The properties of superheated steam approximate those of a perfect gas rather than of a vapor. It behaves much like dry hot air and takes up water with avidity. If superheated steam is used for sterilization purposes there is not only the likelihood of overheating the materials with the abstraction of normal residual moisture from textiles or fabrics followed by a reduction in tensile strength and premature disintegration, but most important is the ever-present danger of ineffective sterilization. It is an inferior sterilizing agent. Minor degrees of superheating are not particularly objectionable, but when the condition approaches a temperature rise of 20° to 30°F (11° to 17°C) or greater, sterilization may not occur.[5] In general, this condition dictates that it should be the goal in sterilizer operation to avoid all superheat. With every degree of superheat added to steam, its microbicidal properties are reduced until temperatures are attained which destroy microbes by actual burning or slow oxidation, as occurs in the dry heat or hot air sterilizer.

DETERMINATION OF TEMPERATURE OF SATURATED STEAM OR AIR-STEAM MIXTURES

By consulting steam tables in engineers' handbooks, the temperature of pure saturated steam at various pressures may be determined. These steam tables can also be used to determine the ultimate temperature of any known mixture of steam and air at any gauge pressure. Air-steam mixtures do not develop the same temperatures characteristic of saturated steam at the same pressures—a fact rarely appreciated by those responsible for sterilizing technics. As a consequence, this condition is a contributing factor to many failures encountered in sterilizing processes. To determine the ultimate temperature of a known mixture of steam and air, apply the following formula:

$$Pl = Po - \left(\frac{30-V}{2} \right) \text{ (From Dalton's Law of Gaseous Pressures)}$$

in which

Pl = absolute pressure in pounds per square inch, the temperature of which is the desired factor. (Determine this by reference to steam tables.)

Po = absolute pressure applied to the sterilizing chamber = gauge pressure plus 14.7 pounds.

V = the degree of vacuum applied to the sterilizing chamber in inches of mercury.

The average operator of sterilizers need not make use of the above formula for other than a proper mathematical background for basic principles upon which sterilization depends. The actual temperatures attained in the sterilizer under ordinary conditions of proper and improper usage are given in Table 5-1.

REMOVAL OF AIR FROM STERILIZER BY MEANS OF PARTIAL VACUUM

The complete evacuation of air from a vessel or chamber defines a perfect vacuum. This is measured in terms of the height of a column of mercury which will be sustained under that condition. This column of mercury is 29.9 inches high. The combination vacuum-pressure gauges commonly used, as shown in Figure 5-1, are graduated for measurement of the degree of vacuum to this scale, in inches of mercury.

TABLE 5-1

STERILIZER TEMPERATURES WITH VARIOUS DEGREES OF AIR DISCHARGE

Gauge Pressure Pounds	Sat'd. Steam Complete Air Discharge		Two-thirds Air Discharge (20" Vacuum)		One-half Air Discharge (15" Vacuum)		One-third Air Discharge (10" Vacuum)		No Air Discharge	
	°C	°F	°C	°F	°C	°F	°C	°F	°C	°F
5	109	228	100	212	94	202	90	193	72	162
10	115	240	109	228	105	220	100	212	90	193
15	121	250	115	240	112	234	109	228	100	212
20	126	259	121	250	118	245	115	240	109	228
25	130	267	126	259	124	254	121	250	115	240
30	135	275	130	267	128	263	126	259	121	250

Prior to 1959, the usual vacuum type sterilizer in hospitals was equipped with an ejector valve by means of which a maximum of about 10 inches vacuum could be attained. Occasionally a more powerful steam ejector was employed and this component made it possible to produce a 15- to 20-inch vacuum in the sterilizer. In a few instances sterilizers were used in industry—still are used—with an initial vacuum of 26 to 28 inches obtained by means of an electrically operated water ring pump. Operating directions accompanying the older and now obsolete vacuum-type sterilizers usually instructed the operator to draw a partial vacuum of 10 to 15 inches as the initial step in the sterilizing cycle. Such a procedure is useless because only one third to one half of the air is removed from the chamber and the residual quantity is sufficient to seriously retard or prevent the attainment of the correct temperature required for sterilization. In fact, an initial vacuum of 26 to 28 inches is still inadequate for removal of sufficient air so as to ensure that the steam will reliably penetrate all portions of a porous load within a practical period of time.

Admittedly, there has been in the past a great deal of misunderstanding relative to the operation of sterilizers equipped with mechanical devices for drawing a partial vacuum on the chamber. Operators have been led to believe that vacuum plays some mysterious part in sterilizing—that it is difficult to sterilize except by first producing some relatively minor degree of vacuum in the chamber. Events of the past few years have clarified this situation considerably. It is now recognized that if an initial vacuum is utilized it must be of such a magnitude as to reduce the partial pressure of air in the

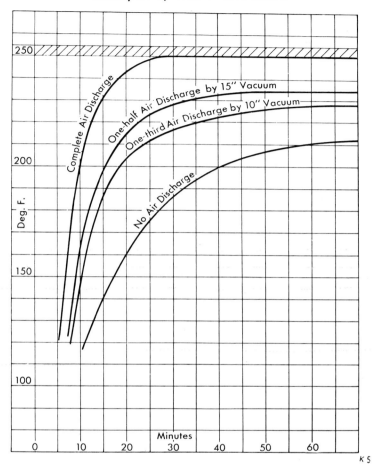

FIGURE 5-6. The temperatures resulting from complete and partial air discharge from a sterilizing chamber operated at 15 pounds pressure.

chamber and the load to a point where the residual will not interfere with steam penetration. From the explanation given above it may be observed that a 10-inch vacuum means 10/30 of a perfect vacuum or, in other words, the exhaust of only one third of the air. A 15-inch vacuum exhausts one half and a 20-inch vacuum, two thirds of the air. Similarly, a 28-inch vacuum means that approximately 93 per cent of the air has been removed from the chamber. The temperatures resulting from such incomplete evacuation of air are not suitable for dependable sterilization, as indicated by the data in Table 5-1 and the temperature curves in Figure 5-6.

THE EFFECT OF GRAVITY ON AIR-STEAM MIXTURES IN A STERILIZING CHAMBER

When steam is admitted to a sterilizing chamber, the relatively cool air present is much heavier than the steam at the normal sterilizing temperature. Steam has a density of 0.07 pounds per cubic foot as compared with 0.12 for air under the same pressure and temperature and they show a marked disinclination to mix. This means that when steam is forced by pressure into a sterilizing chamber containing air, the steam will literally float to the top of the chamber, compressing the air at the bottom. It is known, however, that the air and steam will eventually mix, resulting in a uniform gas made up of steam and air, in which a part of the heat contained in the steam will have been absorbed by the air.

This mixing process which results after a long period of time in a uniform temperature throughout the chamber is a most uncertain condition. The period required for this mixture to occur is affected materially by the character of the load and under no condition can it ever be determined precisely except by actual temperature measurements. However, the important details for consideration are these: 1) The presence of air greatly reduces the ultimate temperature of the steam below that of pure saturated steam at the pressure maintained. 2) Throughout the normal period of sterilization, the temperatures in the lower areas of the chamber will be substantially lower than in the upper areas because of differences in specific gravities and reluctance of steam and air to mix.

This latter fact accounts for radically misleading tests which are often noted in an attempt to prove the adequacy of a sterilizing process. For example, a culture test consisting of a sample of contaminated material placed in the upper part of a sterilizing chamber from which very little air has been removed will frequently show complete sterilization because the test material will have been subjected, for at least a brief interval of time, to nearly pure saturated steam at the operating pressure. Similarly, sterilization indicators located in the upper part of a poorly air-evacuated chamber will often incorrectly indicate sterilizing conditions. Tests made in imperfectly air-evacuated chambers, at the bottom, will invariably show failure in any reasonable period of exposure.

To further illustrate the importance of gravity or stratification of air-steam mixtures in a sterilizing chamber, the reader's attention is called to the temperature curves (Fig. 5-7). They demonstrate effectively the differences in temperature encountered in different areas of a sterilizer from which air has not been evacuated. It is easily conceivable that tests made in the upper portions of the load might have indicated satisfactory conditions for sterilization, but it is certain that any test made in the lower areas must have failed.

HOW STEAM STERILIZATION IS ACCOMPLISHED

Steam sterilization as normally conducted in the autoclave is a product of heat plus moisture in which the moisture factor plays an exceedingly important part. It is generally accepted that the thermal destruction of microorga-

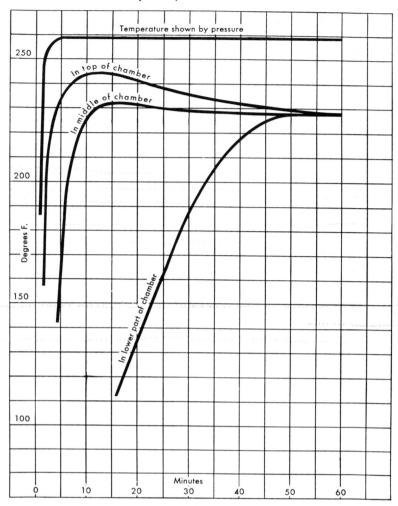

FIGURE 5-7. These radical differences in temperature for different areas in the chamber are representative of a sterilizer from which air has not been discharged. Measurements were made with potentiometer and three thermocouples, one located near the top, the second in the middle, and the third close to the bottom of the chamber.

nisms closely parallels the heat coagulation of proteins. Various workers who have investigated this phenomenon have concluded that death occurs as the result of the heat denaturation of the proteins which make up the microbial cell. When moisture is present this coagulation process takes place at relatively low temperatures, but when moisture is absent a considerably higher temperature is required for microbial destruction.

Steam possesses the singular property of being able to heat materials, and particularly to permeate porous substances by the relatively rapid process of condensation, as opposed to the very slow process of heat absorption as in the case of hot air or any other gas used as the heating medium. Steam gives up its heat in sterilizing only by the process of condensing back into the water from which it came. Specifically this means that every fiber or particle of any porous article undergoing sterilization will abstract, absorb, or contain a quantity of moisture from the steam in exact proportion to the amount of heat absorbed by the article. Knowledge of this principle is of great importance to the student because it explains in many instances how various supplies should be prepared for steam sterilization, i.e., an arrangement of the materials that will provide for thorough, rapid, and complete permeation with steam. If the steam can permeate any mass of materials such as gowns, sheets, towels, or other porous supplies, it will heat that mass through condensation and leave in it the finely dispersed moisture required for sterilization.

CONDENSATION AND LATENT HEAT

The condensation process of heating makes use of the latent heat of steam. The heat required to convert a unit mass of water into steam at the same temperature is called the latent heat of vaporization of water or simply the latent heat of steam. For example, heating one pound of water from room temperature of 70°F and converting it into steam at 212°F requires first the expenditure of (212°—70°) = 142 heat units, to bring the temperature of the water to 212°F. Then there must be added for each pound of water 970 heat units to convert that pound of water at 212°F into steam at 212°F. This factor of 970 heat units is known as latent heat. Then to heat each pound of steam at 212°F into steam at 250°F (15 pounds gauge pressure), the normal sterilizing range, requires only 13.5 heat units. It is obvious that a high percentage of the energy stored in steam, actually over 80 per cent, is accounted for in the latent heat.

In abstracting heat from steam, for every pound that is condensed into water, surrounding objects absorb that latent heat. This feature is highly important in its application to the permeation of dry goods, fabrics, or textiles. As steam contacts the outer layer of fabric, the cooler substance immediately causes a film of steam to condense, leaving in the fabric a minute amount of water, that moisture so necessary for the destruction of microbial life. The next film of steam immediately fills the space created by the volume collapse of the previous film (99 per cent decrease in volume), but it does not condense in the outer layer; rather it passes through and attacks the second layer of fabric—condenses and heats it. So on until the entire mass of fabric has been heated, after which the package will contain an amount of moisture (condensate) exactly equivalent to the amount of heat abstracted from the steam. Continuation of the process will cause no further condensation, but the temperature of the fabric will remain constant at the temperature of the surrounding steam. Condensation takes place at the same temperature as evaporation occurs for any given pressure and is, in fact, the reverse process of evaporation.

DIRECT STEAM CONTACT

All steam sterilization is based upon *direct steam contact*. This is a detail of great importance which must be thoroughly understood in order to prevent attempts to sterilize by steam any article where direct steam contact is difficult or perhaps impossible. All steam sterilization functions are based upon the supposition that the steam can and will contact all surfaces as well as every strand, fiber, or particle of the substance undergoing sterilization. The bulk of the average surgical pack is made up of fabrics of one kind or another (gauze, cotton products, linens). To sterilize these materials, correct performance assumes complete permeation of the entire mass with the heat and moisture of the steam. In fact, it is impossible in any reasonable operation to heat these porous materials in the autoclave without bringing in the moisture factor, since heating is accomplished by the process of condensation as described above.

It follows that the same process of condensation and heating applies to instruments, utensils or other articles undergoing surface sterilization. With these supplies there is no permeation of steam through the metal, the object being only to heat and sterilize the surface. In this case the cold metal condenses the steam until the instrument is heated to the temperature of the steam. Throughout sterilization the metal surfaces are bathed with an abundance of moisture, much greater than in the case of fabrics, which facilitates sterilization. Because of the rapid heating effect and the abundance of moisture, it becomes possible to prescribe a shorter exposure period for instruments than for fabrics or textiles, which require time for permeation.

It is a popular misconception among personnel responsible for sterilization procedures in hospitals that anhydrous materials such as oils, greases, and powders can be sterilized in the autoclave. It is not possible to effect direct steam contact to all portions of these materials. Heat will gradually be absorbed through any such mass; the equivalent condensate will deposit on the exposed surfaces, but no moisture permeates the materials. The correct method for sterilization of anhydrous substances is by means of dry heat in the hot air oven.

Another example of failure to bring about direct steam contact in the autoclave is found in the attempt to sterilize hollow needles or other delicate instruments in test tubes with the ends tightly stoppered and impervious to steam. The heat absorbed through the glass walls is inadequate for the destruction of resistant organisms. The method of protecting an instrument by means of a glass or metal tube is excellent, but the tube must be closed with nothing more restrictive than a cotton plug and the tube must rest on its side in the sterilizer so that air can escape, permitting the steam to enter.

Aqueous solutions are the only exception to the rule of direct steam contact. In this case the moisture factor is present in abundance and it is necessary only to absorb heat from the surrounding steam.

THE ADVERSE EFFECTS OF AIR UPON THE PENETRATING POWER OF STEAM

It has been explained how steam heats porous materials by its peculiar process of condensation. The great opponent to the diffusion of steam is air, and all fabrics as they are placed in the sterilizer have their interstices filled with air at the surrounding temperature and at atmospheric pressure. Unless the steam is able to displace this air it cannot permeate the material and its behavior will then be similar to that of hot air under the same operating pressure. When air is mixed with the steam, obviously only the steam content of the mixture heats by the condensing process. The air has no useful penetrating power. The heating or penetrating power of the mixture is reduced in accordance with the proportion of air present. This point is illustrated graphically in Figure 5-8.

If the sterilizing chamber is well exhausted of air so that the free spaces all about the load are promptly filled with pure steam, then the air pockets within a bulky package of fabrics will dissipate rapidly by gravity to the

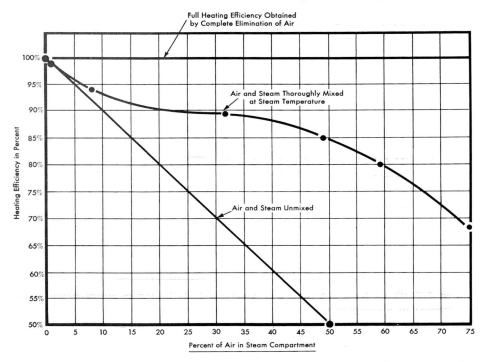

FIGURE 5-8. The effect of air on the heating efficiency of a steam chamber, based on atmospheric pressure inside chamber. (Data from Warren Webster Co.)

bottom of the chamber from which a correctly designed gravity discharge system will permit escape. If, however, the chamber has not been evacuated of air, then there will be no material difference in density between the air pockets within the package and the air which has gravitated to the areas below the package. These air pockets will therefore remain in the load and greatly retard the entrance of steam.

The temperature curves shown in Figure 5-9 illustrate this point rather

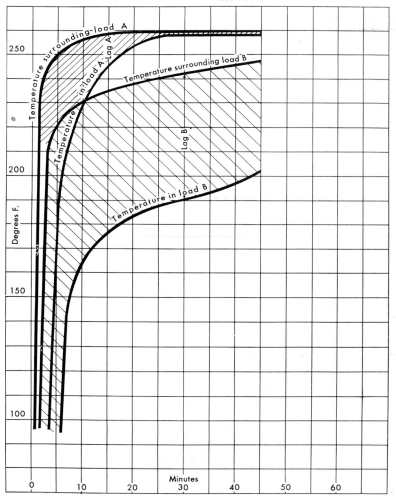

FIGURE 5-9. These temperature curves are typical of the lag in steam penetration to be expected in a sterilizer from which air has not been discharged. Load consisted of large package of Hampton pads. Pressure was maintained at 20 pounds. When air was completely discharged from chamber, temperature in package (Lag A) rapidly approached that of surrounding steam (Load A). When only a small amount of air was discharged, temperature in package lagged approximately 50°F (Lag B) that of surrounding steam (Load B) throughout 45-minute exposure.

convincingly. Also, they further emphasize the necessity for placing any sterilization indicator in the center of the package undergoing study rather than near the surface.

The presence of air in the sterilizer is a grave handicap to effective sterilization for several reasons: 1) it reduces the ultimate possible temperature of steam at any pressure; 2) steam and air are reluctant to mix, resulting in great variations in temperature in various parts of the chamber; 3) the ultimate reduced temperature can be attained only after prolonged periods of exposure, and 4) it has an adverse effect upon steam penetration of porous supplies.

AUTOMATIC AIR ELIMINATION FROM STERILIZING CHAMBERS

The first essential requirement for an efficient steam sterilizer is that some means must be provided for the automatic removal of air and condensate from the chamber without reliance upon skillful manipulation of hand valves or any other precise and confining attention to the sterilizer. To this end, it is generally true that all modern sterilizers are equipped with a thermostatic valve for the automatic control of air and condensate discharge from such chambers, with excellent results. Prior to the introduction of thermostatic valves on sterilizers it was necessary to control the air and condensate discharge by hand regulation of a drainage valve located near the front bottom of the sterilizing chamber. The obvious fault of that system was the necessity for complete reliance upon the individual, the close attention required, and the degree of safety being largely a matter of the care and skill of the operator.

Thermostatic valves are of the general classification commonly known as steam traps. They contain flexible metallic elements filled with a volatile liquid which expands under heat or contracts when cool, opening or closing the discharge orifice of the valve. A sectional diagram depicting the functional parts of a thermostatic valve is given in Figure 5-10. It should not be assumed that the usual steam trap, available from the nearest supply store, can be applied satisfactorily for this delicate operation of automatic air removal. The discharge orifice of the usual steam trap is so small that an abnormal period of time is required to evacuate a sterilizing chamber. Still more objectionable is the fact that some of these traps are designed to shut off before air discharge is complete.

The more sensitive thermostatic valves, specially designed for use with sterilizers, permit rapid and complete evacuation of air. The proper application of such valves affords the opportunity for the automatic discharge of all air from the sterilizing chamber, so that the maximum possible temperature throughout the chamber can be attained quickly. Fortunately these better grades of valves are fairly dependable, not readily subject to structural changes in use which interfere with their performance. The best of them,

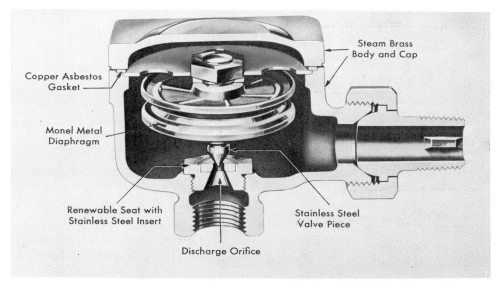

Steam Brass
Body and Cap

Copper Asbestos
Gasket

Monel Metal
Diaphragm

Renewable Seat with
Stainless Steel Insert

Stainless Steel
Valve Piece

Discharge Orifice

FIGURE 5-10. Sectional diagram of thermostatic valve used on steam sterilizers.

however, do fatigue after long service, and it is always necessary to check their performance to avoid the hazards of attempted sterilization with a chamber badly clogged with air. No valve will remain permanently accurate.

METHOD FOR DETERMINING THE EFFECTIVENESS OF AIR DISCHARGE FROM STERILIZING CHAMBER

From the foregoing the reader will have observed that for safe operation some dependable method must be adopted for determining the degree of air discharge from a sterilizing chamber. That has now been made possible by the simple method of measuring the temperature in the chamber discharge line. It has been shown that air or any mixture of steam and air will gravitate to the lower areas of the chamber. It follows as an obvious physical fact that if the discharge line is clogged or if the thermostatic valve is not working properly there will be no material advance in temperature in the discharge line, but if the line is free, the temperature will advance after the air has been eliminated and replaced by steam to the temperature of the steam. Only when this has occurred will the indicated temperature advance to the sterilizing range. Even then this temperature will always lag one to two degrees behind the actual temperature of the medium surrounding the load. The thermometer reading will be, without exception, a measurement of the coldest medium within the sterilizing chamber. A partial clogging of the system will simply retard the movement or clearance of air, all of which will be indicated by the thermometer or temperature sensing element.

At this point, the student might well pose the question as to why is it not desirable to measure temperature within the sterilizing chamber instead of in the discharge system. The purpose is to measure the effectiveness of air discharge, which under all conditions is the fundamental requirement, and to indicate promptly if there is an interruption which must be cleared. A thermometer bulb placed at any fixed point within the sterilizing chamber would measure merely the temperature at that point. It would also reflect the temperature of circulating currents of steam and would not be so clearly indicative of the condition which the operator needs to know. In addition, the bulb of such a thermometer would necessarily be installed permanently at some point close to the steam jacket wall, out of the way of the load—giving free access to the chamber. In this position, the thermometer bulb would always respond to some extent to the temperature of the hot steam jacket surrounding the chamber.

STERILIZING CONDITIONS BASIS—TEMPERATURE RATHER THAN PRESSURE

In spite of all that has been written on this subject during the last seventy-five years the tendency still prevails to think of steam sterilization in terms of pressure rather than temperature. Moist heat is the sterilizing agent. Pressure is only incidentally significant. The common practice of measuring the sterilizing period from the instant that the pressure gauge shows 15 pounds, perhaps 20 pounds, with little regard for anything else, should definitely be discouraged. Often such observations are made with sterilizers from which little air has been exhausted.

Under the presently established system of effective steam sterilization, the period of exposure is measured, without immediate regard for pressure, from the instant that the thermometer in the discharge line shows temperature of 250°F (the equivalent of saturated steam at 15 pounds gauge pressure), the *minimum* standard considered safe for sterilization. This indication also means that the temperature of the steam surrounding the load will range from one to two degrees higher in every part of the chamber.

It is obvious, of course, that pressure must be regulated at the prescribed range in order that suitable temperature can be attained, and for each kind of heat (steam, electricity, or gas) it is a simple matter to provide automatic pressure regulation about which the operator of the sterilizer need not be greatly concerned. The immediate and constant interest of the operator should be centered in the maintenance of "discharge line temperature" which is indicative of these essential factors: 1) proper functioning of the air discharge system and 2) measurement of the temperature of the coldest medium surrounding the load—maintaining that temperature within the prescribed safe range.

For sterilization purposes steam under pressure is used rather than atmospheric or flowing steam for the sole purpose of attaining higher temperatures. Pressure of itself has nothing whatsoever to do with the microbicidal properties of steam. A scale of pressures and equivalent temperatures of saturated steam as employed for sterilization purposes is given in Table 5-2. Saturated steam at a temperature of 250° to 254°F (121° to 123°C) will

TABLE 5-2

SCALE OF PRESSURES AND EQUIVALENT TEMPERATURES OF SATURATED
STEAM FOR STERILIZATION PURPOSES

(*From Perkins*[4])

Pounds Pressure		Temperature		
Gauge	Absolute	Degrees F	Degrees C	Sterilizing Application
80.3	95	324.1	162.2	
75.3	90	320.3	160.1 → Maximum pressure in steam supply lines.
70.3	85	316.3	158.0	(For pressure sterilizers)
65.3	80	312.0	155.6	
60.3	75	307.6	153.0	
55.3	70	302.9	150.6 → Ideal pressure in steam supply lines.
50.3	65	298.0	147.8	
45.3	60	292.7	144.8	
40.3	55	287.1	141.9 → Minimum pressure in steam supply lines.
				(For pressure sterilizers)
39.3	54	285.8	141.0 → Almost instantaneous sterilization
35.3	50	281.0	138.3	
30.3	45	274.4	134.6 → Prevacuum high temperature sterilization
27.3	42	270.2	132.3 → Emergency (high-speed) sterilization of instruments
25.3	40	267.3	130.7	
20.3	35	259.3	126.2	
19.3	34	257.6	125.3	
18.3	33	255.8	124.2	
17.3	32	254.1	123.4 ⎧ Sterilization of hospital supplies—surgical instruments, dressings, solutions.
16.3	31	252.2	122.3	
15.3	30	250.3	121.2 ⎬ Sterilization of laboratory supplies. Commercial sterilization processes.
14.3	29	248.4	120.3	
12.3	27	244.4	118.0	
10.3	25	240.1	115.6 → Sterilization of laboratory supplies. Commercial sterilization processes.
8.3	23	235.5	113.0	
6.3	21	230.6	110.3 → Terminal heating of infant formulas.
4.3	19	225.2	107.1	
2.3	17	219.4	104.2	
0.0	14.70	212.0	100.0 ⎧ Sanitization of instruments and utensils. Terminal heating of infant formulas. Streaming steam (fractional) sterilization. Water boils @ sea level, New York City.
	14.13	210.0	98.8	Water boils @ altitude 1025 ft., Omaha, Nebr.
	13.03	206.0	96.6	Water boils @ altitude 3115 ft., Calgary, Alta.
	12.01	202.0	94.4	Water boils @ altitude 5225 ft., Denver, Colo.
	11.06	198.0	92.2	Water boils @ altitude 7381 ft., Laramie, Wyo.
	10.40	195.0	90.5	Water boils @ altitude 9000 ft., Quito, Ecuador
	8.95	188.0	86.6	Water boils @ altitude 12,700 ft., LaPaz, Bolivia
	8.03	183.2	84.0	Water boils @ altitude 15,771 ft., Mont Blanc, France

destroy the most resistant forms of microbial life in a brief interval of exposure. These temperatures are not destructive of most materials and supplies, and the necessary period of exposure is well within practicable limits.

THE MOST PRACTICAL RANGE OF STEAM PRESSURE AND TEMPERATURE FOR STERILIZERS

Because many sterilizers of the classical or gravity-displacement type are deficient in the attainment of sterilizing temperature in a brief interval of time, there exists an all too prevalent tendency to increase the operating pressure range and the periods of exposure beyond those actually needed. The method of "graduating the pressure and the temperature to the load" is erroneous. It has no scientific background, no logical explanation, because it takes just as much heat to kill an organism in a rubber glove as in a table drape or a gown. The only variable permissible in surgical sterilization should be "duration of exposure," but, for the most part, this can be rigidly standardized. The potency of the applied steam should be, therefore, identical for all loads for a gravity-displacement-type sterilizer.

There is also the false supposition that steam at 20 to 25 pounds pressure heats the load much faster than steam at 15 to 17 pounds pressure. To be sure, higher pressure will certainly result in correspondingly higher temperature in any modern sterilizer, but the rate of heating to the desired range is not sufficiently greater to justify serious consideration. Whereas the pressure carried for the sterilization of routine surgical supplies in the average hospital sterilizer is usually in the range of 15 to 20 pounds, it is also known that in more than a few instances considerably higher pressures are employed, despite the fact that the sterilizers were not designed for use with pressures greater than 20 pounds gauge. In the sterilization of heat-sensitive supplies, rubber gloves and glucose solutions particularly, temperatures higher than those of pure steam at 15 to 17 pounds may prove needlessly destructive.

TABLE 5-3

Boiling Point Water °F	Altitude Above Sea Level Feet	Atmos. Pressure Lbs./Sq. In.	Barometer Reduced to 32°F Inches	Steam Pressure Required Lbs./Sq. In. Gauge
212	Sea Level	14.7	29.9	15–17
210	1025	14.1	28.7	15.6–17.6
208	2063	13.5	27.6	16.1–18.1
206	3115	13.0	26.5	16.7–18.7
204	4169	12.5	25.4	17.2–19.2
202	5225	12.0	24.4	17.7–19.7
200	6304	11.5	23.4	18.2–20.2
198	7381	11.0	22.5	18.7–20.7
196	8481	10.6	21.6	19.1–21.1
194	9579	10.1	20.7	19.6–21.6
192	10685	9.7	19.8	20.0–22.0
190	11799	9.3	19.0	20.4–22.4
188	12934	8.9	18.2	20.8–22.8

When pressure sterilizers are used in areas or localities of high altitude, it becomes necessary to employ proportionally greater steam pressures in order to attain the minimum standard range of temperature required for sterilization, namely, 250° to 254°F. The data given in Table 5-3 clearly show that the boiling point of water varies with the barometric pressure at various altitudes. Hence it becomes necessary to compensate for this reduction in temperature by increasing the pressure when steam is admitted to a sterilizing chamber; otherwise the minimum standard range of temperature could not be maintained at high altitudes. As an approximation, the boiling point of water is reduced 2°F (1.1°C) for each 1000 feet increase in altitude above sea level. From the figures given in the last column of Table 5-3

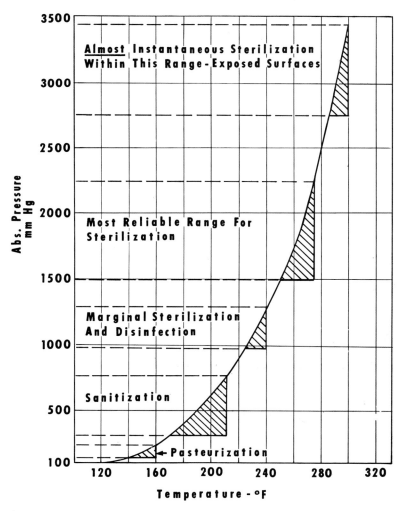

FIGURE 5-11. Pressure-temperature ranges utilized for moist heat sterilization, including less efficient processes.

it may also be observed that for each 1000 feet elevation above sea level the pressure in the sterilizing chamber should be increased approximately 0.5 pound per square inch gauge. When these factors are taken into consideration there is little excuse for not operating surgical supply sterilizers under proper physical conditions to assure the maintenance of minimum standards for sterilization. A diagram to illustrate the pressure-temperature ranges utilized for moist heat sterilization, including less efficient processes, is given in Figure 5-11.

BASIC MECHANICAL COMPONENTS REQUIRED FOR STEAM STERILIZATION

In order to sterilize by steam under pressure, the machine must have the basic elements as shown in Figure 5-12. A pressure vessel equipped with a safety-lock door is a necessity. The pressure vessel should be manufactured in accordance with the Pressure Vessel Code as established by the American Society of Mechanical Engineers or by an equivalent regulatory body for other countries. This code is designed to protect human life and, as such, all people associated with the purchase, operation, and maintenance of autoclaves should see to it that the vessel conforms strictly to the code.

This chapter has dealt with the basic principles or engineering fundamentals of pressure steam sterilization. The factors discussed are those which govern precise, dependable performance. There are other factors equally as important relating to the preparation of materials for sterilization and the

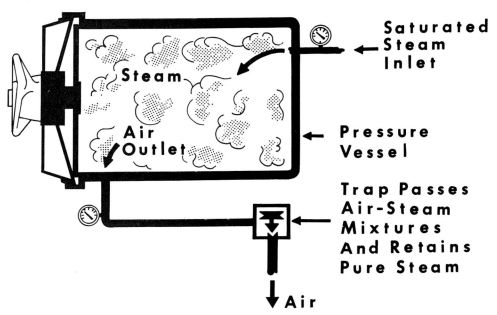

FIGURE 5-12. Basic components required for pressure steam sterilization.

loading of supplies in the sterilizer. Without due regard for these elements, the sterilization process in the most perfect of sterilizers can easily remain uncertain.

REFERENCES

1. GIFFORD, G. E.: Occurrence of morpholine in steam and its solution during autoclaving. *J Bact, 80*:278-279, 1960.
2. HOLMLUND, L. G., and TÄRNVIK, A.: Cytotoxic investigation of cyclohexylamine and decyl-amine—two corrosion inhibitors. *Odont Rev (Malmö), 14*:335-341, 1963.
3. HARVEY, J. L.: Use of octadecylamine in steam lines of food and drug establishments. *Federal Register, 22*:9594, 1957.
4. PERKINS, J. J.: Bacteriological and surgical sterilization by heat. In G. F. Reddish (Ed.): *Antiseptics, Disinfectants, Fungicides, Chemical and Physical Sterilization.* Philadelphia, Lea & F., 1954, p. 664.
5. SAVAGE, R. H. M.: *Principles Underlying Steam Sterilization.* Report of a Symposium, May 9, 1959, Pharmaceutical Press, London, p. 1-11.

Chapter 6

PREVACUUM HIGH TEMPERATURE
STEAM STERILIZATION

REVIEW OF LITERATURE

IN 1958, Knox and Penikett[1] reported to the Medical Research Council
of Great Britain on the influence of initial vacuum on steam sterilization of dressings. A horizontal jacketed autoclave was used for their experimental work with a capacity of 11 cu ft. Steam was supplied to the
jacket and chamber independently from a supply line pressure of 46 psig,
then reduced to an operating pressure of 20 psig. The air was removed from
the chamber with an oil-sealed rotary type piston vacuum pump protected
by a water-cooled condenser. The test load comprised a standard dressing
drum lined (11½" dia. 8½" high) containing 20" × 30" hand towels, each
folded to give twelve thicknesses. Temperature was measured inside
the center of the drum by a recording thermometer. Times were recorded
for the temperature inside the drum to reach 240°F (115°C) after the
chamber reached 20 psig and plotted against the initial vacuum for a series
of forty-three experiments. The time required to reach a minimum sterilizing temperature of 240°F inside the drum was found to be about one minute when the pressure in the chamber, before admitting steam, was reduced
to 20 mm Hg (absolute) or below. When lesser degrees of vacuum were
used the times for temperature to reach 240°F were variable and prolonged. These findings led Knox and Penikett to make the suggestion that if
rapid and predictable sterilization is required in an autoclave fitted with a
pump for drawing a preliminary vacuum, then the pump should be capable
of rapidly reducing the pressure in the chamber to 20 mm Hg or below.

Automatic high prevacuum steam sterilization for surgical dressings and
gloves is the subject of a paper by Alder and Gillespie[2] published in 1959.
These workers gave results of studies on a 25 cu ft capacity downward displacement autoclave upgraded to automatic high vacuum operation. The
upgrading was accomplished by use of an oil-sealed rotary pump (Edwards) coupled with an automatic control mechanism (Drayton) to satisfy
the requirements. The pump was used in conjunction with a condenser system to remove steam from the chamber during the postvacuum period,
without the oil in the pump being contaminated by steam. Observations
showed prevacuum to be consistent in the range of 15 mm, ±1 mm, absolute

in a period of about 4 minutes. Temperature penetration records from the centers of packed test drums (full load) showed chamber drain temperature and test package temperature to be in agreement within 1.8°F (1°C) at sterilizing temperature of 259° to 262°F (126° to 128°C).

Total cycle times ranged between 29 and 31 minutes. Rubber gloves were found to survive at least twelve cycles of sterilization.

The following factors were cited as important in the testing of high prevacuum autoclaves:

> The functioning of the automatic control system must not be dependent on any adjustment by the operator. Any attempt to interfere with the cycle should result in the chamber being returned to atmospheric pressure and the indicator should show that the goods are not sterile.
>
> There should be a consistent prevacuum to absolute pressures of 15 to 16 mm Hg, and without the risk of the pump being influenced by changing vapor pressures caused by fluctuations in temperature of the pump sealing fluid, which could cause prolonged pumping times.
>
> There should be no possibility of faulty sterilization arising from variation in steam pressure during the sterilization period.
>
> A manual take-over system should be provided for emergency use only, and its operation should be independent of the automatic system.
>
> There should be a warning indication if the sequence of events has not been properly carried out. Also, an indicator showing the satisfactory completion of the cycle should be fitted, but this should be cancelled upon opening the autoclave door.
>
> The indicator system should be an integral part of the control mechanism and should the electrical supply fail, an indication of the phase of the cycle should still be given.
>
> A time chart of the procedure should show a combined temperature and pressure record.

Alder and Gillespie also stated that with the high prevacuum method an autoclave can be packed to capacity, thereby increasing the output of sterile goods; a precise automatic control eliminates the human element, and the total process time can be reduced to one quarter or less of the time required by other prevacuum methods. The damage caused to rubber gloves is diminished because very little air is left in the chamber to denature the rubber, and because the total time spent in the chamber is shorter than with older methods.

In May, 1957, the Medical Research Council (Great Britain) set up a working party to examine the question of pressure-steam sterilizing procedures from the standpoint of defining performance of such sterilizers and to consider how it could be attained. The working party presented their findings and recommendations on this subject in 1959.[3] In accord with classical approach, the removal of air was cited as the first essential in the sterilization of textiles. This may be accomplished by either of two methods, the "high-vacuum" method or the "downward-displacement" (gravity air-discharge) method, with corresponding types of sterilizers. In the high-vacuum sterilizer air is removed by a powerful pump which reduces the absolute pressure of air in the chamber to a few millimeters of mercury before steam is admitted. This means removing more than 98 per cent of the air initially present. The point was emphasized that this is the only method of sterilization that can overcome the effects of bad packing or overloading of the sterilizer.[1,4]

In a downward-displacement sterilizer the air is removed from the load by gravity—the difference in density between cool air and steam, of the order of 1 mg per cc, gradually forces the air downward out of the load.[5,6] (One liter steam at 100°C weighs 0.606 gm. One liter air at 20°C weighs 1.206 gm.) Authorities agree that this method will render contaminated material sterile only if the sterilizer is correctly operated, carefully packed, and not overloaded. The working party recommended that the air content of steam in any part of the load should not exceed 5 per cent by volume during the sterilizing period. The point was stressed that this does not mean that only 95 per cent of the air need be removed from the sterilizer at the outset, because *the steam entering a mass of cotton material will push the air ahead of it to form a central "bubble" of nearly pure air, which is slow to diffuse to the outside.* Such a bubble will prevent sterilization of the dressings in contact with it. Under correct conditions of packing and loading it will be displaced slowly by gravity.

With high-vacuum equipment the total sterilization time can be greatly reduced, a complete cycle taking as little as 20 minutes.[4] The penetration time is greatly reduced, because after an almost perfect vacuum has been drawn, steam permeates the load almost instantaneously. Also, with a minimal penetration time a high sterilization temperature may be employed with a consequent reduction in holding time and safety period. At 274°F (134°C), an accurately timed exposure period of 3 minutes is adequate. Evidence by Bowie,[4] Schmidt and Moller,[7] suggests that high-vacuum, high-pressure sterilizers permit brief exposures for gloves at 266°F (130°C) or over with safety and with minimum deterioration.

In the opinion of the working party, the high-vacuum sterilizer should replace many other types. The output of sterile packaged equipment per hour in a high prevacuum sterilizer of 9 cu ft (with automatic control) is equivalent to the most efficient downward-displacement sterilizer of 40-50 cu ft with or without automatic control. For air removal, a pump should be provided which will reduce the absolute pressure to 15 mm Hg or below when the chamber is fully loaded with cotton fabrics containing 4 per cent by dry weight of water, and having a temperature not exceeding 59°F (15°C). The pump should be capable of reducing the pressure to this figure within 5 minutes. At the end of the sterilizing operation the pump must be able to reduce the absolute pressure to 50 mm Hg or less within 5 minutes.

It is the conclusion of the working party that while there are a number of causes contributing to inefficient sterilization, the underlying factor responsible for the situation as a whole is a widespread lack of understanding of the technical requirements involved. This condition exists because no one member of the medical staff is given the final responsibility of ensuring the provision of suitable equipment and its proper use and control by specially trained operators. Until this is done, and until routine supervision of the sterilizing apparatus by a member of the engineering staff is insisted upon, patients in many hospitals will continue to be exposed to the unnecessary hazard of infection caused by the use of imperfectly sterilized articles.

Preliminary to recommendations of the working party, described above, Bowie issued an article, "Requirements for an Automatically Controlled, High Prevacuum Sterilizer."[8] His suggestions were submitted as a basis upon which specifications could be considered for new dressing sterilizers. The sterilizer design, instrumentation, and system of automatic control should be such that the process of sterilization is executed in the following stages:

1. Extraction of air to a chamber negative pressure of approximately 28 inches Hg; this stage to be controlled by a chamber pressure-gauge/pressurestat (contact pressure-gauge).
2. Further extraction of air to attain a chamber absolute pressure of 0 to ¾ inch Hg; this stage to be controlled by a timer and monitored by the contact pressure-gauge of stage 1.
3. Raising chamber steam temperature to 274°F (134°C) under control of a chamber thermometer/thermostat (contact thermometer).
4. Holding temperature at not less than 274°F (134°C); this stage to be under control of a timer and monitored by the contact thermometer of stage 3.
5. Drawing vacuum in chamber to approximately 28 inches Hg under control of a contact pressure-gauge.
6. Holding vacuum at not less than 28 inches Hg under control of a timer monitored by the contact pressure-gauge of stage 5.
7. Breaking vacuum through an adequate air filter element sterilized automatically during each cycle.

With a full load of fabrics in a 9 cu ft chamber, the sterilizer should effect stage 1 in less than 2 minutes; stage 2 in less than 5 minutes; stage 3 in approximately 2½ minutes when the chamber is set for 274°F (134°C) and the supply pressure to jacket and chamber is 35 psig; stage 5 in approximately 2 minutes; and stage 7 in less than 1 minute. Therefore, when the chamber contact thermometer is set for a 3-minute sterilization holding period and the chamber contact pressure-gauge for a 4-minute drying period, the whole process for fabrics should occupy not more than 20 minutes. When using a dry main steam supply of 55 psig, pressure reducing valve set to pass steam at 35 psig to jacket and chamber, and the chamber loaded with four large caskets full of fabrics, the temperature in all parts of the load should reach 274°F (134°C) before or as soon as this temperature is indicated from the bulb of the thermometer located in the chamber discharge channel.

A substantial contribution to the subject of high prevacuum sterilization appeared in 1961, by Bowie[9] of the Royal Infirmary, Edinburgh, Scotland. This paper deals with the mechanics of high prevacuum sterilizers, residual air clearance from within a mass of hydrated fabrics, the hazards of air leaks to chamber, functional tests on sterilizers, time-temperature integrators, and instruments for the control of sterilization. Bowie uses the phrase "proper working order" in connection with high prevacuum sterilizers to indicate that temperatures throughout a challenge load rise at the same speed as the chamber discharge channel and remain at the same temperature as the chamber discharge port during the steaming stage of any automatic run. Provided that the articles making up the load are easily penetrable by steam and that the sterilizer is suitably designed and in proper functioning order, there is no demonstrable time differential between complete steam penetration of large or small, tight or loose caskets or packs making up any chamber load. *The main characteristic in high prevacuum sterilization is the absence of any steam penetration time whatever.*

Bowie contends that if residual air is not cleared from a pack before steam is admitted to the chamber, the air is swept by the steam into the most inaccessible part of the pack—usually the center portion. The same condition occurs if air leaks are present between the end of stage 1 (initial vacuum) and the attainment of zero gauge at the beginning of stage 2 (vacuum break). The instantaneous and complete steam penetration of challenge loads requires maintenance of a chamber pressure below that inside the least accessible parts of the load for long enough time to effect residual air clearance—*the release of molecular air clinging to fibers.* Bowie found that a prevacuum period of 8 to 10 minutes is essential, with the prevacuumstat set for 15 mm Hg. At the end of this time, the absolute pressure in the chamber is usually 4 to 8 mm Hg, and the pressure within the load is less than 10 mm Hg, dependent upon the percentage hydration of the fabrics. A vacuum of 10 mm Hg in the free chamber space is inadequate for loads with a moisture content of 6 to 8 per cent if insufficient time is allowed for the release of physically adsorbed air.

Air leaks may induce the development of a steam penetration *lag-time* in spite of an adequately timed prevacuum period. Leakage must be controlled to the extent that the vacuum loss is no greater than 1.5 mm Hg per minute over a period of 5 minutes immediately after drawing a vacuum of 10 mm Hg absolute pressure in an empty chamber. *In high prevacuum sterilizers, an initial vacuum of inadequate duration or the development of an air leak delays steam penetration in medium and large packs to such an extent that the chamber drain temperature becomes an unreliable guide to the control of sterilization within all parts of the load.*

Rowe, Kusay, and Skelton[10] have reported on the application of vacuum to steam sterilizers. Studies were made on the effect of varying degrees of preliminary vacuum in sterilizers loaded with textiles. A pressure below 15 Torr* was indicated even when textiles were wrapped in fabric and not otherwise contained. Methods of obtaining the vacuum were also investigated from the standpoint of reliability and convenience. In general, an air-ballasted, oil-sealed rotary pump protected by a condenser was found to be a most suitable combination.

Rowe and his associates believe that the mechanism of "high-speed" prevacuum sterilization requires the production of a sufficiently low partial pressure of air throughout the system to the extent that the quantity of air remaining in each individual drum or pack, together with any air in the system which will be shared among the packs, is sufficiently small. The criterion of quantity must take into account the final steam pressure and the size of the packs, so that a core of residual air which can be trapped in each pack is so small, and at a sufficiently low pressure, that no significant interference with the steam sterilizing process can occur. Results from 250 sterilizing cycles led these workers to the following conclusions:

> The significant factor in the process is almost certainly the partial pressure of air remaining in the prevacuum stage.
>
> To ensure the necessary low partial pressure of air in drums, a prevacuum of 15 Torr total pressure is highly desirable and one of 10 Torr is even more desirable.
>
> The low partial pressures of air can be achieved by double evacuation and steam purging, and by two-stage water ring pumps with or without air ejectors. As no convenient instrumentation exists for indicating that the necessary low partial pressure has been reached, this approach is not recommended.
>
> Low *total* pressures can be achieved by two-stage water ring pumps with or without an air ejector, but there is doubt of their ability regularly to obtain a pressure of 15 Torr in actual installation.
>
> An oil-sealed, air-ballasted rotary pump protected by a condenser for the first vacuum and operating via a bleed valve in conjunction with a condenser for the second vacuum appears to be satisfactory and reliable and capable of very high speeds. The condenser can assist the pump in obtaining the first vacuum and in terms of size is probably the fastest steam and vapor removing agent for the postvacuum. High temperature of the cooling water can prolong the prevacuum time if the system is wet but contaminated water does not present a problem.

Another interesting point made by Rowe *et al.*, is to the effect that the

---

* The "Torr" is defined as the pressure necessary to support a column of mercury (Hg) 1 mm high. The Torr is equal to 1 mm mercury pressure absolute (see Fig. 6-1).

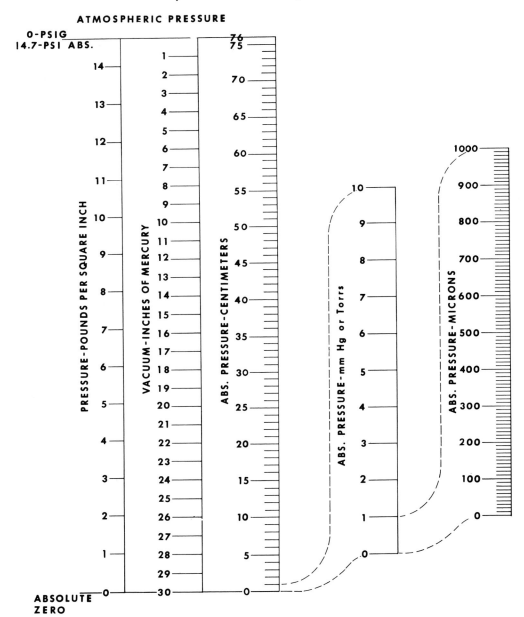

FIGURE 6-1. Absolute pressure scale.

time to evacuate a fully loaded sterilizer to 20 and 15 Torr respectively is approximately 1.13 and 1.3 times that for exhausting an empty chamber. Assumedly this refers to an initial moisture content of the textiles of about 5 per cent by weight.

Any review of the literature on prevacuum methods for the elimination of air from the chamber and the load would be considered incomplete unless some mention were made of early attempts to apply vacuum in the commercial sterilization of packaged surgical cotton. In 1943, research workers of the American Sterilizer Company conceived and developed a refined process for the commercial sterilization of wrapped products which, for the first time in the United States, permitted manufacturers to effectively sterilize bulk loads without serious distortion of cartons or discoloration of labels.

This process employed a prevacuum step in the operating cycle in order to produce an initial vacuum of 26 to 28 inches in the chamber. Steam was then admitted to the chamber from the jacket maintained at 15 to 17 pounds pressure for a brief period of what was termed "preheating." This continued for about 15 minutes during which the load attained a temperature of about 212°F. The vacuum pump was turned on again to discharge the initial (preheating) steam and to draw out the excess moisture deposited on the goods, but leaving them hot. The actual sterilizing steam was then admitted to the chamber, and since the materials were essentially dry and hot, very little additional moisture was deposited in the load. Exposure for 30 minutes to a temperature of 250°F then followed, after which a final vacuum was drawn to dry the load.

THEORY AND PRINCIPLES GOVERNING PREVACUUM STERILIZATION

Surgical dressings comprise a major percentage of the bulk of supplies to be sterilized daily in hospitals. The term "dressings" normally indicates such materials or fabrics as hand towels, skin towels, lap sheets, table drapes, gowns, and a variety of sponges. When these materials in suitable quantity are arranged in an orderly fashion, and an outer cover or wrapper applied, the result is a *surgical pack*. Modern-day practice discourages the use of large dense bundles because of the difficulty in attaining reliable routine sterilization. Standardization has made it possible to limit the size of the largest pack to 12″ × 12″ × 20″, with an average weight of twelve pounds (5.5 kg).

In contrast to synthetics, cotton still remains the dominant fiber from which washable textiles are made. Of the cotton fabrics, medium weight muslin is the type most commonly found in general hospital use. Cost and durability are usually based on thread count which specifies the number of threads per square inch. For purposes of comparison, other grades of muslin with corresponding thread counts are as follows:

Heavyweight muslin—not less than 140 threads/sq in.
Medium muslin—not less than 128 threads/sq in.
Lightweight muslin—not less than 112 threads/sq in.
Backfilled muslin—fewer than 112 threads/sq in.

When viewed microscopically, a cotton fiber gives the appearance of a flat twisted ribbon, but this information is of little value in attempting to explain the structure of the fiber. By means of x-ray diffraction analysis, it has been shown[11] that native cotton fibers consist of crystalline cellulose, but the crystallinity of the individual fiber is discontinuous. In other words, a cellulose fiber is not a single crystal, rather it exists in part as a crystalline aggregate with long-chain molecules which are oriented more or less parallel to one another. The molecules of almost all fibers consist of many similar units joined together in long chains. For example, in native cellulose fibers there may be 2,000 to 3,000 basic units in the chain, whereas in synthetic fibers at least 100 units are recognized. Within these molecules there are certain groups which strongly attract water. In the case of cellulose, there are active hydroxyl groups present in the molecular composition of the fibers to which water molecules can be attached by hydrogen bonds.

Moisture Content of Cotton Fabrics

It is a well-known fact that cellulose (cotton) and cellulose derivatives, when surrounded by an atmosphere containing the vapors of water or of some organic liquid, take up or give off the vapor until an equilibrium condition is reached. This behavior is characteristic of the phenomenon of *sorption*, exhibited by most solid materials. In broad terms, sorption refers to a physicochemical process of attraction and retention of gaseous substances by a liquid or solid medium. It is further recognized that there are two separate and distinct processes involved in sorption. The one, commonly termed *absorption*, applies to the collection of a gas or a vapor by solution in a liquid absorbent. The other, known as *adsorption* is the capture of a gas or vapor by a sorbent that is solid, rather than liquid. In this book, when reference is made to adsorption, the implied meaning shall be the taking up of vapor, and the release of vapor shall be referred to as *desorption*.

Moisture has a profound effect upon cotton fibers. In fact, the strength of cotton fibers varies directly with moisture content, which, in turn, is more or less completely dependent upon temperature and relative humidity. Cotton fiber breaking strengths increase with rising relative humidity and approach a maximum at 60 to 70% relative humidity. The fibers become less rigid, more plastic, and more extensible as they acquire moisture. When fabrics are exposed to unchanging atmospheric (external) conditions, they attain ultimately a moisture content that remains constant just as long as these conditions remain unaltered. This constancy of moisture content is not a static condition but rather one of equilibrium, in which the amount of water evaporating from the fibers in a given time is exactly counterbalanced by the water condensing on the fibers. The rate of evaporation depends on the amount of water in the fibers and on the temperature. The rate of condensation depends on the number of potential adsorbing points (hydrophilic or

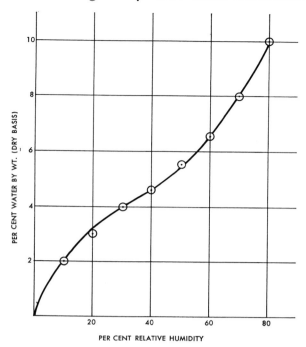

FIGURE 6-2. Equilibrium moisture content (sorption) of surgical cotton at 68°F (20°C).

free hydroxyl groups) still unoccupied on the fibers and also on the concentration of water vapor in the surrounding atmosphere.

The equilibrium relationship of relative humidity to moisture content of cotton material at 68°F (20°C) is shown in Figure 6-2 (data from Filby and Maass[12]). The figures given by the curve are in close agreement with those of other workers, namely, Henry,[13] Penikett, Rowe, and Robson.[14] Most surgical dressings of cotton material will contain 5.0 to 6.5% water by weight when in equilibrium with atmospheres of 45 to 60% relative humidity. It is not unusual, however, to encounter dressings in hospitals with a lesser moisture content. Bowie,[9] for example, has mentioned that freshly laundered towels may show a state of hydration of less than 0.5 per cent. Others[14] have shown that dressings properly dried after laundering will have a moisture content between 2 and 5 per cent. Unfolding and airing of freshly laundered materials for a few hours under normal humidity conditions will restore the moisture content to higher levels. Such action is necessary to avoid superheating of fabrics during the steam sterilizing process.

In summary, one may visualize that the transfer of moisture from the atmosphere to the fabrics or packs occurs in three distinct phases, not differentiated by time:

1. Passage of moisture from the surrounding air to the surface of the pack in which the air is partially denuded of its water content.

2. Diffusion of moisture and air from the surface to the interior of the pack via the air spaces or interstices between fibers.

3. Adsorption of moisture by the individual fibers. Other factors influence the rate of conditioning and uptake of moisture, such as dimensions of the package, weight of the fabrics, and thread count. For all practical purposes, the permeability to water vapor may be considered to be directly proportional to the density of the package.

Removal of Adsorbed Air from Hydrated Fabrics

As in the case of water vapor, cellulose materials exhibit a strong attraction for air (nitrogen, oxygen, and carbon dioxide) and other gases. Air in the molecular state clings tenaciously to each fiber and in this condition it is believed to be adsorbed. There is a great mass of evidence, accumulated over the past eighty years, to show that air is the common foe of all methods of steam sterilization. The new concept of prevacuum sterilization likewise has contributed its share of evidence, as presented here, to show that residual air clearance from within a mass of fabrics is an absolute necessity in the attainment of reliable sterilization.

The physics of air removal from a mass of fabrics is complicated, and it is doubtful if anyone can substantiate fully any plausible theory. Several factors are at work in a dynamic relationship involving vacuum pumping capacity, density of the load, temperature, moisture content of the load, free space in the chamber, difference in pressure between the center of each pack and the free chamber space, air leakage into the chamber, ratio of load volume to chamber volume, and the nature and history of the fibers from which the fabrics are made. In the generally accepted concept of high prevacuum sterilization as advanced by the working party (MRC), it is contended that residual air is removed from cotton material by entrainment (boiling out) when the absolute pressure in the chamber is reduced to a level equal to that of the equilibrium water vapor pressure over the material. If one accepts this theory, then attention must be given to the fact that the pressure of water vapor in equilibrium with cotton containing 4 per cent by weight of water at 77°F (25°C) is about 8 mm Hg. This is typical of a 30% relative humidity condition with respect to fabrics and, in practice, a pumping system capable of drawing this degree of vacuum (with some reserve capacity) would be required to effectively remove adsorbed air from the load. Other values for equilibrium vapor pressures of fabrics versus their moisture content at 77°F are as follows:

Moisture % Dry Wt	% RH	Vapor Pressure
2	10	3.5 mm Hg
3	20	6.0 mm Hg
4	30	8.0 mm Hg
5	45	11.0 mm Hg
6	55	14.0 mm Hg

It is regrettable that the original recommendations of the working party were misunderstood with respect to the degree of vacuum required to remove residual air from materials. Whereas Knox and Penikett[1] reported satisfactory results only when their vacuum reached a level of 20 mm Hg, the figure suggested by the working party was 15 mm Hg *or below* for a chamber fully loaded with cotton fabrics containing 4% water and having a temperature not exceeding 59°F (15°C). The point of confusion seems to have arisen from an element of the British Standards Specification #3220, which states that high prevacuum sterilization shall effect "removal of air from the chamber of the autoclave to within 0.8 inches Hg (2 cm) absolute pressure in not more than 5 minutes." More recently it has been acknowledged by several investigators that this specification is inadequate, since it is doubtful if a critical point exists expressed in terms of absolute pressure, and disregarding the pumping down time, whereby assurance can be given that residual air will have been removed from all types of loads. Findings reported in this chapter tend to support this view.

It has ben argued by Rowe *et al.,*[10] that the concept of "boiling off" (evaporating) moisture to remove residual air is not applicable to high prevacuum sterilization. Their reasoning is to the effect that no abrupt change occurs in the mode of evaporation of water from a load as the external pressure falls; and to permit evaporation, the partial pressure of water vapor in the chamber must be less than at the surface of the pack. Also, it is claimed that, under any external conditions of partial vapor pressure, no significant loss of moisture from the center of the pack will occur over periods of several hours.

Regardless of whether the total pressure attained in the prevacuum stage is critical, and the evidence presented here indicates it is not, the point still remains that both fabrics and paper can be dehydrated under vacuum. Furthermore, if residual air is physically adsorbed on fibers, then the process must be reversible, and it is reasonable to conclude that release of air can be assisted by entrainment with water vapor evolved by the fabrics. At this point it must be admitted that the basic difference between a high prevacuum sterilizer and all other types (systems) is the absolute dependence upon a pumping system with adequate capacity, unassisted by other means, to remove residual air from the load.

Alternate systems may be utilized for the removal of air. Of those studied and reported by the writer the most practical is the application of prevacuum plus steam injection for stage one of the process cycle. *In terms of performance, this system differs markedly from that of high prevacuum in that the selected degree of vacuum is of the order of 25 mm Hg, and throughout the pumping-down period steam in a predetermined volume vs. time is admitted to the chamber and discharged through the pump.*

In principle, the purpose of steam injection in stage 1 is to accelerate the desorption or release of air from the load through the medium of displacement. On the assumption that residual air is adsorbed on cotton fibers, it follows that the process of adsorption is reversible and not unlike that of water vapor. Also, cotton fibers containing a definite amount of adsorbed air or vapor will be in equilibrium with respect to the concentration of air or vapor in the space surrounding the fibers. This equilibrium can be easily disturbed by any change in temperature or in the concentration of gas or vapor in the surrounding space. If then, during the prevacuum stage, steam is admitted to the chamber, the effect is one of immediately reducing the partial pressure of air in the space surrounding the fabrics, and at the same time, steam assisted by the partial vacuum will diffuse rapidly through the fibers thereby releasing adsorbed air through the process of displacement. The rate of diffusion is greater for a gas or vapor with lesser density (specific gravity) and this diffusion is increased considerably by means of the partial vacuum.

EVALUATION OF HIGH PREVACUUM AND PREVACUUM WITH STEAM INJECTION SYSTEMS

Two basic systems utilizing steam under pressure were studied to determine the most desirable one, from a practical standpoint, for application to standard sterilizing equipment. These systems are currently recognized as high prevacuum and prevacuum with steam injection.

The high prevacuum system utilized a vacuum pump (water-ring seal) with an ejector for removing air from the chamber and the load to a degree that the remaining air exerted an absolute pressure of 20 mm Hg or less. The degree of air removal was purposely adjusted to fulfill the objectives of the individual experiments.

The prevacuum with steam injection system utilized a similar pumping arrangement, but steam was admitted to the sterilizing chamber during the time that the vacuum was being drawn on the chamber. To clarify by analogy, one might picture a bucket full of water with a hole pierced suddenly in the bottom which allows the water to escape. At the same time water is poured into the top of the bucket, but at a slower rate than the flow from the bottom. Eventually there would be very little water remaining in the bucket. The same principle was applied to the steam injection system except the air was removed from the chamber and load as a steam-air mixture and steam was constantly admitted to the chamber but at a slower rate.

When using a steam injection system, several factors must be controlled to obtain proper conditions for air elimination. The size of the sterilizing chamber determines to some extent the quantity of steam which must be delivered per unit time in order to rid the chamber and the load of air. Attention must be given to the site of admission of steam and the location of applying vacuum to the chamber. Also, the quantity of steam admitted must be correlated with the capacity of the pumping system used to remove the steam and air mixture. Finally, the time factor for producing the proper vacuum must be taken into account.

EXPERIMENTAL MATERIALS AND METHODS

Test Packs

Dense Sheet Pack (20.6 lbs/cu ft)

Consists of 5 muslin sheets (130 threads/in). Each sheet folded double six times to give 64 layers per sheet. Overwrapper consisted of double muslin.

Dimensions of pack approximately 5″ × 10″ × 14″—weighing 8.2 pounds. (It should be noted that for test purposes, this pack and conditions of loading were designed to represent the most difficult conditions for obtaining proper temperature and time for sterilization. This "challenge load" far exceeds the packaging and loading conditions one would expect to find in hospital use.)

Standard Surgical Pack

Basic linen pack—(6.0 lbs/cu ft)
  2 Wrappers—double thickness muslin, 36″ × 60″ or of adequate size to cover operating table top and allow for 6″ overhang.
  1 Mayo stand cover (drape)
15 Towels
    3 Dry hands of Surgeon and Assistants
    1 Cover tray on Mayo stand
    2 Sutures
    4 Drape patient; Outline operative site
    2 Skin towels
    3 Extra
30 Sponges, R. O.
  5 Tape sponges, R. O.
  3 Gowns
    Surgeon
    Assistants

Varied Loads

1. Glassware (bottles, flasks, cylinders, petri dishes and test tubes).
2. Muslin wrapped metalware (basins, canisters and pails).
3. Rubber gloves (101 pairs per load).
4. Standard surgical packs ranging from 2 to 6 per load.
5. Dense packs ranging from 1 to 20 per load.
6. Huck towels (29 in metal casket) 1 casket per load.
    Each towel folded double, twice, to give a total of 116 layers.

7. European metal caskets holding 10 sheets folded to 32 thicknesses per sheet (4 caskets per load).
8. Metal cylinder (4″ diameter × 18″ long, open at one end) packed with surgical cotton and gauze; placed upright in sterilizer.

The numbered items listed as varied loads were not intermixed. These varied loads were processed as a control on the dense pack or "challenge load." In no instance were the varied loads as difficult to penetrate as the "challenge load."

Test packs were not used more than four times without being laundered and mangled by a commerical laundry. In no instance did the data indicate a difference between freshly laundered and previously sterilized packs.

Temperature Measurements

Temperature measurements were made with a Leeds and Northrup Potentiometer, Serial #1318705. Copper-constantan thermocouple wire (Leeds and Northrup #24-55-1, enamel and glass insulation) entering the sterilizer through the backhead via a Conax adaptor. Temperature measurements were made from the pack center and at the chamber drain line.

Load Lag

Load lag is the difference in minutes and/or seconds between the time the experimental chamber reached 270°F and the time when the load reached the same temperature.

Autoclave Time Temperature Tapes

1. Minnesota Mining and Manufacturing Company—Type 1222
2. Johnson and Johnson—TYLOC® (The test tape used was designed for 270°F operation.)

Tapes were used in addition to the thermocouple readings to indicate whether or not sterilizing conditions had been achieved within the pack.

Timing

All times were taken with manually operated stop watches and were validated with charts from a recording potentiometer.

Vacuum Measurements

1. Mechanical Gauges (absolute)
   a. Wallace and Tiernan
   b. Edwards
2. Other Absolute Gauges
   a. Fisher and Sargent Mercury Manometers
   b. Hastings Thermocouple Gauge

Sterilizer

All tests were conducted in an experimental chamber (24″ × 36″ × 36″ —18 cu ft) equipped with a water-seal pump (Siemen and Hinsch) to which was added either an air ejector or steam ejector as required by the experiments.

Steam Supply

Steam supplied by plant boiler to site of usage with approximate line pressure 60 to 70 psig fed to sterilizer through regulating valve set to give 34 psig within the sterilizer

Steam Injection

Steam for injection was introduced into the bottom of the experimental chamber through the chamber drain line.

Steam for Sterilization

Steam for sterilization was introduced into the experimental chamber through the upper portion of the backhead.

Vacuum

Vacuum was applied to the experimental chamber and load through the upper portion of the backhead.

Leaks

Leaks were artifically produced through a valve into a tube leading from the center portion of the backhead to the lower front of the experimental chamber. These were leaks of a known rate (mm Hg absolute per minute) introduced for experimental purposes.

Leak Check

For those experiments where leakage of less than 1 mm Hg absolute per minute was required, leak checks were performed on the experimental chamber, valves, and associated piping. In all cases, leak checks were performed using manometer calibrated absolute gauges, over a five-minute period, to insure leakage rates of less than 1 mm/min within the vacuum range of the given experiments.

TEST RESULTS

The characteristics of a typical high prevacuum cycle with the load consisting of a single dense pack are shown in Figure 6-3. The findings demonstrate a definite load lag in coming up to the sterilizing temperature of 270°F (132°C). This condition is typical of a high percentage of all experimental tests conducted at 18 mm Hg prevacuum. Figure 6-4 is a represen-

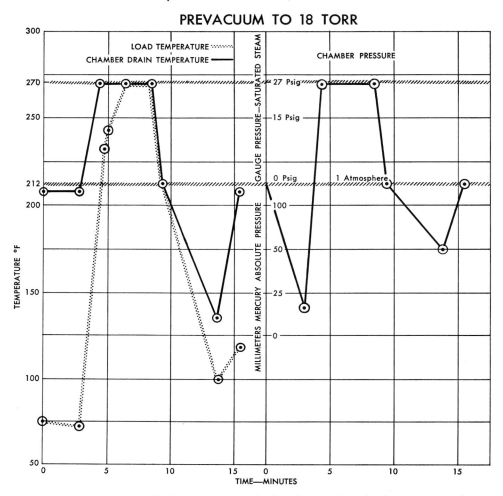

FIGURE 6-3. Typical cycle for experimental chamber with a load consisting of one dense pack.

	CHAMBER Min.-Sec.		LOAD Min.-Sec.	
Prevacuum (18 mm Hg)	2	50	2	50
Come up to 270° F	1	30	3	30
Exposure	4	0	2	0
Exhaust to 0 psig	1	0	1	0
Postvacuum (50 mm Hg)	4	30	4	30
Return to 0 psig	1	30	1	30
Total Cycle	15	20	15	20

tative cycle of a single dense pack load in the chamber when subjected to an initial vacuum of 5 mm Hg. In this case no load lag was observed.

In an attempt to further evaluate the high prevacuum system of sterilization, a series of tests were made on various loads subjected to 18 mm through 5 mm Hg absolute in increments for the purpose of determining the relationship between load lag and the magnitude of prevacuum. Figure 6-5 shows the results of these studies. The findings indicate that as the absolute pressure was decreased in the chamber and the load, the following occurred:

> In the 16 to 18 mm Hg range the greatest percentage of the tests performed showed lags of one minute or more.
> In the 13 to 15 mm Hg range the greatest percentage of load lag was again in the range of one minute or more.
> In the ranges of 9 to 12, 7 to 8 and 5 to 6 mm Hg the greatest percentage of lag was in the less-than-one-minute series.
> More than 50 per cent of the tests performed at the 5 to 6 mm Hg range showed 0 seconds load lag. Less than 10 per cent of the tests in the 7 through 18 mm Hg absolute pressure range showed 0 seconds load lag.

The findings further indicate that pressure of less than 5 mm Hg absolute is necessary to completely eliminate load lag under the experimental conditions used for the tests.

The combination of prevacuum and steam injection was studied experimentally to determine the effect on total cycle time as well as reduction of load lag. A typical cycle utilizing the steam injection system with a load in chamber is shown in Figure 6-6. The quantity of saturated steam, expressed as condensate, injected during the prevacuum phase of the test cycles is shown in Figure 6-7. The steam injection system reduced the total cycle time with a single dense pack load in the chamber to 12 minutes, but of far greater importance was the reduction of load lag to 0 seconds in all of the tests.

In experimentally determining a reliable cycle by using a prevacuum time of 3 minutes and 40 seconds plus steam injection, the load lag and degree of prevacuum were correlated as shown in Figure 6-8. From this graph it is apparent that to approach 0 second load lag the prevacuum must be of the order of 25 mm Hg absolute. All tests relating to Figure 6-8 were conducted with an arbitrarily timed prevacuum of 3 minutes and 40 seconds. During the prevacuum phase of the cycles experimentally studied, the vacuum chamber (sterilizer), connecting valves, and piping had to be virtually leak-free in order for the load to show 0 time lag. This was shown to be true, even when easily penetrable loads were processed in the chamber. Figure 6-9 illustrates the point that leak rates appreciably more than 1 mm Hg solute per minute, demonstrated over a 5-minute period, produce

PREVACUUM TO 5 TORR

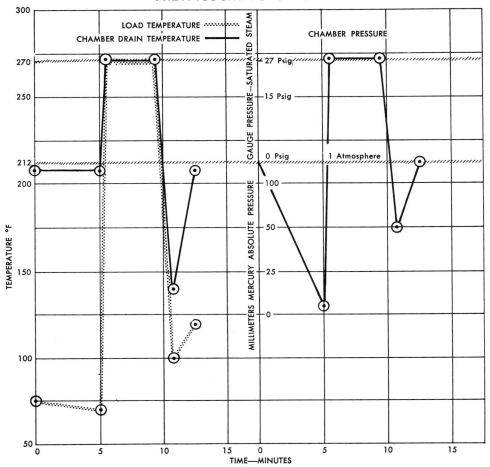

FIGURE 6-4. Typical cycle with a load consisting of one dense pack in the chamber and an initial vacuum of 5 mm Hg. A load lag of 0 seconds was obtained in 50 per cent of the experimental tests.

	CHAMBER AND LOAD	
	Min.	*Sec.*
Prevacuum (5 mm Hg)	5	0
Come up to 270° F	0	20
Exposure	4	0
Exhaust to 0 psig and postvacuum (50 mm Hg)	1	25
Return to 0 psig	1	45
Total Cycle	12	30

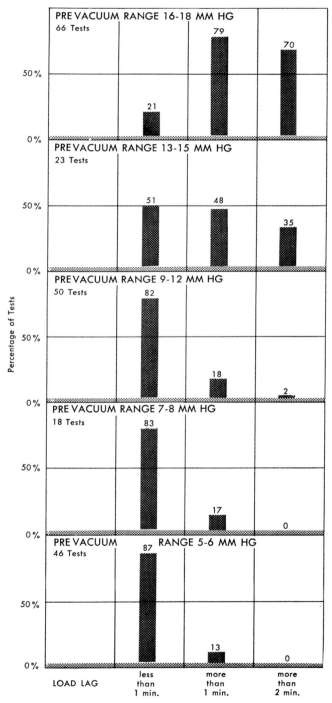

FIGURE 6-5. Results of tests for load lag using varied loads and increments of prevacuum in ranges from 18 to 5 mm Hg absolute.

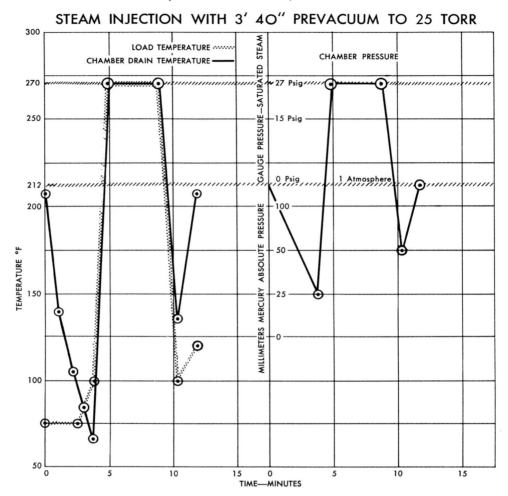

FIGURE 6-6. Typical cycle of a load consisting of one dense pack in chamber with prevacuum of 25 mm Hg and steam injection. This system showed 0 seconds load lag in 100 per cent of the experimental tests.

	CHAMBER AND LOAD	
	Min.	*Sec.*
Prevacuum (25 mm Hg)	3	40
Come up to 270° F	1	15
Exposure	4	0
Exhaust to 0 psig and postvacuum (50 mm Hg)	1	20
Return to 0 psig	1	45
Total Cycle	12	0

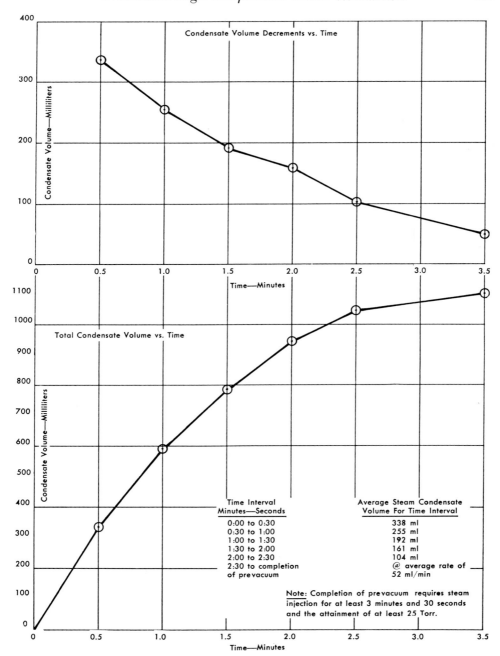

FIGURE 6-7. Quantity of steam, expressed as condensate, injected during test cycles.

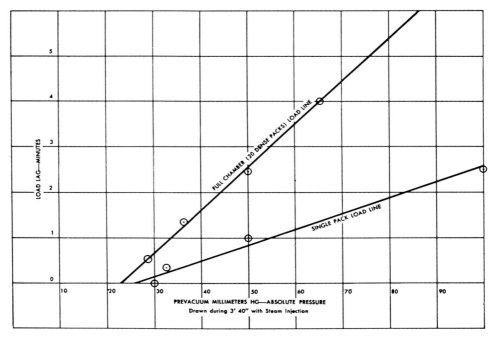

FIGURE 6-8. Correlation of load lag with degree of prevacuum drawn during 3'40" of steam injection.

and definitely cannot be tolerated. This criterion was shown to apply to both the high prevacuum and the prevacuum with steam injection systems.

As a summary statement on the evaluation of the high prevacuum system for sterilization, it can be said that no critical point exists in terms of absolute pressure in the range of 4.5 to 18 mm Hg whereby load lag is reduced to 0 seconds time in test loads. The autoclave should be equipped with means for reducing the air content in the chamber and the load at prevacuum phase to about 1 mm Hg or less partial pressure. Under automatically controlled operating conditions, the prevacuum with steam injection system is a satisfactory process. In addition, it has the advantage of functioning properly in the range of 25 mm Hg absolute and is the more acceptable of the two systems for practical application to steam sterilization.

DETERIORATION OF MATERIALS WHEN SUBJECTED TO PREVACUUM HIGH TEMPERATURE STERILIZATION

Tests were conducted to determine and compare the rate of deterioration in surgical rubber gloves and in fabrics when subjected to 250°F and 270°F using gravity air discharge, and air removal by mechanical means (prevacuum).

Rubber Gloves

In all tests, gloves were subjected to conditions normally encountered in hospitals between sterilization cycles. A complete cycle to duplicate one use of the gloves consisted of handling, soiling, laundering, steam sterilization, and 24-hour quarantine.

GROUP I was sterilized at 250°F for 15 minutes employing the gravity-discharge method.

GROUP II was sterilized at 270°F for 5 minutes employing prevacuum air removal method.

GROUP III served as a control and was subjected to all parts of a routine handling cycle except for processing in the sterilizer.

After 4, 8, 12, and 15 cycles, sample gloves were removed from the test groups and tested for tensile strength loss according to standard methods. As seen in Figure 6-10, there was no significant difference initially in tensile strength loss between the two systems of steam sterilization. After four cycles, 20.9 per cent tensile strength loss was observed in Group I, and 19.7 per cent in Group II.

Beyond eight cycles, gloves sterilized by the gravity discharge method showed a greater loss of tensile strength than gloves sterilized by the prevacuum method. The tensile strength loss after twelve cycles was 54.3 per

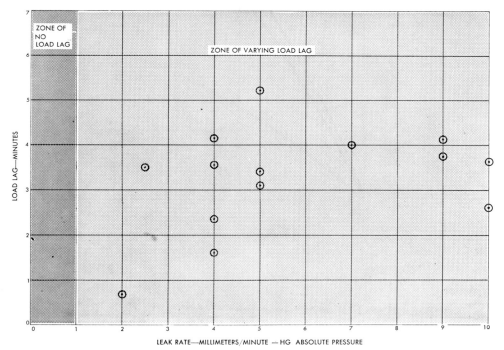

FIGURE 6-9. Load lag produced by controlled leak rates over a 5-minute period.

cent at 250°F, and 44.9 per cent at 270°F. After fifteen cycles, 60.9 per cent and 52 per cent, respectively.

Approximately one half of the damage caused to rubber gloves during the first eight cycles was due to the effects of handling, soiling, and laundering and not to sterlization. Beyond eight cycles, the rate of deterioration due to handling, soiling, and laundering decreased.

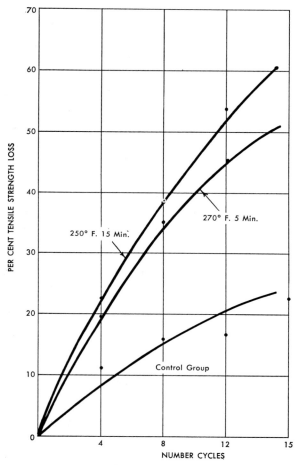

FIGURE 6-10. Deterioration of rubber gloves resulting from sterilizing cycles of 250°F for 15 minutes and 270°F for 5 minutes vs control group subjected to all routine handling except steam sterilization.

Fabrics

A comparison was made between fabrics sterilized at 270°F for 10 minutes employing the prevacuum technique with fabrics sterilized at 250°F for 30 minutes employing the gravity-air discharge technique. The following materials were employed in these tests:

1. A 16″ × 16″ × 24″ pressure steam sterilizer equipped with a vacuum pump.
2. Five (5) linen packs with approximate dimensions—12″ × 12″ × 20″, weight 10 to 12 pounds.

Contents:

2 surgical gowns	1 laparotomy drape
1 stand cover	4 large towels
2 lap pads	3 hand towels
2 small draw sheets	40 A.I.L. test pieces 12″ × 18″
1 double muslin outer wrapper	(American Institute of Laundering)

3. Five (5) groups of 40 A.I.L. test pieces suspended from a rack with paper clips.

Five (5) identical packs were prepared and subjected to the following conditions:

Pack A—control, not laundered or sterilized
Pack B—laundered only
Pack C—sterilized only
Pack D—laundered, sterilized at 250°F and relaundered between sterilizing cycles
Pack E—laundered, sterilized at 270°F and relaundered between sterilizing cycles

Packs were placed in the sterilizer on edge with layers of fabric in a vertical position. With each test pack 40 A.I.L. test pieces, suspended from a rack, were processed to simulate conditions upon the outer surface of the pack. All test packs were equilibrated to room humidity for 2 hours between cycles.

At ten-cycle intervals, four A.I.L. test pieces were removed from the pack and from the outside group of test pieces. Tensile strength loss was determined by the American Institute of Laundering, Joliet, Illinois, according to the formula:

$$\% \text{ loss} = 100\% \times \left(1 - \frac{\text{Breaking strength of test fabric}}{\text{Breaking strength of control (nonprocessed) fabric}}\right)$$

To maintain identical conditions with respect to load capacity, replacement fabrics were substituted for the test fabrics which were removed.

The test results showed a progressive loss in tensile strength when fabrics were subjected to steam sterilization. As seen in Figure 6-11, after fifty cycles of sterilization with relaundering between cycles, the tensile strength loss of fabrics within the pack was 27 per cent at 250°F for 30 minutes, and

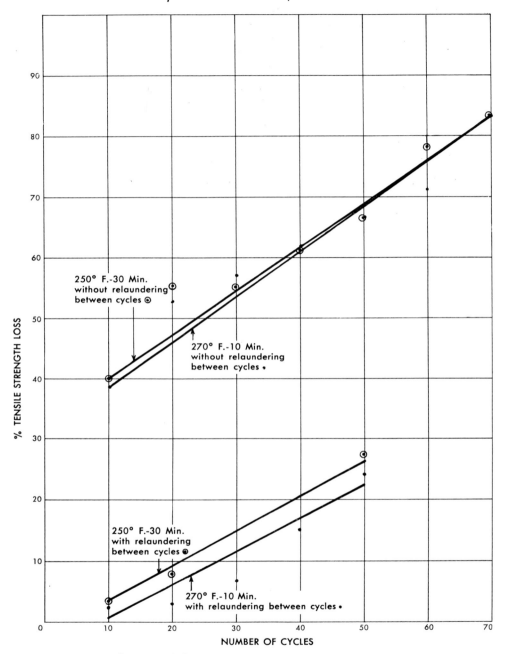

FIGURE 6-11. Tensile strength loss of test fabrics *inside* pack at 270°F for 10 minutes vs 250°F for 30 minutes, with and without relaundering between cycles.

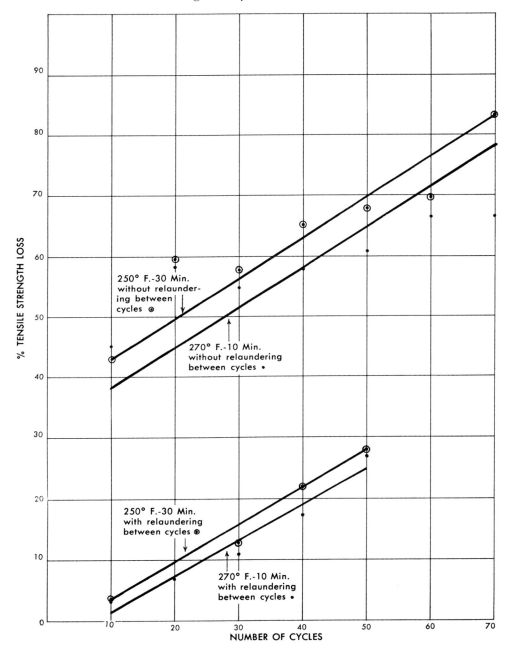

FIGURE 6-12. Tensile strength loss of test fabrics *outside* pack at 270°F for 10 minutes vs 250°F for 30 minutes, with and without relaundering between cycles.

24 per cent at 270°F for 10 minutes. As seen in Figure 6-12, tensile strength loss was slightly higher, 28 per cent and 27 per cent, respectively, when fabrics were freely exposed to steam, that is, not inside the pack.

Fabrics repeatedly sterilized without laundering between cycles (Fig. 6-11) showed a much greater rate of deterioration. After fifty cycles of repeated sterilization, fabrics within the pack lost 55 to 57 per cent of their tensile strength. Fabrics freely exposed to steam (Fig. 6-12) showed similar loss in tensile strength.

Tensile strength loss due to laundering only was approximately 6 per cent after fifty cycles.

The results of experimental work show that steam sterilization will deteriorate fabrics and rubber gloves. Deterioration of fabrics is lessened to a slight degree with the use of high temperatures and short exposures. Laundering between sterilizing cycles reduces the deterioration rate of fabrics regardless of whether sterilizing temperatures of 250°F or 270°F are used.

Damage to gloves, as reflected by tensile strength loss, is essentially the same with either the 250°F or 270°F process for the first eight cycles. Less damage was demonstrated with the 270°F process beyond the eighth sterilization cycle.

STEAM STERILIZER PULSING SYSTEMS

A variety of methods have been advocated for promoting rapid steam penetration and sterilization of dense challenge loads of fabrics. The classical gravity displacement-type sterilizer offers the most common and least expensive means of acomplishing sterilization. The cycle times are long because adequate time must be allowed for steam penetration and effective air elimination from the load. In contrast, the high prevacuum system depends upon a single pressure and vacuum excursion at the start and completion of the cycle. This method of operation results in very short cycle times due to the rapid removal of air from the chamber and the load by the vacuum pump, the higher operating temperature (272°-276°F), shorter exposure time, and accelerated drying of fabric loads. The equipment cost, however, becomes greater in the case of high prevacuum because of the required mechanical components and related control devices. Recently, sterilizer manufacturers have employed more than one excursion or pulse to create a dynamic condition in the chamber and thereby enhance load penetration. A pulse may be defined as the process of increasing the sterilizer pressure to a set pressure with steam followed by venting the sterilizer to a minimal pressure preceding the next pulse. There are basically three kinds of pulsing systems currently applied to sterilizers.

Pressure gravity. This system operates in the positive pressure range and returns the chamber pressure to near atmospheric as soon as the temperature in the chamber reaches a predetermined level.

Ten pulses are usually employed which following the load is exposed to 270°F steam for a short period. The total cycle time is substantially less than that of the standard gravity displacement type sterilizer.

Vacuum pulsing. This system operates in the negative pressure or vacuum range. Two pulses are usually employed at the start of the cycle and then the steam pressure is advanced to about 30 psig for a short exposure time at 272° to 275°F. The total time cycle is much shorter than that developed in the gravity displacement type sterilizer. The sterilizer must, of course, be equipped with a vacuum pump and related control devices.

Pressure-vacuum. The third system employs pulsing both in the positive pressure and vacuum regions. In addition, it measures the quality of the vacuum attained at the end of a given time period for each vacuum excursion. If the predetermined quality is reached at the end of the third pulse, the system omits the next pulse and exposes the load to a sterilization period at 285°F (141°C). The result is the shortest cycle time of the pulsing systems.

The time required to heat the load to sterilizing temperature with a pulsing system depends upon the number of pulses and the time expended for each pulse. The effectiveness of a pulse, and therefore the number of pulses required, is in turn dependent upon the amplitude or excursion of the pulse and the ratio of the maximal and minimal absolute pressures of each pulse. The time expended by a pulse is a function of the rate of delivery and expulsion of steam and of the maximal and minimal pulsing pressures related

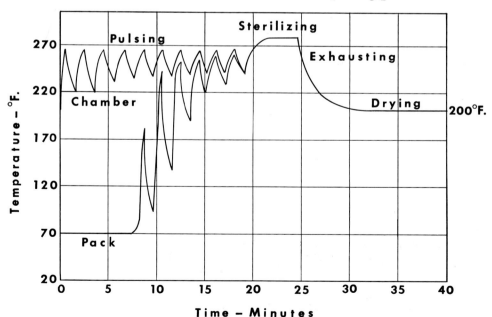

FIGURE 6-13. Characteristics of a pressure gravity pulsing cycle for steam sterilization.

TYPICAL CYCLE - CHALLENGE LOAD - 4 PACKS

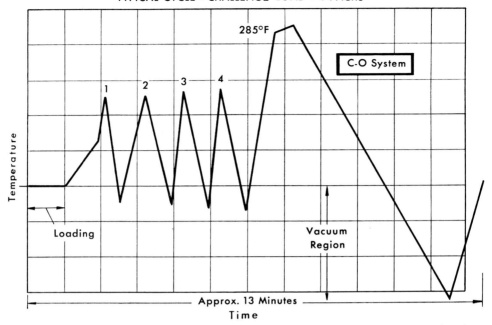

FIGURE 6-14. Characteristics of a pressure-vacuum pulsing cycle for steam sterilization. The ultimate temperature is 285°F (141°C).

to atmospheric pressure. Therefore, pulses of great amplitude in a given system will require more time than pulses of small amplitude. The time-temperature characteristics of a pressure gravity pulsing cycle are shown in Figure 6-13. With a challenge load of 20 test packs in the sterilizer, the total cycle time is 40 minutes or approximately one-half the time required for sterilization in the conventional gravity displacement unit. The characteristics of a pressure-vacuum pulsing cycle are shown in Figure 6-14. With a challenge load of 4 dense packs in the sterilizer, the total cycle time is less than 15 minutes or approximately one-fourth the time required for sterilization in the conventional gravity displacement unit.

REFERENCES

1. KNOX, R., and PENIKETT, E. J. K.: Influence of initial vacuum on steam sterilisation of dressings. *Brit Med Jour, 1*:680-682, 1958.
2. ALDER, V. G., and GILLESPIE, W. A.: *Automatic High Prevacuum Steam Sterilisation for Surgical Dressings and Gloves.* Drayton Regulator & Instrument Co., Ltd., West Drayton, England, May, 1959.
3. WORKING PARTY (MRC): Sterilisation by steam under increased pressure. *Lancet,* Feb. 28:425-435, 1959.
4. BOWIE, J. H.: *Health Bulletin* (Edinburgh, Scotland), *16*:36, 1958.
5. BOWIE, J. H.: *Pharmaceutical Jour, 174*:473, 1955.
6. PERKINS, J. J.: *Principles and Methods of Sterilization.* Springfield, Illinois, Thomas, 1956.
7. SCHMIDT, B., and MOLLER, E.: *Z Hyg Infektionskr, 140*:144, 1954.

8. Bowie, J. H.: Requirements for an Automatically Controlled, High Prevacuum Steriliser, XVI, *No. 2 Health Bulletin,* Edinburgh, 1958.

9. Bowie, J. H.: The Control of Heat Sterilisers, Symposium on Sterilisation of Surgical Materials, London, Pharmaceutical Press, 1961, pp. 109-142.

10. Rowe, T. W. G.; Kusay, R., and Skelton, E.: The Application of Vacuum to Steam Sterilizers, *Paper submitted to 2nd Intern, Congress of I.O.V.S.T.,* Washington, Oct. 1961.

11. Sisson, W. A.: X-ray examination. From *Cellulose and Cellulose Derivatives.* Ott, E. (Ed): New York, Interscience, 1946, pp. 203-252.

12. Filby, E., and Maass, O.: The sorption of water vapor on cellulosic materials. *Canad J Res, 13, B:*1-10, 1935.

13. Henry, P. S. H.: Physical aspects of sterilizing cotton articles by steam. *J App Bact,* 22:159-172, 1957.

14. Penikett, E. J. K.; Rowe, T. W. G., and Robson, E.: Vacuum drying of steam sterilized dressings. *J Appl Bact, 71:*282-290, 1959.

Chapter 7

MINIMUM STANDARDS FOR STERILIZATION

DOWN THROUGH the years various standards have been proposed and established for the sterilization of surgical supplies. Certain of these standards were obviously based upon expediency, taking into consideration the often extreme inaccuracies resulting from the use of highly inefficient sterilizers. For many years the common practice for sterilizing bulk loads of supplies was "20 pounds pressure for 1 hour." This was a purely arbitrary rule which had little or no scientific background, for which apparently no one could formulate a logical excuse or reason—except in average usage it seemed to suffice. It must be remembered, however, that the old style sterilizers were operated with "pressure" as the sole indication of regulation. There was no means for measuring the degree of air evacuation, other than the vacuum gauge, and there was no means for measuring the temperature developed by the steam in the chamber.

With the introduction in 1933 of temperature control for sterilizers, it became immediately apparent that detailed investigations were needed to more clearly define minimum requirements and exposure periods for adequate sterilization without waste of time and undue destruction of fabrics from the oversterilization. W. B. Underwood,[1] a leading investigator in the field of sterilization, was largely responsible for the initial atack on this problem. He frequently demonstrated by means of potentiometer tests on sterilizers in daily use in hospitals that far better sterilizing influence in 30 minutes' exposure could be attained with a temperature-controlled sterilizer than was shown in routine performance under pressure control in one full hour exposure. The results of these early studies by Underwood are shown in Figure 7-1. That such hazardous conditions continue to exist through the use of highly inefficient sterilizers has been the subject of several investigations by authoritative groups.[2,3,4,5,6]

Bowie's[6] devastating report published in 1955 indicated that about 90 per cent of the sterilizers in use in Britain's hospitals and pharmacies were obsolete. It is hoped that this situation has since been rectified and in large measure. Reports continue to appear, however, on the low standards of sterilizing practice in hospitals. One of these investigations into bacterial standards in hospital ward practice showed that between 9 per cent and 50 per cent of the equipment stated to be sterile was in fact contaminated.[7] The finding of

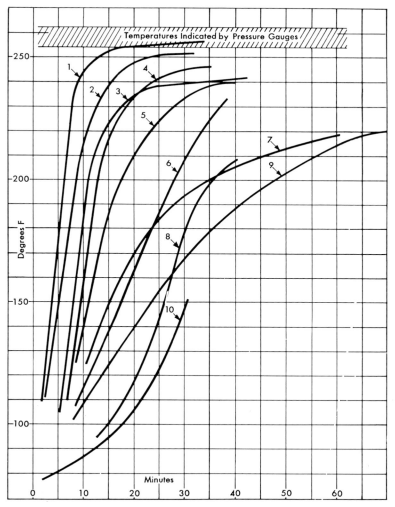

FIGURE 7-1. These curves record actual temperatures attained within the loads of ten surgical supply sterilizers found in six hospitals. Sterilizers were operated under pressures of 17-22 pounds, with no means of measuring the degree of air elimination or the true temperatures developed. Shaded area denotes temperatures which were indicated by pressure gauges for saturated steam.

bacteria in 27 per cent of surgical packs is a disturbing example of the inefficiency of the sterilization process.[8] Findings of this nature would seem to lend support to the claim made by Dandy[9] many years ago that most wound infections resulted from contaminated gauze sponges and that infections did not occur following prolongation of the sterilizing process. Extension of the sterilizing time is not necessarily the answer to the problem of a fewer number of nonsterile articles in the hospital. Other factors enter into the probability of achieving sterilization of inanimate things and each of these factors must be dealt with respectfully and comprehensively.

STERILIZATION DEFINED

Sterilization means the act or process of destroying completely all forms of microbial life, including viruses. This is a rigid, uncompromising, absolute term. There is no such condition as "partial sterility"—the article is either sterile or nonsterile. Terms like "almost sterile," "practically sterile," and "degree of sterility" are incorrect and they only serve to confuse the issue, particularly in the minds of students. The actual practice of sterilization in the hospital must be established on an "all or none" basis with no allowance made for even one demonstrable living organism on an article or in a solution at the end of the process. It should be recognized, of course, that a product is sterile only insofar as one is able to demonstrate sterility by approved laboratory methods. Also, in order for anyone to give a guarantee that a product is sterile demands, first, that the test methods used be infallible in their ability to detect single organisms of all known types, including viruses. Unfortunately, sterility test methods possessing this degree of reliability are not available.

The terms and conditions mentioned above add up to the accepted fact that achievement of true sterilization is a function of probability and the process is influenced by the laws of chance. Of the many factors known to have a bearing on the end result of the sterilization process the following are believed to be the most important:

- —Number of organisms on the material and their resistance to the sterilizing agent.
- —Protection afforded organisms by extraneous matter—unable to establish direct steam contact to all surfaces. Examples: oils, greases, protein soil, soap curds, blood, pus, feces, tissue debris.
- —Exponential death rate. Numbers of organisms dying per unit of time are proportional to numbers present at start of time interval. An increase in exposure time results in an increase of kill.
- —Functional efficiency of sterilizer and reliability of mechanical components. What is the overall factor of safety for the entire process cycle? A sterilizer may be capable of sterilization but it also may recontaminate the load.
- —The human element. From raw materials to purchased articles to packaged supplies ready for sterilization there is one all-encompassing factor to control—people. The performance of people is based on their knowledge and ability to follow instructions. If their actions are inadequate, incorrect or the result of emotional conflicts, established sterilization standards will be invalidated. Those who have the responsibility for producing sterile supplies should be constantly alert to behavioral characteristics associated with human error in the sterilization process. Examples are as follows:

- Antagonistic cooperation instead of voluntary cooperation. Noncommunicative with other workers who share responsibility for producing sterile supplies.
- Disregard for precautions and for adherence to sound principles in preparation and packaging of supplies. Inculpable ignorance excludes fault.
- Refusal to follow the principles of sterilization; no interest in learning anything new or in teaching others the right way or in developing a sterile technic conscience.
- Shortcuts of sterilization cycles by manual control so as to avoid working overtime.
- Resistance to change—did it that way for twenty years without trouble. Example: a 27-pound surgical pack.
- No judgment and tact in correction of errors, thereby inviting resentment on the part of others.

SPEED—A MILITANT FORCE AGAINST STERILIZATION

More than a decade ago the author made the statement that "it is unwise to establish any standard for surgical sterilization without due regard for the economic factors involved." The purpose of the statement at that time was to discourage the use of an unnecessarily long time-temperature relationship for sterilization which, in many instances, was costing hospitals needless expense through destruction of materials and the waste of time and fuel. Today, we are living in an era typified by speed, and productivity in most fields of endeavor has had to move forward by leaps and bounds. With respect to speed, the field of sterilization is no exception, and if present terminology ("flash sterilization," "ultrashort cycle time," "fastest cycle ever") is any indication of the future pattern then the end is not in sight. To many individuals a 30-minute exposure period for steam sterilization is much too long; an exposure of 2 hours in the hot air oven has become an absurdity and an outmoded process, irrespective of whether the substitute processes carry substantial factors of safety.

Most people responsible for the purchase, operation, and maintenance of sterilizers are unaware that speed is a militant force working against sterilization. It reduces the overall factor of safety; it becomes an accomplice of trapped air, and it demands a high degree of reliability in functional and mechanical controls. It is unfortunate indeed that in certain types of sterilizers minimum standards have been tampered with as the result of overzealous manufacturers who fight the "battle of the minutes" to see which one can offer the fastest operating cycle. Contrary to popular opinion, most hospitals are not organized and automated for central materiel processing to the extent that a difference of a few minutes in the total sterilization cycle detracts from patient care or is of any real economic concern. It is important to remember that sterilization is an event. It requires the maximum control of all variables so as to effect a minimum margin of doubt in the end result.

LEVELS OF CONTAMINATION

In developing realistic standards for sterilization the question must be asked as to how great the microbial populations are on articles selected for sterilization or decontamination. Data relating to accurate estimates of numbers of organisms on clean and used medical-surgical instruments and supplies are seemingly not available. With the exception of environmental sanitation studies, the information recorded in the literature does not deal specifically with population densities, but rather the presence or absence of clinically important microbial species. This is to be expected inasmuch as the actual counting of organisms on inanimate objects in the hospital is not a highly rewarding activity. The criterion of success has been, and probably will continue to be, the lowering of infection rates, not microbial counts.

It seems to be well established that the majority of hazardous organisms in the hospital stem from patients with infected lesions. Observations made by McDermott[10] showed that population densities of lesions infected with staphylococci, streptococci, or tubercle bacilli may be as great as 10^8 or 10^9 organisms per milliliter of emulsified tissue. This should be of vital concern to those who are responsible for the decontamination of surgical instruments. Another prolific source of contamination is the eschar from burns. Hurst[11] reported a level of 3,750,000 *Pseudomonas aeruginosa* per square centimeter of eschar. Hospital dust and lint may have counts ranging from 150,000 to 3,500,000 per gram, with some resistant spores present. A level of 180,000 staphylococci per surgical glove was reported by Wise *et al.*[8]

There appears to be little information available on the number of organisms in a freshly prepared surgical pack, ready for sterilization. A recent study made by Lloyd[12] showed that surgical packs from two hospitals made up in clean surroundings had an average microbial population of 3000 per square foot, or approximately one million organisms per pack. These figures are somewhat lower than those reported by Church[13] on freshly laundered bed linens in which the mean total count amounted to 5854 organisms per square foot. With the exclusion of laboratory apparatus, contamination of hospital medical and surgical supplies with high populations of resistant bacterial spores is unlikely. It is believed that anticipated levels would rarely approach 1000 spores per article. This does not lend support to a less rigid standard for sterilizaton because small quantities of garden soil containing highly resistant spores may invade the hospital and eventually contaminate instruments and other materials prior to sterilization. In addition, pathogenic clostridia are frequent textile contaminants and the use of tourniquets and bandages on orthopedic operations carries a risk of infection with *Cl. tetani* or *Cl. perfringens.*

Another point affecting standards for sterilization is the false sense of security in the minds of many people that all materials destined to undergo sterilization will have been thoroughly cleaned beforehand. It is doubtful if the average worker understands the meaning of "thoroughly clean." Moreover, the step of preliminary cleaning may be cursory or omitted entirely on articles destined for the decontamination process, since it is the prime purpose of decontamination to render materials safe for human (employee) handling. In the case of the cleaned article, we may be dealing with a few hundred viable organisms, while in the uncleaned the population may be of the order of several million per article, with the probability that some protection is afforded the organisms by a protein film or lubricant. It would be unwise, therefore, to expect that any practical working standard for hospitals could ensure that all contaminated articles such as surgical instruments, gloves, and inhalational therapy equipment are cleaned either manually or mechanically prior to sterilization or decontamination. Where a centralized decontamination service exists, this situation can be effectively controlled.

A third factor directly linked to minimum standards is the need to evaluate the efficiency of the sterilization process. Here it is necessary to decide on what constitutes a rigid challenge in terms of kill of a specified population of resistant test organisms, including a reasonable margin of safety beyond the maximum level of contamination anticipated in practice. For the evaluation of moist heat sterilizing processes, the organism known as *Bacillus stearothermophilus* is commonly used. The resistance of this organism is considerably greater than that of the pathogenic clostridia and bacilli.

MINIMUM REQUIREMENTS OF TIME AND TEMPERATURE

One of the most difficult problems encountered in attempting to define safe sterilization is to determine from reliable data the minimum time-temperature relationship needed to ensure destruction of the most resistant forms of microbial life. Unless this relationship can be stated positively, it is useless to attempt to discuss the subject intelligently or to make specific recommendations on the preparation and sterilization of various materials and supplies. Much of the information written on the subject is either vague in meaning, inconclusive or avoids the issue entirely. Certain of the standards proposed for surgical sterilization have been based upon a time-temperature relationship adequate for the destruction of pathogenic spores but not entirely adequate for the destruction of nonpathogenic sporebearing organisms. Others propose the use of a time and temperature sufficiently great to cause unnecessary destruction of materials and to be wasteful of time and fuel.

In establishing minimum standards for surgical sterilization, careful attention must be given to the prescribing of exposure periods for the various types of loads that will ensure a time-temperature relationship adequate for the destruction of the most resistant forms of microbial life. Adequacy in sterilization means that the process must subject the microbial flora to the stage in which any vital organisms that remain will not be able to germinate. Any exposure period that is selective in its lethality to microorganisms is not in keeping with the concept of absolute sterility—the goal of all surgical sterilization. In other words, it should be expedient always to prescribe a performance which carries a reasonable factor of safety in terms of temperature or time or both, based upon reliable experimental data relating to the destruction of the pathogenic spores, but also great enough to provide for the destruction of the still more resistant nonpathogenic sporebearing organisms.

In developing a safe minimum standard for surgical sterilization, several workers have proposed the use of garden soil which contains a variety of heat resistant aerobic and anaerobic sporebearing and non-sporebearing organisms as a control. Walbum,[14] for example, in using soil as a control in steam sterilizaton gives the following times and temperatures as necessary for sterilization of materials loaded in the autoclave:

222.8°F (106°C)	4-5 hours
233.6°F (112°C)	1 hour
249.8°F (121°C)	30 minutes
273.2°F (134°C)	10 minutes
291.2°F (114°C)	5 minutes

In a similar study, Ecker[15] determined that one-gram samples of air-dried, powdered garden soil inserted in the center of laparotomy sets and in maternity supplies were found to be sterile after exposure at 240°F (116°C) in the autoclave for periods of 60, 45, 30, and 15 minutes. When samples of the same soil were placed in carefully packed dressing drums, it was found that an exposure of 45 minutes at 240°F (116°C) was necessary for sterilization. Ecker also found in a long series of experiments that the spores of pathogenic anaerobes were destroyed at 240°F (116°C) for 15 to 20 minutes, whereas a temperature of 250°F (121°C) for 30 minutes was sufficient to destroy the highly resistant nonpathogenic sporebearing organisms of garden soil. The spores of *Cl. novyi* survived 5 minutes at 230°F (110°C) but were destroyed in 10 minutes at this temperature. The spores of *Cl. welchii* survived exposure of 15 minutes at 215°F (101.7°C) but were destroyed at 220°F (104°C) in 5 minutes. Spores of *B. subtilis* were killed at 215°F (101.7°C) in 10 minutes. These results relating especially to the resistance of soil seem to agree with the work of Bang and Dalsgaard,[16] who observed that when garden soil was autoclaved at 248°F (120°C) for 20 minutes, effective sterilization took place, but when heated for only 10 minutes, the bacterial content was 200,000 organisms per gram of soil.

In an attempt to accurately define the minimum limits of saturated steam temperature requirements for surgical sterilization, Underwood[17] conducted a long series of tests by planting dried spores of *Cl. welchii* and *B. subtilis* in gauze packs, approximating actual conditions of surgical sterilization. His findings revealed that an exposure period of 5 minutes to saturated steam at

225°F (107°C) gave evidence of sterility in all test packs upon incubation of the cultures. These data were apparently confirmed by the work of Ecker, referred to above.

Walter[18] has made the recommendation that 13 minutes' direct exposure to saturated steam at 250°F (121°C) is a safe minimum standard for surgical sterilization. This time and temperature conform closely to the thermal death time of the most resistant bacterial spores, and in the opinion of this writer it represents one of the safest and most practical standards that has yet been developed for reliable routine sterilization.

Generally speaking, authorities are in agreement that in direct contact with saturated steam at a temperature of 250°F (121°C), a period of 5 to 10 minutes is sufficient to ensure destruction of most resistant forms of microbial life (see Table 4-4). However, to define minimum standards of time and temperature required for steam sterilization of the wide variety of surgical supplies used in hospitals today is a difficult matter. The time-temperature relationship selected must not only be microbiologically safe, but it must also permit the prescribing of practical exposure periods for the various supplies, including reasonable margins of safety, with due regard for economic factors. On the basis of carefully conducted studies strengthened by experience in many hospitals and laboratories, it has been shown that minimum standards of time and temperature substantially greater or less than the following are either incompatible with approved sterilizer design (requiring steam pressure in excess of maximum operating pressure), unnecessarily destructive of materials, or unsafe from the standpoint of effective sterilization:

Degrees F	Degrees C	Time (Minutes)
280	138	0.8
270	132	2
257	125	8
250	121	12
245	118	18
240	116	30

The times and temperatures given above do not denote prescribed exposure periods for the sterilization of the various kinds of surgical supplies. Rather, they indicate the absolute minimum standards of time and temperature to be maintained throughout all portions of a load in direct contact with saturated steam in order to accomplish effective sterilization. They do not provide the additional time factor required for steam penetration of porous supplies such as fabrics nor do they attempt to compensate for the rate of heat transfer through solution containers.

These standards were first introduced to hospitals and laboratories by the author in 1954.[19] Since that time they have been adopted for hospital sterilization by many countries throughout medically advanced parts of the

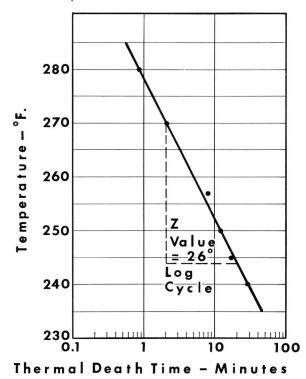

FIGURE 7-2. Thermal death times recommended for moist heat sterilization. For a tenfold change (one log cycle) in thermal death time there is a 26°F (14°C) change in temperature.

world. As basic standards, they have been subjected to a broad spectrum of sterilization processes. Figure 7-2 shows thermal death times and temperatures for moist heat sterilization based upon the minimum standards. For a tenfold change in thermal death time there is a 26°F (14°C) change in temperature. This is within the range of z values given in Table 4-4. *Extrapolation of the curve to temperatures substantially below 240°F (116°C) or above 280°F (138°C) is not recommended.*

Heat-Up Time

Heat-up time is the same as steam penetration time. It means the time required for the entire load to reach the selected sterilizing temperature after the chamber has reached that temperature. When steam is admitted to the chamber, the temperature as shown by the thermometer will advance in a few minutes to the selected range, depending upon the size of the sterilizer and the nature of the load. From this point the heat-up time is determined. In prevacuum and pulsing-type sterilizers the heat-up time is short, of the order of one minute.

Holding Time

Holding time means that after the entire load has reached the selected sterilizing temperature, a holding time not less than the minimum standard for that temperature shall be imposed on the load.

Exposure Period

Exposure period is the total time required for sterilization of the load. The period begins from the moment that the indicating or controlling thermometer in the chamber discharge line reaches the selected sterilizing temperature. It continues thereafter for the prescribed period of time. The exposure period represents the sum of the heat-up time, the minimum standard holding time, and a prescribed factor of safety. The latter does not attempt to compensate for human errors in the preparation of supplies or in the operation of the sterilizer. Most of the medical-surgical supplies prepared for sterilization in hospitals can be classified as hard goods (unwrapped), hard goods (wrapped), fabrics, or liquids. Table 7-1 gives minimum exposure periods for the sterilization of these supplies with times and temperatures dependent upon the type of sterilizer and the characteristic method of air removal.

DEFINING THE PROPER RANGE OF TEMPERATURE AND PRESSURE

In establishing precise standards for surgical sterilization, it becomes necessary to define the most suitable range of temperature and pressure for the sterilization of all types of supplies. This means that we must predetermine

TABLE 7-1

Minimum Exposure Periods (minutes) for Sterilization of Hospital Supplies

Load	Temperature	Holding Time	Air Removal Method	Heat-up Time	Factor of Safety	Exposure Time
Hard goods (unwrapped)	250–254°F	12	Gravity	1	2	15
	270–274°F	2	Gravity (High Speed)	<1	0.5	3
	270–274°F	2	Pulsing	<1	1	4
	270–274°F	2	Prevacuum	1	1	4
Hard goods (wrapped)	250–254°F	12	Gravity	5	3	20
	270–274°F	2	Gravity	7	1	10
	270–274°F	2	Pulsing	<1	1	4
	270–274°F	2	Prevacuum	1	1	4
Fabrics—packs	250–254°F	12	Gravity	12	6	30
	270–274°F	2	Pulsing	<1	1	4
	270–274°F	2	Prevacuum	1	1	4
	285–287°F	0.5	Pulsing	<1	0.5	2
Liquids	250–254°F	12	Gravity	Dependent upon liquid volume and container		

and measure within fairly close limits the quality of steam maintained in the sterilizer, to the end that any sterilizing process can be reproduced repeatedly, with the least possible variation. Today most sterilizers built for installation in hospitals are designed for a dual range of operation: 250° to 254°F (121° to 123°C) and 270° to 274°F (132° to 134°C). There is a definite trend toward standardization of the higher temperature, shorter time method for sterilization of fabrics, instruments, and utensils, whereas solutions, including flasked surgical fluids, are sterilized at the lower temperature. Exposure to temperatures in the range of 270° to 274°F does not necessarily cause a more rapid deterioration of textiles and rubber goods, providing that the exposure time is accurately controlled and oversterilization prevented.

Wherever possible, one fixed range of temperature and pressure should be be employed. With modern sterilizing equipment featuring automatic control of pressure, it is not difficult to maintain the prescribed range with a total variation of no more than 1 to 2 pounds. The most practical reason for one fixed range of temperature and pressure for all supplies, with the exception of solutions, is the ability to standardize procedures, to have all pressure sterilizers controlled in exactly the same manner. In many hospitals this has been done most effectively and to the advantage of the institutions. There is the mistaken supposition that steam at the higher operating pressure of 27 to 30 pounds heats or permeates the load much faster than steam at 15 to 18 pounds pressure. To be sure, the higher pressure will result in a correspondingly higher temperature and the chamber may build up to the operating pressure level somewhat faster, but the rate of heating the load to the higher temperature is not substantially greater.

As a rule, the smaller capacity sterilizers of the gravity displacement type are constructed with an inner and outer shell to withstand an internal pressure of 36 psig. The medium rectangular and large industrial sterilizers usually have an inner shell designed to withstand an internal pressure of 55 psig and an external pressure of 55 psig (40 psig in jacket with simultaneous vacuum of 30 inches Hg gauge in chamber). The outer shell is designed to withstand an internal pressure of 40 psig. The sterilizer must have an approved (ASME) safety valve set at the approved maximum operating pressure of the vessel. It should blow down at least 2 pounds per square inch before closing and should be so sized that the pressure in the vessel will not rise more than 10 per cent over the set pressure.

STANDARDIZATION OF STERILIZING TECHNICS

Standardization can be accomplished through the applied integration of five factors: 1) conscientious, dependable, skilled personnel; 2) correct methods of preliminary cleaning, assembling, and packaging of supplies to ensure direct steam contact; 3) proper loading of the sterilizer; 4) approved sterilizer with demonstrated reliability, and 5) adequate exposure period that will provide for complete penetration of the load and ensure destruction of microbial life with a liberal margin of safety.

Developments of the past ten years have provided hospitals with highly productive automatically controlled pressure steam sterilizers. They are precision instruments, but their value will be minimized or perhaps lost altogether unless hospitals cooperate to the extent of assigning responsibility for the production of sterile supplies to only those individuals who can be adequately supervised, skilled in their jobs, and, in brief, have control over all variables entering into the process. In the standardization of sterilizing technics, there is no substitute for intelligent, painstaking supervision.

Of the various factors upon which effective sterilization of surgical supplies depends, there is none more important than the exposure period. This does not mean that other factors are less important, but rather that for every item undergoing sterilization there is a minimum period of exposure based upon adherence to a specific procedure for the preliminary preparation of the item, the method of packaging or wrapping, and the manner of placing the item in the sterilizer. Unless the principles of correct technique are rigidly enforced, the exposure period becomes little more than an attempt toward sterilization. With intelligent application of these requirements, the proper exposure periods at the selected temperature range provide minimum time for heat penetration and sterilization (see Table 7-2).

TABLE 7-2

EXPOSURE PERIODS FOR STERILIZATION OF SPECIFIC ARTICLES

Article	*Minimum Time Required (in minutes)* *Sterilizer Type and* *Temperature*			
	Gravity *250° F*	*Gravity* *270°*	*Prevacuum* *270°*	*Pulsing* *270°*
Ampoules, spinal, heat-stable, in test tubes (on sides)	15	—	—	—
Brushes, synthetic fibers, in dispensers or individually wrapped	30	15	4	4
Dressings, wrapped in paper or muslin	30	15	4	4
Dressings, loosely packed, in canisters (on sides)	30	15	4	4
Glassware, empty, inverted	15	3	4	4
Inhalational therapy equipment (heat stable)	30	—	—	—
Instruments, metal only, any number in perforated tray, unwrapped	15	3	4	4
Instruments, metal, unwrapped, combined with sutures, tubing, or other porous materials	20	10	4	4
Instruments, metal only, in lightly covered or padded tray	20	10	4	4
Instruments, metal, combined with other porous materials in lightly covered or padded tray	30	15	4	4
Instruments, wrapped in muslin—four thicknesses—for storage	30	15	4	4
Linen, packs, maximal size (12″×12″×20″) and weight (12 lbs.)	30	—	4	4
Needles, hollow, individually packaged in glass tubes, lumen moist (on sides)	30	15	4	4

TABLE 7-2—(*Continued*)

EXPOSURE PERIODS FOR STERILIZATION OF SPECIFIC ARTICLES

Article	*Minimum Time Required (in minutes)* Sterilizer Type and Temperature			
	Gravity 250° F	*Gravity* 270°	*Prevacuum* 270°	*Pulsing* 270°
Needles, hollow, individually packaged in paper wrappers, lumen moist	30	15	4	4
Rubber gloves, wrapped in muslin or paper	20	—	4	4
Rubber catheters, drains, tubing (lumen moist), unwrapped	20	10	4	4
Rubber catheters, drains, tubing, individually packaged in muslin or paper (lumen moist)	30	15	4	4
Rubber or plastic sheeting (heat-stable) interleaved with layer of muslin	30	—	4	4
Treatment trays, wrapped in muslin or paper	30	—	4	4
Solutions (Square-Pak bottles)				
75 ml–250 ml	20	—	—	—
500 ml–1000 ml	30	—	—	—
1500 ml–2000 ml	40	—	—	—
Sutures, silk, cotton or nylon, wrapped in paper or muslin	30	15	4	4
Sutures, wire, on metal reel, wrapped	30	15	4	4
Syringes, disassembled, individually packaged in muslin or paper	30	15	4	4
Utensils, on edge, unwrapped	15	3	4	4
Utensils, on edge, wrapped in muslin or paper	20	10	4	4

All supplies requiring a common exposure period may be safely and economically sterilized in the same load, with the exception of rubber gloves and solutions. In fact, for all bulk loads of supplies in a gravity displacement sterilizer a continuous exposure to saturated steam at 250° to 254° F for 30 minutes provides a technique which is practicable, safe, and does not destroy the materials. For the higher temperature and shorter times, it is necessary to know precisely the functional characteristics of the individual sterilizer. Rubber gloves should always be sterilized separately in order to avoid the possibility of retarding the immediate passage of steam to the gloves. Solutions must also be sterilized separately, never in mixed loads, because the method of exhausting pressure and cooling of solutions after sterilization is not applicable to the drying of fabrics and other supplies.

REFERENCES

1. UNDERWOOD, W. B.: *A Textbook of Sterilization,* 2nd ed. Chicago, Lakeside, Donnelley, 1941, p. 2.

2. JOHNSON, D. W.: *Handbook of Sterilization Procedures.* Brisbane, Australia, A. H. Tucker, Govt. Printer, 1953, p. 9-11.

3. ADAM, W.: Unsere Erfahrungen bei der Prüfung von Sterilisations-Apparaten mit bestimmter Dampfführung. *Arch Hyg Bakt,* 138(5):364-372, 1954.

4. NUFFIELD PROVINCIAL HOSPITALS TRUST: *Present Sterilizing Practice in Six Hospitals.* London, Whitefriars Press, 1958.

5. MEDICAL RESEARCH COUNCIL: Report by working party on sterilisation by steam under increased pressure. *Lancet,* 1:425-435, 1959.

6. BOWIE, J. H.: Modern apparatus for sterilisation. *Pharm J,* 174:473, 1955.

7. DARMADY, E. M.; HUGHES, K. E. A.; JONES, J. D., and VERDON, P. E.: Failure of sterility in hospital ward practice. *Lancet,* 1:622-624, 1959.

8. WISE, R. I.; SWEENEY, F. J. JR.; HAUPT, G. J., and WADDELL, M. A.: The environmental distribution of *Staphylococcus aureus* in an operating suite. *Ann Surg,* 149:30-42, 1959.

9. DANDY, W. E.: The importance of more adequate sterilization processes in hospitals. *Bull Amer Coll Surg,* 16:11, 1932.

10. McDERMOTT, W.: Microbial persistence. *Yale J Biol Med,* 30:257-291, 1958.

11. HURST, V., and SUTTER, V. L.: Survival of *Pseudomonas aeruginosa* in the hospital environment. *J Infect Dis, 116*:151-154, 1966.

12. LLOYD, R. S., and VOGEL, D.: Microbial content of surgical packs prior to sterilization and its relation to laundering and preparation procedures. Tech Report No. 1967-3. Unpublished. American Sterilizer Co., Erie, Pa.

13. CHURCH, B. D.: Hospital Laundry Hazards Leading to Recontamination of Washed Bedding. *Proc. Natl Conf. on Institutionally Acquired Infections, Sept. 4-6, 1963.* Atlanta, Ga., U. S. Dept. HEW, Publ. No. 1188, p. 70.

14. WALBUM, L. E.: Sterilization of surgical instruments. *Hospital, 76*:57, 1933; *Z Hyg Infektionskr, 112*:281, 1931.

15. ECKER, E. E.: Sterilization based on temperature attained and time ratio. *Mod Hosp, 48*:86, 1937.

16. BANG, O., and DALSGAARD, A. T.: Symposium on sterilisation. *Arch Pharm Chem (Kobenhavn)* 25:699, 1948. Reprinted from *Pharm J, 162*:236, 1949.

17. UNDERWOOD, W. B.: *op. cit.,* p. 3-4.

18. WALTER, C. W.: *Aseptic Treatment of Wounds.* New York, Macmillan, 1948, p. 76.

19. PERKINS, J. J.: Bacteriological and surgical sterilization by heat. In G. F. Reddish (Ed.): *Antiseptics, Disinfectants, Fungicides, and Chemical and Physical Sterilization.* Philadelphia, Lea & F., 1954, p. 672.

Chapter 8

MODERN HOSPITAL STERILIZERS

THE TERMINOLOGY used in describing modern hospital sterilizers is frequently misleading. The more common expressions noted in designating equipment of this type are "autoclave," "dressing sterilizer," "pressure steam sterilizer," "steam pressure sterilizer," "vacuum sterilizer," and "sterilizer-decontaminator." The term *autoclave* naturally takes precedent over all other names because of its historical background and relationship to a pressure vessel. However, by way of definition, the word *autoclave* means self-closing, as in the case of a vessel made close by the pressure of steam within against the lid. To use the word *autoclave* indiscriminately when speaking of the various types of pressure steam sterilizers being manufactured today, steam jacketed chambers, single-wall laboratory sterilizers, vacuum-pressure chambers and washer-decontaminators, is inaccurate and confusing to say the least. Basically, there are two distinct kinds of pressure steam sterilizers—the steam jacketed (double wall) type, which constitutes the almost universal standard for sterilization of surgical supplies, and the single wall (nonjacketed) sterilizer used only in the laboratory or in highly specialized industrial applications.

STRUCTURAL FEATURES

A modern hospital sterilizer, small rectangular, gravity air removal type, for processing heat- and moisture-stable materials, and equipped with automatic controls is shown in Figure 8-1. The structural and piping features as provided by different manufacturers will vary to some degree, but the essential elements of control over component operating systems are the same. Although this sterilizer is properly designated a "pressure steam sterilizer," its performance is gauged not by pressure but by temperature as measured by a thermal-sensing element located in the chamber drain line. Pressure gauges are provided, one for the jacket that surrounds the chamber and another for the chamber in which supplies are sterilized. These gauges are, however, of minor significance because the sterilizing power of steam is a function of its temperature integrated with time rather than its pressure.

In Figure 8-2 is shown a longitudinal cross section of the same sterilizer as illustrated in Figure 8-1. The body of the sterilizer consists of the rectangular chamber surrounded on the sides by a steam jacket which is enclosed by

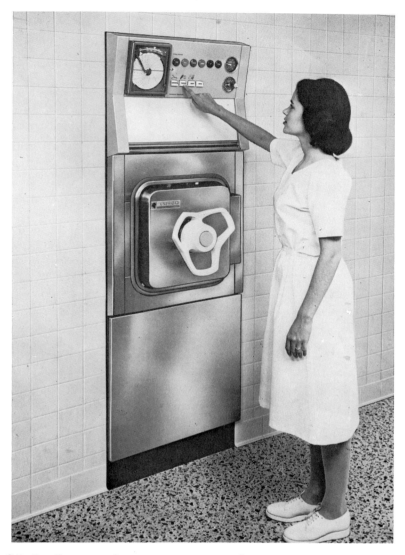

FIGURE 8-1. Small rectangular pressure steam sterilizer, general purpose, gravity air removal type, equipped with automatic program control.

the outer shell and the whole installed within a stainless steel cabinet. The standard material of construction for the inner chamber, outer chamber, backhead, and door frame is Monel metal. The chamber is welded to an end ring thus forming a seamless unit without the use of rivets or solder. This feature of all-welded construction has become the standard of the industry and it provides greater structural strength, smooth surfaces devoid of crevices, and long-time resistance to the corrosive and erosive action of steam, water, and solutions. Each inner and outer shell is constructed to withstand

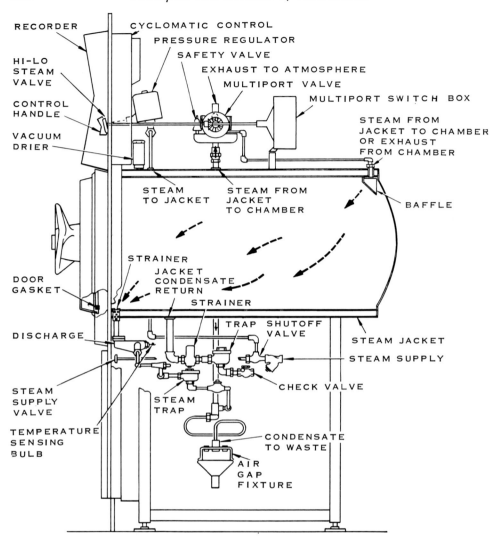

FIGURE 8-2. Longitudinal cross section of sterilizer shown in Figure 8-1.

an internal pressure of 36 psig. The exterior of the outer shell is normally insulated with glass fiber and aluminum foil. A safety steam-lock door closes the front end of the chamber and it is made steam tight by compression through the door mechanism against a flexible heat-resistant gasket. The gasket is held firmly in place by means of a dovetailed groove around the periphery of the door.

Steam Jacket

In Figure 8-2 it may be seen that the sterilizing chamber has a steam jacket which surrounds the side walls of the chamber only; it does not cover the backhead. Pressure is first generated in the jacket space prior to the admission of that steam to the chamber, and this pressure is maintained throughout the performance. In fact, many sterilizers in hospitals are maintained in operating state with steam in jacket for an average of 20 or more hours per day. This means that the walls of the sterilizing chamber are heated by the steam jacket, no condensate forms on them, and they are always dry. It is not necessary to provide jacketing for the backhead or door because the condensate that forms on these surfaces drains directly downward behind a baffle or deflector plate to the bottom and it is then discharged from the chamber. The jacket serves another purpose in that it functions as a gravity steam separator to remove entrained droplets of water from the steam prior to its admission to the chamber.

When the sterilizer is set in operation, steam is first turned on until pressure at the proper range has been developed in the jacket only. Then, with the load in the chamber, steam is admitted and promptly contacts the walls of the chamber and the load. The only condensate that contacts the load is that formed by heating the load itself. After the materials have been heated to the temperature of the surrounding steam, no more condensate will form in them and the entire mass will contain finely diffused moisture, the exact equivalent of the amount of heat abstracted from the steam. Even though the load is distinctly moist, it contains no excess moisture, and as such, drying is not difficult.

When the pressure in the chamber is then suddenly exhausted, the heat that has previously been transferred to the load begins to take effect in drying. The moisture in the fabrics is vaporized by the residual heat, and if this vapor is permitted to escape freely, the load will be satisfactorily dried within a brief interval of time. This drying effect is possible only with the steam jacketed sterilizer. Otherwise, in the case of a single wall sterilizer, the vapor excaping from the load would recondense on the chamber walls and be reabsorbed by the load.

Safety Door

From the standpoint of engineering design the potentially weakest point on a pressure steam sterilizer is the door. Far too few people responsible for the purchase and operation of sterilizers in hospitals today recognize the importance that correct design and construction play in insuring safety of the operator. To illusrate the point, a sterilizer such as that shown in Figure 8-1, with door dimensions of 20 × 20 inches, has a total pressure of 6000 pounds (3 tons) exerted on the door when the sterilizer is operated under 15 pounds per square inch pressure. Knowledge of this fact alone should command the respect of the most careless of operators and also stress the importance of a pressure-locked safety door to prevent explosive or premature opening while the chamber is under pressure.

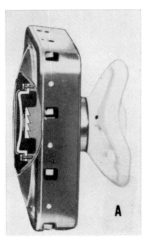
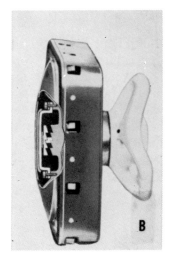

SAFETY LOCK
PROTECTS OPERATOR

FIGURE 8-3. Detail of the locking mechanism of a typical pressure-lock safety door for sterilizers.

The locking mechanism of a truly pressure-locked safety door should be a positive one, automatically actuated when chamber pressure is applied, unlocked only by exhaust of pressure. A sectional view of this type of door is shown in Figure 8-3. On the inside of the door there is an opening which is closed by a flexible diaphragm about 5 inches in diameter, shaped like a shallow pan, and made of corrosion-resistant metal. This diaphragm expands outward under internal pressure and causes the engagement of two clutch plates which, when engaged, prevent the turning of the center plate that controls the movement of the radial locking arms from the locked position to the unlocked position. The internal pressure of the sterilizer holds these two clutch plates engaged through the action of the flexible diaphragm. The lock can be released only when the chamber pressure is reduced to approximately atmospheric. The door can be tightened, but not loosened, while the chamber is under pressure.

Thermostatic Steam Trap In Chamber Discharge System

The valve designated "steam trap" in Figure 8-2 controls the flow of air and condensate from the sterilizing chamber automatically. When the valve is cool, the thermostatic element inside contracts, leaving the orifice wide open for free discharge. When steam is admitted to the chamber for sterilizing, air is forced out by way of the screened outlet (strainer) leading to the discharge line and then through the thermostatic valve by the pressure of the incoming steam. The valve remains open until steam following the air heats the valve, then the element gradually expands and closes the orifice. Valves are made to operate within 2°F of steam saturation temperature. The thermostatic element is extremely sensitive and throughout sterilization, as condensate or air pockets gravitate to the valve, it will open slightly until the cooler fluid has been discharged.

Occasionally the thermostatic valve may become clogged with lint or sediment so that it cannot function properly. Also, after long service the thermostatic element (Fig. 8-4) may fatigue or lose its fluid content upon which it depends for thermostatic action. In either case the valve will close off entirely or in part, slowing down or completely interrupting air and condensate discharge.

If the sterilizer becomes sluggish or lags appreciably in attaining the proper temperature, the chamber drain line should be flushed out with a hot solution of trisodium phosphate. Should the sluggishness persist, it is advisable to remove the thermostatic element and check it for clogging. If the orifice is unobstructed, shake the element to check the fluid content. If there

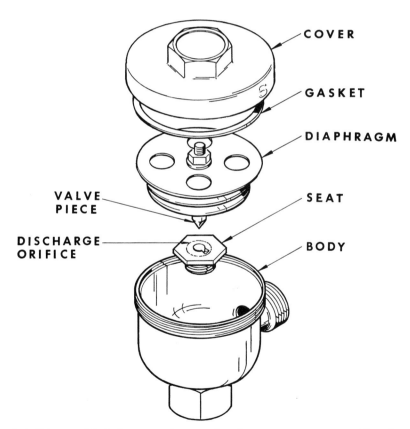

COVER

GASKET

DIAPHRAGM

VALVE PIECE

SEAT

DISCHARGE ORIFICE

BODY

Figure 8-4. Disassembled thermostatic trap showing component parts. The thermostatic diaphragm contains a fluid which expands under heat to close the orifice in the body.

is no fluid in the element, it should be replaced by a new element at once. Usually this procedure will be found to remedy the difficulty.

One should not confuse the thermostatic valve which controls the chamber discharge system with the return trap from the jacket of steam heated sterilizers. Usually these two valves have the same bodies, but the orifices and the thermostatic elements are different. The chamber discharge valve is adjusted primarily for the rapid discharge of air and condensate while the jacket trap is adjusted primarily for condensate drainage. The orifice in the chamber discharge valve is much larger than in the jacket (return line) trap. It is standard practice to place on the cover of each valve an identifying number which should be used when requisitioning new elements for use with any make of sterilizer. Each trap should be pressure-balanced for operation at a maximum pressure of 60 psig.

Return System

For all pressure steam sterilizers of the jacketed type it is necessary to provide a "return" system for the purpose of receiving the discharge from the steam jacket, a more or less continuous flow of condensate which is controlled by the return line trap shown in Figure 8-2. This trap is also thermostatic in its action and when cool its orifice will remain open for free discharge. The thermostatic element responds to heat and it will close off nearly, but not quite completely, when contacted by steam following the water or condensate discharge. Directly back of the return line trap is located a check valve. It opens freely for the discharge of condensate from the jacket but closes against any back pressure which may occur in the return line system. This feature is necessary because occasionally the return line piping beyond the sterilizer is so small that appreciable back pressure may be developed from other equipment located on the same line. If steam were to back up to the location of the trap, the heat might cause the trap to close off and thus interfere with the performance of the sterilizer.

A point which many people fail to comprehend is that no steam jacket can function properly unless the return system is so controlled that condensate is disposed of just as rapidly as it forms. Interference with this discharge is always a serious matter. Primarily the discharge is controlled by the trap, but obviously the trap cannot function unless the piping into which it feeds is not closed off or restricted. Oftentimes sterilizers are unjustly criticized when the fault lies entirely with the steam supply or the return system.

Automatic Pressure Control Valve

Before the initial operation of the sterilizer, the automatic pressure control valve should be carefully adjusted to insure that it will deliver to the jacket the prescribed amount of pressure (16 to 18 pounds for low tempera-

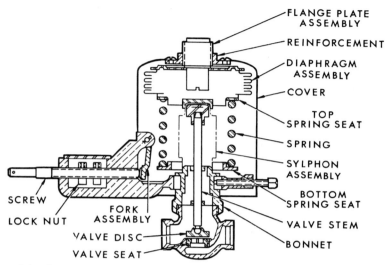

FLANGE PLATE
ASSEMBLY

REINFORCEMENT

DIAPHRAGM
ASSEMBLY

COVER

TOP
SPRING SEAT

SPRING

SYLPHON
ASSEMBLY

BOTTOM
SPRING SEAT

VALVE STEM

BONNET

SCREW

LOCK NUT

FORK
ASSEMBLY

VALVE DISC

VALVE SEAT

FIGURE 8-5. Cross-section diagram of pressure control valve used on sterilizers.

ture operation or 28 to 30 pounds for high temperature operation). The valve (Fig. 8-5) is strictly a pressure regulator. It is so constructed that an internal expansion diaphragm (flexible bellows) expands or contracts, as pressure varies in the jacket of the sterilizer, reacting against a regulating spring, thereby opening and closing the orifice in the valve proper. Regulation for any desired pressure in the range of 3 to 30 pounds (0.21 to 2.1 kg/cm^2) is accomplished by a secondary adjusting screw at the side which, when turned, increases or lessens the tension on the valve spring. The valve should be constructed for operation on maximum supply line pressure of 80 psig.

While the pressure gauge must be used for the initial adjustment to the operating range, it should be borne in mind that commercial pressure gauges at best are highly inaccurate. After use they frequently become distorted due to fatigue, often reading several pounds high. For this reason, it becomes necessary to regulate the sterilizer pressure with direct reference to the temperature produced in the chamber. This may be accomplished in the following manner:

> With or without a load in the sterilizer, turn steam to the jacket, and wait until the pressure has become stable at the maximum range. Then turn steam to the chamber and wait until the temperature, as indicated by the thermometer or indicator-recorder, has become stable at its maximum range. If the stabilized temperature is below 250°F, turn the regulating screw on the pressure control valve clockwise half a turn or so; wait until the temperature has become stable again at the higher range. If the maximum temperature is still too low, repeat the procedure until the temperature remains constant at slightly above 250°F

If the temperature is above 254°F, reverse the process, turn the regulating screw counterclockwise a little at a time until the maximum temperature is within the prescribed limits. Once adjusted, the valve should require no further regulation unless the steam supply line pressure fluctuates badly. If this does occur, the maintenance engineer should be consulted so that proper arrangements can be made to stabilize the supply line pressure.

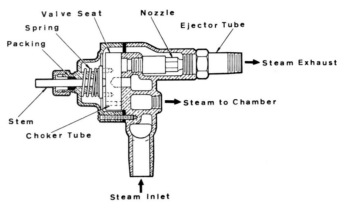

FIGURE 8-6. Cross-section diagram of a multiport valve. This forms vital part of automatic control system on many pressure steam sterilizers.

Multiport Valve

The device shown in Figure 8-6 and located on top of the sterilizer in Figure 8-2 is known as a multiport valve. It forms a vital part of the automatic control system on many pressure steam sterilizers. The multiport valve possesses this highly advantageous feature: the one valve, when motorized, controls all the functions, admits steam to chamber, exhausts steam from chamber, and creates a mild degree of vacuum for drying the load following sterilization. It is coupled directly to the automatic control by means of a flexible shaft. This assembly serves as a universal joint, transmitting rotation from one shaft to another. The valve operates sequentially as follows:

When in the STERILIZE position, steam from the jacket flows through the valve and through a connecting pipe which leads to the rear of the chamber where the steam enters behind a baffle plate. At the close of the sterilizing period, the valve moves to the EXHAUST position. This opens an outlet to the exhaust piping and steam passes from the chamber to the atmosphere. Also, the flow of steam from jacket to chamber is cut off. Following the sterilization of solutions, the valve moves to the SLOW EXHAUST position where steam is directed from the chamber to the atmosphere through a choker tube.

When the chamber pressure has been exhausted to zero gauge, the valve proceeds to the DRY position, thereby permitting steam from the jacket to escape through an ejector tube built into the valve. This exerts a slight degree of suction on the chamber to expedite the escape of vapor, which is discharged to the vent. To further enhance the drying of the load, a small stream of filtered air is admitted to the chamber through the vacuum drier as the result of the influence of the ejector.

OPERATION OF THE STERILIZER

In tracing the course of steam through the sterilizer, the reader should keep in mind that the same essential features will apply to any modern surgical supply sterilizer, providing the principles of gravity air discharge and thermometric control are incorporated. Steam from the main supply line or source is admitted at the top of the steam jacket. In the diagram (Fig. 8-2), the sterilizer is heated by direct steam from the supply line and the pressure is reduced to the proper range by initial adjustment of the pressure control valve. If the sterilizer is heated by electricity, a steam generator or boiler is mounted under the sterilizer, and steam is delivered directly to the jacket from the generator. Control of pressure then is governed by automatic regulation of the heat.

In beginning operation with a cold sterilizer, steam is first admitted from the source to the jacket, with the connection to the chamber closed, until the jacket pressure becomes constant at the correct operating range. This constitutes the reservoir from which the chamber steam will be drawn. In sterilizing, the load is placed in the chamber and the door locked immediately after the jacket has attained the correct pressure. Then the operating valve is turned to the LO position for 250°F sterilization or to the HI position for a 270°F cycle. This permits the jacket steam to flow through the multiport valve and piping on top of the sterilizer and into the chamber at the top rear adjacent to the backhead. At this point the steam is deflected upward by means of a baffle to prevent undue wetting of the load.

It is important to remember that when steam is admitted to the chamber, the chamber and the load of more or less porous supplies are filled with air. This air must be evacuated in order to attain the sterilizing temperature and to facilitate thorough permeation of the load with steam. The method of evacuation is accomplished as follows:

Air is more dense than steam, and as steam enters the chamber it gravitates above the air, fills the upper areas of the chamber and compresses air at the bottom. Since steam is admitted under pressure, air in the lower areas is forced out through the screened outlet or strainer at the extreme bottom near the front end, through the thermometer case and the pipe that leads to the thermostatic valve, then on to the vertical pipe which is vented to the atmosphere at the top and drained to the waste through the open (sanitary) funnel at the bottom. This air gap above the open funnel leading to the waste connection is highly important. It prevents possible back flow of contaminated waste to the sterilizer.

When the sterilizer is cool, the thermostatic valve is open, offers no restriction to the flow of air and condensate to the vent or waste. Only when air evacuation is complete and steam finally contacts the thermostatic valve does it close, interrupting the discharge. Thereafter it will open intermittently to discharge condensate as it accumulates. This method of air evacuation is known as the "gravity" system and it has been almost universally employed on pressure steam sterilizers produced since 1933.

From the foregoing, it is obvious that some method must be provided for definite measurement of the degree of air discharge and quality of steam in the chamber. This is the specific function of the recording thermometer. The thermal sensing element of this device is located in the discharge line that drains air and condensate from the chamber, and it will immediately respond to any interruption of air discharge from the chamber. Under any condition of performance, the thermometer will never indicate less than the temperature of the coolest medium surrounding the load. This is due to the fact that air or any mixture of steam with air will invariably gravitate below pure steam. The thermometer, therefore, when properly located in a correctly designed discharge system serves as a reliable means of measuring the sterilizing quality or lethality of the steam in contact with the load.

The majority of pressure steam sterilizers manufactured today are equipped with a combination temperature indicator, recorder, and controller as shown in Figure 8-7. The temperature-recording component of this device is an electrically driven, 24-hour-clock mechanism with a 6-inch-diameter chart and an easily reversible indicating scale. The recording pen is of the capillary type for inking. The thermometer system of the recorder consists of a helical pressure element connected to the sensing bulb

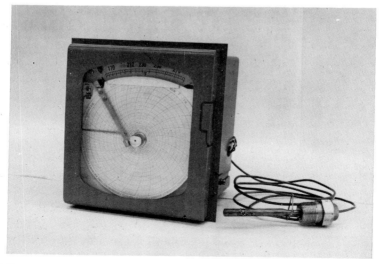

FIGURE 8-7. Combination temperature indicator, recorder, and controller. Thermal sensing bulb is located in chamber discharge line of sterilizer.

by a flexible capillary tube. The bulb, tubing, and pressure element are filled with a fluid approved by the Scientific Instrument Makers Association, and they form a sealed system. This system must never be broken because even the most minute leak will render it inoperative. The accuracy is $\pm 2°$F over the range of 160° to 280°F (71° to 138°C).

Bimetallic, dial-type, indicating thermometers continue to be used on some of the lesser sophisticated models of sterilizers. With the bimetal thermometer, the circular dial and pointer method of indicating temperature permits the use of easily read, widely spaced scale graduations. The temperature-sensitive element consists of a strip of bimetal wound into a continuous multiple helix. Thermometers of this type are fairly consistently accurate to within $\pm 2°$F in the sterilizing temperature range. Occasionally one may find a mercury thermometer installed in the chamber discharge line of a sterilizer. It offers the disadvantage of being more difficult to read, and it responds more slowly to temperature changes than the bimetallic type. The latter condition is not necessarily true but is due in large measure to the protection afforded the thermometer by the case and/or housing employed in the chamber discharge line.

When the sterilizer is functioning properly, temperature will advance to the selected sterilizing range within 10 to 20 minutes. (Sterilizers arranged for a steam pulsing system may require 15 to 20 minutes to come up to temperature, but the total cycle time is much shorter). At this point the period of exposure begins on the automatic timer. When the sterilizing period is complete, steam is exhausted from the chamber, but the jacket pressure is maintained. The steam from the chamber then escapes through the venting system.

PROGRAMMING CONTROLS FOR STERILIZERS

Sterilizer manufacturers have made a valuable contribution toward advancement of the art through development of automatic control mechanisms designed to minimize the human element in sterilizer operation. Serilizers equipped with efficiently designed and reliable automatic controls overcome many of the problems and inaccuracies attendant with the manual method of control. Typical of a class of automatic controls used on modern hospital sterilizers is the instrument shown in Figure 8-8. The principal function of this control is not limited to automatic timing of the exposure period, but rather it extends to all phases of the sterilizing process, to the end that all steps in the cycle previously carried out manually by the operator are performed automatically according to the program selected. The control allows the operator to select the proper programming cycle for wrapped goods, unwrapped goods, or liquids by pressing the appropriate button on the main control panel. The selector buttons lock automatically when pushed so that alternate selections cannot be made without first pressing a reset button or completing the selected program.

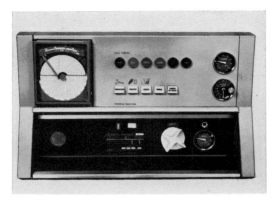

FIGURE 8-8. This modern version of hospital-proved cyclomatic control is typical of class of automatic controls for sterilizers used in Central Service processing.

After the sterilizer has been placed under automatic control, no further attention is necessary until an audible alarm and visual signal indicate that the following cycle is complete:

—Charging the chamber with steam from the jacket at not less than the selected sterilizing temperature for a predetermined period.
—Timing the exposure period in accord with minimum basic standards.
—Exhausting the chamber either slowly or rapidly, as dictated by the program selected.
—Providing a drying action for the load if the cycle is for wrapped goods.

The program selector buttons glow when actuated and the separate indicators glow during each phase of the processing cycle. Visual aids such as shown in Figure 8-8 enable inexperienced personnel to understand the functions of an automatic control as applied to sterilizers.

In order to permit sterilization of a large variety of materials, it is necessary to have an adjustable timer. The one shown on the control panel is adjustable between 3 and 90 minutes and is graduated in increments of 5 minutes. It is imperative that the timer shall reset automatically when any one of the following conditions occurs: completion of the sterilizing cycle, electric power failure, temperature drop of 2°F below the set sterilizing value.

The purpose of the MANUAL selector button is to make the automatic master control inoperative. This permits manual operation by a single programming wheel with an indicator to show each phase of the processing cycle. Return to the automatic cycle is impossible until the manual cycle has been completed or the reset button has been pressed and another cycle selected.

Drying System

Sterilizers to be used for the sterilization of wrapped materials, fabrics, or textiles must be equipped with an efficient drying system. The device designated Vacuum Drier in Figure 8-2 is typical of one way of attaining satisfactory drying of porous loads following sterilization. It operates in conjunction with the multiport valve which creates a reduced pressure in the chamber and at the same time filtered air is admitted to the chamber by means of the vacuum drier. By this method steam and moisture are replaced with filtered air while the door is still closed. The circulating filtered air will entrain and then exhaust vapors and odors from the chamber following sterilization of wrapped goods. Also, the heat in the jacket assists in the evaporation of moisture for discharge into the vent stack or condenser exhaust. Located just above the sterilizer door in Figure 8-1 is an elongated vent designed to allow heat from the chamber and door to escape behind the upper front panel.

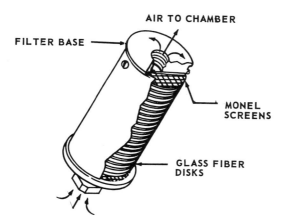

FIGURE 8-9. Bacteria-retentive filter as used on prevacuum high temperature sterilizers. It contains replaceable filter cartridge comprising many disks of superfine glass wool.

The prevacuum high temperature sterilizers must also be equipped with a reliable system for drying fabrics and hard goods. Following the terminal vacuum (48 to 50 mm abs) of the exhaust phase, it is necessary to admit air to the chamber through a bacteria—retentive filter to relieve the vacuum and to return the chamber to atmospheric pressure. Representative of a class of bacterial air filters used on prevacuum sterilizers is that shown in Figure 8-9. This contains a replaceable filter cartridge that is made up of 16 filter disks separated by screens. The filter disks are made of superfine glass wool and this serves as the primary medium for removal of bacteria from the incoming air. Inefficient filters which admit air after steam has been evacuated constitute a hazard. The filter cartridges should be replaced at least twice each year. Furthermore, periodic tests should be made in the sterilizer as near as possible to the air entry port to check on the efficiency of the filtration system.

PREVACUUM STERILIZERS

The past few years have witnessed a mounting pressure by consultants and hospital staffs to design more function per square foot of space in the Central Service Department of new or modernized hospital projects. This motivating force, coupled with sterilizer developments in Great Britain and continental Europe, ushered in a new era of steam sterilization—the prevacuum high temperature system—where speed, greater productivity, and compact equipment design dictated to manufacturers the course to follow in developing new automated sterilizers to meet the demands of the market place.

Basically, prevacuum sterilizers differ from the classical gravity displacement type only in the manner in which air is eliminated from the chamber and the load. The purpose of prevacuum is to provide a more effective method for the removal of air so that when saturated steam is admitted to the evacuated chamber it will penetrate uniformly and completely the most dense pack—thus assuring sterilization. It is now recognized that to make this a reliable process the degree of initial vacuum must be controlled and coupled with simultaneous steam injection. By conditioning the load in this manner it is possible to eliminate temperature lag in the load when the exposure period starts.

A schematic diagram to illustrate the principle of prevacuum plus steam injection as applied to a Vacamatic® sterilizer is given in Figure 8-10. The function of the water ring pump with steam ejector is as follows:

> The vacuum pump features an off-center impeller which rotates clockwise within the housing. Centrifugal force creates a ring of water between the impeller and housing forming a seal.
>
> Air to be evacuated from the chamber is drawn into the pump through an opening (A) and its exits through opening (B). As air is being evacuated "conditioning steam" is injected into the chamber through (C) thus diffusing the air in the space surrounding the fabrics. Also, conditioning steam, assisted by the partial vacuum, diffuses rapidly through the fibers, thereby completely releasing the adsorbed air by displacement. Conditioning the load assures fast heating to the sterilizing temperature.
>
> The water-ring pump creates a vacuum of about 50 mm Hg absolute at the base of the steam ejector (D)—the further vacuum is created by the steam ejector itself.
>
> Steam from the sterilizer jacket enters the ejector through (E). Incoming steam expanding through nozzle (F) creates a tremendous velocity which draws with it air from the sterilizer chamber out to the condenser and through the pump.

A prevacuum steam sterilizer with fully automatic program cycling is shown in Figure 8-11. The basic automatic control system employs various sensing and timing mechanisms which regulate the sterilizer in predeter-

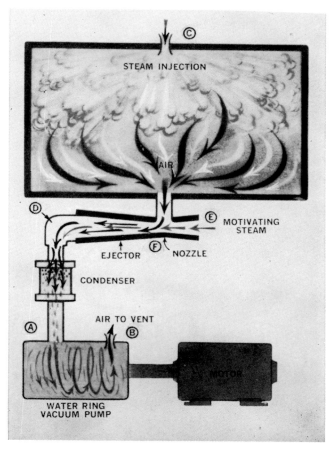

FIGURE 8-10. Schematic diagram to show one method of operation of a prevacuum sterilizer when simultaneous vacuum and steam injection are employed to rid the chamber and load of air.

mined operational stages. When an automatic cycle has begun, the sterilizer will proceed through the various steps in the cycle without further attention, shutting off when the cycle has been completed. This particular sterilizer is furnished with a power-operated door, and all operations of opening, closing, and positioning the locking arms are accomplished by means of an electric motorized control system.

Depending upon the type of load, three programs are available to the operator on a typical prevacuum sterilizer: fabrics, hard goods, and liquids. The sequential phases of each cycle are as follows:

Fabrics

—Drawing an initial vacuum and, simultaneously, injecting steam into the sterilizing chamber until an absolute pressure of 18-20 mm Hg is attained

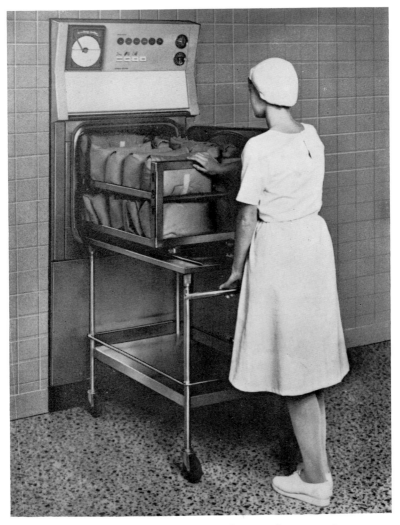

FIGURE 8-11. Prevacuum high temperature sterilizer with automatic program control, mechanical air removal, and power operated door. The monitor-controlled system controls and records both temperature and absolute pressure (barometrically compensated). It also records tests for airtightness on the chamber.

within the chamber; maintaining the evacuation and steam injection for a predetermined period of time.

—Charging the chamber with steam from the jacket to 274°F (134°C) and maintaining this temperature for a predetermined continuous period of time.

—Exhausting the chamber quickly to atmospheric pressure.

—Drawing a terminal vacuum until an absolute pressure of 48-50 mm Hg is attained in the chamber; admitting filtered air into the chamber to relieve the vacuum and return chamber to atmospheric pressure.

Hard Goods

—The automatic cycle for hard goods consists of the same phases as for fabrics with the exception of the vacuum drying phase, which is extended to a period of 8-10 minutes.

Liquids

—Charging the chamber with steam from the jacket to 251° to 258°F (122°-126°C) and maintaining this temperature for a predetermined continuous period of time.
—Timing the exposure period.
—Exhausting the chamber slowly to atmospheric pressure.

Performance Capabilities

The capability of a given piece of equipment to perform its intended function is of the utmost importance in sterilization. Any sterilizer in use today—the prevacuum is no exception—must have a demonstrated and continuous reliability to produce sterile supplies. This demands reliable components, good basic design, and above-average workmanship in features of construction. For greater productivity, speed is important but it is not the only criterion upon which sterilization depends. Claims such as "the fastest cycle ever," "in less than 20 minutes," and others used in advertising literature have no place in protecting the patient and employee against the ravages of infection. The performance capabilities of a series of prevacuum sterilizers in terms of average cycle times is given in Table 8-1.

MONITORING THE EFFICIENCY OF STERILIZERS

The sterilizers described herein or others with similar characteristics must be tested frequently and in an exact manner to determine if they conform to basic standards for sterilization. For prevacuum sterilizers a temperature-recorder-controller for the determination of positive pressure, vacuum, temperature, and time is a necessity. A monitoring instrument control panel of this type is shown in Figure 8-12. In addition, the presence of an absolute pressure gauge reading directly from the chamber provides evidence of chamber tightness and measures the magnitude of air leakage. The accuracy of all gauges and thermometers employed on monitor-controllers should be checked every three months as a minimum by a qualified service engineer. A continuous operational control reflecting precisely the saturated steam temperature in the center or in the most inaccessible parts of a load would be an ideal instrument for monitoring of sterilizers. To the author's knowledge, no such instrument exists, although attempts have been made to approach the true load condition with respect to temperature and the partial

TABLE 8-1

PERFORMANCE CAPABILITIES OF PREVACUUM STERILIZERS

Average Cycle Phase Times (in Minutes)

Cycle Phase	Empty Chamber 24" × 36"			Fabrics (Full Load) 24" × 36"			Hard Goods 24" × 36"		
	36"	48"	60"	36"	48"	60"	36"	48"	60"
Time Required to Achieve Jacket Pressure: 30 to 32 psig									
Initial Vacuum 15–20 mm Hg Absolute	5–10	7–11	8–12	4.5–5	5–6	5–6	4.5–5	5–6	5–6
Charge Chamber 15–20 mm Hg Absolute to 270° F	4.5–5	5–5.5	5–5.5	2.5–3	3.5–4.5	4.7–5	1.5–2	2.5–3	3–3.5
Exposure 270° F to 275° F	0.5–1	0.5–1.5	1–2	4–5	4–5	4–5	4–5	4–5	4–5
Final Vacuum 32 psig to End of Final Vacuum	4–5	4–5	4–5	6–7	7–8	8–9	8–10	8–10	8–10
32 psig to 48 mm Hg Absolute	1–1.5	1–2	1.5–2						
Admit Air to Chamber To zero psig	1–1.5	1–2	1.5–2	1–1.5	1–2	1.5–2	1–1.5	1–2	1.5–2
Average Cycle Time Range	12–14	14–16	15–17	18–22	21–26	25–27	21–24	22–26	24–27

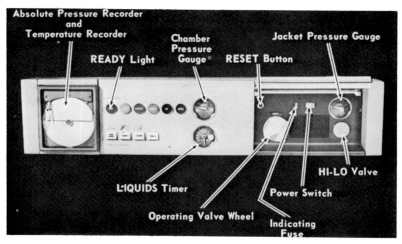

FIGURE 8-12. Automatic control panel of prevacuum high temperature sterilizer as shown in Figure 8-11.

pressures of air and steam through devices known as *load simulators*. Attention should be given to the temperature sensor or controller located in the chamber discharge line of the sterilizer. Some prevacuum sterilizers are equipped with sensors having a mean time value ranging from about 30 to 60 seconds. Unless the sensor responds almost immediately to temperature changes it may be unsafe as a controller for the sterilizing phase of the cycle, particularly if the steam supply is interrupted and a pressure drop occurs in the sterilizer.

The most accurate physical means, readily available, for determining the efficiency of the sterilizing process is to measure the temperature in the center of a challenge pack by means of a thermocouple(s) used with a potentiometer. The challenge pack and test procedure described on pages 135-137 may serve as a model for functional acceptance tests applied to prevacuum sterilizers. It should be remembered, however, that the thermocouple is not sensitive to moisture and it will give temperature readings only, regardless of whether saturated steam is present. Instances occur at times whereby superheat is present in a load for indefinite periods of time, and judgment must be used when interpreting temperature readings obtained with thermocouples.

AIRTIGHTNESS OF THE PREVACUUM CHAMBER

Undetected air leaks constitute a threat and a real hazard to sterilization in any prevacuum chamber. A survey on prevacuum steam sterilizers made by Darmady, Drewett, and Hughes[1] showed that of ten sterilizers of different makes tested not one was able to produce and maintain the conditions advocated by authorities for effective sterilization. This situation demands the utmost in respect from everyone whose responsibility centers in the operation, control, and maintenance of sterilizers. At the present time there is no alternative to safety other than to perform daily an airtightness test on the prevacuum high temperature sterilizers. The test should be carried out under the supervision of the hospital engineer and in accord with the sterilizer manufacturers instructions. A satisfactory test will conform to the following:

> By means of an absolute pressure gauge, determine the rate of air leakage into the chamber. The maximum permissible leakage rate should not exceed 1 mm per minute extended over a period of 5 minutes for a maximum increase of 5 mm pressure, starting with 12 mm or less in chamber. If these conditions cannot be met and if the leaks cannot be located for correction, then resort should be made to a Freon leak-test procedure.

DAILY CARE OF STERILIZERS

It should be the routine duty of someone to clean the interior of the sterilizer every day, before it is heated. This may be easily accomplished by washing the surfaces with a mild detergent solution such as Calgonite®, and then rinsing the chamber with plain water. If this is not done the walls of the chamber frequently become coated with greasy substances originating from the materials sterilized and also due to the entrainment with steam of volatile compounds used in the treatment of boiler water. The loading car, the tray in the bottom of the chamber, and any other wire mesh or perforated metal shelves used in the sterilizer should be cleaned in a like manner. CAUTION: never use abrasive cleaning compounds, wire brush, or steel wool on the sterilizer.

All modern sterilizers have a freely removable plug screen or strainer located in the opening to the chamber discharge line. This strainer should be removed daily (Fig. 8-13) before operating the sterilizer, while it is cool, and thoroughly cleaned so that the pores are free from lint and sediment. If this detail is neglected the sterilizer cannot be depended upon for prompt and efficient performance.

In the interest of preventive maintenance, it is excellent practice to clean out the chamber discharge system as suggested in Figure 8-14. This should be established as a weekly procedure. It only involves removing the strainer as indicated in Figure 8-13, inserting a funnel into the opening, and then pouring into the pipe one quart of hot trisodium phosphate solution, containing about one ounce of the trisodium phosphate. Follow this step by flushing the line with one quart of hot tap water. The periodic flushing of the discharge system will keep the channel free of clogging substances, greasy or resinous, which, if allowed to accumulate, may offer some retardation to free discharge of air and condensate from the chamber.

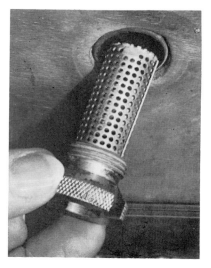

FIGURE 8-13. Remove this strainer daily before operating the sterilizer. Clean it thoroughly so that openings are entirely free from lint and sediment.

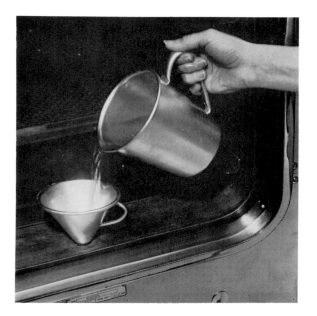

FIGURE 8-14. Method of cleaning chamber drain line.

MINOR MAINTENANCE ON STERILIZERS

Gravity Air Discharge Type

Problem	Probable Cause	Correction
Steam pressure in jacket does not rise to correct operating range.	Pressure control valve setting is not correct.	Adjust setting on valve.
	Steam supply valve is closed.	Open steam supply valve.
	Thermostatic trap in return line from jacket is inoperative.	Replace element in steam trap.
	Strainer in steam supply line to jacket is plugged.	Clean strainer.
Chamber temperature does not rise to 250° F or 270° F as se-selected.	Setting on automatic controller is not correct.	Consult a trained service man.
	Pressure control valve setting is not correct.	Adjust setting on pressure control valve.
	Chamber drain line strainer is plugged.	Remove and clean strainer.
	Thermostatic trap in chamber drain line is inoperative.	Replace element in steam trap.
	Thermometer inaccurate.	Replace thermometer.
When correctly set, the pressure control valve yields too much or too little steam pressure in jacket.	Worn seat and disc assembly in valve.	Replace seat and disc assembly.
	Valve has ruptured bellows.	Replace bellows in valve.
	Faulty pressure gauge.	Correct or replace gauge.
Ready light on control panel does not come on.	Power switch not turned on.	Check to see if power is flowing to sterilizer.
	Control fuse burned out.	Replace fuse.
	Ready light pressure switch on automatic control not adjusted properly.	Adjust switch.
	Ready light bulb burned out.	Replace bulb.
Excessive steam in the area of sterilizer while it is in operation.	Water valve on condenser vent device is closed during manual operation.	Open water valve on sterilizer equipped with condenser vent.
	Strainer in cold water line plugged.	Clean water strainer.
	Not enough water is flowing through condenser vent device.	Adjust water flow regulator.
	Steam is leaving sterilizer through safety valve.	Usually caused by too much pressure in jacket of sterilizer. Adjust pressure control valve.
Steam pressure in chamber will not rise during the Sterilize phase of cycle.	Not enough steam pressure in jacket.	Adjust pressure control valve.
Steam enters the chamber when sterilizer door is open.	Phase indicator not in off position.	Turn operating valve wheel to off.
	Steam is blowing into chamber from building vent stack or exhaust system.	Eliminate back pressure in building vent stack or exhaust system.
Pools of water on floor of chamber after sterilization cycle is completed.	Condensate has collected in lower part of jacket.	Replace element in thermostatic steam trap.
	Thermostatic trap in jacket return line has defective element.	

Problem	Probable Cause	Correction
	Chamber drain line strainer is plugged.	Clean strainer.
	There is back pressure from the building steam return system.	Eliminate back pressure from building steam return system.
	Chamber floor not pitched toward the chamber drain line opening.	Raise floor flanges so as to tilt sterilizer chamber forward and to permit water to flow freely from rear to front drain opening.
Goods are wet following fabrics cycle; or there is excessive steam in chamber upon opening sterilizer door.	Ball check in vacuum drier not functioning properly.	Clean ball and seat in vacuum drier.
Solution loads are exhausted too quickly; containers boil over and bottle closures blow off.	Thermostatic trap in chamber drain line is not functioning properly.	Replace element in trap.
	Exhaust valve is not functioning properly.	Reduce rate of exhaust.
	Containers too full.	Reduce volume of liquid to correct level in each bottle or flask.
Buzzer does not sound at end of cycle.	Defective buzzer on automatically controlled sterilizer.	Replace buzzer.
Steam escapes through safety valve.	Pressure control valve is not adjusted properly.	Adjust valve or replace it.
Steam leaks around sterilizer door during STERILIZE phase of cycle.	Worn door gasket.	Replace gasket.
	Door closed improperly.	Close properly. If problem continues notify maintenance.
Sterilizer door will not open.	Vacuum in chamber.	Place controls in OFF position and wait for equalization of pressure.
	Door lock clutch is jammed.	Notify maintenance.
	Gasket is sticking to end ring.	Notify maintenance.
	Old gasket or dirty end ring.	Recoat end ring.

PREVACUUM HIGH TEMPERATURE STERILIZERS

Problem	Probable Cause	Correction
Steam pressure in jacket does not rise to 35 psig.	Pressure control valve setting is not correct.	Adjust setting on valve.
	Steam supply valve is closed.	Open steam supply valve.
	Thermostatic trap in steam return line from jacket is inoperative.	Replace element in steam trap.
	Strainer in steam supply line to jacket is plugged.	Clean steam strainer.
	Faulty pressure gauge.	Replace gauge.
Chamber temperature will not rise to selected temperature.	Control valve setting is not correct.	Adjust setting on valve.
	Thermometer is inaccurate.	Replace thermometer.
	Chamber drain line strainer is plugged.	Clean strainer.
	Thermostatic trap in chamber drain line is inoperative.	Replace element in trap.

Problem	Probable Cause	Correction
When correctly set, the control valve yields too high pressure in jacket.	Worn seat and disc assembly in valve. May have ruptured bellows.	Replace seat and disc assembly and/or bellows in valve
Automatic control READY does not come on.	Power switch not turned on. Control fuse burned out. READY light pressure switch on control not adjusted properly. Light bulb burned out.	Turn power switch on Replace fuse. Adjust switch. Replace bulb.
Excessive steam in the area of sterilizer when it is in operation.	Strainer in cold water line is plugged. Not enough water is flowing through the condenser. Steam is leaving sterilizer through the safety valve.	Clean water strainer. Adjust water flow regulator on condenser to increase flow of water. Too much pressure in jacket of sterilizer. Adjust control valve.
Steam pressure in chamber will not rise during the STERILIZE phase of the cycle.	Not enough steam pressure in jacket.	Adjust pressure control valve.
Buzzer does not sound at end of cycle.	Defective buzzer.	Replace buzzer.
Steam escapes through safety valve.	Control valve is not properly adjusted. Defective safety valve.	Adjust control valve. Replace safety valve.
Steam leaks around the door during the STERILIZE phase of the cycle.	Worn door gasket.	Replace door gasket.
Vacuum pump motor will not start.	Motor overload switches have cut out. No power to vacuum pump motor.	Push reset button on automatic control panel. Check fuses in branch circuit box.
Vacuum pump will not start.	Pump to motor coupling sleeve broken.	Replace coupling sleeve.
Insufficient chamber vacuum.	Door gasket leaks. Insufficient water to vacuum pump.	Replace gasket. Check water supply valve and flow control.
Hard goods load comes out wet.	Inadequate drying time and/or load is positioned incorrectly in sterilizer.	Check drying time and arrange load so that moisture can drain off.
On solution loads the caps on bottles blow off.	Solution exhaust accelerator valve is improperly adjusted.	Adjust accelerator valve to cut in at 8 psig.

NOTE: Repairs and adjustments to sterilizers, other than those described above and perhaps a few more of a minor nature, should be attempted only by experienced mechanics fully acquainted with all details of the equipment.

REFERENCE

1. DARMADY, E. M., DREWETT, S. E., and HUGHES, K. E. A.: Survey on prevacuum high pressure steam sterilizers. *J Clin Path*, 17:126-129, 1964.

Chapter 9

PREPARATION AND STERILIZATION OF DRESSINGS, DRY GOODS, AND RUBBER PRODUCTS

LINEN PACKS

CONVENTIONAL use of the term "dressings" implies the application of various materials for the protection of a body wound. It may apply to any type of covering regardless of the style, size, texture, or weave; and the materials may be either gauze, cotton, cellulose, cloth, wool, paper, plastic, or sponge. The term "packs" generally refers to all linen materials processed for sterile usage in surgical, delivery, and nursery procedures. References to linen as a material usually mean a muslin, bleached or unbleached, a plain closely woven cotton fabric.

The processing of sterile linen supplies begins in the laundry. As a rule, the washing procedures are efficient in removing microorganisms from used textiles. However, the extraction and ironing procedures do not necessarily contribute to the reduction in microbial populations. In fact, studies[1] indicate that washed textiles can be recontaminated in the extractors, and subsequent ironing heat at a temperature of 350°F (177°C) is ineffective in destroying organisms if they are surrounded by an extraneous dried mucous coating.

From the moment that the washed textiles are removed from the machines, placed upon a folding table, handled perhaps by unclean hands, moved to another area for a temporary period, exposed to germ-laden air, then transported to other areas of the hospital with further handling and rehandling, there is a gradual buildup in the numbers of organisms in the textiles. Eventually when the linens are assembled into surgical packs ready for sterilization the mixed microbial flora may have reached a level ranging from several million to a billion or more organisms per pack. This point is rarely appreciated by those responsible for the production of sterile linen.

Effective sterilization of surgical supplies is not only dependent upon conscientious operation of the sterilizer but also upon correct methods of packaging and proper arrangement of loads in the sterilizer. Operators should constantly bear in mind that reliable performance demands complete permeation of every strand and fiber of the materials with the moisture and heat of the steam. This permeation will occur rapidly or slowly, depending upon the size and density of the packs, the positioning of the load in the sterilizer, and the method employed for air elimination in the sterilizer.

Steam Penetration Through Porous Materials

The movement of air and steam through the sterilizer has a direct bearing on the preparation of packs for sterilization. All modern sterilizers of the downward displacement type employ the gravity system for air elimination in which steam enters the chamber at the back end, moves promptly to the top of the chamber, compresses air in the bottom areas, forcing the air from the chamber through an opening in the extreme front bottom. This assures movement of steam from one end of the chamber to the other and from top to bottom. In the case of prevacuum sterilizers, the air is removed from the chamber by means of a vacuum pump prior to full admission of steam. When steam enters the evacuated chamber, it undergoes considerable expansion and immediately fills the space. Permeation of the load is remarkably rapid because essentially no air remains in the chamber to retard the flow of steam to all parts.

Except during the initial stage of the sterilizing process, there is no rapid movement of steam or air. When the free air in open spaces surrounding the load has been eliminated, there is an approach to a static condition of the gases. Since the pressure is relatively uniform, the only movement of the gases will be occasioned by the slow release of air from the load itself. This is brought about by gravity. Air, being heavier than steam, will gravitate downward out of the packs and steam will replace it as rapidly as the air can escape. This movement will be fast or slow depending upon the density and depth of the mass through which the discharge must occur.

It should be obvious that a textile pack 6 inches in depth will present twice as much resistance to steam permeation as a similar pack 3 inches in depth. With the same reasoning, if two packs each 6 inches in depth are placed in the sterilizer in close contact, one directly above the other, the effect will be the same as if both were wrapped in one package 12 inches in depth. On the other hand, if the upper pack is separated from the lower one by a short distance, steam will quickly fill the intervening space and permeate the lower pack essentially the same as if the two were placed side by side in the sterilizer.

It is important to remember that the vital discharge of air from the load always occurs in a downward direction, never sidewise. Knowledge of this movement pattern provides the background for this basic rule:

> Prepare all packs and arrange the load in the sterilizer so as to present the least possible resistance to the passage of steam through the load, from the top of the chamber toward the bottom.

Assume for analysis a simple package consisting of ten pieces of muslin

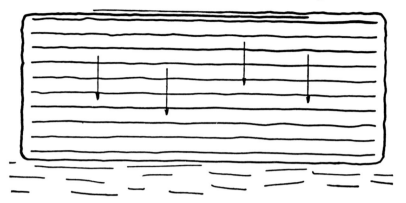

Figure 9-1. Packs made up of many layers of fabric placed in sterilizer horizontally, as shown, are difficult to sterilize because air within pack must travel downward through successive layers to escape. Each horizontal layer adds to resistance and as outer layers become moist from steam, resistance is further increased.

cut into 10-inch squares and wrapped together without folding. If this pack were placed in the sterilizer flat side down as in Figure 9-1, air within the pack would have to pass through ten layers of muslin, plus the cover, in its downward passage. The resistance of the dry pack will be increased by the moisture of the steam in contact with the outer layers, further retarding the evacuation of air. Also, the closer the weave of the fabric, the greater the resistance. If this same pack is now placed in the sterilizer vertically (on edge) as shown in Figure 9-2, even though the pack be wrapped fairly tightly, there will remain minute spaces between layers through which air can gravitate toward the bottom with comparative freedom.

The above rule should guide the operator in preparing every pack or drum of bulk supplies to be subjected to sterilization and also in the arrangement of the load which will normally consist of several packs. This point can not be overemphasized, especially when heavy packs are encountered as illustrated by the two temperature curves in Figure 9-3. The pack tested in this case (Fig. 9-4) was abnormally large and dense, but it serves as a good example to show the importance of proper positioning in the sterilizer and to indicate the hazards encountered when packs are too large and dense.

Hazards of Abnormally Large or Dense Packs

While the temperature curve in Figure 9-3 shows that 33 minutes exposure at 250°F (121°C) would have been adequate for sterilization of the pack when placed on edge in the sterilizer, this by no means justifies acceptance of the pack as suitable. The day of the old-fashioned laparotomy set containing far more materials than actually required for the surgical procedure and with little consideration for the internal arrangement of the pack

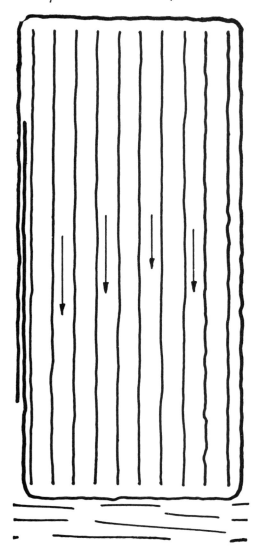

FIGURE 9-2. When packs are placed on edge with layers of fabric in vertical position, air will escape quickly through minute spaces between layers.

should be over. Unfortunately it is not over. Some hospitals continue to ignore basic principles by preparing and attempting to sterilize packs that weigh as much as 27 pounds. The practice of preparing large dense bundles of textiles is hazardous. Rigid standardization of packaging should be enforced. The largest pack should not exceed 12 × 12 × 20 inches in size for routine work, and it should weigh no more than 10 to 12 pounds. The factors which seem to indicate the desirability of much larger surgical packs do not offset the safety factor in sterilization.

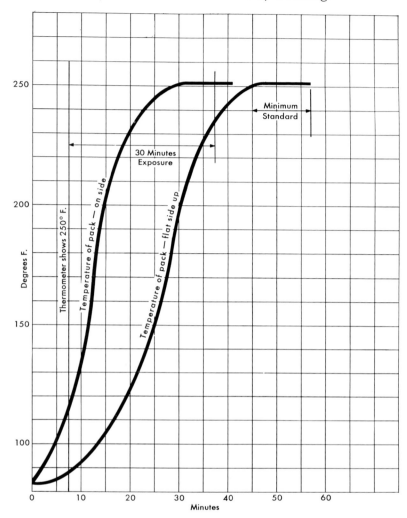

FIGURE 9-3. These two curves show load temperatures attained with pack illustrated in Figure 9-4. With pack flat side up, 50 minutes exposure is required for sterilization. When pack is placed on edge in chamber, 33 minutes exposure is needed to meet minimum standard for sterilization.

When tests show that any pack, sterilized by itself, resting either vertically or horizontally in the sterilizer, requires more than 30 minutes exposure to 250°F to meet the minimum standard of 12 minutes plus a liberal margin of safety, that indicates the pack is too large and it should be broken down into smaller packs. Reliable routine sterilization of surgical supplies correctly prepared can be accomplished in 30 minutes exposure to saturated steam at 250°F (121°C) in the modern gravity displacement sterilizer or for an equivalent period of time in a prevacuum high temperature sterilizer.

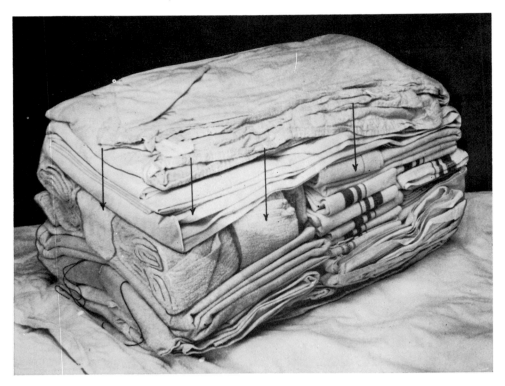

FIGURE 9-4. This is the pack referred to in Figure 9-3, an abnormally large and dense pack. The practice of using large and heavy packs should be discouraged.

Many operating room supervisors and central service supervisors have long since discovered this fact, but the practice of using abnormally large or dense packs still persists in some hospitals. With all of our refined knowledge of the subject of sterilization, it still is not unusual to find recording thermometer charts on surgical supply sterilizers showing exposure periods ranging from 10 to 90 minutes. The hospital pays heavily for such inconsistencies, not to mention the probability of sterilization failures.

The economic factor should not be ignored, because the hospital has a considerable investment annually in replacement of textiles and other materials. It is indeed possible to effect a substantial savings on materials subject to repeated sterilization simply by establishing standardized methods for their preparation and sterilization. If the operating room or central service department supervisor blindly persists in preparing large, overstuffed packs such as shown in Figures 9-4 and 9-5, then the periods of exposure must be prolonged to 60 minutes or more, with resultant deterioration of outer fabrics.

To further explain the hazardous element involved in the use of abnormally large or dense packs, suppose there are several of these to be sterilized

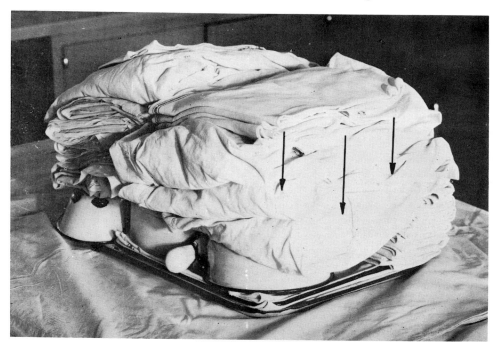

FIGURE 9-5. Another example of faulty arrangement of individual pack. Inclusion of basins with fabrics in one package should not be permitted. Basins seriously interfere with steam permeation and retard drying following sterilization.

in one load. If through carelessness the load is arranged as in Figure 9-6, the upper packs would retard passage of steam to the lower packs so seriously that 60 minutes exposure might not be adequate for sterilization. But if these packs are broken down into moderate sizes, some degree of carelessness in loading could be tolerated without jeopardizing the end result in a 30-minute exposure period. By establishing methods of packaging that permit safe sterilization in 30 minutes, definite economies will be effected: more work can be done with the sterilizers in a given time; less steam and fuel will be required, and materials will need to be replaced less frequently.

Protective Covering for Surgical Packs

The protective covering or wrapper for surgical packs logically precedes any discussion on what constitutes the ideal pack from the standpoint of bulk and density. The wrapper must provide protection against contact contamination in handling, guard against the entry of insects or vermin (cockroaches, ants, silverfish), and it must also serve as a dust filter. When packs of porous supplies are removed from the sterilizer, they are more or less filled with vapor; and, as this vapor condenses, it creates a negative pressure condition within the goods. This results in a definite intake of room air from

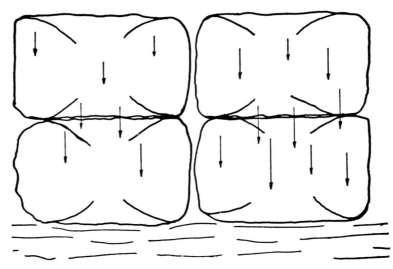

FIGURE 9-6. Abnormally heavy packs arranged in sterilizer as shown here become doubly hazardous. In effect, pack is double its normal depth and an exposure period of 60 minutes or longer might still be inadequate for steam penetration through lower packs.

which dust particles and microorganisms must be removed in the covering envelope or the contents may be contaminated.

When selecting a wrapper for sterile supplies, it is necessary to consider the characteristics of the product and to determine how closely they conform to those of the ideal wrapping material. Points for comparison are the following:

—The material should not inhibit or retard appreciably the passage of water vapor, steam, or ethylene oxide gas to the contents of a package. It should present no barrier to air elimination and it should not be affected by the sterilizing process.

—The material should have a proven record as an effective, reliable filter for dust particles and microorganisms. Extremes in ambient temperature and humidity as encountered in human-occupied areas should cause no adverse change in the material. Water repellency is a desirable characteristic.

—It should be a durable material, preferably reusable, with known tensile strength to both wet and dry conditions. It should not tear, crack, or puncture easily when exposed to necessary handling from the point of wrapping through sterilization, storage, delivery, and end use.

—The material should offer no resistance or hazard to the practice of asepsis. It must permit opening of the package without danger of contaminating the contents.

—The material should be consistent in quality, not subject to a high percentage of rejects, and require a minimum of inspection time on the part of hospital personnel.

—It should be economically priced, readily available, and supplied by a reputable manufacturer.

Broad experience has shown that a *minimum* of two thicknesses of good quality muslin, 140 thread count, serves well as wrapping material. Two thicknesses are used to guard against possible minute flaws in the muslin. The porosity of muslin is determined by the thread count. This means that the cloth has a minimum number of 68 threads in the warp and 72 in the filling per square inch. Unbleached muslin is about 10 per cent stronger than bleached. Badly worn muslin should not be used because the thin portions may not filter out dust particles effectively. Some hospitals prepare covers for surgical packs from two ordinary bed sheets (63×90 inches), folded crosswise so as to form four thicknesses of fabric. With this procedure the finished wrapper is about 63 inches long and 45 inches wide. It will serve to cover adequately a large pack with dimensions of about $22 \times 15 \times 8\frac{1}{2}$ inches. A list of suggested wrapper sizes and their uses follows.

Size (inches)	Use
12×12	for small articles
22×22	for gloves
10×20	single thickness, for inner glove wrapper
30×30	for treatment trays
36×36	for basin sets
48×48	for small linen packs
60×60	for large linen packs in major surgery

Canvas covers or other heavy woven fabrics should not be used because the tightly woven structure seriously retards the passage of steam. For the same reason canvas should not be used for table covers or any other requirement where sterilization is necessary. Heavy woven fabrics should be wrapped individually for sterilization, never with other goods.

Paper Wrappers as a Substitute for Muslin

During the last few years there has developed a fairly widespread usage of paper products as a substitute for muslin in the wrapping of supplies. Coarse, brown wrapping paper (30 or 40 pound Kraft) is used rather extensively in hospitals for the wrapping of gloves and other small articles. This type of paper will pass steam quite freely, but not as rapidly as muslin. Assuming that it is devoid of holes, it will also filter out dust particles satisfactorily. It is an inexpensive material, noisy, not too pliable, and certainly not as durable as textiles or plastic films. The principal objection to its use for surgical supplies is the obvious hazard of contamination through rupture in handling.

Many institutions use small paper bags for packaging cotton balls, dressings, syringes, and similar items, with apparent success and economy. However, a single paper bag is not recommended as a wrapping for sterile articles because of the risk of contamination of the contents during extraction. During the process of opening the bag contamination can occur as the result of the release of organisms into the air from the outer surface of the bag.[2,3] Also, it is not commonly recognized that many papers are degraded by the steam sterilizing processes with a loss in tensile strength. This degradation can be associated with an increase in microbial penetration. Evidence has been presented which suggests a porosity rating of 175 to 180 for paper wrappers used for sterility maintenance.[4] The porosity of a paper is the time required for 100 milliliters of air to flow through a fixed area at a given pressure, usually determined by means of the Gurley Densometer.

Beck, Shay, and Purdum[5] examined fifty-five samples of paper to determine their value as a wrapping material for articles sterilized by steam under pressure or by hot air. Their results showed that the Kraft-type papers were the most suitable and most economical. The conclusions drawn in this study were later criticized by Walter[6] on the basis that the data were not valid because conditions of the test were not critical. More recently, Alder and Alder[7] reported on the efficiency of a water-repellent sterilizing paper used as a wrapper for dressing packs. It proved to be highly satisfactory in protecting packs against contamination when exposed to a dirty atmosphere for twenty-one days.

Whittenberger[8] reported on the steam sterilization of paper wrapped packages by comparing the effectiveness of standard muslin, one and two layers, with a 2-way crepe paper (Dennison Wraps). Measurements were made in terms of the temperature attained at the core of a 10-inch cube of muslin. The results showed that layer for layer the barrier to steam was about the same for both materials. A detailed study of muslin versus paper wrappers was made by Christie.[9] Her findings stressed the superior characteristics of the 2-way crepe paper. The point should not be overlooked that the degree of springiness or elasticity present in certain types of paper makes it difficult to obtain a flat sterile field when the wrapper is opened.

As a substitute for muslin, certain hospitals use the vegetable parchment paper known as Patapar, 27-2T.® This material permits passage of steam at a useful rate through a single layer. It possesses high wet strength and does not tear or puncture easily. Tests indicate that objects wrapped in Patapar should be subjected to the normal period of exposure required for sterilization of muslin wrapped articles in a gravity discharge type sterilizer. It is advisable, however, to add an additional 5 to 10 minutes to the drying time following sterilization because the moisture vapor transmission rate of the parchment is slower than that of muslin.

Plastic Films

The use of plastic films for packaging and wrapping of articles is becoming increasingly popular, especially for those supplies destined for ethylene oxide gas sterilization. Films such as polyethylene, polypropylene, and polyvinyl chloride exhibit the desirable qualities of resistance to tearing, impermeability to dust particles, pliability, and transparency, and they are heat sealable. With the exception of Nylon or polyamide, the films are impermeable to steam and they must be heat-sealed following sterilization. This is a disadvantage. In addition, the majority of films are practically impermeable to air and this condition is incompatible with steam sterilizing processes. In order to avoid failures in sterilization, the characteristics of the material must be known and it should be used accordingly.

Certain films, like polyethylene, serve a useful purpose as a protective dust cover for muslin or paper-wrapped packs applied after sterilization. Any package placed in storage will, sooner or later, collect a layer of dust particles on the wrapper making it difficult if not impossible to open the package without danger of contamination to the contents. *A double wrapper is essential for packs destined for the operating room or any other specialized area in the hospital where asepsis is practiced.* The outer dust protective wrapper should be removed before the pack is admitted to the clean zone. The porosity of a plastic film is influenced by the thickness which is measured in mils or fractions of an inch. One mil is equal to 1/1000 of an inch. Film wraps are normally available in the range of 1 to 3 mils in thickness. Pinholes may be present in plastic films.

Moisture Vapor Transmission of Films and Papers

At the present time there are no standard requirements for moisture vapor transmission rates through films and papers which would assist in selecting suitable wrapping materials. Table 9-1 gives water vapor permeability

TABLE 9-1

MOISTURE VAPOR PERMEABILITY OF COMMON FILMS AND PAPERS

Material	Thickness (inches)	Permeability*
Cellophane (sterilizable)	0.0015-0.008	High
Cellophane (moistureproof)	0.0009-0.0017	0.2-0.6
Kraft paper	0.002-0.009	High
Ethyl cellulose film	0.001-0.2	High
Glassine (plain)	0.00075-0.002	High
Glassine (lacquered)	0.0008-0.002	0.2-1.0
Glassine (waxed)	0.0008-0.003	0.2-1.0
Pliofilm®	0.0008-0.002	0.5-1.0
Polyamide film	0.0005-0.001	High
Fluorocarbon film (Aclar®)	0.001-0.002	0.15-0.55
Polyethylene film	0.004	0.25
Polyethylene (low density)	0.001	High
Polypropylene film	0.001	0.46
Nylon 6	0.0005-0.001	High
Saran film	0.001-0.002	0.2 or less
Vegetable parchment	0.0017-0.0075	High
Vinyl chloride film	0.001	High
Vinyl coated paper	0.001 (film thickness)	High

* Measured as grams of water transmitted per 100 square inches, per 24 hours, at 100°F and 95% relative humidity.

values for a variety of common films and papers. Some films exhibit very low water vapor transmission rates and others are sufficiently high that they could be classified as free vapor breathing. Films and papers with less than a "high" permeability rating should not be used as basic wrapping materials for sterilizing processes involving moisture transfer through the film. A typically high permeability rate would be not less than 3.0 grams of water transmitted per 100 square inches, per 24 hours, at 100°F and 95% relative humidity.

There is no absolutely vaporproof barrier. Even metal foils free from pinholes and other defects transmit minute amounts of water vapor due to the nonhomogeneity of their structure. The transmission of water vapor and gases depends upon several factors, including the temperature of the gas and of the barrier; the difference in pressure on the two sides of the barrier; the type, thickness, composition, and crystallinity of the barrier; and the area exposed to transmission. For plastic films there is no apparent relationship between microbial permeability and moisture permeability.

Single Use Wrappers

There is a trend toward increased usage of paper as a wrapping material. This may be due, in part, to the large scale use of disposables in many hospitals. It does not necessarily follow, however, that the act of using disposables in any hospital will automatically result in a higher standard of patient care. The very fact that certain disposables are promoted and reused for a limited number of times represents a deplorable condition, totally unfair to the patient.

TABLE 9-2

PACKAGING MATERIALS FOR ARTICLES TO BE STERILIZED

Material	Nature	Type of Product	Thickness or Grade	Suitable for: Steam	Suitable for: Dry Heat	Suitable for: Eto Gas
Muslin	Textile	Wrappers	140 thread count	YES	YES	YES
Jean cloth	Textile	Wrappers	160 thread count	YES	NO	YES
Broadcloth	Textile	Wrappers	200 thread count	YES	NO	YES
Canvas	Textile	Wrappers	—	DO NOT USE		
Kraft brown	Paper	Wrappers, Bags	30–40 lb	YES	NO	YES
Kraft white	Paper	Wrappers, Bags	30–40 lb	YES	NO	YES
Glassine	Coated Paper	Envelopes, Bags	30 lb	YES	NO	YES
Parchment	Paper	Wrappers	Patapar 27-2T	YES	NO	YES
Crepe	Paper	Wrappers	Dennison Wrap	YES	NO	YES
Cellophane	Cellulose Film	Tubing, Bags	Weck Sterilizable	YES	NO	YES
Polyethylene	Plastic	Bags, Wrappers	1–3 mils	NO	NO	YES
Polypropylene	Plastic	Film	1–3 mils	*	NO	YES
Polyvinyl Chloride	Plastic	Film, Tubing	1–3 mils	NO	NO	YES
Nylon	Plastic	Film, Bags	1–2 mils	*	NO	YES
Polyamide	Plastic	Film, Wrappers	1–2 mils	*	NO	YES
Aluminum	Foil	Wrappers	1–2 mils	NO	YES	NO

* Not recommended. Difficult to eliminate air from packs.

The repeated use of paper wrappers is typical of false economy in handling disposables. It is an unsafe practice that deviates from and discourages sound aseptic technique. Moreover, any article used on a patient must be cleaned or decontaminated and then sterilized prior to use on the next patient. This principle applies no less to paper wrappers that are subjected to reuse. The human element associated with the handling and processing of paper-wrapped packages, both before and after sterilization, offers ample opportunity for violating the integrity of the wrapper. Another point to consider is that reuse of paper or plastic film entails inspection procedures and monitoring controls with added costs of labor. The indiscriminate use of paper lowers present day standards for sterilization of supplies. Table 9-2 shows a list of packaging materials for articles to be sterilized by steam, dry heat, or ethylene oxide gas. The ideal wrapping material probably does not exist.

Correct Methods of Packaging

The preparation and packaging of sterile linen comprises a series of operations. They are as follows:

- Inspection
- Folding
- Assembly
- Wrapping and labeling
- Sterilization
- Storage

All linen used for sterile supplies should be carefully inspected for holes, tears, lint, stains, and other defects. This work is usually conducted over an illuminated glass table top to assist in locating the defects. When holes are found, they can be encircled with pencil and immediately repaired by the sewing room with thermopatching equipment. During the course of inspection, particular attention should be given to the linting of fabrics. Lint and dust particles contribute to an insanitary environment, promote hospital sepsis, and provide a vehicle for the transfer of organisms from one location to another. Small particles of lint from gauze sponges induce adhesions, granulomata, and foreign body reactions in tissues.[10]

Arrangement of Contents of Linen Packs

In promoting correct methods of packaging, the first requirement is to restrict the size and density of the individual pack so that 30 minutes exposure at 250°F (121°C) with gravity air discharge, or 4 minutes at 270°F (132°C) in a prevacuum sterilizer will ensure uniform steam permeation with an adequate margin of safety in sterilization. This can be accomplished by limiting the largest pack to dimensions of 12 × 12 × 20 inches. Do not attempt to mix trays or basins with fabrics, all in one package, as shown in Figure 9-5. The basins interfere with air elimination, cause excess condensate, and also retard effective drying of the fabrics following sterilization.

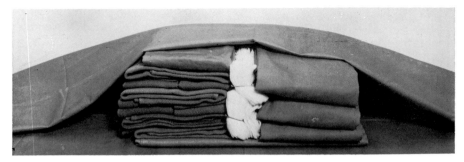

FIGURE 9-7. This major pack, arranged for muslin wrapping, is suggested as model for all heavy packs. Note how alternate layers are crossed to promote steam permeation. Table drape is folded once and spread out to form ultimately an inner covering of pack. This provides convenient method of draping table as pack is opened. After pack has been covered with table drape, an outer double-thickness muslin cover is put on and secured by pressure sensitive tape.

The contents of the pack should be arranged in an orderly manner so that the item to be used first in the sterile area is the last item to be placed on the pack. The basic pack shown in Figures 9-7 and 9-8, arranged for muslin wrapping, is suggested as a model for all major packs. The materials are ideally arranged, alternate layers of linen are crossed in order to promote rapid and complete permeation of steam through the mass. The pack includes the following items:

    2 wrappers double thickness muslin—(large enough to provide
                                              at least a 6-inch
                                              overhang on all sides of table)
    3 gowns   —for surgeon and assistants
    14 towels   —3—drying hands
                                      1—sutures
                                      4—skin towels
                                      4—operative site
                                      1—cover for Mayo tray
                                      1—extra
    10 sponges, radiopaque
    5 tape sponges
    1 Mayo stand cover

Drape sheets are not included in the basic pack because of the intent to reduce the density and to increase the flexibility of the pack. The patient's drape sheet should be wrapped individually in a double thickness muslin wrapper. The same procedure should be followed for the nurse's gown.

To facilitate the work when this pack is opened in the surgical suite,* the

* The opening of packs in the operating room proper is not recommended due to the release of dust and fiber particles. An ancillary room or area should be made available for this activity.

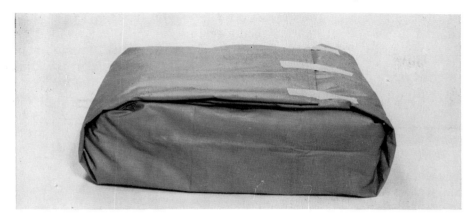

FIGURE 9-8. Example of a linen pack properly wrapped.

table cover is folded once only and spread on the work table in two thicknesses only. It will be used to form the inner covering of the pack. More than two thicknesses of the table cover over the rest of the pack should not be permitted because of the resistance of heavier covering to the passage of steam. The gauze sponges are located near the center of the pack to break up the close contact between the other more closely woven fabrics. Gauze, being light and porous, admits steam through the center of the pack for prompt contact with the heavier articles on either side. All other articles are folded flat and each succeeding layer is placed crosswise of the one below, to promote free circulation of steam.

When the materials are all assembled as shown, the extended sides of the table drape are used to cover the pack, then the double-thickness muslin covers are applied. The covers should not be drawn up too tightly, only enough to hold the materials together for a reasonable amount of handling. The outer wrapper and package can be secured with a substantial cord or pressure-sensitive tape. The latter offers a convenient means for labeling or identification of the individual packs. The use of pins for holding wrappers in place should not be permitted. They shorten the life of fabrics, increase the tendency of tearing or tight wrapping, and above all, they permit contamination to gain access to the interior.

Walter[11] has described another highly efficient method for the preparation of a laparotomy kit. He recommends the use of a wooden trough with dimensions of 22 × 13 × 8½ inches to serve as a guide in limiting the size and shape of the package to standard dimensions which permit uniform steam penetration. In this procedure the wrapper consists of two sheets (63 × 90 inches) folded crosswise and interleaved pamphletlike to form four thicknesses 63 inches long and 45 inches wide. The sheets are then draped in the trough as the first step in preparing the package.

Table Drapes, Sheets, and Gowns. Of the various kinds of dry goods encountered in the operating room, the table drapes and sheets are the most difficult to sterilize. These fabrics are closely woven with few interlacings and when they are ironed, folded together several times, and again ironed, the result is an exceedingly compact mass through which steam can permeate only very slowly. If such materials are wrapped with other supplies, the interference in the passage of steam to other articles may constitute a hazard. For this reason, it is advisable wherever possible to wrap such articles separately or in packs containing no more than two drapes or sheets each. Such packs are easily sterilized and they may be included in the same load with the major packs. Towels, on the contrary, present no special problem when included in the major pack. The towel fabric is relatively coarse and even when ironed it offers little resistance to the passage of steam.

When it is found necessary to reduce the size and density of large packs, gowns may also be removed and wrapped separately. The gown pack usually includes four gowns in a muslin wrapper. These packs can also be sterilized with the major load in 30 minutes exposure, with a liberal margin of safety. As a rule, it is not necessary to remove gowns from a major pack, provided all of the other articles have been properly arranged in the pack. The loose arrangement of the gown fabric, even when folded, offers little resistance to the passage of steam.

Infant Linen

All linen for the nursery should be sterilized following the laundering process. It should be brought from the laundry in a closed cabinet which may also serve as the linen storage unit. If this system is not used, the linen should be stored in specifically designated cabinet drawers in a clean area of the nursery. Rules for handling nursery linen, making up of packages, etc., should be worked out with the medical, nursing, laundry, and administrative staffs of the hospital.[12]

Use of Dressing Drums, Jars, or Cans

It has long been known that the use of drums in sterilizing necessitates considerably greater exposure time, particularly when the drums are heavily loaded—as they almost invariably are. Regardless of the number and arrangement of portholes in the drum, passageways for the escape of air and intake of steam are restricted far more than when goods are put up in packs. To illustrate this point see Figure 9-9. The obsolete forms of drums with sliding bands for closing and opening ports are definitely hazardous. Operators are prone to forget to open the ports prior to sterilization. Also the idea that closure of the ports following sterilization will render the drum essentially dust-proof is erroneous. The loose fitting cover will always admit air and dust quite freely. Other types have no sliding bands but do have more

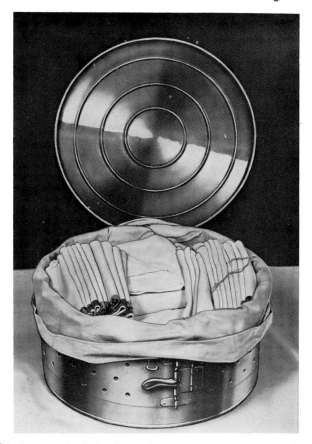

FIGURE 9-9. This is typical of the hazardous condition encountered in use of drums. Compact arrangement of materials, crowded against ports in sides, necessitates prolonged exposure. This load was sterilized in half the time when removed from drum.

and better distributed portholes around the walls for the escape of air and the entrance of steam. Even with these improvements the metal surface of the drum still very seriously retards passage of steam to the contents, especially when the drum is fully loaded. For these reasons the use of drums can not be recommended. Metal caskets of the type shown in Figure 9-10 are popular in hospitals in European countries. They are susceptible to damage by abuse, encourage overpacking, and make sterilization more difficult.

If drums must be used, it is of extreme importance to limit the size and density of the load. Under no condition is it safely permissible to crowd the contents against the inside walls of the drum. Place the flat packages of sheets, table covers, towels and other articles in the drum but do not fill it completely. Do not attempt to fill in the open spaces at the sides, rather leave them open for steam circulation. When the cover is closed, it must not compress the goods. The contents are completely surrounded by two thick-

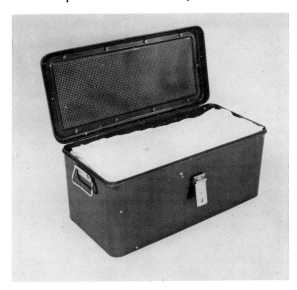

Figure 9-10. Rectangular metal casket popular in many hospitals in European countries. There is a filter insert in cover and base; also a gasket seal between cover and body of casket.

nesses of muslin covering. This covering of muslin serves as an air filter to eliminate dust when air is drawn in following removal of the drum from the sterilizer. Loaded in this manner, sterilization should occur in 30 minutes exposure of 250°F (121°C).

Stainless steel, enamelware or other metal jars and cans are commonly used in hospitals for containing gauze squares, cotton balls, and small dressings for floor use. This type of container is suitable only for loose dressings, and it should never be filled with tightly compressed materials. Figure 9-11 shows the correct and incorrect way to place jars or other nonporous containers of dry material in the sterilizer. When placed in the sterilizer upright, with or without the loose fitting cover in place, air cannot escape, and it will be difficult, if not impossible, to effect sterilization in any reasonable period of exposure. By placing the jar on its side in the sterilizer, with the cover removed or held loosely in place by means of pressure-sensitive tape, the air will drain out slowly and steam will take its place as indicated by the arrows. Tightly wrapped articles should never be placed in jars or other nonporous containers because the admission of steam during sterilization is retarded by having to enter at the open end and traverse the depth of the jar. Any container of the type shown in Figure 9-11, used for the storage of materials, and which is opened for withdrawal of the contents many times during the day, is nothing more than a communal device. Each time the jar is opened contamination is admitted. It contributes to the hazard of cross-

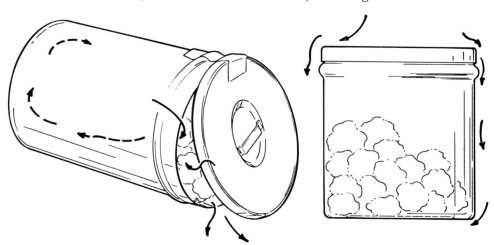

FIGURE 9-11. Correct and incorrect ways to place metal jars or cans containing dressings in sterilizers. Right side up, even with cover removed, air is trapped in container. Resting on its side, with cover held loosely in place, air will drain out and steam will take its place as indicated by arrows. Continued usage of such containers should not be permitted.

contamination and works against the interest of better patient care. The patient deserves the individually packaged and sterilized article, not something that has been exposed to a variety of contaminants a dozen or more times per day.

The problem of jar sterilization furnishes the background for another important principle governing sterilization of several articles, e.g. delicate instruments or hollow needles placed in glass or metal tubes. If the tube or jar is closed, steam cannot enter, and the only sterilizing effect will be that of dry heat developed from the surrounding steam. *An excellent rule to follow when sterilizing any dry material in a jar or tube is to imagine that the container is filled with water. Then place it in the sterilizer in a horizontal position so that the water would drain out freely.*

Arrangement of Load in Sterilizer

The fundamental rule in loading the sterilizer is to prepare all packs and arrange the load in such a manner as to present the least possible resistance to the passage of steam through the load, from the top of the chamber toward the bottom. Packs containing sheets, table covers, towels, which constitute the difficult-to-permeate-with-steam group must be placed in the sterilizer so that they rest on edge, rather than flat side down, in order to permit prompt and complete permeation of the materials with the moisture and heat of the steam.

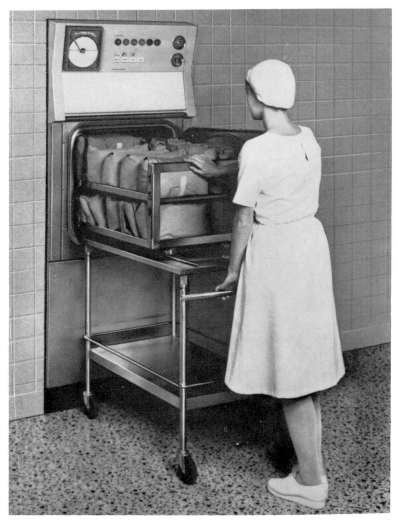

FIGURE 9-12. Good example of proper arrangement of load for moderate-size sterilizer. All packs rest on edge in loose contact with each other.

Figure 9-12 is a good example of proper arrangement of the load for a moderate size sterilizer. All packs are resting on edge, in loose contact with each other. When placing two layers of packs on one shelf, the upper layer should be placed crosswise on the lower layer. This is recommended as routine practice in order to promote free circulation of steam to the lower packs. Avoid compressing and jamming of the packs into a tight mass, and above all, do not overload the sterilizer.

In loading small cylindrical or square-shaped sterilizers with bulk goods, the operator should be aware of the purpose of the perforated or wire-mesh tray in the bottom of the chamber. As air is released from the load, it gravitates downward to the space underneath the tray and then flows into the chamber discharge outlet. If this tray is omitted or if it becomes flattened so that it conforms to the shape of the sterilizer, the back end of the chamber will become air clogged. Sterilization will then be seriously retarded and, in addition, the goods resting on the bottom will become saturated with water. Examine the tray frequently and make sure that it does elevate the load slightly above the bottom of the chamber.

Another example of good loading practice for a large sterilizer is shown in Figure 9-13. Here it will be observed that there are no oversized packs and all are placed on edge, without crowding, to facilitate free access for steam penetration. Properly arranged loads in large sterilizers can be sterilized just as effectively as in small chambers. In some respects, the large chamber equipped with shelf-type loading car does not present the problem apparent in small sterilizers. The shelves automatically provide an open space between tiers or layers of packs as a passageway for steam.

The size of the sterilizer or the amount of material placed in it is not the determining factor in fixing the period of exposure. The exposure must be determined initially by the size of the largest and most compact pack in the load. Then if these packs are arranged properly, it matters not whether the sterilizer contains one pack or fifty. The only factor subject to change under that condition will be the time required for the temperature to reach the sterilizing range, as indicated by the thermometer. With heavy loads, in a gravity displacement sterilizer, the temperature will rise more slowly.

Superheating of Fabrics During Sterilization

The effect of steam sterilization on desiccated cotton fabrics produces a condition known as superheat, causing deterioration of the materials and the attendant possibility of failure to sterilize. This subject is little understood by those responsible for the sterilization of surgical dressings. Before explaining the causes of this condition, it is necessary to define the meaning of superheat. The term comes from our knowledge of the properties of steam. *Superheated steam is steam the temperature of which exceeds that of saturated steam at the same pressure.* It is produced by the addition of heat to saturated steam which has been removed from contact with the water from which it was generated. A similar condition occurs when dehydrated or thoroughly dried fabrics are subjected to steam sterilization, or when water is adsorbed by cellulose fibers. The temperature of the fabric exceeds that of the surrounding steam, rising as much as 15° to 20°F (8° to 11°C) higher than the temperature of the steam in the sterilizer. When this occurs, it exerts a destructive effect on the strength of the cloth fibers which, of course, hastens deterioration of the material. Historically, it is interesting to

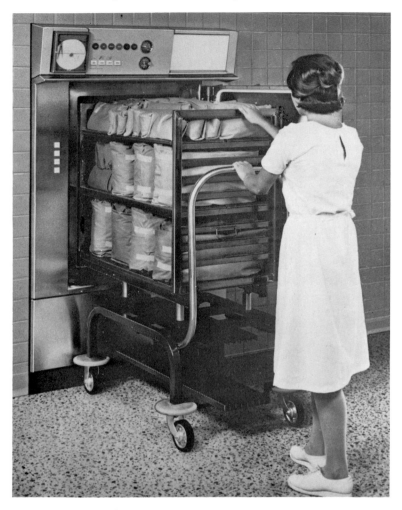

FIGURE 9-13. Another example of good loading practice for large surgical supply sterilizer. All packs are resting on edge with some space between them for free circulation of steam.

note that superheating of dressings occurred to a much greater degree when materials of low moisture content were preheated in the autoclave with steam in jacket only for long periods of time before sterilization.

Freshly laundered fabrics, if sterilized promptly, do not undergo superheating. The reason for this is that the fibers are in a relatively normal state of hydration prior to sterilization. On the other hand, if fabrics are stored in areas of low humidity for even brief periods of time, they give up some of their normal residual moisture content to the atmosphere. Then, when subjected to sterilization, the fibers adsorb additional water from the steam, thereby releasing excess latent heat (heat of adsorption) which results in superheating of the fabrics. Henry[13] has discussed the physical processes occurring when cotton materials are sterilized within an autoclave. He claims that the amount of moisture which a textile contains at equilibrium with its surroundings is dependent upon the relative humidity. Also, the ability of dressings to adsorb further moisture diminishes as their temperature exceeds that of steam, and there soon comes a point where a temporary state of *quasi-equilibrium* is reached and the temperature ceases to rise. Findings by Knox, Penikett, and Duncan[14] showed that dressings containing 1 per cent or less of moisture may superheat as high as 14° to 16°F (8° to 9°C).

The cumulative effect of superheating of textiles has been carefully studied by Walter.[15] His findings showed that samples of freshly laundered (hydrated) textiles lost 50 per cent of their tensile strength after seventy trips through the laundry and sterilizer, while identical samples which were repeatedly sterilized without laundering lost 73 per cent of their tensile strength. The control samples which were laundered only, lost 20 per cent of their tensile strength. Johnston[16] has presented further evidence on this subject to the effect that fabrics which were sterilized twenty times without laundering lost 50 per cent of their tensile strength. Results from a more recent study conducted in the author's laboratory are shown in Figure 9-14. Samples of new textiles subjected to a routine laundering process only for a total of fifty cycles showed an average loss in tensile strength of 7 per cent. Identical samples subjected to fifty cycles of laundering and sterilization at 250°F (121°C) for 30 minutes showed an average loss in tensile strength of 27 per cent. Simultaneously, a third series of identical textile samples were subjected to repeated sterilization only and, after fifty cycles, the average loss amounted to 68 per cent. These data indicate the economic advantages attendant with the use of freshly laundered fabrics.

To effectively guard against the problem of superheating, the hospital should institute control measures to ensure several points:

—Freshly laundered fabrics are used only for supplies undergoing sterilization.
—Freshly laundered fabrics are not subjected to storage in areas of low humidity prior to sterilization.
—Surgical packs and other wrapped supplies are not subjected to preheating in the sterilizer, with steam in jacket only, prior to sterilization.
—Sterilizers are not operated with steam at a higher pressure and temperature in the jacket than in the chamber.

Drying of Load Following Sterilization

While dressings are undergoing sterilization, the fabrics become saturated with moisture, the condensate left in the goods as heat is adsorbed from the steam which permeates them. This moisture, finely distributed through the

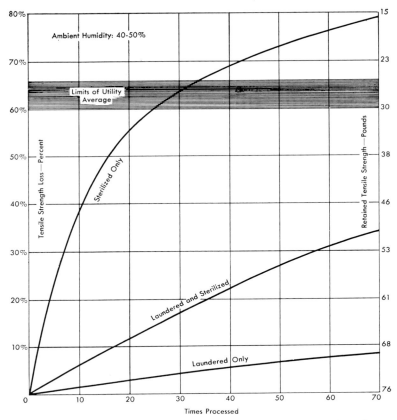

FIGURE 9-14. Loss in tensile strength of textiles subjected to routine laundering process, laundering plus sterilization, and sterilization only.

load, is at the same temperature as the surrounding steam, namely 250°F (121°C). The same condition prevails at the close of exposure time, but immediately when pressure reduces, with the exhaust of steam, the moisture flashes into steam or vapor, brought about by the residual heat in the goods —above the boiling point of water—and the heat conducted to them from the hot steam jacket. The real drying process then resolves itself into the detail of getting rid of the vapor as fast as it forms.

There are three well-known systems of drying in common use, any one of which will give good results if performed correctly.

The simplest method known is to exhaust the steam from the chamber to zero gauge pressure, leaving the jacket pressure on to keep the walls of the chamber hot. When chamber pressure has been exhausted, unlock the door and open it slightly, about ¼ inch, just enough to permit vapor to escape. This will provide a chimney effect in which room air will enter at the bottom of the door, while vapor mixed with this air will escape at the top of the door. An interval of 15 to 20 minutes will usually suffice to dry the load satisfactorily. Objectionably, this method permits all vapor to escape into the room. It is commonly employed on the classical gravity displacement type sterilizers.

The second method involves principles common to older systems with the added feature of being able to exhaust practically all vapor to the vent. The system employs a venturi (suction device) in the multiport valve which creates a reduced pressure in the chamber following the sterilizing phase of the cycle. It is used in this manner: Following sterilization, pressure is exhausted to zero gauge, then the multiport valve moves to the dry position. Instead of creating a partial vacuum the venturi device functions as a pump to circulate filtered air to the chamber where it entrains with the vapor and odors and all are then discharged to the vent (see Fig. 9-15). This method has the advantage of disposing of all vapor before the door is opened. The filter is so designed as to be self-sterilizing with each cycle. The minimum drying time is 20 minutes for the average load of fabrics. There is very little difference in drying efficiency by either of the above methods. The latter system possesses the advantage of preventing vapor from escaping into the room, a detail worthy of consideration, especially in the interests of air-conditioning.

The third system is associated with sterilizers equipped with efficient vacuum pumps for the mechanical removal of air from the chamber and the load. At the conclusion of the sterilizing phase the chamber is exhausted quickly to atmospheric pressure, followed by evacuation of the chamber to

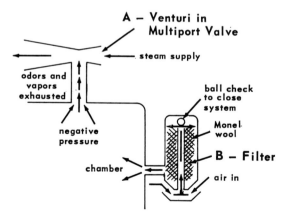

FIGURE 9-15. In gravity air removal sterilizers, a venturi in the multiport valve (A) creates a reduced chamber pressure following sterilization of fabrics or wrapped goods. This reduction in pressure allows air to be admitted to chamber through the Monel wool-packed filter (B). Resulting circulating air entrains and exhausts vapors and odors from chamber. System permits effective drying with sterilizer door(s) closed. Filter is self sterilized with each cycle.

approximately 50 Torr. At this point the cotton materials are almost as dry as when they were placed in the sterilizer. The final chamber vacuum is relieved to atmospheric pressure by means of air drawn through a bacteria-retentive filter. This system is capable of drying an average load of fabrics in 6 to 8 minutes.

State of Dryness

Dryness of the load following sterilization is a function of the equilibrium established between the vapor pressure over the load and the pressure in the chamber. In other words, the lower the chamber pressure the more rapid will be the release of moisture from the goods. Also, the dryness of the load at the end of the cycle will be related to the initial moisture content of the materials. This means that if surgical packs are wet when placed in the sterilizer, or if they are made wet by poor quality steam, they will continue to be wet when removed from the sterilizer. Most fabrics stored under normal atmospheric conditions show a moisture content of 3 to 6 per cent.

It has been determined that a large surgical pack, weighing 12 pounds, adsorbs 18 ounces of moisture as condensate from the steam in the normal sterilizing process. This is representative of a 9 per cent increase in weight and this amount of moisture must be removed during the drying process in order to restore the material to its original condition. The application of a terminal vacuum to 100 Torr reduced the moisture content to about 2 per cent of the original weight. At 40 Torr the moisture content of the pack was reduced to less than 1 per cent—a satisfactory value. Surgical dressings in the subjectively dry state contain about 5 per cent moisture. Observations by Penikett, Rowe, and Robson[17] indicate that towels begin to feel damp when they contain as little as 6 per cent moisture. For practical purposes, experience dictates that a terminal vacuum of 40 to 50 Torr produces dry dressings. This value should be attained in about 6 to 7 minutes in a fully loaded average capacity (12 cu ft) sterilizer.

Recontamination of Sterilized Goods

Surgical supplies may become contaminated during their removal from the sterilizer, in transport from one area to another, and during subsequent storage in operating rooms or nursing units. Darmady[18] *et al.* for example, found 23 per cent of the dressings to be contaminated in some wards.

The proper handling of sterilized packs as they are removed from the sterilizer demands that they never be stacked up in close contact with each other, but rather maintained in such a position that air can circulate freely around them, on all sides. When loading carriages are used, it is good practice to leave the load on the carriage, after removing from the sterilizer, for 15 or 20 minutes. If no loading carriage is used, the packs should be laid out on edge, preferably on a wire mesh or slatted wooden surface covered with several layers of muslin to absorb the sweating moisture.

Dressings delivered from the sterilizer in a wet or soggy condition present a definite hazard and they should never be sent to the operating room. Even when dressings are well dried out in the sterilizer sufficient vapor remains in the goods so that sudden cooling may result in condensate forming objectionably—perhaps dangerously. It is unwise to place freshly sterilized packs or other wrapped supplies on any cold surface such as a metal table top. The sweating that occurs on the cool table top will accumulate in little pools of water which may pick up contamination. In turn, this contaminated water may be reabsorbed by the fabric rendering it unsterile. Probst[19] has demonstrated clearly that once sterile cloth becomes damp, even if the water source is sterile, it allows contamination to take place provided it is in contact with an unsterile object. Beck and Collette[20] also proved that bacteria readily pass through two layers of wet cloth whereas two layers of dry cloth prevent such migration. The permeability of wet surgical drapes to *Staphylococcus aureus* has been studied by Karlson, Riley, and Dennis.[21] Two layers of wet linen are unlikely to prevent passage of organisms to the surgical field. Three layers were found to offer substantially greater security against the passage of organisms.

In discussing recontamination of sterilized articles, it is well to keep in mind that the floor of any room presents a highly contaminated surface, regardless of sanitary precautions which may prevail. Resistant bacterial spores are carried to work rooms on the feet of visitors and hospital personnel. For this reason any sterilized pack which may have fallen to the floor accidentally should be rejected for use. Moreover, it should become standard practice to avoid any unnecessary handling of sterilized packs and arrange for the nearest approach to "sterile" storage that conditions will permit.

Causes of Wet Dressings

In addition to faulty methods of packaging and loading, there are other conditions responsible for wet dressings. Most of these require the attention of a trained serviceman or maintenance engineer for correction. Those of major importance are the following:

—*Clogging of chamber discharge line on sterilizer.* If the air and condensate discharge line becomes clogged with sediment and lint, or if the thermostatic valve or check valve fails to open properly, water will collect in the bottom of the chamber and the lower portion of the load will not dry satisfactorily. This fault will be indicated by the presence of water in the bottom of the chamber when the door is opened. If no water is found in the chamber, but if the lower portion of the load is perceptibly wet, that will indicate sluggish performance of the discharge system. In either case, the remedy is to clean out the line and check the operation of the thermostatic valve.

—*Improperly drained steam supply line.* An improperly drained steam supply line may deliver water to the sterilizer instead of steam. If this fault is pronounced, both jacket and chamber will fill with water and the load will be saturated. There is only one remedy for this difficulty. The steam supply line must be adequately drained before it reaches the sterilizer by a correctly trapped bleeder line. An indication of water in the supply line or a clogged return trap from the jacket of the sterilizer is a loud hammering noise which occurs when steam is turned on to the sterilizer.

—*Overfilling steam generator with water.* On electric or gas heated sterilizers, wet dressings are sure to occur as the result of overfilling the boiler or steam generator with water. This usually occurs through carelessness of the operator in not shutting off the filling valve when the proper level has been reached. It may also occur by slow leakage of the water filling valve.

—*Faulty sterilizer installation.* An occasional cause of wet dressings is the incorrectly installed sterilizer with the back end lower than the front end. In this case, condensate will drain to the rear and the vapor forming from it will saturate the goods. This can be easily corrected by adjusting the supports on the sterilizer so that the front end is slightly lower than the back end.

CARE AND STERILIZATION OF RUBBER GOODS

The handling, washing, and sterilizing of rubber goods presents special problems to the hospital. As a rule, rubber goods do not wear out—they are destroyed. Rubber will deteriorate with age, exposure to light, heat, and chemicals, but the life of any rubber article is materially shortened by abuse and careless handling. With the exception of the synthetic products, rubber is of vegetable origin, and sunlight, heat, oils, greases and solvents are natural enemies of rubber. While contact with these substances, including light, cannot be avoided in normal hospital routine, it is suggested that care be exercised to remove any oils, greases, or solvents thoroughly and as soon as possible.

Disposable and Reusable Surgeon's Gloves

The purchase and one-time use of prepackaged disposable surgeon's gloves continues to increase in popularity in hospitals. This development is the natural outcome of a systematic search for methods of making more efficient use of nursing time and skills. The greatest contribution of disposables, in general, in the voluntary hospital system is not in saving money but in providing a higher degree of patient safety and comfort and in effecting standardization. At present, there is no evidence to show, beyond the opinion stage, that adoption of disposables in American hospitals helps in the control of cross-infection. Hospital *practices* more than hospital *supplies* determine the incidence of cross-infection. The outlook for the future of disposable medical products is one of definite optimism for increased usage. The use of a disposable, whether a surgeon's glove, a plastic device, or some other article, does not necessarily imply an intrinsically safe product. Hospital personnel, particularly the professional staff, must accept the responsibility as to "where is the greater risk of human error in faulty processing—in the hospital or in the factory?"

Rubber Gloves

Many institutions continue to reprocess in fairly large numbers the reusable gloves for use in the operating room and for examining purposes. It is for this group that the following details are directed.

Before new gloves are put into use, they should be washed to remove any powder or residue which may be on them. The irritants occasionally present in rubber gloves can be removed by soaking in a 5% solution of sodium carbonate for 15 minutes, followed by rinsing and sterilization. The life of the gloves can be prolonged by permitting them to rest for 48 hours after steam sterilization and before recirculation into general use.

Immediately following an operation, the gloves should be washed off under cold water before removal from the hands. This step should be performed with caution in order to prevent splattering and to avoid the release of aerosols into the environment. If a brush is used to loosen any adhering particles of blood or debris, the action should take place with the hands and brush submerged under water. After removing the gloves from the hands, place them in a plastic container, and deliver to the central service department or the laundry for machine washing. The soaking of gloves for long periods of time is not recommended because water is absorbed, the gloves become tacky, and the drying cycle is prolonged. From this point onward the processing of gloves involves the following sequence of operations:

—*Washing and Drying.* Thorough washing and rinsing to remove all traces of soil and detergent is essential. A commercial rotary washer offers many advantages over home models. A water temperature of 90° to 105°F (32° to 41°C) is satisfactory with a mild, low-sudsing detergent. NOTE: If gloves are soiled with blood, the temperature of the wash water must be raised to at least 180°F (82°C).[22] The drying temperature should not exceed 100°F (38°C), otherwise tackiness may occur. To reduce tackiness during drying, glove powder should be added to the final rinse at the rate of 8 ounces to 5 gallons of water. The drying time depends largely on the number of gloves in the dryer.

—*Resting Period.* Gloves should be held for a minimum of 8 hours after washing, rinsing, and drying for regain of tensile strength. Latex rubber is weakest when wet, and defects will occur if testing is carried out prior to adequate dry and rest.

—*Testing and Sorting.* Gloves should be inspected for defects and sorted as to quality and size: *good* (no defects and of good tensile strength) and *rejects* (defects such as holes, tears, or poor tensile strength). Gloves may be tested by inflating them by hand or by using a machine to distend them with nitrogen. Since many new gloves contain minute holes, an adequate testing method should be available in the hospital for evaluating new gloves before use.

—*Powdering.* Gloves should be powdered according to the manufacturer's recommendations. The hazards of glove powder are well documented and, if it must be used, it should be used as sparingly as possible.

—*Packaging.* Sort according to size and type, right and left. Place paper or muslin inserts within palm and cuff of gloves to facilitate air removal and steam intake. Use inner wraps for surgical gloves. Then wrap in steam permeable paper or double thickness muslin. Label.

—*Sterilizing.* Glove packages should be sterilized by exposure to saturated steam at 250°F (121°C) for 20 minutes. If sterilization is to be conducted in a prevacuum high temperature sterilizer the manufacturer's operating instructions should be followed. Ethylene oxide gas may also be used for sterilization of gloves, followed by an aeration period of 96 hours. Affix sterilization control number and date to each package.

—*Quarantine.* After sterilization gloves should be held in temporary storage for a minimum of 24 hours, preferably 48 hours, before distribution for general use. This permits regain of tensile strength and prolongs life of the gloves.

—*Storage.* Gloves should be stored where they will be protected from excessive light, natural or artificial, and from excessive heat.

The manual washing of gloves, one-at-a-time, hanging them individually on racks or glove trees to dry, and powdering each one inside and outside, by hand, are elements of an outmoded technique which has given way to a mechanized process, utilizing labor-saving machines and devices.

Today most hospitals are aware of the advantages of mechanical aids in the processing of gloves. Automatic washers, glove conditioners, and dryers are used in many hospitals with a high degree of efficiency and economy. Some of the larger institutions send all of their gloves to the main hospital laundry for processing. However, experience has shown that the key to a successful mechanized operation for the average hospital is the establishment of a glove-processing room as a part of the central service department. All of the above operations can then be performed in a centralized area and the various related tasks can be turned over to nonprofessional workers. A typical layout for a modern glove reprocessing room is shown as part of the central service layout (see Fig. 15-3). The individual mechanical equipment items shown on this plan include an automatic washer, glove dryer, powderer, and a surgical glove tester. It has been estimated[23] that the processing of 1000 pairs of reusable gloves requires about 53.3 hours of personnel time. To process 30,000 pairs of gloves a year would require the services of one full-time employee just for this task.

Following the washing, drying, and resting period, the gloves are tested for miniscule holes or defects. Each glove is inflated with compressed air supplied by the glove tester in order to detect a leak. Alternate methods for testing of gloves are available. Beck and Carlson,[24] for example, described a simple glove tester for the central service units which operates on the principle of magnifying the size of a hole or defect in the glove by producing a difference in the air pressure inside ond outside of the glove. Under this difference in pressure, the hole is stretched to the point where the flow of air quickly shows up as a loss of vacuum on the exterior of the glove. A few seconds suffice for the test. Russell *et al.*[25] have described recently an electrical glove-testing instrument. This operates on the principle of a loss in electrical resistance when a hole is present in a glove.

The glove tester shown in Figure 9-16 requires air and electricity for operation. When a glove is placed over the manifold, air is pumped in to a point where the pressure of the expanding glove makes contact with a microswitch beneath the screen. If during a period of about 4 seconds there is sufficient air loss to relieve pressure on the microswitch, a light appears on

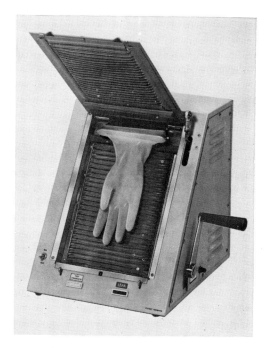

FIGURE 9-16. Glove tester. Air is pumped into glove to a point where pressure of distended glove makes contact with microswitch and then air supply is cut off. If during period of few seconds there is reduction in pressure on microswitch due to air loss, glove is rejected as a "leaker."

the front of the tester and the glove is rejected as a "leaker." Gloves found to be punctured should be discarded. An attempt to mend defective gloves with liquid glove patch or by other means is economically not feasible.

Hazards of Glove Powder

The hazards of powdering the hands of surgeons and using powder on surgical gloves, drains, and tubing prior to sterilization are not fully appreciated. The problem is of dual significance to the hospital. First, there is the ever-present danger to the patient of postoperative complications of powder granulomata; second, the fallout of powder from the hands and gloves provides a prime vehicle for dissemination of microorganisms throughout the institution. The organisms become attached to dust particles as they sediment to the floor and they are then transmitted from one area to another by air currents and on the soles of shoes of people.

As early as 1933, Antopol[26] called attention to the hazard of using lycopodium powder on gloves and other rubber articles because of the possibility of postoperative complications. Later, Seelig and his coworkers[27,28] pointed out to surgeons the irritating and dangerous properties of talcum powder. In 1949, starch powder was introduced to the surgical profession as a glove lubricant.[29] It had excellent physical properties, and it was described as relatively innocuous. Since that time several reports[30,31,32,33] have appeared in the literature showing that starch or a starch-derivative powder is not inert and its use may result in severe granulomatous lesions and adhesions in the abdominal cavity. A recent report by Yunis and Landes[34] emphasizes the importance of avoiding contamination of catheters, syringes, and contrast media by glove powder while assembling equipment for renal angiography.

The use of powder as a lubricant for gloves and the hands in the operating room should be abolished. The propensity of powder to contaminate wounds and to adversely influence environmental sanitation should be of concern to all professional personnel. Liquid and cream lubricants have been developed as substitutes for glove powder with the added feature of maintaining a low bacterial count in the glove.[36,37] There is still room for further developments in this field.

If powder must be used it should be distributed sparingly over the object with the thought in mind of the future fallout pattern. In addition, a scrupulous preoperative lavage of gloves should be mandatory. Other latex articles such as Penrose drains and tubes should be treated in the same manner. If a glove is punctured or torn, it should be immediately replaced and the fresh glove washed before the wearer returns to the surgical field.

Packaging and Sterilization

Although not commonly recognized, rubber gloves constitute one of the most difficult of all items to be sterilized in the hospital. The reason is obviously not one of steam penetration through successive layers of material but rather ineffective air removal from the fingers of the gloves. Care must be used in the packaging and wrapping of the gloves to insure that all surfaces shall be freely exposed to the steam as shown in Figure 9-17. Where the wrist section of the glove is folded back to form the cuff, it is important to keep the two surfaces separated from each other. This can be done by placing a band of gauze or muslin under the fold when the wrist section is turned back. It is also suggested that a pad of gauze or muslin be inserted in the palm of each glove, as far in as the fingers, to hold the apposing surfaces apart and to promote egress of air and intake of steam. The chief factor to keep in mind in packaging is to prepare the glove so that no pressure is applied which might force any two surfaces into tight contact with each other.

Gloves are preferably sterilized alone, not in combination with other bulk loads of supplies. The gloves should rest on edge (horizontally) in the sterilizer with the thumbs uppermost, and the packs well away from the sidewalls of the chamber. A large wire basket makes an ideal container for glove packs (Fig. 9-18). It is imperative that the gloves be stacked loosely, never more than one tier deep. They cannot be sterilized on top of each other because compression of the bottom of the pile prevents access of steam. The baskets should always be placed in the upper two-thirds of the sterilizing chamber, not on the bottom shelf. Residual air present in the lower portion of the chamber, even as little as 0.1 per cent, will hasten the rate of deterioration of rubber. For sterilization, an exposure period of not less than 15 minutes and no longer than 20 minutes at 250° to 254°F is recommended, followed by a minimum of 15 minutes drying. After sterilization the gloves should be held in storage for a period of 24 to 48 hours before dispensing for use. This will help the rubber to regain its tensile strength, prevent tackiness

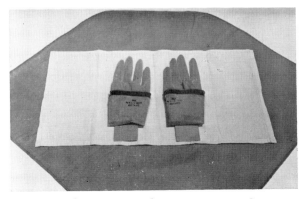

FIGURE 9-17. In wrapping gloves for sterilization, it is good practice to insert paper or cloth separators under turned-back cuffs and inside palms (as far in as fingers) of gloves. This permits exchange of air for steam. Billfold-type muslin cover is commonly used for wrapping gloves. Outer wrapper, 18 inches square, is used for added protection.

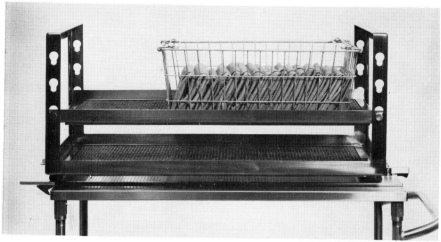

FIGURE 9-18. Wire basket ideal container for gloves. Packs should rest on edge in sterilizer with thumbs uppermost. Place basket in upper two-thirds of the chamber.

and the useful life will be prolonged. Gloves sterilized by ethylene oxide gas are not subject to noticeable tackiness, and their rate of deterioration as the result of resterilization is much less.

Glove Punctures

The leakage of skin bacteria through a punctured glove into the surgical wound is recognized as one of the agents with high potential for causing wound infections. Cole,[37] for example, has demonstrated that as many as 40,000 organisms can pass through a single hole made by a #18 neeedle in a 20-minute period. This possibility gains significance when it is remembered that under best conditions the incidence of glove punctures may range from 10 to 35 per cent.[38,39,40,25] Another point deserving of mention is that no matter how long one scrubs or what agent is used, it is virtually impossible to remove all bacteria from the hands. In practice, this means that the only effective barrier between bacteria on the surgeon's hands and the wound is the intact surgical glove.

A recent study by Gad[41] on glove damage as a route of wound infection indicated that one-third of all glove punctures occurred in the thumbs and index fingers. Surgeons were responsible for 46 per cent of the damaged gloves; nurses were second with 32 per cent. His findings also showed that 1.4 per cent of new gloves, still in the manufacturer's packaging, were defective. Others [25] have found approximately 12 per cent of the gloves to have holes in them before use in the operating room. This latter point stresses the importance of thorough testing of all presterilized, disposable gloves immediately before use. It also indicates that the introduction of a glove-testing device in the operating room to periodically check for glove defects during the course of an operation could be a practical adjunct to aseptic surgery. For those concerned with the processing and use of surgical gloves the requirement is clear—conscientious checking of all gloves (reusable or disposable) for punctures or defects. Also, the sooner leaks are discovered, the less will be the number of bacteria which gain entrance into surgical wounds via this route.

Catheters, Drains, and Tubes

All articles made of rubber, especially latex and red rubber, are highly susceptible to attack and deterioration by chemical agents. No rubber article should be subjected to cleaning agents made of or containing hydrocarbons, oxidizing acids, or oils. The following substances are known to cause deterioration and they will destroy the usefulness of all articles made of rubber.

- Mineral and vegetable oils (petroleum jelly, mineral oil) and oil containing cleansing agents, particularly green soap, cause swelling, tackiness, and final deterioration.
- Hydrocarbon solvents, chlorinated hydrocarbons, ethers and esters (acetone, benzene, cleaning fluids) cause swelling and rapid deterioration.
- Oxidizing agents (sulfuric and hydrochloric acids, lye, sodium hypochlorite) cause rapid deterioration.
- Copper and manganese (ionic concentration of 0.001%) causes rapid catalytic decomposition. Avoid permanganate solutions.
- Phenols, cresols, and terpenes (Lysol, carbolic acid, hexachlorophene, essential oils, soaps containing phenol or phenyl compounds) cause stickiness and disintegration.
- Quaternary ammonium compounds such as benzalkonium chloride cause tackiness and decrease resistance to steam sterilization. If the article has been disinfected in a quaternary ammonium compound, it should not be autoclaved later. The pores of the latex absorb the quaternary.
- Volatile amine compounds (morpholine, benzylamine, and cyclohexylamine) contribute to rubber deterioration. Some hospitals add volatile amine compounds to their steam boilers to protect the supply lines against corrosion. Since the compounds are volatile, they will be present in the steam during sterilization and thereby contribute to deterioration of rubber.
- Ozone—generated by fluorescent lights, electric motors and diathermy apparatus. Rubber articles should be stored in the dark and remote from sources of ozone generation.

Prior to sterilization, rubber catheters should be cleaned with an alkaline detergent such as trisodium phosphate or household Oakite®, followed by copious rinsing with water. (Do not use harsh cleaning methods with stiff brushes.) To cleanse the lumen, water should be forced through the catheter with a syringe. This permits the rubber to become hydrated, and if sterilized promptly superheating will not occur. A dry catheter upon contact with steam will undergo deterioration as the result of superheating. Catheters may be packaged in muslin, sterilizable cellophane tubing, or in long paper envelopes, several of which are commercially available. When catheters are packaged in this manner, one end of the tubing is left open to provide ready access for steam, and to prevent bursting of the tubing which is not uncommon when the package is sterilized with both ends closed. When sterilized by saturated steam the exposure period should be 20 minutes at 250°F. All catheters and tubing require moisture in the lumen to convert to steam and thereby purge the air. This can be accomplished by flushing with distilled water, leaving a few drops of water in the lumen, just prior to steam sterilization. In the case of soft, flat drains, care should be taken to ensure that they are not folded when packaged, steam must circulate through the lumen. In the case of prevacuum high-temperature sterilizers the exposure period is usually fixed for 4 minutes at 270°F.

The above conditions regarding preparation and sterilization of rubber catheters apply equally to vinyl catheters and perfusion tubing, with the exception that sterilization should be restricted to the lower temperature range. Care should be taken in coiling and wrapping to prevent kinks and crushing. Vinyl catheters should be laid out perfectly straight because if curled or bent, they may take a set and not straighten out. Moisture will temporarily cloud vinyl tubing after sterilization, but its original clarity can be restored by storage at room temperature for 24 hours. Gas sterilization by ethylene oxide may also be used, provided that ample preuse storage time is allowed for dissipation of the residual gas from the material. Polyethylene tubing is a heat-labile plastic. It can not be sterilized in the autoclave. Ethylene oxide gas or gamma irradiation are the only satisfactory sterilizing agents for this material.

Catheters, T tubes, drains, thoracotomy tubes, and other articles that are stored in the operating suite for occasional use should be individually packaged. The practice should be discouraged of keeping such articles in jars or boats into which the circulating nurse must reach repeatedly with pickup forceps. The repeated opening of these containers increases the chance for contamination. This is another example of a communal container—an outmoded technique.

Woven Catheters, Bougies, and Filiforms

Woven catheters are used primarily for either diagnostic or treatment purposes. The coating on the catheters is composed of synthetic resinous materials which absorb water, especially in the presence of heat. The principal chemical agents which cause deterioration of woven catheters are alcohol, cresols, phenols, glycerin, and *alkali detergents*.

Before sterilization, the catheters should be thoroughly cleaned in a solution free from alkali or organic solvents. Water containing a mild liquid soap is recommended. Green soap containing glycerin or phenol or solutions of trisodium phosphate should not be used. The cleaning agent should be forced through the lumen either by means of a syringe or siphon. Copious rinsing should be avoided because of the possibility of forcing too much moisture into the catheter surface. After cleaning, the catheter should be wrapped in muslin, without bending or coiling, and sterilized with steam under pressure at 250°F for 20 minutes. After the catheter has been used for the first time, it should again be cleaned and thoroughly dried out before being sterilized the second time. This may be accomplished by placing the catheter in a warm dry area and leaving it there for 3 or 4 days, or by drying it out in the sterilizer with steam to jacket only for 15 minutes. Once a catheter has been properly dried out after the first sterilization and use, the physical structure of the coating changes so that subsequent sterilizations will not develop blisters or cracks. Do not autoclave catheters which have been boiled or soaked in any quaternary ammonium compound.

Tubing—Rubber and Heat-resistant Plastic

Sterilization of rubber tubing is not difficult, provided proper attention is given to the preliminary details of the process. Thorough preliminary cleaning is essential for safe preparation of new tubing to remove impurities and also for used tubing which may contain traces of blood or residual drugs. In the case of transfusion tubing, drainage or suction tubing, the practice should be rigidly enforced of thorough rinsing in cold water immediately after use to prevent blood or body secretions from drying in the lumen. Effective cleaning may be accomplished by immersing the tubing in a large basin containing a 0.5% solution of sodium hydroxide or 5% sodium carbonate and boiling for 15 minutes. The tubing should be coiled slowly into the solution to avoid the formation of air pockets, or better yet, the alkali solution should be circulated slowly through the tubing during the period of boiling. A large irrigating syringe may be used for this purpose or a reservoir of the alkali solution may be attached to a ring stand above the basin, connected to the tubing, and the solution slowly trickled through the lumen. After cleaning, the tubing should be rinsed with freshly distilled water until all traces of alkali have been removed.

For sterilization, and just before wrapping, flush out the tubing and all connectors or attachments with distilled water, but do not drain completely. Rather, leave the interior distinctly moist and wrap in double thickness muslin. The tubing should be carefully coiled but not kinked in the package as in Figure 9-19. The residual moisture in the tubing plus the heat of the steam conducted to the interior will be sufficient for sterilization when exposed for 30 minutes at a temperature of 250°F (121°C) in a gravity displacement sterilizer.

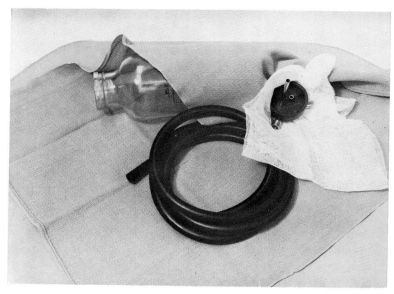

FIGURE 9-19. Stoppers and tubes should be separated from drainage bottles before sterilization. All parts of drainage sets should be protected by an inner wrapper.

Stoppers and tubes should be separated from drainage bottles. All parts of drainage sets should be protected by an inner wrapper. Irrigating (Asepto) syringes should be taken apart. Here also an inner wrap is necessary to hold the parts together and to prevent breakage. For the processing of plastic tubing and other molded plastic articles made of polyvinyl chloride, nylon, or polypropylene the manufacturer's recommendations should be followed.

SUMMARY OF DIRECTIVES GOVERNING STERILIZATION OF SURGICAL SUPPLIES

Packaging

· Use freshly laundered fabrics to guard against superheating.
· Use double-thickness muslin or other approved wrapping material for supplies.
· Limit the size and density of individual linen packs to ensure uniform steam permeation with a liberal margin of safety for sterilization. Contents of the pack should be arranged so that layers of fabrics are all parallel to one another.

Loading of Sterilizer

· Remove all shelving from loading car. Load from bottom up, adding shelves above each layer of supplies. If some items are higher than others, they may be placed on half of the car and a half-shelf placed over lower objects.

· Place all packs (linen, gloves, and others) on edge and arrange the load in the sterilizer so as to present the least possible resistance to the passage of steam through the load.
· Place all jars and other nonporous containers of dry material on their sides in the sterilizer so as to provide a horizontal path for the escape of air and to facilitate drying.
· Place treatment trays and utensils on edge so they will dry properly.
· Instrument sets assembled in trays with mesh or perforated bottoms may be placed flat on shelves of loading car to keep contents in order.
· When fabrics and hard goods are combined in the same load, the hard goods (jars, utensils, and treatment trays) should be placed on bottom or lower shelves of loading car. This will prevent wetting of fabric packs from condensate formed on hard surfaces. The drying phase of the sterilizing cycle must be adequate for a combination load.
· Rubber gloves should be sterilized separately, not in combination with other bulk loads of supplies, unless the operating instructions of the particular sterilizer indicate otherwise. In any event, the glove packages should rest on edge in trays placed in the upper two-thirds of the chamber, not on the bottom shelf.
· Plastic utensils should not be stacked, nested, or have other articles leaning against them; they may become misshapen.
· Liquids should always be sterilized in a separate load with a gravity air discharge method of operation.
· Small items are best handled in baskets.

Exposure Period

· Establish a standard exposure period for all bulk supplies that will provide for complete air elimination, complete steam penetration of the load, and ensure destruction of all microbial life with a liberal margin of safety.
· For sterilizers equipped with automatic controls and program selector, the actual exposure time and temperature must be known and recorded for a specific type of load. For manual operation of gravity displacement sterilizers, the exposure period should be timed from the moment that saturated steam at 250°F (121°C) fills the chamber as indicated by the thermometer in the chamber discharge line.

Drying of Load

· Establish a minimum drying period of 20 minutes for all bulk loads of supplies processed in gravity displacement type sterilizers. When utilizing prevacuum high-temperature sterilizers, the manufacturer's operating instructions should be followed and the degree of terminal vacuum recorded.
· Guard against the placement of freshly sterilized packages on cold surfaces. Avoid unnecessary handling of all sterile supplies.

REFERENCES

1. CHURCH, B. D.: Hospital laundry hazards leading to recontamination of washed bedding *Proc Nat Conf Institutionally Acquired Infections, Minneapolis, Sept. 4-6, 1963.* U S Dept H E W, Atlanta, Ga.
2. SPEERS, R., JR., AND SHOOTER, R. A.: Use of double-wrapped packs to reduce contamination of the sterile contents during extraction. *Lancet, II:*469-470, 1966.
3. FALLON, R. J.: Wrapping of sterilized articles. *Lancet, II:*785, 1963.
4. HUNTER, C. L. F.; HARBORD, P. E., AND RIDDETT, D. J.: *Packaging Papers as Bacterial Barriers. Symposium on Sterilisation of Surgical Materials, April 11-13, 1961.* London, Pharmaceutical Press.
5. BECK, C. E.; SHAY, D. E., AND PURDUM, W. A.: An evaluation of paper used for wrapping articles to be sterilized. *Bull Amer Soc Hosp Pharm 10:*421-427, 1953 (see also *Bull Amer Soc Hosp Pharm, 12:*511, 1955).
6. WALTER, C. W.: *Bull Amer Soc Hosp Pharm, 11:*317, 1954.
7. ALDER, V. G., AND ALDER, F. I.: Preserving the sterility of surgical dressings wrapped in paper and other materials. *J Clin Path, 14:*76-79, 1961.
8. WHITTENBERGER, J. L.: *Steam Sterilization of Paper-wrapped Packages.* Framingham, Mass., Dennison Mfg. Co., Sept., 1949.
9. CHRISTIE, J. E.: Muslin vs. paper autoclave wrappers—a hospital study. *Hospital Topics,* PT. I, 35:117-121; PT. II, 35:111-116, (March-April), 1957.
10. STURDY, J. H.; BAIRD, R. M., and GEREIN, A. N.: Surgical sponges: A cause of granuloma and adhesion formation. *Ann Surg, 165:*128-134, 1967.
11. WALTER, C. W.: *Aseptic Treatment of Wounds.* New York, Macmillan, 1948, pp. 97-98.
12. AMERICAN ACADEMY OF PEDIATRICS: *Hospital Care of Newborn Infants,* rev. ed. Evanston, Ill., 1964, p. 56.
13. HENRY, P. S. H.: Physical aspects of sterilizing cotton articles by steam. *J Appl Bact, 22:*159-173, 1959.
14. KNOX, R.; PENIKETT, E. J. K., and DUNCAN, M. E.: The avoidance of excessive superheating during steam sterilization of dressings. *J Appl Bact, 23:*21-27, 1959.
15. WALTER, C. W.: *Op. cit.,* p. 64.
16. JOHNSTON, L. G.: Personal communication, June 3, 1947.
17. PENIKETT, E. J. K.; ROWE, T. W. G., and ROBSON, E.: Vacuum drying of steam sterilized dressings. *J Appl Bact, 21:*282, 1958.
18. DARMADY, E. M.; HUGHES, K. E. A.; JONES, J. D., and VERDON, P. E.: Failure of sterility in hospital ward practice. *Lancet, I:*622-624, 1959.
19. PROBST, H. D.: The effect of bactericidal agents on the sterility of surgical linen. *Amer J Surg, 86:*301-308, 1953.
20. BECK, W. C., and COLLETTE, T. S.: False faith in the surgeon's gown and surgical drape. *Amer J Surg, 83:*125,1952.
21. KARLSON, K. E.; RILEY, W., and DENNIS, C.: A quantitative evaluation of the permeability of wet surgical drapes to *Staphylococcus aureus. Surg Forum, Vol. IX:*568-571, 1959.
22. EXPERT COMMITTEE on HEPATITIS: World Health Organization Tech. Report, Series No. 62, March 1953.
23. STRUVE, M., and LEVINE, E.: Disposable and reusable surgeons' gloves. *Nurs Res, 10:*79-86, 1961.
24. BECK, W. C., and CARLSON, W. W.: Aseptic barriers. *Arch Surg, 87:*288-295, 1963.
25. RUSSELL, T. R.; ROQUE, F. E., and MILLER, F. A.: A new method for detection of the leaky glove. *Arch Surg, 93:*245-249, 1966.
26. ANTOPOL, W.: Lycopodium granuloma. *Arch Path, 16:*326, 1933.
27. SEELIG, M. G., and VERDA, D. J.: Talcum powder problem. *J Mount Sinai Hosp NY, 12:*655, 1945.
28. SEELIG, M. G.: The talcum powder evil. *Amer J Surg, 76:*272, 1948.
29. ALDRICH, E. M.; LEE, C. H., and LEHMAN, E. P.: Further experiment with non-irritating glove powder. *Surgery, 25:*20, 1949.
30. MYERS, R. N.; DEAVER, J. M., and BROWN, C. E.: Granulomatous peritonitis due to starch

glove powder. *Ann Surg, 151*:106, 1960.

31. ISING, U.: Foreign body granuloma resulting from the use of starch glove powder at surgery. *Acta Chir Scand, 120*:95, 1960.

32. McNAUGHT, G. H. D.: Starch granuloma—A present-day surgical hazard. *Brit J Surg, 51*:845, 1964.

33. HARDER, H. I., and CHRIST, N. M.: The peril of glove powder. *Amer J Nurs, 66*:761-764, 1966.

34. YUNIS, E. J., and LANDES, R. R.: Hazards of glove powder in renal angiography. *JAMA, 193*:304-305, 1965.

35. MINSTER, J. J.; NOVAK, M. V.; PARKHURST, B., and COLE, W. H.: Use of liquid glove lubricants in the operating room to minimize wound contamination from glove powder. *Surgery, 52*:424-429, 1962.

36. WALTER, C. W.: Disinfection of hands (editorial), *Amer J Surg, 109*:691-693, 1965.

37. COLE, W. R., and BERNARD, H. R.: Inadequacies of present methods of surgical skin preparation. *Arch Surg, 89*:215, 1964.

38. WISE, R. I., *et al.*: The environmental distribution of *Staphylococcus aureus* in an operating suite. *Ann Surg, 149*:30, 1959.

39. SHOULDICE, E. E., and MARTIN, C. S.: Wound infections, surgical gloves, and hands of operating personnel. *Canad Med Ass J, 81*:636, 1959.

40. WALTER, C. W.: *The personal factor in hospital hygiene.* Report of conference, 19 June, 1963. London, Roy Soc Health, p. 40.

41. GAD, P.: Glove damage as a route of wound infection. *Danish Med Bull, 12*:1-4, 1965.

Chapter 10

PROCESSING OF SURGICAL INSTRUMENTS

STERILIZATION FACILITIES FOR THE OPERATING SUITE

THE ESTABLISHMENT of high quality standards for the care and sterilization of surgical instruments should be of vital concern to every hospital. It is fundamental to the practice of aseptic surgery that safe, rapid and effective methods be provided for the sterilization of instruments and other supplies. Also, the physical facilities comprising the operating suite should be adequate in terms of design and clinical function so as to reduce to a minimum the exposure of patients to risks of infection. Furthermore, reliable methods and equipment should be instituted for mechanically contained decontamination of instruments with a minimum of risk to staff employees.

These requirements can best be met initially through the medium of intelligent and efficient planning of the operating suite with special attention given to the necessity of providing ancillary facilities which will permit directional control over the movement patterns of staff personnel, patients, supplies, and air. In practice this means that the movement of people and supplies through changing accommodations is from "dirty" to "clean" to "sterile" zones. Air movement is from "clean" to "dirty" and from "dirty" to "exhaust", with provision for positive pressure, sanitary ventilation for each operating room.

There are two schools of thought on the system of distribution and disposal of supplies for the operating suite.[1] The first group believes that all sterile supplies should be delivered *direct* to a clean supply area or "sterile" room adjoining the operating room. This method of delivery and service requires that all operating rooms be grouped around and in direct contact with the central core of supply. With such an arrangement, it may be difficult to provide a separate exit route or corridor for the return of contaminated articles for reprocessing or disposal.

The other group believes that there should be a separate exit route for release and disposal of articles from the operating room and that these articles should not come in contact with patients or staff assigned to the operating rooms. Obviously, there are points worthy of consideration in both methods, but the one significant element that is lacking is the facility for controlled decontamination of instruments immediately following each case, without traversing intermediate space. In other words, the basic issue is the safety and practicality associated with a decontamination facility adjacent to each operating room versus the transport of all instruments by automation or otherwise to a centralized decontamination service at some other location in the hospital.

The one-time popular substerilizing room with facilities for serving each pair of operating rooms is now recognized as an inadequate and obsolete plan. In its place there has emerged the central instrument room with modern facilities, including the sonic instrument cleaner, for serving a number of operating rooms as shown in Figure 10-1. This arrangement may be expanded for centralized decontamination of instruments and supplies with the aid of a washer-sterilizer. With this plan, the processing of instruments involves completely wrapped trays prior to sterilization.

A new approach to the planning of sterilization facilities for the operating suite is illustrated in Figure 10-2. Schematically, this arrangement comprises a four-room surgical complex served by a clean supply area and adjacent (subservice) decontamination rooms. In describing the directional flow pattern, it should be noted that clean and packaged sterile articles coming from

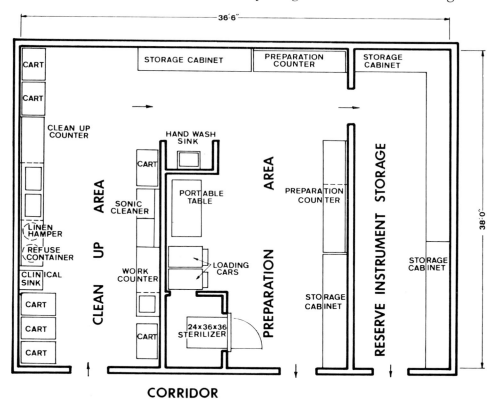

FIGURE 10-1. Central Instrument Room. Facilities, including sonic cleaner, are adequate for serving a number of operating rooms.

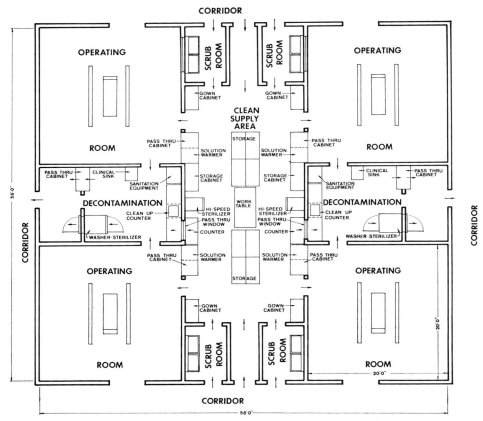

FIGURE 10-2. Schematic arrangement of four-room surgical complex. One important feature of this concept is close proximity of decontamination facilities to operating rooms and sources of contamination.

the central service department are admitted to the "clean supply area" from restricted corridors on either end of the complex. These are clean entrances. Cabinets are provided for storage of special or infrequently used instruments and supplies. Two high speed sterilizers make it convenient to carry out emergency sterilization. A pass-thru window is located between the clean supply room and each decontamination room. If an instrument is dropped during a surgical procedure, it can be washed and degreased in the decontamination room, transferred to clean supply via the pass window, sterilized in the high speed sterilizer and returned to the respective operating room in approximately 5 minutes time.

The sterile supply table for each operative case is prepared in the clean supply room. The service table is moved into the area where linen, instruments, and other supplies are unwrapped and placed upon the table according to a prescribed pattern. After the basic setup is completed, the table is moved into the operating room. NOTE: This method avoids the hazard of opening packages in the operating room. At the close of the procedure, all soiled material, linen, and waste are collected and transferred to the decontamination room. Instruments, utensils, glassware, and other such items are decontaminated in the washer-sterilizer. Other articles which cannot be subjected to steam sterilization may be sanitized or disinfected at the cleanup counter prior to discharge from the decontamination room. The decontaminated articles may then be held in the access room with entrance to corridor, until an employee assigned to pickup service is able to transfer them to the central instrument room, the laundry, or some other department for further processing.

The important feature of the concept expressed in Figure 10-2 is the close proximity of decontamination facilities to the operating rooms and the sources of contamination. It is not necessary to convey the articles to some distant point before decontamination is accomplished. The arrows show the progressive movement pattern of supplies through the complex. Dirty materials can be removed without passing through a clean area. Personnel working within the suite can move from one clean area to another without having to pass through unprotected areas. It is also possible to directionally control the air-movement pattern with properly maintained differential air pressures from room to room or from the cleaner to less clean areas.

There is probably no one plan, automated or otherwise, with centralized or decentralized decontamination facilities that will really satisfy any one hospital. The evidence indicates that, by and large, we are dealing with the problem of balancing certain recognizable hazards. A variety of disciplines are involved. Some are microbiological, some are medical-surgical, others are nursing, engineering, administration, and equipment suppliers. To ignore any of these is to invite disaster in planning.

Manual Cleaning of Instruments

Instruments must be cleaned as soon as possible after use, to avoid rusting or pitting, and to remove soil before it can dry and harden in the serrations and crevices. If stainless steel instruments are permitted to lie around for several hours before cleaning they may acquire a tarnish which is difficult to remove (Fig. 10-3). Likewise, plated instruments may show evidence of rusting at points where the plating has been damaged or worn through by previous cleansing processes. Therefore, immediately after use the instruments should be rinsed in cold water to assist in the removal of blood and debris. Then, if the instruments must be exposed for a period of time before routine cleaning, they should be immersed in warm water containing an effective blood solvent or detergent.

The final washing should be conducted with care and each step should be thoroughly understood by the person performing the duty. It is essential to remove all particles of adhering tissue, dried blood, scale, and accumula-

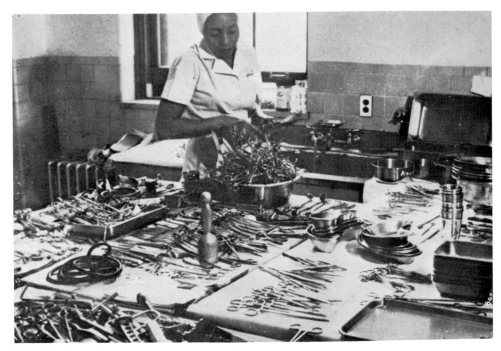

Figure 10-3. This illustrates why fast, effective cleaning of instruments is necessary. In excess of 90,000 instruments per operating room per year have to be cleaned.

tions of lime salts in the serrations, ratchets, and box locks of the instruments. In the scrubbing process, a hand brush with fairly stiff bristles may be used to advantage. It is important to remember that all brushes should be washed in detergent after use and sterilized. Under no circumstances should ordinary soap be used in the cleaning process because of the formation of insoluble alkali earth films (soap curd) in hard water which enmeshes and protects bacteria. This is a hazard. The use of abrasives or other sharp cleaners should be avoided because continued use of such compounds may roughen the surface, thereby minimizing the "stainless" properties of instruments.

The selection of a detergent for use in the cleaning process is not a simple matter. Surgical instruments are delicate, easily damaged, and susceptible to chemical attack. The challenge then is to choose the detergent and the use solution which will clean effectively with a minimum of scrubbing and with minimum damage to the instrument surface. In general, moderately alkaline, low-sudsing detergents such as Edisonite,® Reliance Solvent,® or Haemosol® are satisfactory. Before selecting a detergent or changing brands, the instrument manufacturer should be consulted. Caution should be exercised in accepting claims made for the "all purpose" detergent. There is no such **thing.**

To assist in the removal of inaccessible soil, it is necessary to establish a routine consisting of preliminary soaking of the instruments in warm water at a temperature of about 125°F (52°C), to which has been added the recommended quantity of an effective detergent. Adequate soaking time is required for the detergent solution to penetrate and loosen soil films. On the other hand, too much time may be detrimental and the solution may damage the instrument surfaces. Thorough cleaning is extremely important because organisms concealed and protected by dried blood and scale in inaccessible parts of the instruments render sterilization more difficult.

Immediately after washing, the instruments should be rinsed with hot water for a brief interval and then dried thoroughly. Rinsing with hot water is essential in the hand washing of instruments because the residual heat assists greatly in drying. If any moisture remains on the instruments, they may rust in storage. When spots, stains, or areas of discoloration appear on instruments, they may be the result of the wrong detergent, too much detergent, mineral content of the water, laundry residue from cloth instrument wraps, or chemicals released from paper wrappers. The corrosion problem in some hospitals is complicated by the fact that a few surgeons supply their own instruments. Some of these favorite instruments are in poor condition, the basic metal having long been exposed, thereby making these instruments extremely susceptible to corrosion.

At best, the manual cleaning of instruments is a difficult and time-consuming process. It is almost impossible to remove all traces of soil from inaccessible areas of box locks, serrations, and ratchets. In addition, manual cleaning contributes to the dissemination of microorganisms through the release of aerosols and droplets during the scrubbing process. For the operator, the potential hazard of direct contact with the virus of serum hepatitis is ever present. The mechanical cleaning process, utilizing the pressure instrument washer-sterilizer makes it possible to establish a superior technique with decontamination as an integral part of the operating cycle.

Instrument Washer-sterilizer

The need for a safe and rapid mechanical process for the routine cleansing and terminal sterilization of instruments in the operating room has been recognized for many years. It was not until 1938 that Walter[2,3] described such a process together with appropriate illustrations of an instrument washer-sterilizer. The first apparatus was designed along the lines of a vertical autoclave, constructed to withstand an operating pressure of 27 pounds. It utilized a stainless steel bucket as a receptacle for the soiled instruments. The bucket was placed in the washer-sterilizer directly over a baffle which forced the water to circulate through perforations in the bottom of the bucket. A steam coil in the bottom of the chamber supplied heat for sterilization and produced convection currents in the water to carry oil and grease released from the instruments to the surface and then to an overflow at the rear of the chamber. The addition of a suitable detergent to peptonize proteins and saponify greases was necessary for proper cleansing. After the water reached a temperature of 273°F (133°C), the steam was shut off and the water drained into a flash tank equipped with atmospheric vent. The instruments could then be removed from the washer-sterilizer in a clean, dry, and sterile condition, ready for immediate use if so desired.

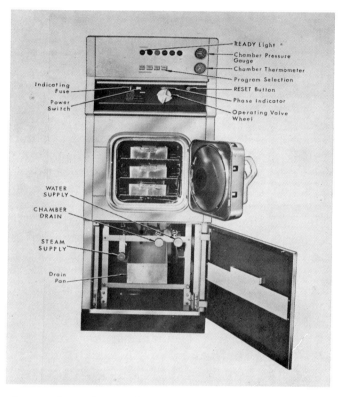

FIGURE 10-4. Automatic washer-sterilizer, for the cleaning and decontamination of instruments and utensils.

The latest development in the design of an instrument washer-sterilizer is shown in Figure 10-4. The horizontal (cabinet type) design makes it possible to utilize standard instrument trays which, in turn, permit easier and more efficient loading and unloading of instruments. The sliding, pull-out shelves permit the withdrawal of trays aseptically. The complete cycle of washing and sterilizing is governed solely by an automatic, programmed control. Three cycles are available to the operator, each having its own selector button and interlocking safety device:

• Wash and sterilize in 25-minute cycle.

- Sterilization of unwrapped metal or glass instruments or utensils (3 minutes at 270°F).
- Sterilization of unwrapped instruments or utensils with nonmetal components, including tubing and sutures (10 minutes at 270°F).

After any one of the cycles has been activated, a cycle lock prevents its being changed unless the reset button is first depressed. When the door is closed and locked, the cycle starts. Colored discs on the control panel illuminate to indicate progress through various stages of the cycle. An audible signal indicates completion.

The washing process is accomplished by means of a vigorously agitated detergent bath, the result of a combination of high velocity jet streams of steam and air which develop a violent under-water turbulence as illustrated in Figure 10-5. During the washing phase the water temperature automatically rises to 145° to 155°F (63° to 68°C). The agitated detergent solution disengages blood, grease, and tissue debris from the instruments and carries the soil to the surface. As the heated water expands in the chamber, the level rises and the released soil and scum overflow into the waste line. The automatic program control then activates the steam inlet and water outlet valves (Fig. 10-5) and steam is admitted into the top of the chamber,

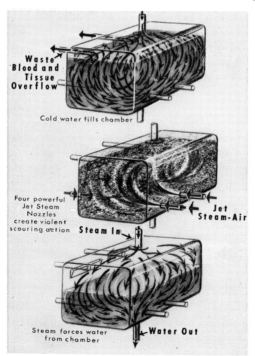

FIGURE 10-5. Cleaning of instruments and utensils is accomplished by means of vigorously agitated detergent bath. Combination of high velocity jet streams of steam and air develop violent underwater turbulence.

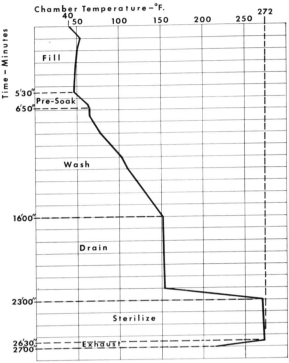

FIGURE 10-6. Process chart showing time elapsed and temperature attained for each phase of operating cycle of washer-sterilizer.

forcing the wash water out through the bottom drain. Steam under pressure floods the chamber and the temperature of 270°F (132°C) is maintained for not less than 3 minutes. Finally, the steam is exhausted through an automatic condenser exhaust and an audible signal indicates the washer-sterilizer is ready for unloading. The high residual heat in the instruments is sufficient to flash any adherent moisture. The clean, dry, sterile instruments are then ready for immediate use upon removal from the washer-sterilizer or they may be placed in storage until needed. A typical process chart showing time elapsed and temperature attained for each phase of the operating cycle is shown in Figure 10-6.

Factors Influencing Removal of Soil from Instruments

In the washing of surgical instruments, there are certain basic factors which must be considered in order to evaluate the functional efficiency of the process. As a practical approach to the problem the functions of all the components in the washing system should be studied. In the case of the instrument washer-sterilizer these components are as follows:

• Kind of soil.

- Quality of water.
- Type of detergent.
- Concentration of detergent.
- Types of instruments.
- Time detergent solution is permitted to act.
- Efficiency of washer.

Certainly one of the most important factors is the kind and amount of soil present on the instruments. Blood, feces, tissue fats, and extraneous debris constitute the common types of soil encountered on surgical instruments. The amount of blood and organic matter present, as well as the total number of instruments soiled, is greater in certain operations than others. Consequently the efficiency of the washing process is influenced by the total number of soiled instruments in the load. If the blood has been permitted to dry on the instruments for a period of hours it will be difficult to properly clean them in any mechanical washer. Good results can only be expected when instruments are washed promptly following completion of the surgical procedure. If this is not possible, then the instruments should be placed in a basin of water to prevent excessive drying of blood in serrations, depressions, and other inaccessible surfaces.

Water is perhaps the most important single component of the washing process. In many cases it can be demonstrated that the solvent action of water alone will remove a high percentage of soil from the instruments. This action is obviously enhanced by the factor of agitation and cutting action when correctly applied in the washing machine. Water also serves as the medium for carrying the detergent to all surfaces of the instruments and for taking away the separated soil. Unfortunately the quality of tap water in many localities is not well suited for use in any mechanical washer. Over half the United States is plagued with problems traceable to hard water. In view of this condition, it may be necessary to soften the hospital's water supply or to select a detergent which will properly condition the water for cleaning purposes.

It is probably no exaggeration of fact to state that there is no one detergent best suited for use in the instrument washer-sterilizer under any and all conditions. The principal function of the detergent is to render nonwettable surfaces wettable. By virtue of its chemical and physical properties, the detergent lowers the surface tension of water, permitting more intimate contact of the water with the instrument. In addition, it assists in the solubilization of albuminous soil, emulsifies grease and suspends soil particles in the solution. Most detergents are chemical mixtures of crystalline substances comprising a surface-active or wetting agent in combination with one or more builders such as the sodium phosphates, carbonates, or silicates.

Sequestering or chelating agents may also be added to prevent precipitation of hard water salts. Representative of this group are the detergents known as Haemosol, Edisonite, Calgonite, Alconox,® and many others. All of these products have been evaluated for use in the washer-sterilizer. They have been found relatively unsatisfactory in that they leave a residue or film of powder upon the instruments after the washing and sterilizing cycle has been completed.

Some of the common phosphate detergents recommended for use in mechanical dishwashers have been tried in the instrument washer-sterilizer. Not only were the results disappointing from the standpoint of cleaning but the instruments underwent a severe metallic staining. The brassy tarnishing of the instruments was due to the copper solubilizing action of the polyphosphated detergent upon internal parts of the washer-sterilizer. The dissolved copper was then deposited upon the instruments by electrolytic action. Bacon and Nutting[4] have described a similar condition which occurred from the use of polyphosphate detergents in mechanical dishwashers. A special detergent* has been developed for use in the washer-sterilizer. It is all-liquid in composition and is made from a coconut-oil base. It has remarkably good surface-active properties with a special affinity for metallic surfaces. When used in a concentration of one to two ounces in the washer, it leaves an invisible protective film on the instruments which resists corrosion.

Under the most careful operating conditions there are certain instruments difficult to clean by the mechanical process. Because of the accumulation of soil in the serrations, box locks, and ratchets, hemostats are especially difficult to clean.

Other instruments of importance are those shown in Figure 10-7. The flat ground surfaces of scissors may occasionally present a problem if blood has been permitted to dry on them. Instruments used in bone surgery such as curettes and files may contain extremely adherent particles of tissue in the depressions and teeth which resist removal and cleansing in the washer-sterilizer. Likewise, multiple-action bone-cutting forceps and Rongeurs may offer difficulty in cleansing because of the multiple joints, inaccessible and tightly apposing surfaces. For these instruments a special treatment is recommended consisting of a preliminary soaking period in warm water containing 1 ounce per gallon of an approved detergent-sanitizer. Following this procedure the instruments may be subjected to the normal washing and sterilizing process given above.

The economic advantages of the instrument washer-sterilizer are recognized and accepted by many hospital administrators and professional personnel. The study made by Prickett[5] in 1953 laid the foundation for acceptance of mechanical methods for the processing of instruments. The point so frequently overlooked and apparently little understood is the safety protection that this equipment affords to employees assigned to the task of routine

---

* A product of American Sterilizer Co., Erie, Pa.

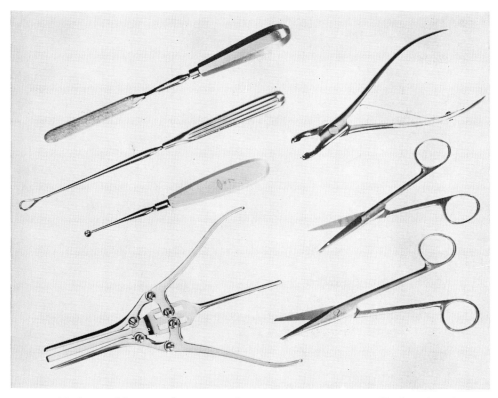

Figure 10-7. In addition to hemostats, these instruments are usually found to be difficult to clean by mechanical process. Careful attention to prevent excessive drying of blood on their surfaces will enhance considerably the mechanical cleaning process.

cleaning and processing of surgical instruments. The uninformed individual does not appreciate the hazard attached to the cleaning of instruments. Perhaps this is due to a lack of understanding on the part of many as to the meaning of "decontamination." It is hoped that the gap between a "dirty" and a "clean" case, a "pathogen" and a "nonpathogen" may be rapidly closing.

ULTRASONIC CLEANING OF INSTRUMENTS

Theory

The term *ultrasonic* is used to describe a vibratory wave of a frequency above that of the upper frequency limit of the human ear. It generally embraces all frequencies above 15,000 cycles per second according to the American Standards Association.[6] Sound is a series of wave motions which compress and rarefy the medium through which they pass (Fig. 10-8A). The medium may be air, water, metal, or any other elastic medium. The longer the wave, the lower the frequency or pitch of the sound (Fig. 10-8B). The higher the amplitude of the wave, the greater is the loudness

RAREFIED WAVE

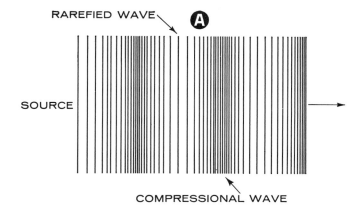

SOURCE

COMPRESSIONAL WAVE

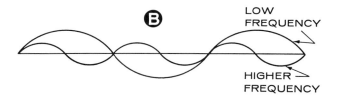

LOW
FREQUENCY

HIGHER
FREQUENCY

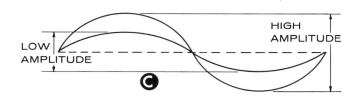

HIGH
AMPLITUDE

LOW
AMPLITUDE

COMPLEX WAVE
SUCH AS SPEECH

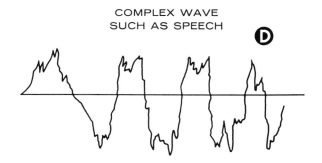

SINE WAVE
SUCH AS USED IN ULTRASONICS

ONE CYCLE - 360°

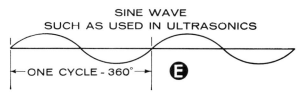

FIGURE 10-8. Characteristic sound waves.

(Fig. 10-8C). A sound wave may be complex as represented in Figure 10-8D, or sinusoidal as shown as Figure 10-8E. The latter is employed in ultrasonic cleaners. One of two discrete frequencies is normally used in ultrasonic cleaners for hospitals: 20,600 (20.6 kc) or 38,000 (38 kc) vibrations per second. The frequency of 20.6 kc is usually associated with sonic cleaners which utilize metallic transducers. The 38 kc energy commonly employs one of the crystal transducers.

Ultrasonics is an effective cleaning method because it initiates *cavitation,* a precise definition of which is necessary for an understanding of the theory. Gas-filled, vapor-filled, or empty cavities ranging in size from submicroscopic to very large may be produced in a liquid by varying methods such as chemical, thermal, or mechanical actions, and they may have a short or prolonged life. The production of these cavities and the effect that they induce on the medium or environment in which they are produced is known as

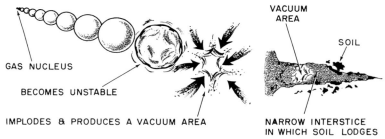

FIGURE 10-9. Schematic diagram of cavitation as induced by sonic energy.

cavitation.[7] Minute bubbles are generated by ultrasonics from gas nuclei. The bubbles expand until they are unstable, then they collapse. A schematic diagram of the phenomenon of cavitation is shown in Figure 10-9.

At the onset of cavitation, the gas nuclei vary in size, depending upon the surface tension of the liquid, temperature, wetting action of the detergent, and the frequency of the applied ultrasonic energy. The implosion (bursting inward) generates minute vacuum areas which are responsible for the cleaning process. The forces of cavitation are initiated at the instant of implosion, and the binder or matrix which causes adherence of the soil to the instrument surface is dislodged, dispersed, or dissolved. Soluble binders go into solution in the bath water and the heavier insolubles settle to the bottom of the cleaning tank.

Many hospitals have been cleaning their instruments daily with ultrasonics for more than a decade. Superior cleaning has been experienced in the majority of these institutions; but in others, the quality of cleaning has been erratic. A study of "problem" installations has indicated that when cleaning is substandard, the procedures are wrong, personnel are inadequately instructed, or the equipment is not adjusted for optimum performance. When sonic cleaners are correctly adjusted and the operators adhere to manufacturer's instructions, the quality of cleaning surpasses that of hand scrubbing by a wide margin. Ultrasonic energy through cavitation penetrates areas that the bristles of a brush are much too coarse to contact and remove soil.

The Cleaning Process

Quantitative tests using radioactive isotopes and a Geiger-Müller counter indicate that most of the soil on instruments is removed in the first 15 seconds; after which, the process slows down. This is explainable on the basis that a high percentage of the soil is on exposed surfaces and not tightly adhered. The removal of soil which defies the solvency of specific cleaning agents and which cannot be contacted by the filaments of a brush reveals the superiority of ultrasonic cleaning.

The mechanics of cavitation, and the action of detergent plus heat combine to rapidly loosen tenacious soils in hidden recesses of instruments. Mechanical agitation supplied by the onslaught of cavitation unleashes energy of several hundred atmospheres.[8] This combination of forces disrupts the bonds which hold particulate matter to instruments. As the result, the larger and more dense particles fall to the bottom of the cleaner tank and some of the more finely dispersed soils rise to the surface of the water. This means that loosened particulate matter and detergent remain on the instruments after ultrasonic cleaning and they must, therefore, be thoroughly rinsed off. *Sonic cleaning is not a brightener, and the process will not remove stains on instruments.*

The optimum bath temperature for cleaning surgical instruments soiled with blood and tissue debris ranges between 80° and 110°F (27° to 44°C). If the temperature rises above 140°F (60°C) protein will coagulate and be more difficult to remove. Coagulated protein absorbs sound, thereby reducing its effective action. The most effective removal of proteinaceous soil is accomplished by controlling the bath temperature to forestall coagulation.

If excess gas is present in the cleaning water, it will decrease cleaning efficiency because the cavitation bubbles fill with gas and the energy released during implosion is reduced by the "cushioning" effect. Water can be readily degassed by applying ultrasonic energy to the cleaning bath. However, there is no definitive time for degassing other than to state that tap water should be degassed for not less than 5 minutes each time it is changed. Also, conditions arise where degassing may not be required, such as water held in a dormant state overnight.

Rinsing and Drying

Rinsing is an important phase of the ultrasonic cleaning process. A water temperature of 180°F (82°C) is normally used for rinsing when heat-labile articles are not being processed. Some plastic items may soften, deform, or undergo permanent physical change at this temperature. These items should be rinsed and dried separately from metallic instruments and at a temperature not exceeding 130°F (55°C). The injection of a wetting agent into the final rinse enhances its effectiveness by breaking the surface tension of the water droplets, permitting more intimate contact between water and the particulate matter to be removed. The more sophisticated sonic cleaners are equipped with wetting-agent injectors as shown in Figure 10-10. A final rinse with distilled water is essential for removing residual

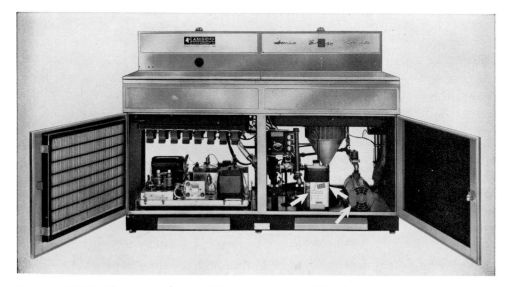

FIGURE 10-10. Ultrasonic cleaner. Upper arrows in right hand compartment point to wetting agent container and injector. Lower arrow indicates pump which pressurizes distilled water for rinsing.

chemical agents imparted to the instruments in the cleaning cycle. Distilled water is rarely available under pressure, and a pump is required to pressurize the water to 30 pounds or more for effective rinsing.

Several factors influence the time required for drying of instruments. The most important are the temperature of the instruments and of the drying air, the velocity and the moisture content of the drying air, and the quantity and arrangement of instruments. If all of the instruments are metal or if they contain plastic parts known to be thermosetting, the drying temperature should be at least 190°F (88°C). If thermoplastics are being dried, the thermostat setting on the unit should not exceed 130°F (55°C). The dryer should use air from an air-conditioned room, otherwise the drying time may be prolonged and thereby interfere with a balanced production operation between cleaning, rinsing and drying.

Instrument Cleaning Trays

Instrument trays for use in ultrasonic cleaners should be specifically designed for this purpose. There is an important relationship among wire gage, size of openings, and the sonic frequency. A large mesh with small wire size transmits more energy than heavy wire with narrow spacing. An acceptable woven wire mesh for ultrasonic cleaning trays is eight openings per inch woven from 0.031 inch stainless or Monel® wire. Solid bottom trays fabricated from sheet steel of less than 0.025 inch thick are effective, but they should be designed so that air is not entrapped beneath them. An air-water interface does not transmit ultrasonic energy. The piercing of large air-escape holes in the bottoms of trays is poor practice. This permits small objects to fall through the tray.

When assembling instruments in a tray for processing, care should be exercised to guard against overloading. Jointed instruments with box locks should be opened wide to expose the maximum surface area. Sharp instruments should be carefully spaced in the tray in order to prevent contact with the easily damaged surfaces. A tray of instruments properly loaded is shown in Figure 10-11. The instruments are stacked less than 3 inches high, which is considered maximum for optimum cleaning, rinsing, and drying. Use care to ensure that stainless steel instruments are not mixed with aluminum, or with brass or copper. Also, be certain that detergents used in the cleaning process are nonharmful to the instruments.

Testing the Ultrasonic Cleaner

If cleaning does not appear to be as thorough as when the system was first installed, there are certain tests which can be made to determine the level of operating efficiency of the equipment as well as to indicate the need for service. Several manufacturers of ultrasonic cleaning equipment maintain laboratories devoted solely to research on cleaning processes and test methods for evaluation of these processes. In general, manufacturers rely upon the ceramic ring test as an indicator of product quality and any sonic cleaner which fails to pass this test is rejected. The test is simple and fast and requires no special equipment except the ceramic rings. The test can be performed at any site where a sonic cleaner is installed.

The test consists of rubbing pencil lead into the microscopically porous surface of one face of a ceramic ring (Fig. 10-12) which is then cleaned by ultrasonics for a specific time under controlled conditions. Tests used by manufacturers are usually conducted with ten rings, the water temperature and other parameters being accurately controlled. The residual lead on the rings is compared to a grouping of rings, each a little cleaner than the other, each assigned a number corresponding to the nearest matching ring (Fig. 10-13). A total score of 75 or higher indicates a properly functioning

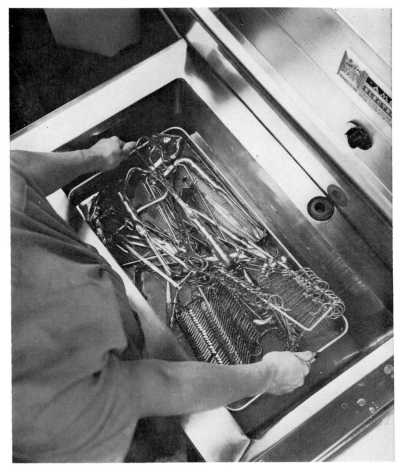

FIGURE 10-11. Tray of instruments assembled for effective processing in sonic cleaner.

cleaner. A test conducted in this manner is fairly conclusive; however, it is more elaborate than is generally required to determine whether or not a hospital-type ultrasonic cleaner requires servicing.

A simpler field test involves placing two rings, heavily coated on one side, in a tray, coated side up. Apply ultrasonics for one minute. If more than 75 per cent of the lead is removed, the cleaner is adjusted nearly enough to optimum for practical purposes. The ceramic rings required for the test are generally obtainable from ultrasonic cleaner manufacturers.

Erosion of Ultrasonic Cleaner Tanks

Ultrasonic cleaner tanks, usually the bottoms, are eroded by cavitation, in a normal aging process. If ultrasonic power is reduced to minimize this cavitation erosion, cleaning is substandard. If excess power is applied, cavitation

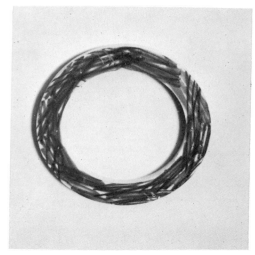

FIGURE 10-12. Ceramic ring rubbed with pencil lead in preparation for test.

erosion is accelerated, and a vapor blanket at the tank-water interface above the transducers reduces cavitation in the cleaning bath. An optimum power level of ultrasonic energy, determined by experimentation, produces the most effective cleaning with the least erosion of the tank. At this time, there is no known method for measuring ultrasonic energy in a liquid medium. Cleaning, of course, is the main objective, and tank rehabilitation or replacement is of secondary importance.

To prolong the service life of an ultrasonic cleaner, it should be designed so that the tank may be removed and rehabilitated after a few years of ser-

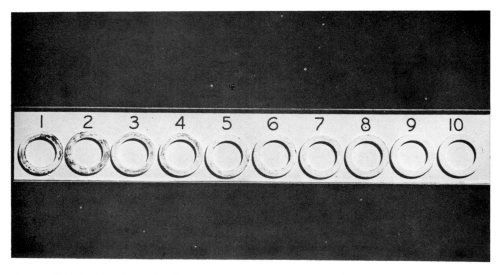

FIGURE 10-13. Set of standard comparison rings by means of which cleanliness of test ring can be measured.

vice. The more sophisticated ultrasonic cleaners incorporate designs which permit the transducers or tank bottoms to be removed for rehabilitation. Tank bottoms with hard smooth surfaces, in contact with the cleaning solution, are less prone to cavitation erosion because soft metal and surface blemishes act as starting points for this destructive process. Tank bottoms on new cleaners will usually exhibit a matte finish in many places on their polished surfaces. This does not indicate a used cleaner, but is merely the erosion induced by tests conducted by the manufacturer prior to shipment. Substantial cavitation erosion is evident after the first few weeks of operation; then the process slows down considerably, and there is no simple explanation of this phenomenon.

Decontamination by Means of Sonic Energy

From time to time the question arises as to whether sonic activation can be considered a substitute for sterilization. To be sure, it is known that under proper process control, sonic energy can bring about a major and significant reduction in the bacterial count. Also, ultrasonic methods for injuring or disrupting microorganisms or animal cells are now widely used, but there is as yet no generally accepted theory to explain the disruptive effect. Some workers[9,10,17] believe that the initial event in cellular disruption involves the abrasive cleavage of the cell wall or envelope by high speed microbubbles of gas. Presumably this action results in a release of cellular contents which contain both soluble and insoluble fragments.

In some hospitals sonic energy cleaning is a part of decontamination techniques.[12,13] The process depends upon the proper combination of sonic agitation, detergent, and an effective germicide. The claim is made that sonic decontamination eliminates the possibility of accidental infection of personnel involved in cleaning postoperative equipment. The point to be stressed, however, is that the adequacy of the process for inactivation of the virus of serum hepatitis is not known. So for one to say that the process eliminates the possibility of accidental infection is a half-truth at best. This, of course, constitutes one reason why *all* surgical instruments should be decontaminated in a pressure instrument washer-sterilizer. Also, the problem of preventing contaminated aerosols from escaping to the surrounding work area is difficult to overcome in any sonic bath.[10] For the present, the evidence is convincing that sonic activation is not a substitute for sterilization. Moreover, any apparatus or device worthy of the name "sterilizer" must be capable of doing much more than reducing the count of microorganisms.

LIFE EXPECTANCY OF SURGICAL INSTRUMENTS
Quality Instruments

The skill of the surgeon may frequently be impaired as the result of the quality and condition of the instruments at his command. No instrument is better than the steel from which it is made. For perfect instruments the tempering and workmanship are of great importance and care should be exercised in the selection of a reliable brand of instrument, not overlooking, of course, the reputation and integrity of the supplier. Because of the superior properties of certain alloys of stainless steel, the majority of present-day instruments are made from this metal. Several kinds of stainless steel are used and the difference lies in the formulas of the steel, providing a different quality for different purposes.

The term "stainless" is a misnomer in that metallurgical science has not yet developed any steel which is completely stainproof under all conditions. Basically, stainless steel contains much less carbon than ordinary steel and, in addition, it contains other metals such as chromium and nickel in order to produce high corrosion resistance. With surgical instruments it is far more important to have the proper hardness and elasticity than to have absolute corrosion resistance, providing the corrosion resistance is kept sufficiently high.[14] The carbon content is of vital importance. If the percentage of carbon is too low, then the resulting steel is too soft. If it is too high, it forms a steel which is too brittle and hard to forge. Stainless steel containing about 12 to 14% chromium and about 0.2% carbon is generally considered one of the most satisfactory for surgical instruments.

It is apparent that in the manufacture of instruments, workmanship may vary considerably. It is good practice, therefore, to examine all new instruments. Observe if the points of scissors and forceps are equally long on each instrument; that the jaws of forceps are equally thick; that curved jaws are bent to a smooth, even curve; that serrations mesh properly and are beveled at the edges of the jaws; and that the jaws close evenly, starting at the point and being fully closed when the last ratchet has been reached. It is also important to note if the teeth of all forceps are even, of proper shape and sharpness, and mesh uniformly. There should be no sharp points or edges which may scratch or tear the surgeon's gloves. Scissors should close smoothly and cut well at the points, also along the entire edges. The box lock of forceps should work smoothly, yet show no evidence of looseness. The shanks should be springy and soft enough to permit closing to the last ratchet without undue effort. The ratchets should glide smoothly over each other, hold firmly, open easily, even from the last ratchet. All thumb and tissue forceps should be tested for the proper tension.

Corrosion of Instruments

It is highly improbable that ultrasonic cleaning can crack, break, distort, rust, or stain a surgical instrument made of good quality stainless steel which has been manufactured by expert craftsmen and which has no latent defects. In certain instances, in the past, ultrasonic cleaning has been unjustly cited as being responsible for damaged instruments. Investigations indicated that the damage resulted from defective instruments, incorrect handling techniques, use of incompatible detergents, or some combination of the three causes.

The forging of stainless steels induces built-in stresses, and if the instrument has not been stress relieved, acid detergents can produce stress corrosion. This may cause the instrument to break at a pivot, fulcrum, or at a point of high mechanical stress during use.[15] Excess peening of rivets used at the fulcrums also introduces stresses or invisible cracks and accounts for some broken instruments.

Instruments with latent defects or forged instruments which have not been stress relieved are likely to crack when used even if they have never been cleaned by ultrasonics. On instruments which have been plated and the plating has been ruptured, flaking off or crazing of the chrome may be accelerated by the ultrasonic cleaner. This is because corrosion has started at the interface between the chrome plate and the parent metal. Corrosion and cosmetic effects are promoted by physicochemical actions when instruments are not thoroughly cleaned and dried. Sharp instruments are damaged more readily than others since they are subject to accidental striking of cutting edges or points against hard objects.

The surface of a stainless steel instrument may be "active" or "passive." An active surface is highly susceptible to corrosion. A passive surface is formed by a thin, self-healing, inert, and impervious oxide film. Only stainless steels containing approximately 12% chromium develop passivity. The passivation of stainless steel is accomplished by subjecting the instruments to a dilute solution of nitric acid. Instruments from reliable manufacturers are invariably passivated in the production process.

Rust on the surface of an instrument may result from chemical action of cleaning agents or other environmental exposures on the metal. It may have nothing to do with the steel itself as in the case of a deposition of mineral salts from the tap-water rinse. Rinsing with distilled or deionized water is extremely important in geographical areas where the tap water contains excessive amounts of dissolved metals. Florida, Arizona, and California are typical of states where this problem is acute. It is impossible to completely restore instruments after rusting or pitting has eroded the hard, smooth surface. Once the surface of an instrument has become pitted, it is far more susceptible to further corrosion than is a highly polished surface. In summary, it is fair to say that a substantial amount of evidence exists to show that surgical instruments are not likely to be damaged by ultrasonic energy. The thoroughness of the cleaning process results in smoothly operating instruments with a longer life expectancy.

Lubrication of Instruments

The inconsistency of oiling instruments prior to sterilization, as practiced in some hospitals, is a hazardous procedure and it should not be permitted.

The presence of a film of oil on an instrument simply serves as a protective barrier for any organism that may reside under the film.[16] It should be understood that sterilization is dependent upon moisture and that even a thin coating of oil will prevent moisture contact with instrument surfaces. In many cases the apparent need for lubrication is indicative of the presence of accumulated soil or foreign matter in the joints of the instruments. To relieve this stiffness so they will operate smoothly, it is recommended that a small amount of water-soluble grinding and lapping compound* (Grit No. 180) be placed in the box lock or joint and worked in by opening and closing the instrument several times. This will remove the rough spots from the joints and, after cleaning, the instruments should operate satisfactorily. As a rule, instruments processed routinely in an ultrasonic cleaner do not require this kind of special attention.

One cannot deny the fact that some delicate instruments with moving parts must be lubricated. Also, various drills and dental instruments including handpieces and contra-angles require lubrication. For these special applications the silicone oil compounds, such as Surgeo-Sil®** have been found acceptable. Most of these preparations do not inhibit sterilization by autoclaving. Oil-in-water emulsion preparations†,‡ are commonly used to precoat instruments prior to sterilization for the purpose of preventing corrosion and to provide lubrication.[17] Some liquid germicides such as benzalkonium chloride may be used to impart lubricity to certain instruments. If lubricating oil is placed on an instrument, sterilization must be carried out by means of dry heat.

STERILIZATION OF INSTRUMENTS
Routine Sterilization

In the sterilization of instruments, care must be taken to insure that all instruments have been thoroughly cleaned beforehand and free from oil or grease. In no sense can the sterilizing process be considered as a substitute for adequate preliminary cleaning or to partially compensate for inadequate cleaning of instruments. The technic selected for sterilization must be adequate for the destruction of heat-resistant spores. This requires the use of saturated steam under pressure at a temperature of 250°F (121°C) for a minimum of 12 minutes, or 270°F (132°C) for a minimum of 2 minutes, with direct steam contact to all surfaces.

In assembling instruments for sterilization a serious attempt should be made to standardize on a basic set. Investigations have shown that in many operating rooms there is practically no standardization and very little agree-

---

* A product of Clover Mfg. Co., Norwalk, Conn.
** V. Mueller & Co., Chicago, Ill.
† Proclave Emulsion—Kerr Mfg. Co., Detroit, Mich.
‡ Preplube—The Lawton Co., New York, New York

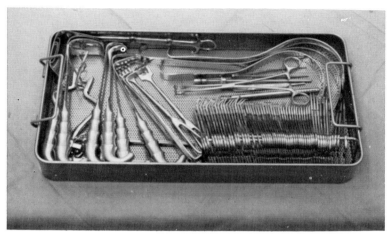

FIGURE 10-14. A perforated or wire-mesh bottom tray is necessary for effective sterilization. All jointed instruments must be open to permit prompt contact of steam to all surfaces.

ment as to the content of the basic set. In fact, the so-called basic sets have a tendency to grow to such an extent that personnel complain about the large number and kinds of instruments which are being processed but not used. The number of unused instruments at the end of a case may serve as a guide in determining if the sets can be safely and advantageously reduced. This information should be reviewed with each surgeon in order to solicit his cooperation in establishing instrument sets which will meet his needs, yet will eliminate the unnecessary.

For the routine sterilization of instruments, the method shown in Figure 10-14 has proved highly satisfactory for many hospitals. The first step in the procedure is to select a conventional instrument tray with wire mesh bottom. The openings in the wire mesh should be small enough to prevent the tips of most instruments from sliding through. Never use a solid bottom, watertight tray or basin because they will trap air. The instrument sets are then arranged in the tray in a definite and fixed pattern. This is important if the tray is to be located later as a unit on the nurse's table from which the instruments are removed as needed. *All jointed instruments must be open or unlocked to permit prompt contact of steam to all surfaces.* This requirement is oftentimes ignored in operating rooms on the grounds that the open instrument is difficult to handle and control. Experience has shown that this argument is not necessarily true. There are several devices (Fig. 10-15), available from instrument suppliers, designed to hold hinged instruments in an open position during sterilization. *Do not hold instruments together by means of rubber bands.*

Instruments composed of more than one part or with sliding members should be disassembled for sterilization. The Balfour retractor and Tydings

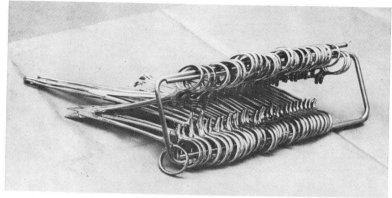

FIGURE 10-15. One method of holding jointed instruments open during sterilization.

tonsil snare are examples of instruments intricate in design and difficult to sterilize unless they are disassembled beforehand. If it is not possible to take the instrument apart or if it must remain assembled during the sterilizing process, then dry heat at a temperature of 320°F (160°C) for one hour is the method of choice for sterilization. Unless provision can be made for direct steam contact to all surfaces of the instrument, it is hazardous to attempt sterilization in the autoclave.

When it is desired to hold sterilized instruments in temporary storage or if they are to be transported from one area to another, the entire tray should be wrapped with double-thickness muslin. The tray should be positioned upright on the sterilizer loading car as shown in Figure 10-16. This helps to maintain an orderly arrangement of the contents. The exposure period should be 30 minutes at 250°F (121°C) when using the gravity discharge type sterilizer. At the end of the exposure period the instruments should be allowed to remain in the sterilizer for 15 minutes with the door slightly open, about ¼ inch, to ensure thorough drying. In sterilizers equipped with automatic controls, the drying phase is a part of the normal cycle of operation.

If wrapped trays of instruments are to be sterilized in the high-speed pressure instrument sterilizer, adjusted for 27 pounds pressure, the minimum exposure period should be 15 minutes at 270°F (132°C). The time required for killing of heat-resistant spores in direct contact with steam at this temperature is 2 minutes. The additional time of 13 minutes allows for penetration of steam through the wrapper plus a reasonable factor of safety. The exposure period also takes into consideration the possibility that non-metal materials such as suction tubing, electrosurgical cords, asepto syringes, suture material, and padding may be added to the tray of instruments. Prevacuum high temperature sterilizers operating at 272° to 275°F (133° to 135°C) have a fixed exposure period of 4 minutes.

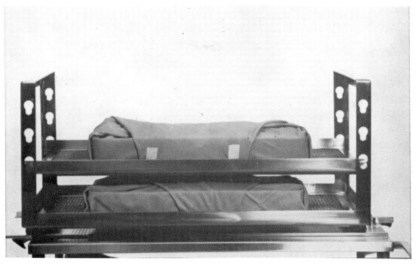

FIGURE 10-16. Place wrapped trays of instruments flat on shelves of loading car in order to maintain an orderly arrangement of contents.

Occasionally it is found that instruments are wet following routine sterilization and drying. The condition occurs more frequently in the electrically heated instrument sterilizer equipped with steam generator. Many times, the cause is the same as that responsible for wet dressings, discussed on page 219. If the sterilizer is operating properly and the principles of good technique have not been violated, the difficulty of wet instruments may be overcome by preheating prior to sterilization. This can be accomplished by simply placing the trays of instruments in the sterilizer, closing the door, and maintaining steam in jacket only for 15 minutes. At the end of the preheating period, steam may be admitted to the chamber and the instruments sterilized in the usual manner. The process of preheating reduces to a minimum the amount of condensate formed on the instruments during sterilization, thereby making drying less troublesome. The preheating of glass constriction tubes containing needles is an effective way of avoiding excess condensation in the tubes.

Emergency Sterilization

In the emergency sterilization of instruments, no compromise with safety can be tolerated. The method selected must be adequate for the destruction of resistant spores and it should be sufficiently rapid so as not to greatly inconvenience the surgeon. These requirements can be met through the use of a high-speed pressure instrument sterilizer, adjusted for operation at 270°F (132°C) and 27 to 28 pounds pressure. When an instrument is urgently needed, as for one that has been accidentally dropped or inadvertently left out of a kit, it is possible for the nurse to wash, degrease, sterilize the instrument, and return it to the operating table in 5 to 6 minutes with no compromise in safety. The detailed steps of the technic are given below.

Steam should be maintained in the jacket of the high-speed pressure instrument sterilizer prior to and during the entire surgical procedure.

- Scrub the instrument with warm water containing detergent for about 15 seconds, followed by another 15 second wash in fat solvent (Stoddard Solvent or its equivalent).
- Place the opened instrument in a tray with wire mesh or perforated bottom, insert tray in sterilizer, close and tighten door securely.
- Turn operating valve wheel to STER. When chamber temperature reaches 270°F begin timing the sterilizing period for 3 minutes. If the sterilizer is equipped with automatic control, push the 3-minute STERILIZE button and the automatic cycle will begin.
- At end of the sterilizing period, turn the operating valve wheel to EXH. When the chamber pressure has exhausted to zero gauge, turn operating valve wheel to OFF, open door, and remove instrument.

Sterilization of Utensils

The most reliable method for the sterilization of utensils, basin sets, and other containers is by means of steam under pressure. In most hospitals the procedure is fairly well standardized. The utensils are wrapped in muslin, sterilized in Central Service, and stored for use, just the same as for dressings (fabrics) and other dry goods. It is important to observe certain details with respect to wrapping and loading in the sterilizer. If several utensils are nested, snugly fitting into each other, they should be separated by a layer of muslin to prevent tight contact of the metal surfaces and to allow some space for direct steam contact to all surfaces. An alternate method of arranging utensil sets is shown in Figure 10-17. Here the bottom of each utensil is parallel to the one below it. This arrangement ensures that all basins in the set will be on their side when the pack is positioned on edge in the sterilizer. Whenever possible, use a variety of basin sizes for the set. This makes fabric separators unnecessary.

Utensils should be wrapped in double thickness muslin. In the case of the standard basin set, the wrapper may then serve as the sterile drape for the basin stand. Always place the wrapped kits of utensils in the sterilizer on edge so that any water contained in them would drain out completely. This facilitates both sterilization and drying. The utensils can be sterilized separately from other supplies in a minimum exposure of 20 minutes at 250°F (121°C). If desired, they may also be sterilized as a part of the bulk load of dry supplies, provided the utensils are not placed above or below other packs. In close contact with packs of dry goods, the basins may interfere with sterilization of the other materials, and they are almost certain to cause some wetting of the packs in contact with them. It is good practice to ar-

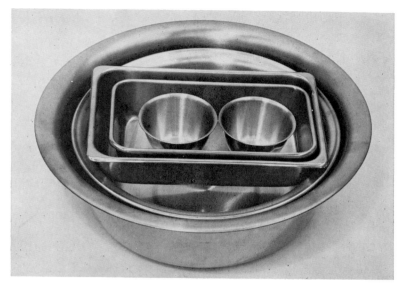

FIGURE 10-17. An alternate method of arranging utensil sets. This arrangement ensures that all basins in the set will be on their side when pack is placed on edge in sterilizer.

range the utensils at one end of the sterilizer, when included as a part of the bulk load of fabrics.

Sterilization of Sutures

Surgical Gut

Basically, there are two kinds of sutures: *absorbable* and *nonabsorbable.* An absorbable suture is one that is digested and absorbed by the tissue enzymes during the process of wound healing.[18] The only commonly used absorbable suture is surgical gut, formerly known as catgut—a misnomer. It is available in the plain or untreated form, having a rapid absorption time, and as chromic gut (treated in a chromic salt solution), having a slower absorption time. The manufacturers of surgical gut furnish the material sterile either in sealed glass tubes or in plastic envelopes. If the exterior of the tube is marked "boilable gut," it may be sterilized by steam under pressure, in the same manner as surgical instruments. On the other hand, if the product is marked "nonboilable gut," it should not be heated and the exterior of the tube must be sterilized by chemical means.

Silk, Cotton and Nylon

A nonabsorbable suture is one that is made from material which is neither digested nor absorbed during the process of wound healing.[18] The buried suture becomes encapsulated with fibrous tissue and remains permanently in the tissues except when surgically removed. The most important nonabsorbable suture materials include silk, cotton, nylon, linear polyethylene, silver, and stainless steel. When silk, cotton, and nylon sutures are purchased nonsterile, they must be sterilized before use. This is best accomplished by subjecting the materials to saturated steam at 250°F (121°C) for 30 minutes or 270°F (132°C) for 15 minutes. Freshly laundered muslin covers serve ideally as wrappers.

Suture materials are subject to the condition of superheating as are all fabrics and textiles. When this occurs, the tensile strength is affected. To avoid superheating, it is necessary to hydrate the suture material by moistening the strands lightly with water before placing them in the sterilizer. Because the fibers have a tendency to shrink slightly when moist, they should not be sterilized on spools, boards, or in direct contact with metal instruments.[19] The latter is conducive to charring of the material. Wooden spools should be avoided because of possible contamination of the suture material with resins extracted from the wood during the heating process. The resinous substances may be imperceptible to the eye, yet may cause irritation and foreign-body reaction in wounds. Repeated sterilization of suture materials, particularly silk and cotton, should be limited to three times in the interest of maintaining high quality sutures.

Monofilament stainless steel sutures can be effectively sterilized by saturated steam under the conditions mentioned above. The material is better sterilized in pre-cut lengths or wrapped around a metal reel to prevent kinking.

Sterilization of Dental Instruments

The significance of cross-contamination in the dental operating room or clinic has not been studied in any great depth. Perhaps this is due in part to a popular misconception that the oral flora is relatively stable and harmless rather than a potentially dangerous source of infection.[20] In 1956, Foley and Gutheim[21] reported twenty-two cases of serum hepatitis of which fifteen were due presumably to exposure at the dentist's, with three deaths. An epidemic of eight cases of acute hepatitis was described by Dull[22] in which transmission of the virus was attributed to repeated use of inadequately sterilized needles and syringes in a physician's office.

Few people realize that microbial aerosols are generated in and discharged from the mouths of dental patients during instrumentation in concentrations exceeding those reported for the normal human activity of breathing and speaking. The microbial content of these aerosols may reach the proportion of a sneeze (77,000 to 200,000 organisms) directed into one's face.[23] Also, the splattering of the environment with blood and tissue debris appears to be a fairly common occurrence in oral surgery operations where high-speed rotating cutting instruments are used.

The Council on Therapeutics of the American Dental Association[24] mentions that sterilization of dental instruments is best accomplished through

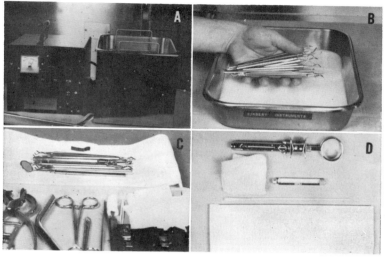

FIGURE 10-18. This techniques makes it possible to program sterile dental instruments and supplies in packs or trays. A, Ultrasonic Cleaner; B, silicone emulsion used to coat instruments before sterilization; C, instruments assembled in packs; D, anesthetic pack. (Courtesy H. G. Green, Captain, Dental Corps., U.S. Navy and Association of Military Surgeons.)

the agency of heat, with saturated steam under pressure as the first choice. All instruments should be scrubbed thoroughly with detergent and water and rinsed prior to sterilization. The terminal sterilization or decontamination of instruments may be accomplished by immersing them in a tray containing a trisodium phosphate solution (1 tablespoonful per quart of water), followed by adequate exposure in the autoclave so as to raise the temperature of the instruments and the solution to at least 250°F (121°C) for a minimum of 12 minutes. At the end of the exposure period, the steam should be *exhausted rapidly* from the chamber, the instruments withdrawn and wiped with sterile towels to maintain brightness and to remove adherent debris.[25]

The use of presterilized disposable needles and syringes should be encouraged in view of the hazard of transmission of serum hepatitis. Disposable equipment must be discarded after each use and not reemployed. Low-speed dental handpieces may be sterilized by means of dry heat in the hot-air oven for 60 minutes at 320°F (160°C) or for 30 minutes at 356°F (180°C). Corrosion of low-speed handpieces and other instruments may be prevented or reduced significantly by the use of an oil-in-water emulsion dip prior to autoclaving.[26,27] The oil-in-water film on the instruments does not hinder the steam sterilization process. Cyclohexylamine and decylamine added to steam have been found useful as corrosion inhibitors on carbon steel instruments (dental burrs) during sterilization.[28]

The application of central sterilization to dental practice was the subject of a recent investigation by Green, Dennis, and Pellen[29] at the U.S. Naval Dental School. Central sterilization and supply for the large dental clinic has many advantages over decentralized sterilization as commonly practiced in individual operatories. The technique described in Figure 10-18 makes it possible to program instruments and other materials in packs or trays, sterilize them in a central area, and store them in a clean cabinet. Instruments are processed through the ultrasonic cleaner, rinsed in water, and dried. They are then coated with an oil-in-water emulsion and assembled in packs. The anesthetic pack includes the carpule, the syringe, and the sterile disposable needle. Cotton rolls, gauze, paper covers, and other disposable items are added to the packs prior to wrapping. At no time are sterilized instruments stored unprotected in cabinets.

SUMMARY

Procedure for Routine Processing of Surgical Instruments

The primary goal of any procedure for processing surgical instruments should be to produce sterile instruments in good working condition. In order to do this, a procedure must be developed for cleaning that is functionally efficient and nondamaging to the instruments.

The following outlined procedure is a guide for implementation in situations where sonic cleaners are available for use in routine cleaning of surgical instruments.

Procedure	Directives to be Incorporated in Technique	Explanation of Directives
I. PRE-PREPARATION		
Preclean—point of use	Remove gross soil from difficult-to-clean instruments as soon as possible after they are used.	Dried or hardened soil is difficult to remove from inaccessible surfaces
	Use moist gauze sponge to wipe soil from surfaces	Friction loosens adherent tissue.
	or	
	Immerse in water and allow to soak.	Prevents soil from drying on instruments.
Sort—point of use	Separate general operating instruments for routine cleaning from delicate instruments which require special handling.	General operating instruments (hemostats, needle holders, retractors) can be processed as a unit without damage to the tools.
		Delicate instruments (cataract knives, sharp pointed scissors, sharp hooks) are very easily damaged and should be processed separately.
Collect—point of use	Replace general operating instruments in instrument tray.	In preparation for decontamination process.
	Arrange in orderly pattern:	
	Place heavy instruments in bottom of tray	Less damaging to small or lightweight items
	Turn instruments with concave surfaces (curettes, rongeurs) with bowl side down.	Facilitates draining of concave surfaces.
	Open all hinged instruments and replace on pin or rack.	Cleaning medium must contact all surfaces.
	Disassemble all instruments consisting of two or more removable parts.	All surfaces should be exposed.

Procedure	Directives to be Incorporated in Technique	Explanation of Directives
Decontaminate	Place tray of instruments in pressure instrument washer-sterilizer.	Instruments and tray should be decontaminated to prevent contamination of sonic cleaner, to prevent spread of infectious material, and to protect working personnel during cleaning process.
	Add suitable detergent.	Low-sudsing, free-rinsing detergent.
	Set selector for complete washing and sterilizing cycle.	
	Remove tray from sterilizer after completion of cycle.	Instruments can be safely handled by working personnel and without danger of spreading infectious material.
	Transfer tray of instruments to cleaning station.	Places them in proper location for cleaning operation.
II. CLEANING OPERATIONS		
Prepare sonic cleaner	Fill cleaning tank to a level one inch above top of instrument tray.	Instruments should be completely immersed in cleaning solution.
	Temperature should be about 70° to 80°F.	Temperature will rise during degassing process.
	Add suitable detergent to bath; amount specified by manufacturer.	Low-sudsing, free-rinsing detergent should be used; too much or too little reduces cleaning efficiency.
	Degas bath:	Removes gas present in most tap water.
	Turn on unit; allow to run for approximately 5 minutes.	Gas impedes the transmission of sonics through bath.
	Temperature will rise.	Optimum temperature 80°–110°F.
Wash	Place tray of instruments in bath.	
	Set timer for 5 minutes.	Cleaning cycle.
	Remove tray; move tray up and down 2 or 3 times rapidly in bath.	Sloshing action will remove some of loosened particles of soil; aids in rinsing.
Rinse and dry	Transfer tray to rinsing and drying chamber.	Combined operation.
	Set timer for 2 minutes rinse at 140°F.	Rinsing cycle.
	Optional—Rinse with distilled water for 15 seconds.	Removes residual chemicals left by tap water; eliminates spotting.
	Set timer for 5 minutes.	Drying cycle.
III. INSPECT AND SORT		
Inspect	Combine inspection and sorting of instruments.	Minimizes handling.
	Examine each instrument for cleanliness and working condition.	Instruments must be completely clean to insure effective sterilization and to function properly.
	Check hinged instruments (clamps, forceps) for stiffness and alignment of jaws and teeth.	Joints should work smoothly; tips of jaws and teeth should meet perfectly; ratchets should close easily and hold firmly.
	Test edges of sharp or semisharp instruments (scissors, shears, chisels, curettes) for sharpness.	There should be no dull spots, chips, or dents on sharp or semi-sharp edges.
	Check plated instruments for chips, sharp edges, and worn spots.	Chipped plating may harbor soil; sharp edges will damage tissue and rubber gloves; worn spots will corrode (rust).
	Examine malleable instruments (retractors, probes) for dents and bends.	Bent instruments are difficult to mold; they should be flat and smooth.

Procedure	*Directives to be Incorporated in Technique*	*Explanation of Directives*
Sort	Return unclean instruments to cleaning station for recleaning.	Must be clean to insure effective sterilization.
	Remove instruments in poor working condition from circulation; hold for repair.	Instruments in poor working condition are a handicap to the surgeon and hazardous for the patient.
		Instruments should be repaired at the first sign of damage or malfunctioning.
	Separate basic instruments from special instruments.	Basic instruments include hemostats, tissue forceps, needle holders.
		Special instruments include those designed for a specific use such as a stomach clamp, kidney clamp, bone rongeur.
	Replace basic instruments in instrument tray.	For reuse.
	Replace special instruments in tray or return to storage.	Instruments not needed should be kept in assigned storage.
IV. PREPARATION FOR STERILIZATION Select	Instruments needed for one operative procedure should be selected and assembled in one unit or set.	Sets must be made up according to the schedule of operative procedures; varies from day to day.
	Content depends on kind of operative procedure for which it is to be used and the preferences of the operating surgeon.	Assembly is simplified by using basic sets and adding special instruments as indicated by schedule and operating surgeon.
Assemble	Arrange instruments in tray.	Instrument trays are designed for effective sterilization and for orderly arrangement of instruments.
	Follow predetermined pattern.	A standardized arrangement simplifies identification and handling at time of use.
	Hinged instruments must be opened; place on pin or rack.	Sterilizing agent must contact all surfaces to insure sterilization; pin or rack will hold instruments in open position and facilitate handling. Sterilizing agent must contact all surfaces.
	Instruments with movable parts (other than forceps) which can be taken apart should be disassembled.	
	Place heavy instruments in bottom of tray.	Lightweight and small items should be protected.
	Avoid overloading; do not attempt to include items for every eventuality.	Extras or questionable items can be sterilized as separate units and held in sterile storage ready for use.
Instrument sets	Instrument sets which are to be sterilized in advance, or transferred through an unrestricted traffic area, must be wrapped before sterilization.	To protect instruments from contamination during storage and transit.
	Wrap instrument sets in one double-thickness muslin wrapper.	Muslin wrappers are strong and pliable, will withstand weight, are easily manipulated at time sterile instruments are removed.
	Secure pack with autoclave tape.	Identifies instrument pack that has been exposed to sterilizing process from one that has not.

Procedure	Directives to be Incorporated in Technique	Explanation of Directives
	Label—identify type of set.	Instrument set must be matched to the operative procedure.
Single instrument	Wrap single or small group of instruments in one double-thickness muslin wrapper.	Pliability and strength of muslin facilitate wrapping of irregularly shaped instruments and minimize puncturing or tearing of wrapper during handling.
V. STERILIZE	Use heat, preferably steam under pressure, to sterilize heat resistant instruments whenever possible.	Method of choice; fast and economical.
Steam under pressure	Expose to steam under pressure: Metal instruments only, unwrapped, 15 minutes at 250° to 254°F or 3 minutes at 270°F	Only surface sterilization is involved.
	Metal instruments combined with other materials or with padding or covering added 20 minutes at 250° to 254F° or 10 minutes at 270°F.	Rubber, plastic, and/or fabrics require longer exposure.
	Metal instruments wrapped in double-thickness muslin. Metal instruments combined with other materials and with pading or covering on tray 30 minutes at 250°–254°F 15 minutes at 270°F.	Addition of wrapper requires a longer exposure period.
Dry heat	Any instrument with tight fitting, movable parts and which cannot be disassembled should be wrapped in heavy duty aluminum foil and sterilized by exposure to dry heat for 1 hour at 320°F.	Steam may not contact all surfaces of tight fitting, movable parts.
	At completion of sterilizing cycle, remove instrument packs from sterilizer and date.	Date is used to determine shelf age; helpful for packs held in storage ready for use.
	Allow instrument packs to cool before storing on cold, metal shelves.	Moisture in pack may condense on cold surface and cause wetting of wrapper and contamination of contents.

Decontamination of Operating Room Materials

Item	Preparatory Steps	Directives	Decontamination Process
Linens	Inspect for instruments. Roll wet portions inwardly so they will not soak through.	Collect in laundry bag. Place in second clean laundry bag and close on removal from operating room.	
		Identify as infectious and send to laundry in routine manner.	Launder.
Gauze sponges	Collect in waterproof bag.	Keep outside of bag clean. Close securely. Discard in receptacle for burnable waste.	Incinerate.
Tape sponges	Collect in waterproof bag.	Keep outside of bag clean. Close securely. Discard in receptacle for burnable waste.	Incinerate.
Instruments General operating	Open all hinged instruments. Disassemble instruments with more than one part.	Collect in instrument tray.	
		Transfer to washer-sterilizer.	Expose to total washing and sterilizing cycle. This includes a 3-minute exposure to saturated steam under pressure at 270°F.
	Alternative #1 Open all hinged instruments. Disassemble instruments with more than one part.	Collect in water-tight basin. Cover instruments with 2% solution of trisodium phosphate. Transfer to pressure steam sterilizer.	Exposure to steam under pressure for 30 min. at 270°F or 45 min. at 250°F. Use *Fast Exhaust* on sterilizer.
Endoscopic (Lensed)	Disassemble.	Soak in chemical disinfectant. Rinse thoroughly. Dry. Transfer to gas sterilizer.	Expose to ethylene oxide gas following manufacturer's recommendations of concentration, time exposure, temperature, and humidity.
Surgeon's needles	Collect in needle box.	Include with instruments.	
Hollow needles		Include with instruments.	
Cautery cords and electrodes	Collect electrodes with surgeon's needles.	Include with instruments.	
Syringes	Disassemble.	Include with instruments.	
Utensils Basins, bowls, trays	Discard liquid waste. Discard solid waste.	Empty into clinical sink. Discard in lined floor bucket.	Incinerate.
		Position utensils on edge in washer-sterilizer.	Expose to total washing and sterilizing cycle. This includes exposure to saturated steam under pressure for 3 minutes at 270°F.
	Alternative Discard liquid waste. Discard solid waste. Remove gross soil.	Empty into clinical sink. Discard in lined floor bucket. Use cloth and chemical disinfec-	Incinerate

Item	Preparatory Steps	Directives	Decontamination Process
		tant to remove gross soil. Discard cloth with linen or waste.	
		Remove rack from pressure steam sterilizer. Position utensils on edge.	Sterilize by exposure to steam under pressure for 3 minutes at 270°F or 15 minutes at 250°F.
Suction bottle	Discard waste.	Empty into clinica sink. Position on side in washer sterilizer.	Expose to total washing and sterilizing cycle. This includes exposure to steam under pressure for 3 minutes at 270°F.
	Alternative Discard waste.	Empty into clinical sink. Rinse with chemical disinfectant. Position on side in pressure steam sterilizer.	Sterilize by exposure to steam under pressure for 3 minutes at 270°F or 15 minutes at 250°F.
Rubber goods Gloves	Collect in waterproof bag.	Keep outside of bag *clean*. Close securely—discard in receptacle for burnable waste.	Incinerate.
Catheters		Include with gloves.	Incinerate
	Alternative Remove gross soil.	Include with instruments.	Same as general operating instruments.
Suction tubing Prox mal segment	Detach from collection bottle.	Place in lined floor bucket.	Incinerate.
	Alternative Remove gross soil.	Flush by drawing chemical disinfectant through tip and tubing while still attached to suction bottle.	
	Detach from suction bottle. Detach tip from tubing.	Include with instruments.	
Distal segment	Detach.	Include with suction bottle.	
Floor buckets	Remove waterproof liner containing waste. Close on removal from operating room. Identify as infectious.	Place in second clean bag. Discard in receptacle for burnable waste.	Incinerate.
		Position floor bucket on side in pressure steam sterilizer or Clean buckets with furniture.	Expose to steam under pressure for 3 minutes at 270°F or 15 minutes at 250°F
Furniture Tables, stools, Mayo stand	Apply a detergent-germicide to any areas soiled with blood or pus—let stand 10 minutes or more, then remove with cloth.	As soon as possible after area is soiled. Place cloth in lined floor bucket or	Incinerate.
	At completion of case.	Include with contaminated linen. Clean all accessible surfaces with a detergent-germicide capable of destroying vegetative cells, plus tubercle bacilli. Place cleaning cloths in lined floor bucket or	Launder. Incinerate.
Walls	Spot clean known contaminated areas with a detergent-germicide solution.	Include with contaminated linen.	Launder.
	Allow residual to dry on surfaces.	Place cleaning cloths in lined floor bucket or	Incinerate.
Floors	Apply a detergent-germicide to any areas soiled with blood or pus—let stand 10 minutes, then remove with cloth.	Include with contaminated linen. As soon as possible after area is soiled.	Launder.
		Place cloth in lined floor bucket or	Incinerate.
		Include with contaminated linen.	Launder.

Item	Preparatory Steps	Directives	Decontamination Process
	At completion of case.	Clean thoroughly with a detergent-germicide capable of destroying vegetative cells, including tubercle bacilli. Place mophead in waterproof bag. Close securely. Identify as infectious	Incinerate.
		or	
Shoes	Remove boots.	Include with contaminated linen. Include with contaminated linen.	Launder. Follow with autoclaving. Launder.
	Alternative		
	Floor mat at door of operating room saturated with a detergent-germicide.	Wipe soles of shoes on mat upon leaving operating room. Place mat in waste receptacle	Incinerate.
		or	
		Place mat in laundry bag with contaminated linen.	Launder.

Note: It is not considered necessary to quarantine an operating theater following a septic procedure.

REFERENCES

1. GRAY, T. C. (Ed): *Operating Theatres and Ancillary Rooms.* Proc Symposium. London, John Sherratt & Son, Altrincham, 1964, p. 225.
2. WALTER, C. W.: Technique for the rapid and absolute sterilization of instruments. *Surg Gynec Obstet,* 67:244, 1938.
3. WALTER, C. W.: Sterilization. *Surg Clin N Amer,* New York Number, April, 1942, p. 350.
4. BACON, L. R., and NUTTING, E. G., JR.: Polyphosphate detergents in mechanical dishwashing. *Ind Eng Chem,* 44:146-150, 1952.
5. PRICKETT, E.: Processing of Surgical Instruments. From a Study of the Operating Room, School of Nursing, Univ. of Pittsburgh and Methods Engineering Council, May 7, 1953.
6. DAVIS, H., PARRACK, H. O., and ELDREDGE, D. H.: Hazards of intense sound and ultrasound. *Ann Otol,* 58:732-738, 1949.
7. CRAWFORD, A. E.: *Ultrasonic Engineering* London, Butterworth's Scientific Publications, 1955, p. 26.
8. GOLDMAN, R. G.: *Ultrasonic Technology* New York, Reinhold, 1962, p. 144.
9. HUGHES, D. E., and NYBORG, W. L.: Cell disruption by ultrasound. *Science,* 138:108-114, 1962.
10. DAVIDSON, E. A., and ROSETT, T.: *Ultrasonic Disruption of Bacteria and Other Microorganisms.* Bulletin S-835, Stamford, Conn, Branson Instruments, Inc.
11. EL'PINER, I. E.: O mekhanizme deistviia ul'trazvukovykh voln na mikroorganizmy (Mechanism of action of ultrasonic waves upon microorganisms). *Mikrobiologiia,* 24:371-381, 1955.
12. BULAT, T. J.: Decontamination techniques using sonic energy. *JAORN,* 2:74-80, 1964.
13. SLEPECKY, R. A.: Sonication—Germicide treatment in surgical instrument cleaning. *Hosp Topics,* 44:133-134, 1966.
14. GLASSMAN, P.: Proper care enables longer trouble-free use of stainless steel instruments. *Hosp Topics,* August, 1964, p. 107-109.
15. HOYT, S. L.: *Metal Data* New York, Reinhold, 1952, p. 336.
16. ECKER, E. E., and SMITH, R.: Sterilizing surgical instruments and utensils. *Mod Hosp,* 48:92-98, 1937.
17. PERKINS, J. J.: Sterilizing Methods. U. S. Patent No. 2, 628, 887.
18. *Suture Manual.* Danbury, Conn, Davis & Geck, 1963, p. 11.
19. MEADE, W. H., and LONG, C. H.: The use of cotton as a suture material. *JAMA,* 117:2140-2143, 1941.
20. BURTON, W. E.: Changing requirements for sterilization. *J Prosth Dent,* 14:127-139, 1964.
21. FOLEY, F. E., and GUTHEIM, R. N.: Serum hepatitis following dental procedures: a presentation of 15 cases, including three fatalities. *Ann Intern Med,* 45:369-380, 1956.
22. DULL, H. B.: Syringe-transmitted hepatitis: a recent epidemic in historical perspective. *JAMA,* 176:413-418, 1961.

23. Miller, R. L., Burton, W. E., and Spore, R. W.: *Aerosols Produced by Dental Instrumentation. Proc First Intern Symp Aerobiol.* Oakland, Calif. Naval Biological Laboratory, 1963, p. 97.

24. Council on Dent Ther Amer Dent Ass: *Accepted Dental Remedies.* Chicago, Ill, 1966, p. 36.

25. Perkins, J. J.: Preparation and sterilization of surgical instruments. *The Surgical Supervisor,* 8:15-22, 1948.

26. Charbeneau, G. T., and Berry, G. C.: A simple and effective autoclave method of handpiece and instrument sterilization without corrosion. *J Amer Dent Ass,* 59:732-737, 1959.

27. Crowley, M. C.; Charbeneau, G. T., and Aponte, A. J.: Preliminary investigation of some basic problems of instrument sterilization. *J Amer Dent Ass,* 58:45-49, 1959.

28. Holmlund, L. G.: On Steam Corrosion and Steam Corrosion Inhibition with Special Reference to the Autoclave Sterilization of Dental (and Surgical) Steel Instrument Materials. Trans. Royal Schools Dentistry, No. 9, 1963. Umea Research Library, Umea, Sweden.

29. Green, H. G., Dennis, H. J., and Pelleu, G. B.: Central sterilization for the dental clinic. *Milit Med,* 131:1483-1489, 1966.

Chapter 11

WATER STERILIZERS

IN THE HOSPITAL sterile water is as essential to clean surgery and aseptic technic as sterile instruments and dressings. It obviously should be protected from recontamination with the same care. Through the aid of modern methods it is not a difficult procedure to render water sterile. To maintain water in the sterile state is not, however, easily accomplished except through the use of equipment designed specifically for this purpose.

Since water as normally supplied to hospitals and institutions contains but few bacterial spores, and because the organisms present are wet, they are easily destroyed upon heating the water to 250°F (121°C) for a brief period of exposure. The real difficulty encountered is in effectively guarding the sterility of the water against airborne, insect, and contact contamination following the sterilization process, especially at the point of draw-off from the storage reservoir or tank.

THE MEANING OF "STERILE WATER"

General use of the term *sterile water* should be discouraged chiefly because it does not denote any particular quality of water from the standpoint of mineral impurities, freedom from pyrogens, chemical or physiological compatibility. In order to avoid possible misunderstanding or confusion as to the acceptability of the water for a particular surgical requirement it is desirable to designate the product as "sterile tap water," "sterile water for external use" or "sterile distilled water," whichever the case may be. Ordinary water as supplied for drinking purposes is usually designated "tap water," meaning that it has undergone only the common purification process of chlorination required of a public water supply so as to make it safe for human consumption. While tap water is generally recognized as being free of pathogenic organisms it is definitely not sterile. After sterilization it will still contain most of the original chemical impurities, including dead bacteria and pyrogens which render it unsafe for use in the preparation of parenteral solutions, isotonic fluids, or for other surgical application where a physiological environment for wound healing must be maintained.

Sterilized tap water produced in water sterilizers of the pressure type is still employed in hospital operating rooms and delivery rooms for routine use in hand basins, irrigations, hot packs. Many surgeons feel that sterile tap water is satisfactory for such applications. However, other surgeons, increasing in number within the last few years, recognize that sterile tap water does not fulfill the requirement for an ideal irrigating fluid, and this group advocates the use of strictly isotonic solutions in the operating room.

The use of nonpressure reservoirs for water sterilization is no longer recognized as a reliable method. Long experience has proved that water in this type of container may not always be rendered sterile because the highest temperature attainable is 212°F (100°C); and it is almost immediately exposed to contamination occurring through unfiltered air contact and through unsterile gauge glasses or draw-off faucets. Loose fitting reservoir covers make it impossible to provide for air filtration and, lacking steam under pressure, there is no means for flushing out gauge glasses or draw-off faucets. If a water filter is provided it is impossible to sterilize it or the pipe connections leading to the filter. These factors constitute the principal objections to the nonpressure method for water sterilization.

Because of more dependable operation, the pressure method for the sterilization of water eventually became the accepted standard of hospital practice. Progress within the past decade shows that the pressure method has given way to an even more reliable process, namely, the individual flask method for the preparation, sterilization, and dispensing of sterile water and other solutions in the hospital (see Chap. 16).

WATER STERILIZERS SHOULD PROVIDE FOR EFFECTIVE WATER AND AIR FILTRATION

The essential features of construction and operation of a pair of modern water sterilizers are shown in Figures 11-1 and 11-2. Other units, whether heated by gas or electricity, are similar in design and operation. Steam is the preferred source of heat because it is fast, economical, and safe. The steam supply for each reservoir is controlled by a single valve, and the return line from each heating coil is equipped with a thermostatic trap and check valve. Automatic pressure regulators, one for each reservoir, maintain the correct steam pressure and temperature of 15 to 17 pounds and 250° to 254°F (121° to 123°C) throughout the sterilizing period. The left-hand (cold) reservoir contains a cooling coil, and the flow of cooling water is controlled by a dialed regulator adjustable for varying water pressures.

Each reservoir is also equipped with an individual, self-sterilizing, combination water and air filter—controlled by a single valve. In filling the tanks, the flow of water is visible through the glass front of the filter case. A percolating system is also provided for each water-level gauge which automatically circulates water through the gauge while the reservoir is undergoing sterilization. Each gauge connection to the reservoir includes a valve which closes automatically if the gauge glass is broken when the reservoir is under pressure.

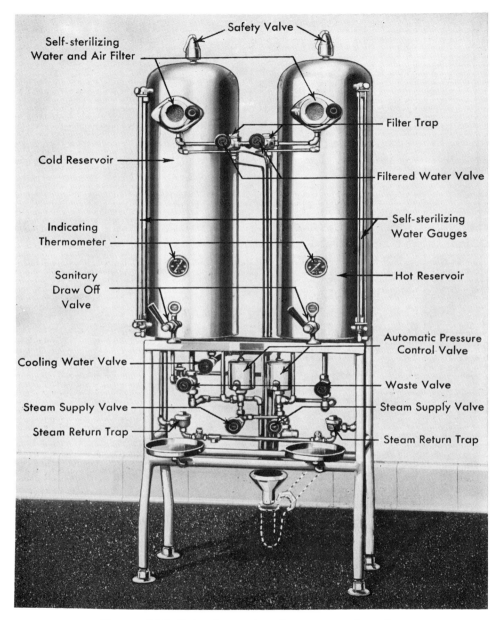

FIGURE 11-1. Pair of water sterilizers—steam heated.

When water is sterilized in any vessel, opportunity for recontamination immediately begins when the water cools and continues until the reservoir has been emptied. Hot water, upon cooling, absorbs air until it is in equilibrium with the atmospheric (room) temperature and with every withdrawal

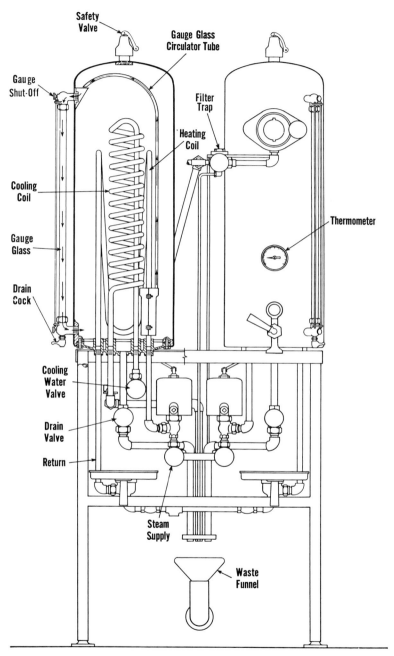

FIGURE 11-2. This diagram shows essential features of construction and operation of the steam heated water sterilizers.

of water from the reservoir, an equal amount of air is drawn in to replace it. To illustrate, a 25-gallon reservoir of water was heated to 250°F (121°C) and then allowed to cool to atmospheric temperature. The reservoir was so arranged that all air was taken in through a glass water trap. Twenty-four hours after the heat was turned off, air bubbles were still being drawn in visibly through the water trap in appreciable quantity. This air absorption and air contact definitely permits contamination, unless the air is passed through an effective bacteria-retentive filter. All room air carries a certain amount of dust, a considerable portion of which is laden with microorganisms which may or may not be pathogenic.

Some of the older water sterilizers, still in use today, are equipped with air filters similar to that shown in Figure 11-3. This device consists of a small metal cup containing cotton wool as the filter medium, mounted above an automatic valve on the dome of the reservoir. The valve closes approximately tight but rarely completely tight, when the reservoir is subjected to internal pressure during sterilization. It opens freely to relieve vacuum when the water cools and when water is withdrawn, for the intake of air. The cotton in the cup serves poorly as a filter because it becomes moistened by steam escaping through the valve during sterilization. This causes the cotton to shrink away from the walls of the cup. When moist, the cotton be-

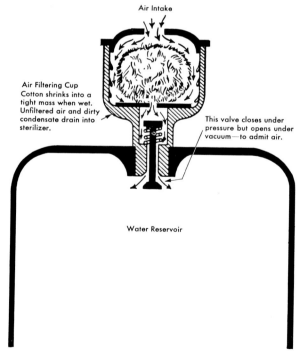

FIGURE 11-3. A common type of vacuum release valve and air filtering cup found on older water sterilizers. It is worthless as an air filter.

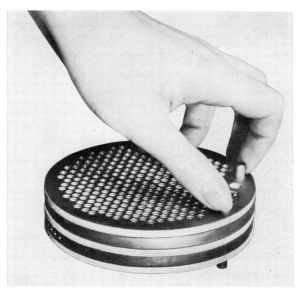

FIGURE 11-4. This is typical of one type of water filter used on water sterilizers. It consists of three removable filter discs made from a compressed fibrous material.

comes so dense that air can be forced through it only with difficulty. As the result, there is little filtration of air but a definite intake of dust particles and condensate from the cup back into the reservoir. This type of filter on a water sterilizer is worthless.

The combined water and air filter used on sterilizers shown in Figures 11-1 and 11-2 is so constructed that it can be automatically sterilized by steam each time the water is sterilized. The water filtering element (Fig. 11-4) consists of three removable filter discs made from a specially prepared fibrous material which will withstand the action of steam without serious loss of efficiency. The water filter is mounted in the filter case behind a glass cover, through which the operator can see the passage of water as the reservoir is being filled.

Air intake to the reservoir occurs through the same filter case and might be drawn back through the water filtering element except that it is so dense that air will pass through it only by considerable pressure. For the filtration of air a secondary element is provided consisting of tightly compressed non-corrosive metal wool, maintained in a moist condition. The air filtering element is backwashed by steam every time water is sterilized. It possesses a fair degree of efficiency in the removal of bacteria and dust particles. No air filter will assure complete protection. In fact, the sterilization of air by filtration through a fibrous medium means nothing more than the establishment of a permissible probability for passage of a contaminant.

The valve controlling raw water supply to the filter is a double-action valve, which, when opened, admits water to the filter and automatically closes the rear connection on the valve leading to the drain. When the valve is closed, water flow is shut off and the rear connection to the drain is opened. Then, should the valve leak slightly, leakage is conducted directly to the drain instead of the water reservoir. During sterilization, steam from the reservoir passes through the filter to the drain and this flow continues until the filter (thermostatic) trap is heated and closes, holding the entire filtering system under pure steam pressure as long as sterilization continues.

An air intake tube connects the air filtering compartment directly to the air-vented waste. A ball check in the filter case prevents flow from the filter to the waste but admits air freely under slight back pressure as when water is withdrawn from the reservoir or when the sterilized reservoir cools down. In this manner modern water sterilizers give fairly reliable protection against the hazards of recontamination.

STERILIZATION OF GAUGE GLASSES

Of the water sterilizers in use today, there are some with no provisions for the automatic sterilization of gauge glasses. These units present special problems because the water contained in the gauge glasses is not subjected to the sterilizing influence of the heat applied to the reservoir. If the gauge glasses are not flushed out during sterilization, the unsterile water will later contaminate the reservoirs. Fortunately many of these older sterilizers have valves on the gauge fittings permitting the gauge to be closed off from the reservoir and the unsterile water then drained from the pet cock in the bottom fitting. Following this, steam is permitted to blow through the gauge glass for about 15 seconds in order to provide for sterilization. Then when the pet cock is closed and the valve to the reservoir opened, the gauge will refill with sterile water to the level in the reservoir.

The system employed for the automatic sterilization of gauge glasses operates on the principle of a coffee percolator, as shown in Figure 11-2. A metal tube is attached to the source of heat so that a small volume of water is heated sufficiently in advance of the main body of water to force it through the tube, the other end of which leads to the top of the water gauge. This circulation, indicated by a film of water flowing into the top of the gauge, continues, vigorously at first, but slowing down as the water in the gauge and the water in the reservoir approach the maximum temperature. This circulation eliminates accumulation of sediment in the bottom of the gauge glass and subjects the water in the gauge to the same sterilizing effect as the water in the reservoir.

DRAW-OFF FAUCETS

One of the most serious criticisms in the use of water sterilizers is that no positive method has ever been devised for the sterilization of the draw-off faucet. This is a most vulnerable location for the deposit of airborne bacteria and it is extremely difficult to completely protect the draw-off faucet against insect or contact contamination. Present day faucets all have bell-shaped mouthpieces, designed to protect, insofar as possible, the water outlets from contact contamination. Probably the most effective method for the cleansing of faucets is as follows:

At the end of the sterilization period, before turning off the heat, place a wide-mouth pitcher or other large container under each draw-off faucet and permit the hot water and steam to flow through vigorously for at least 15 seconds. This will serve to sanitize the critical surfaces of the mouthpiece and to flush out the connection leading to the reservoir as effectively as can be done by any practical procedure. If care is taken to insure that this detail is carried out each time the reservoir undergoes sterilization the draw-off faucet will remain reasonably free of contamination.

Some hospitals require the mouthpieces of faucets to be flamed before use. This is a troublesome detail and the practice should be discouraged, especially if the sterilizers are located close to the operating room where explosive anaesthetic gases are used. It is also questionable if the flame as usually applied ever contacts the critical surfaces of the faucet with sufficient intensity to sterilize.

RESTERILIZATION OF WATER

The question frequently arises as to the maximum length of time water can be considered to remain sterile in water sterilizers. If the sterilizers are equipped with modern protective features and in good repair, there is evidence to show that the water in the reservoirs will remain sterile for at least 24 hours. However, other factors justify the recommendation that the water should not stand more than 12 hours before resterilization. As must be acknowledged, the draw-off faucets can be contaminated easily and they may be covered with dust particles after standing many hours.

The degree of contamination within the reservoir, if it does occur, will likely increase with time. A slow leak in the cooling coil in the cold tank or a faulty air filter may contribute little, if any, contamination in a few hours, but the accumulated leakage or possible passage of contaminants during an entire day would definitely become a serious matter. The best procedure is to establish a routine for the sterilization of water on an 8 to 12 hour basis. This assures an added measure of protection in guarding against recontamination.

SAMPLING WATER FOR STERILITY TESTS

The collection of samples from water sterilizers for sterility testing should become a standard procedure in hospitals with properly equipped laboratories and trained personnel qualified to conduct this type of work. The first step in collecting the sample of water is to see that both reservoirs (hot and

cold tanks) have been sterilized in the routine manner according to the operating instructions. This should be done in the afternoon preceding collection of the sample the following day in order that the sterilized water may
stand for at least 12 hours. The purpose in permitting the sterilized water to
cool overnight is to afford ample opportunity for contamination to enter the
reservoir whether from a faulty air filter or a slow leak in the cooling coil in
the cold tank.

The next step is to draw off approximately three-fourths of the volume of
water in the reservoir and discard it. Then hold a previously sterilized bottle
or flask of about 200 ml capacity under the faucet and collect the sample
from the remaining water. The flask should be immediately covered with a
sterile stopper and delivered to the bacteriological laboratory. By following
this procedure it is possible to collect a sample from the upper portion of
water in the reservoir. This is desirable because a low order of contamination may not always be uniformly dispersed throughout the entire volume of
water.

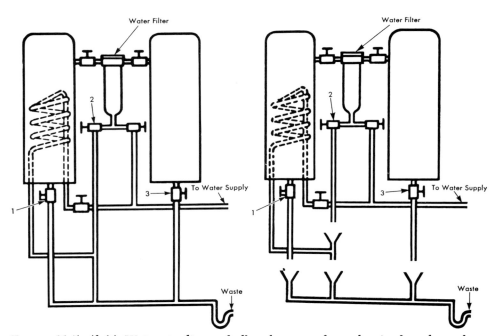

FIGURE 11-5. (*left*) Water sterilizers of all makes were formerly piped as shown here,
with drainage connections leading direct to sewage system with no intermediate air
breaks. Leaky valves 1, 2, or 3 would permit reservoirs, under negative pressure, to draw
in sewage, or this might be occasioned by the backing up of sewage due to clogged
waste line. Present sanitary codes condemn this system of piping.

FIGURE 11-6. (*right*) This shows how air breaks can be applied to piping (Fig. 11-5) to
guard against pollution from waste. Air gaps in all such connections should be 1½
inches or more.

Another method which gives equally satisfactory results is to run the sample of water directly into a tube of sterile culture medium. However, this method requires extremely careful technique in order to collect no more and no less than the required aliquot of water for the volume of medium in the tube. When this method is used, the medium should be contained in large test tubes with dimensions of 30 × 200 mm, each containing 40 ml of fluid thioglycollate or other approved sterility test medium. The sample of water undergoing test should then be limited to about 10 ml. All tests should be conducted in duplicate and the tubes incubated at a temperature of 32° to 35°C.

HAZARDS OF OBSOLETE TYPES OF WATER STERILIZERS

A dangerous source of sterile water contamination is found in obsolete equipment where the connections on the sterilizers are made directly to the waste, with no intermediate air breaks. This system, still occasionally encountered in hospitals, is shown in Figure 11-5. With such a system of piping there is no protection against the backflow of water from the waste to the sterile reservoirs. It is definitely hazardous and sanitary codes condemn the method of piping and require rearrangement to conform to the system shown in Figure 11-6. Here every drainage line is protected against backflow from the waste by means of open funnel air breaks.

Any water sterilizers in use today lacking the latest protective features should be considered obsolete, and prompt action should be taken to replace or to modernize them. Whatever the circumstances may be, it is essential that the waste line piping conforms with modern plumbing codes. Each tank should be equipped with an individually controlled water and air filter, subject to automatic sterilization. Provision should also be made for automatic sterilization of gauge glasses. In addition, methods should be instituted for the routine inspection and control of water sterilizers, with special emphasis given to steam flushing of draw-off faucets each time the sterilizers are operated.

REMOVAL OF SCALE FROM WATER STERILIZERS

The water supply in many localities contains large amounts of lime, responsible for hard water conditions. Application of heat to hard water causes the lime salts to deposit in the form of scale on the heating coils and on the bottom and side of the reservoir. Frequently this scale will accumulate on the bottom of the reservoir, building up into a mass of considerable volume. As soon as any discoloration of water is noted, or if particles of scale appear when water is withdrawn, that is an indication that the tanks need to be cleaned.

The process of cleaning or removal of scale should not be attempted by nursing personnel, rather the work should be carried out by a trained mechanic or maintenance man after routine working hours. At weekly intervals or once each month, depending upon the quality of the raw water, the sterilizer should be filled to about one-third of its capacity and heated to sterilizing temperature. Cover the open funnel in the waste line with towels draped about it to prevent escape of steam and water into the room, then open the waste valve and permit the reservoir to blow down until it is empty. Then, while the coils are still hot, fill the reservoir completely and, without heating, permit the water to drain out. This will remove the loose scale quite effectively but will not remove the hard deposit on coils and other surfaces.

If the sterilizers are electrically heated, the accumulation of scale on the heaters will eventually cause burn out because the mass of scale becomes so dense that the heat builds up to a degree that will actually melt the metal sheath of the heaters. Usually it will be found necessary to dismantle the sterilizers for efficient cleaning, whether heated by direct steam or electricity. This is a major task and the following points should be kept in mind when performing the work: It is impractical to apply an acid or scale solvent to the interiors of tanks. Since comparatively little scale forms on these surfaces the use of a wire brush or coarse knife for scraping the scale loose will usually suffice. Before reassembling, the tanks should be thoroughly rinsed out with water. Coils or heating elements require soaking in warm muriatic acid (1 part acid to 9 parts water) until the scale has softened sufficiently for easy removal. The removal of scale from the interior of a coil can be accomplished by repeatedly filling the coil with the dilute acid while it is being subjected to moderate heating. Terminals on electric heaters must be protected from the acid, and care should be exercised to prevent the acid fumes from contacting highly finished or plated surfaces. After soaking the coils or heaters in the acid solution for about an hour, the residual can be removed by scraping with a coarse knife edge. The parts should be thoroughly rinsed in tap water before reassembling in order to remove all traces of acid.

WATER FOR TRANSURETHRAL SURGERY

For many years it has been common practice for the surgeon to employ two reservoirs or Valentine flasks suspended from a standard, and filled with the desired irrigating fluid for use during urology operations. When the operating room is used exclusively for transurethral surgery, it has been found convenient to install a large capacity water sterilizing tank in a horizontal position near the ceiling of the room from which the irrigating reservoirs may be filled. This arrangement, as shown in Figure 11-7, permits adequate pressure and volume of water for gravity irrigation purposes. The normal installation requires a ceiling height of approximately 10 feet in order to give a drop of about 8 feet from the draw-off outlet to the floor. Usually provision is made for transmitting the sterile water through suitable piping from the draw-off outlet of the tank to a point directly over the operating table. If further reduction in hydrostatic pressure is required, the sterile water may then be conducted into a standard irrigation container, adjustable to the proper height above the level of the patient.

To some degree, professional opinion varies as to the type of irrigating medium to be employed in transurethral surgery. However, since the initial work of Creevy,[3] it has been conclusively demonstrated that operative and postoperative complications occur less frequently when nonhemolyzing solutions are used than when distilled water is employed. The latter may cause intravascular hemolysis of the patient's serum. Popular irrigating media include the amino acid, glycine; an inert sugar, mannitol; and Cytal,® a mixture of the two inert sugars, mannitol and sorbitol.

LIMITATIONS OF WATER STERILIZERS

The continued use of water sterilizers in hospitals has been seriously attacked by several authorities in the field of sterilization. Walter,[1] for example, has stated that "there is no practicable way of guarding the sterilizers against contamination and that the water is likely to be contaminated when it is drawn off. . . . In summary, water sterilizers are decided luxuries that contribute little to aseptic technic." A more recent statement against the use of water sterilizers has been issued by the Advisory Committee on Sterilization Procedures for Queensland Public Hospitals.[2] This group is of the opinion that "sterility of the water can never be relied on—the only safe water is water that has been autoclaved." In a survey of tank sterilizers, including piped systems, used for supplying sterile water for operating theaters, Kelsey[4] found that more than 40 per cent of the devices failed bacteriologically at least once during three 3-month periods of weekly examination by a quantitative method designed to distinguish genuine failure from chance contamination.

There is valid evidence to support the above statements when one considers the many elements of faulty design and the obvious neglect of protective sanitary features on water sterilizers installed in hospitals during the past fifty years. It must be acknowledged then that water sterilizers have definite limitations and whenever such equipment is purchased by a hospital, the facts should be honestly presented and clearly understood. The following features are known to contribute to faulty operation and contamination of the water.

- Ineffective air filters.
- Single water filter serving both reservoirs—always a potential source of contamination.
- Cooling coil in cold tank. This may develop a slow leak.
- No provision for automatic sterilization of side arm gauge glasses.
- Leaky valves permitting raw water to enter sterile reservoirs.

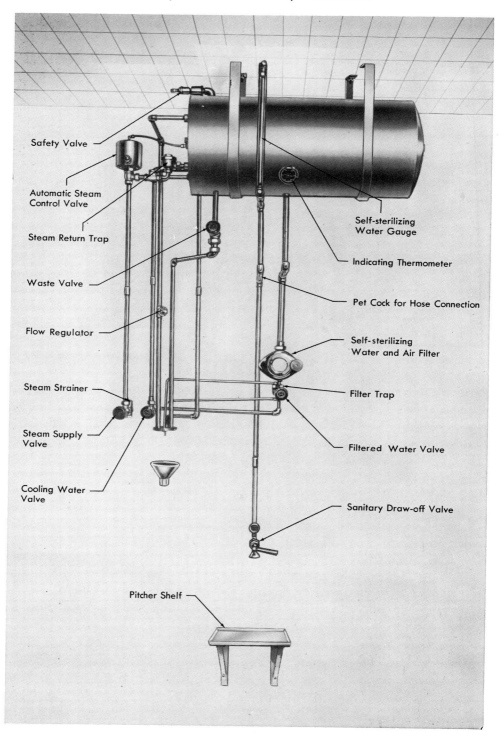

Safety Valve

Automatic Steam Control Valve

Steam Return Trap

Waste Valve

Flow Regulator

Steam Strainer

Steam Supply Valve

Cooling Water Valve

Self-sterilizing Water Gauge

Indicating Thermometer

Pet Cock for Hose Connection

Self-sterilizing Water and Air Filter

Filter Trap

Filtered Water Valve

Sanitary Draw-off Valve

Pitcher Shelf

- Drainage connections piped directly to the waste line, with no intermediate air breaks. This system of piping constitutes a violation of sanitary codes.
- No practicable method for the positive sterilization of draw-off faucets.

REFERENCES

1. WALTER, C. W.: *Aseptic Treatment of Wounds.* New York, Macmillan. 1948, pp. 302-307.
2. COMMITTEE ON STERILIZATION PROCEDURES: *Handbook of Sterilization Procedures.* Brisbane, Australia, A. H. Tucker, 1953, p. 70.
3. CREEVY, C. D., and WEBB, E. A.: A fatal hemolytic reaction following transurethral resection of the prostate gland. *Surgery, 21:*56, 1957.
4. KELSEY, J. C.: Sterilisation—theory and practice. *Brit Hosp J Soc Serv Rev,* 75:2095-2099, 1965.

FIGURE 11-7. Water sterilizer tank commonly referred to as cystoscopic water sterilizer. Usually installed in horizontal position, suspended from ceiling or wall-bracket mounted in operating room. Reservoir of 15 or 25 gallons capacity is equipped with cooling coil, safety valve, thermometer. Sterilization is accomplished by means of steam heat. Reservoir may be supplied with distillate from water still mounted some distance above unit.

Chapter 12

DRY HEAT STERILIZATION

I T IS IMPORTANT for the student of sterilization to clearly understand
the limitations of dry heat as a sterilizing agent. It should be used only
where direct contact of the material or substance with saturated steam is
impractical or unattainable. Dry heat in the form of hot air is difficult to
control within narrow limits, except in a specially designed sterilizer. It
penetrates materials slowly and unevenly and long exposure periods are required for sterilization. Because of the poor penetrability and the destructive effect of the high temperatures employed, dry heat or hot air is entirely
unsuited for the sterilization of fabrics and rubber goods. On the other
hand, it is well suited for the sterilization of keen, cutting edge instruments,
needles, and syringes. Dry heat does not exert a corrosive effect on sharp
instruments as is commonly observed with steam, nor does it erode the
ground glass surfaces of syringes.

The action of dry heat on objects is that of conduction. The heat is absorbed by the exterior surfaces of an article, eventually heating the interior,
but the factor of moisture is lacking. It is a false assumption to believe that
all substances normally in the liquid state, or those which become liquid
upon heating, such as petroleum jelly (Vaseline®), can be rendered sterile
by the usual autoclaving process. Petrolatum, oils, oily suspensions, fats, and
powders have no appreciable water content and the moisture of the steam
cannot be depended upon to permeate the substances. Heat resistant organisms concealed in these materials would, of course, be heated to the temperature of the surrounding steam, but lacking the moisture factor, the temperature would be inadequate for complete bacterial destruction in any
practicable exposure period. Therefore, it is necessary for the sterilization of
anhydrous oils, greases, and powders to utilize a dry-heat method, or its
equivalent, with a safe time-temperature relationship, taking into account
any appreciable time lag characteristic of heating a particular load.

RESISTANCE OF BACTERIA TO DRY HEAT

The phenomena responsible for the widely different temperatures required in dry and moist heat sterilization have been explained on the basis
of the changes in the coagulability of proteins brought about by the abstraction of water. In the classic work of Lewith,[1] frequently cited, it was found
that various proteins are coagulated by heat at lower temperatures when

they contain an abundance of water than when water has been abstracted from them. The following data demonstrate this point.

Egg albumin + 50% water coagulates at 133°F (56°C)
Egg albumin + 25% water coagulates at 165° to 176°F (74° to 80°C)
Egg albumin + 18% water coagulates at 176° to 194°F (80° to 90°C)
Egg albumin + 6% water coagulates at 293°F (145°C)
Egg albumin + 0% water coagulates at 320° to 338°F (160° to 170°C)

Barker[2] repeated and extended the work of Lewith by relating the denaturation temperature to the relative humidity of water vapor with which the protein is in equilibrium rather than to its absolute water content. He found that the temperature of denaturation is a linear function of the relative humidity with which the protein is in equilibrium. If the heat coagulability of proteins as influenced by moisture is the determining factor, it is logical to state that a temperature of at least 320°F (160°C) should be used in dry-heat methods of sterilization. It also follows that bacteria exposed to hot air may be dehydrated greatly before the temperature rises sufficiently to cause death by coagulation, complete dehydration necessitating their destruction by actual burning. For this reason most authorities agree that death by dry heat is primarily an oxidation or a slow burning up process.

A review of the literature shows that there is a lack of systematic study on death time temperatures of dry heat or hot air. Certainly kinetic data are lacking on the inactivation of spores by dry heat. The early findings of Robert Koch[3] and his co-workers demonstrated that the spores of *Bacillus anthracis* required a hot air temperature of 284°F (140°C) for 3 hours in order to insure their destruction. The resistance of both vegetative bacteria and spores varies considerably with different species, some being killed more readily than others. Mold spores appear to be intermediate in resistance between vegetative and sporulating bacteria in that they require a temperature of 230° to 240°F (110° to 115°C) for 90 minutes for their destruction.[4] In the author's laboratory it has been found that dry spores of *Bacillus stearothermophilus* which show maximum resistance to moist heat will survive dry heat at 250°F (121°C) for 2 hours, but they are destroyed at 320°F (160°C) for 1 hour. The data summarized in Table 12-1 are descriptive of the findings of various investigators in determining the time-temperature ratios required for the destruction of bacterial spores by means of dry heat. The author has intentionally omitted the introduction of published D, F, and z values in Table 12-1. Our knowledge of the various biological and physical factors which influence dry heat sterilization is quite inadequate, and this would indicate that current death rate values are not especially helpful in the applied sterilization of medical and surgical supplies. In dry heat sterilization an exposure time of 60 minutes at 320°F is approximately the equivalent of 15 minutes at 250°F in moist heat.

TABLE 12-1

DESTRUCTION OF BACTERIAL SPORES BY DRY HEAT AT DIFFERENT TEMPERATURES

(*From Perkins*[29])

Organism (Dry Spores)	Time—minutes							Investigator
	248°F (120°C)	266°F (130°C)	284°F (140°C)	302°F (150°C)	320°F (160°C)	338°F (170°C)	356°F (180°C)	
B. anthracis	45	20						Murray[5]
B. anthracis			180					Koch et al.[6]
B. anthracis				60				Stein and Rogers[7]
B. anthracis			180					Park and Williams[8]
B. anthracis	60				9			Oag[9]
B. subtilis				60				Perkins and Underwood[10]
Cl. botulinum	120	60	60	25	25	15	10	Tanner and Dack[11]
Cl. septicum						7		Oag[9]
Cl. tetani		35	15					Murray and Headlee[12]
Cl. tetani				30	12	5	1	Darmady, Hughes, and Jones
Cl. welchii	50	15	5					Headlee[14]
Cl. welchii						7		Oag[9]
Garden soil				30	15			Ecker and Smith[15]
Garden soil				90	70	15		Darmady, Hughes, and Jones[13]

The microbicidal action of dry heat is markedly influenced by the nature of the fluid or substance surrounding the organism. In the presence of organic matter, such as a film of oil or grease, the organism is definitely protected or insulated against the action of dry heat. Walter[16] has emphasized the importance of this factor, particularly in the case of surgical instruments, which, if properly cleaned beforehand, may be sterilized in one hour at 320°F. If oil or grease is present on the instrument, safe sterilization calls for 4 hours exposure at 320°F. Rodenbeck[17] has studied the thermal death time temperatures of resistant dry spores in anhydrous oil. The findings of this investigator are deserving of serious consideration in the establishment of safe exposure periods for dry heat sterilization of oils, fats, or other anhydrous fluids. For example, it has been determined that at a temperature of 320°F (160°C) a period of 160 minutes is required for the destruction of resistant spores in anhydrous oil or fat. If the oil is hydrated or contains a small amount of water, as little as 0.5 per cent, sterilization may be accomplished in approximately 20 minutes at this temperature. Rodenbeck also found that the addition of 1% water to fats, oils, or paraffin made sterilization possible in the autoclave after 30 minutes at 120°C or 10 minutes at 130°C. Fortunately most oils do contain a small amount of moisture, less than one per cent, unless subjected to a specific dehydration process.

REQUIREMENTS FOR DRY HEAT STERILIZATION

In setting up standards for dry heat sterilization, it is difficult and somewhat impractical to attempt to establish one time and temperature entirely suitable for all types of supplies. Several factors influence the time-temperature relationship required. The nature and properties of the article or material undergoing sterilization must be reckoned with, strict attention must also be given to the method of preparation, packaging, or wrapping, as well as loading of the sterilizer. If these factors are ignored the exposure time selected may be inadequate for destruction of the most resistant and least accessible organisms.

Instruments represent the ideal for dry heat sterilization because of the heat-conducting properties of the metal, but the maximum temperature employed must be restricted to a safe range beyond which the temper of the metal may be drawn. For heat-stable articles such as glassware, it becomes possible to use a higher temperature for a shorter period of time, than when sterilizing certain powders which may undergo physical or chemical change unless the temperature is maintained below the critical point of the substance. In dry heat sterilization the basic point to keep in mind is that the time required to heat a quantity of one material to sterilizing temperature may differ markedly from that required to heat another material to the same temperature. Allowance must be made for any such differential in the exposure time.

For dry heat sterilization of hospital supplies the most widely used temperature is 320°F (160°C) for 1 hour, preferably 2 hours. This requirement refers to the actual temperature of the load. It does not make allowance for any appreciable time lag characteristic of a particular load after the sterilizer has reached this temperature. In establishing reliable methods for dry heat (hot air) sterilization, the following time-temperature ratios are considered adequate:

```
356°F (180°C)................30  minutes
340°F (170°C)................ 1  hour
320° F(160°C)................ 2  hours
300° F(150°C)................ 2½ hours
285° F(140°C)................ 3  hours
250° F(121°C)................ 6  hours, preferably overnight
```

HOT AIR STERILIZERS

There are two kinds of hot air sterilizers in common use, the gravity convection type and the mechanical convection (forced air circulation) type. For both units, the preferred method of heating is by electricity because it affords accurate and dependable temperature control within the desired range. For routine work the temperature range should be 320° to 325°F (160° to 163°C), but the automatic regulator should be readily adjustable for lower temperature sterilization if the need occurs. When it is desired to sterilize glassware only, as in the laboratory, close temperature control is not so essential, and the temperature may advance to as much as 400°F (204°C) without harming the glassware. For this reason the laboratory hot air sterilizer is frequently just a plain, uninsulated, gas-fired oven, without accurate thermostatic control. To be sure, gas cannot be controlled with the same accuracy as electricity, and the use of gas involves a definite fire hazard. Such equipment has no place in the modern laboratory or hospital, and it should not be used for the sterilization of materials that require accurate temperature control or are known to be combustible in nature.

Gravity Convection

In the gravity convection hot air sterilizer shown in Figure 12-1 the air circulates in accord with existing temperature differences between various portions of the chamber. When air is heated, it expands with a corresponding decrease in density. The cooler air descends in the chamber and the heated air rises to displace it. The ascending warm air gives up some of its heat to the load in the chamber and also contracts in volume. At the same time, the descending cool air is heated as it passes over the heating elements. In this manner the cycle is repeated, setting up "gravity convection" circulation in the chamber. The speed of circulation is dependent upon the ventilation provided through the adjustable air vent or exhaust located on top of the sterilizer, and also the temperature differential between the region of the heaters and the exhaust port.

The design characteristics of the gravity convection hot air sterilizer influence the functional efficiency. The design should not oppose the natural flow of air currents by directing the air stream around corners, through baffles or other places that would impede the currents. The heater bank should be located beneath the chamber, separated from it by a perforated metal plate, which serves not only as the chamber floor, but as a diffusing surface to produce uniform heating effect over the full horizontal plane of the chamber. Preheated fresh air can then rise through the perforated plate, pass up through the chamber, flow through the perforated diffusing panel which forms the ceiling, and finally exhaust itself through the adjustable ventilating port on top of the cabinet. At best, the gravity convection type sterilizer is much slower in heating, requires longer time to reach sterilizing temperature, and is less uniform in temperature control throughout the

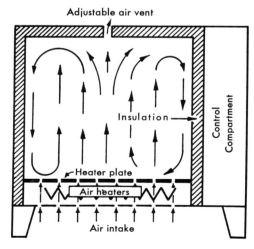

Adjustable air vent

Insulation

Control Compartment

Heater plate

Air heaters

Air intake

FIGURE 12-1. Schematic diagram of air circulation in gravity convection hot air sterilizer.

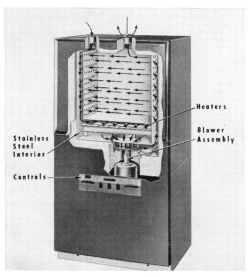

Figure 12-2. Hot air sterilizer, electrically heated, mechanical convection type. Forced air circulation is accomplished by a motor-driven turbo-blower.

chamber than the mechanical convection type. It should be used only for applications where rapid and precise heating, unrestricted loadability of chamber, and accelerated air circulation are not decisive factors.

Mechanical Convection

For hospital use, particularly in the laboratory and the central service department, the mechanical convection hot air sterilizer (Fig. 12-2) offers the maximum in functional efficiency at minimum cost. This type is usually equipped with a motor-driven turbo-blower which produces rapid movement of a large volume of heated air, to convey heat directly to the load under controlled temperature conditions. The heater bank is mounted in a compartment separated from the working chamber by a diffusing wall, directly in front of the turbo-blower. An adjustable air inlet opens into the heater compartment. As the incoming air is heated, it enters the turbo-blower where it is mixed and diffused with recirculating air. The heated air then passes through a duct, where a high static pressure is built up, forcing the air over to a compartment on the opposite side of the chamber. Here it passes through another perforated diffuser wall and the air is discharged uniformly over the entire vertical plane area of the chamber. This insures a positive airflow in the horizontal plane, thus maintaining uniform temperature and equal transfer of heat to all regions. As the heated air flows across the chamber and passes through the diffusing wall in front of the heaters, it is recirculated by the turbo-blower and the cycle repeated. Any portion of the circulating air can be exhausted to the outside through the adjustable vent on top of the sterilizer.

With the mechanical convection sterilizer, air velocity, direction of circulation, and heat intensity are controlled to produce uniform temperature in the chamber regardless of the type of load. To meet the requirements of heavy usage in hospital work, an efficient hot air sterilizer should have performance characteristics as follows:

Power consumption—approximately 520 watts per cu ft of chamber capacity.
Come up time to 320°F in chamber (no load)—no longer than 30 minutes.
Maximum temperature deviation throughout chamber (no load)—±2°F.
Come up time to 320°F with fully loaded chamber of glassware—no longer than 75 minutes.

In addition to the above characteristics, the sterilizer should have positive means for exhaust of gases or vapors liberated during the sterilizing process. Automatic controls are also a desirable feature, including a temperature recorder, a 5-hour timer, and an alarm.

INFRARED RADIATION OVEN

Conveyor ovens heated by infrared radiation or by gas with forced convection are in use in some hospitals. Darmady and others[18] have described a moving belt infrared sterilizer applicable to a Syringe Service operating on a large scale. Infrared heating is preferred because it does not depend upon air conduction. The apparatus consists of an insulated tunnel in which a series of infrared heaters has been placed at predetermined positions. The syringes in sealed metal containers are carried through the oven on a moving belt at a speed geared to a holding time of 7½ minutes at 356°F (180°C) and a sterilization time of 22 minutes. It is claimed that one sterilizer of this kind can do the work of four ordinary hot air ovens and its continuous flow operation permits the processing of at least six hundred syringes a day.

USE OF AUTOCLAVE AS HOT AIR STERILIZER

Supervisors frequently inquire as to the advisability of using the ordinary pressure steam sterilizer (autoclave) with steam in jacket only as a substitute for the hot air or dry heat sterilizer. Certainly this can be done, is being done in many hospitals, but the method is not deserving of recognition as a standard procedure, unless the sterilizer is equipped with proper controls. When operated with steam in jacket only at 15 to 17 pounds pressure, it is true that the chamber walls of the dressing sterilizer are uniformly heated to 250°F, and that conditions in the chamber are moderately suited to hot air sterilization. However, the thermometer located in the chamber discharge line does not function as an indicator of the chamber temperature when steam is applied to the jacket only. Moreover, it is just as important to record the true conditions of time and temperature for dry heat sterilization as it is for saturated steam under pressure. This constitutes the first serious objection to the method—there is no reliable means of checking temperature conditions in the chamber, without modification of the sterilizer.

Another disadvantage in the use of the autoclave as a dry heat sterilizer is that the standard steam pressure maintained in the jacket is 15 to 17 pounds, equivalent to 250° to 254°F (121° to 123°C). With this dry heat temperature in the chamber, safe sterilization calls for 6 hours exposure, preferably overnight. An exposure period of this order is indicative of a relatively inefficient process, especially when safe sterilization can be accomplished in a much shorter time at a higher temperature in a dry heat oven. In the interest of economy and for the hospital that does not have a dry heat sterilizer, there is some merit to loading the dressing sterilizer with syringes and needles for an overnight exposure at 250°F. During this period the dressing sterilizer would not normally be required for other purposes.

In the case of oils, greases, and lubricated gauze, it is not uncommon to experience spillage or leakage of these materials in the sterilizer chamber. When this occurs in the autoclave, it necessitates careful cleaning to remove all traces of oil or grease from the chamber surfaces. Otherwise, supplies undergoing steam sterilization later may possibly become contaminated with a film of oil which serves as a protective barrier against moist heat sterilization. Oil or grease in the chamber eventually leads to partial clogging of the discharge line, which then requires cleaning and service by an experienced mechanic to insure efficient operation of the sterilizer. The obvious answer to all of these shortcomings is not to use the autoclave as a substitute for the hot air sterilizer, except in an emergency or until such time as suitable equipment designed for dual-purpose sterilization can be procured.

PREPARATION OF SUPPLIES

The importance of thoughtful attention to details cannot be overemphasized in preparing supplies for dry heat sterilization. Instruments, syringes, and needles must be free from traces of oil or grease. Wherever practicable, the quantity of a liquid or a powder should be limited to that required for a single-use application. An attempt should be made to standardize on types of containers, methods of packaging and loading to insure that when the sterilizer reaches the proper temperature the load also will be at this temperature or very close to it.

Cutting Edge Instruments

Selection of a satisfactory method for sterilization of cutting edge instruments frequently poses a problem for the operating room supervisor. Surgeons require both sharp and sterile instruments. Chemical disinfection is commonly resorted to, particularly for scalpel blades, but great care must be used to insure that the instruments are thoroughly cleaned before immersion in the germicide and that sufficient time be allowed for disinfection to take place. Then, if the germicide contains formaldehyde or any other irritating substance, it is necessary to rinse the instruments in sterile water and dry them under sterile conditions before use. In many cases it is apparent that chemical disinfection methods are employed for convenience rather than bacteriological efficiency or surgical safety.

Dry heat sterilization of sharp instruments, including cataract knives and keratomes, can be carried out conveniently in the hot air sterilizer at 320°F (160°C) for 1 hour. The first requirement is that the instruments be clean, free from oil or grease, otherwise this exposure time may be inadequate. It is preferable to place the instruments on shallow aluminum trays in the sterilizer to enhance the rate of heating through the heat-conducting properties of the metal. Caution must be exercised to guard against overheating. Exposure to temperature appreciably higher than 320°F may destroy the keenness of the cutting edge. Carbon steel cutting instruments are heat treated to produce maximum hardness. They should not be sterilized routinely at

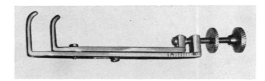

FIGURE 12-3. Instruments of this type can best be sterilized by means of dry heat. The features of construction prevent direct steam contact to all surfaces.

temperatures above 325°F. Repeated heating at temperatures above this level will result in loss of hardness. If the autoclave is used as the dry heat sterilizer with steam in jacket only at 250° to 254°F the exposure period should be no less than 6 hours for clean instruments prepared as above (Fig. 12-3).

Walter[19] has described a dry heat sterilizer for cutting-edge instruments in which the instruments are heated by direct contact with a metal surface maintained at 320°F. This method provides rapid and uniform heating. Hawn and Walter[20] have also described a unique method of packaging scalpel blades for dry heat sterilization. The scalpel blade is hermetically sealed in an aluminum foil packet prior to sterilization. Blades packaged in this manner are commercially available.

Suture Needles

When suture needles are sterilized by saturated steam, serious rusting occurs which is difficult to overcome. Experience has shown that dry heat sterilization is the method of choice. The needles should first be cleaned by soaking in a detergent solution and then dried. If polishing is required, they can be passed through a bag of fine emery powder. For packaging, it is de-

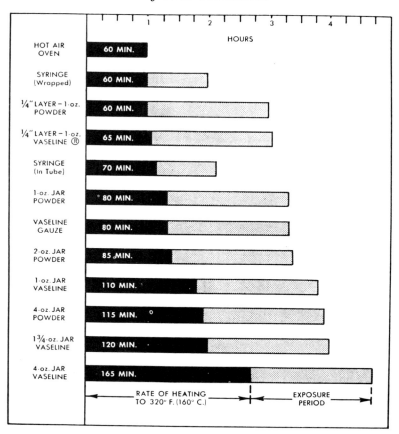

FIGURE 12-4. Time required to heat specific quantities of materials from room temperature of 75°F to 320°F in hot air sterilizer. Lightly shaded section of each bar represents exposure period after material has reached temperature of 320°F. Total time consumed in heating process is equal to entire length of each bar.

sirable to insert the needles in a lightly folded gauze pack and wrap with muslin. Sterilization may then be accomplished at a temperature of 320°F for not less than 1 hour.

Powders

The slow rate of heat transfer through jars or canisters of powder makes it necessary to employ abnormally long periods of heating to ensure sterilization. This point is illustrated graphically in Figure 12-4. A 4-ounce jar of powder of the type shown in Figure 12-5 requires 115 minutes to reach the sterilizing temperature of 320°F in the hot air sterilizer. From the time that the sterilizer itself reaches this temperature, the powder still requires 55 minutes longer. Then, for safe sterilization it is necessary to add an exposure period of 2 hours which makes the total heating time about 4 hours. Similar

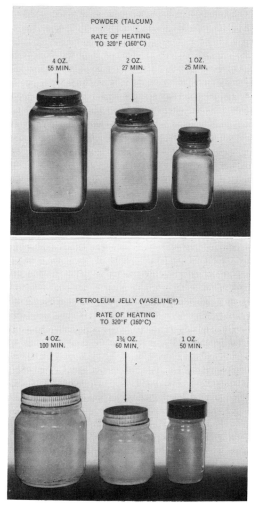

FIGURE 12-5. Comparative rates of heating different quantities of material to 320°F in hot air sterilizer. Time recorded for each container is actually the additional time needed for material to reach 320°F, after sterilizer has attained this temperature.

conditions of slow heating prevail for the smaller 2-ounce and 1-ounce jars of powder. The poor heat-conducting properties of the glass jar, the layer depth of powder, and the surface area exposed are the chief factors which contribute to the slow rate of heating of powder. The use of containers for bulk powder involving quantities much greater than one ounce should be discouraged. Also, wherever possible, the quantity of powder should be restricted to a ¼ inch layer in a Petri dish or similar type of container. If these conditions are ignored the exposure period of 2 hours at 320°F may be inadequate.

SULFONAMIDE POWDERS. The sulfonamides, including sulfanilamide, sulfadiazine, sulfathiazole, and sulfamerazine, are relatively heat-stable chemicals. In powder form they may be heated to a temperature of 311°F (155°C) for 1½ hours without decomposition. This temperature is, however, close to the melting point of sulfanilamide (165°C), and for a greater margin of safety, it is recommended that the powders be sterilized at 285° to 300°F (140° to 150°C) for 3 hours. A convenient method of preparation is to place small amounts of the powder, not exceeding 4 or 5 grams, in double envelope paper containers. Test tubes with cotton plugs, individually wrapped, also serve as suitable containers. In order to prevent "caking," the sulfanilamide powders should be dried at 212°F prior to sterilization.

Zinc peroxide is another substance which should be dry heat sterilized at 285°F (140°C) for four hours. This time and temperature is required to activate or mobilize the oxygen and at temperatures higher than 285°F it begins to decompose. To be effective this material must conform to certain minimum standards which have been outlined in detail by Meleney.[21]

Other chemicals such as kaolin, zinc oxide, mercurous chloride, and bismuth subnitrate can be dry heat sterilized at 340°F (170°C) for 1 hour or 320°F (160°C) for 2 hours.

Oils and Nonaqueous Vehicles

The slow rate of heating evidenced in the sterilization of powders is even more marked in the case of oils. For example, the time required to heat a 4-ounce jar of petroleum jelly (Vaseline) from room temperature of 75°F to 320°F in the hot air sterilizer is 165 minutes, as shown in Figure 12-4. From the time the sterilizer reaches this temperature, the petroleum jelly requires 100 minutes longer heating to reach 320°F. If the exposure period of 2 hours is then added, the total heating time becomes 4¾ hours for sterilization of this quantity of petroleum jelly.

The time required to heat small quantities of petrolatum to sterilizing temperature is far greater than commonly observed in hospital practice. This statement is supported by the times given in Figure 12-4 which show that a 1¾-ounce jar requires 120 minutes and a 1-ounce jar 110 minutes to heat to 320°F. This means that when the sterilizer reaches 320°F, an additional period of 60 minutes and 50 minutes respectively is required for the two smaller containers to reach sterilizing temperature. As in the case of powder explained above, the depth of the layer of oil and the surface area exposed greatly influence the rate of heating. To illustrate, a ¼-inch layer of petrolatum (1¾ ounces) was placed in a Petri dish and then heated in the hot air sterilizer. With potentiometer and thermocouple it was determined that after 30 minutes heating the temperature rise in the petrolatum almost paralleled that of the sterilizer, and that at the end of 60 minutes the petrolatum required only 3 minutes longer heating to reach 320°F. Again, this condition approaches the ideal, and the results support the recommendation that for safe sterilization the quantity of oil should be limited to approximately 1 ounce.

Admittedly the Petri dish is not the most suitable container for oils because of its shallow depth and the possibility of spillage. It can serve as a convenient receptacle for petroleum jelly, ointments, or other preparations not normally liquid at room temperature. A stainless steel needle jar (3⅛ × 2½ inches) with cover, is a suitable container for oils; also the small glass jars shown in Figure 12-6. Since the commonly used oils such as petrolatum,

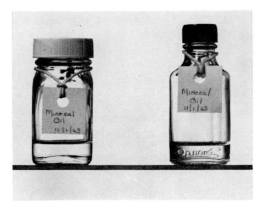

FIGURE 12-6. Small glass jars or bottles with screw caps are suitable containers for oils. Layer depth should be restricted to about ¼ inch.

paraffin, olive oil, and peanut oil are thermostable, they may also be sterilized at 340°F (170°C) for 1 hour. At this higher temperature small bottles with heat-resistant screw caps, containing no more than 1½ ounces of the material, are quite satisfactory. If larger quantities are required, then it becomes necessary to determine beforehand the additional time needed for the material to reach sterilizing temperature, after the sterilizer has attained that temperature. Failing this, it is useless to try to establish a minimum safe-exposure period, especially where the operator must rely upon the chamber temperature indicated by the thermometer as the beginning of the exposure period.

Glycols and Glycerin

It is not commonly recognized that certain glycols, particularly polyethylene and propylene, and also glycerin pose a problem with respect to sterilization. If these compounds are to be sterilized in the autoclave, a minimum water content of 10 to 20 per cent is essential.[22] When there is little water present, sterilization by means of dry heat is recommended according to the following conditions:

Propylene glycol (100%)............................ 285°F for 2 hrs
Polyethylene glycol 400 (100%)................... 285°F for 2 hrs
Polyethylene glycol 4000 (100%)................. 300°F for 2 hrs
Glycerin, 80%..................................... 265°F for 2 hrs
Glycerin, 90%..................................... 285°F for 2 hrs
Glycerin, 95%..................................... 300°F for 1 hr

Caution should be exercised when attempting to sterilize mixtures of glycerin and water in a hot air oven. According to Geist[23] an explosion may occur dependent upon the water content and boiling point of the mixture. Nonaqueous glycerin has a boiling point of 554°F (290°C), whereas glycerin with a water content of 13 per cent boils at 267°F (130.5°C).

Petrolatum Gauze

The preparation and sterilization of petrolatum gauze has long been a troublesome procedure. Observations in many hospitals have revealed the all-too-frequent error of preparing too much material, with large excess of petrolatum, inadequate exposure for sterilization, or overheating at too high a temperature with consequent charring or partial destruction of the gauze strips. If proper attention is given to the details of preparation and heating, the product easily can be controlled within safe limits. The procedure is as follows:

Prepare about twenty strips of bandage gauze, each 6 to 8 inches long and 2 inches wide. Place the strips in a stainless steel catheter tray with dimensions of 2½ inches wide x 8 inches long x 1¼ inches deep. Cover the strips with 4 ounces of petrolatum, previously liquefied by heating. This should form a layer ½-inch deep in the tray with a thin layer of petrolatum over the topmost gauze strip (see Fig. 12-7). Sterilize in the hot air sterilizer at 320°F for 2½ hours.

In the sterilization of petrolatum gauze prepared as above, a longer exposure period is required than in the case of oils, because of the greater depth of the layer in the tray. If the temperature is maintained within the range of 320° to 330°F, there should be no evidence of charring or discoloration of the gauze. Repeated tests have shown that a temperature of 340°F will produce some discoloration, while a temperature of 360°F for a short period of time produces definite charring of the gauze.

Gershenfeld[24] made a thorough investigation of methods of preparation and sterilization of petrolatum gauze in hospitals. His findings showed no uniform satisfactory technique employed in the various institutions. He stated that "the homemade techniques vary widely as to details of preparations; and one cannot help but feel dubious of the efficiency of the procedures of preparation and sterilization, as to their yielding at all times a sterile product and one possessing pharmaceutical elegance." Yarlett, Gershenfeld, and McClenahan[25] have also reported on methods for sterility testing and the preparation and sterilization of petrolatum gauze. Their findings

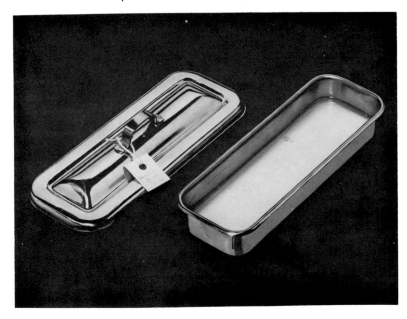

FIGURE 12-7. Petrolatum gauze can be conveniently prepared in catheter tray. Gauze strips should be limited to about 20 and petrolatum to no more than 4 oz, making layer ½ inch deep in tray. Thin layer of petrolatum should cover topmost gauze strip.

indicate that steam processing of gauze impregnated with white petrolatum cannot be relied upon to produce a sterile product. In fact steam treatment at 259°F (126°C) for 60 minutes failed in every instance to kill spores of an organism belonging to the *subtilis-pumilis* group of the genus *Bacillus*, even when the petrolatum gauze was processed in thin layers.

Gauze Impregnated with Furacin®

This product is prepared with an ointment base consisting of polyethylene glycols. As marketed, the material contains from 1 to 5% water and, for this reason, it may be sterilized by autoclaving. "A stack of ten layers of impregnated gauze are rendered sterile in 15 minutes at 250°F saturated steam."[26]

OPERATION OF HOT AIR STERILIZER

For efficient operation of any hot air sterilizer, the characteristics of the individual unit must be known. Close regulation of temperature is important to avoid over-exposure of the less heat-stable articles and to prevent under-exposure with the possibility of an unsterile load. Never load the chamber to the limit. Allow some space between each packaged article and between each basket or container of supplies. Keep all articles well away from chamber sidewalls, so that the free circulation of air is not cut off.

After placing load in sterilizer, check the thermometer to see that it is properly inserted in top of chamber. Adjust the air flow damper to MEDIUM position and partially open the air inlet and exhaust vents. The heat should then be turned on and the thermostat set to maintain the desired temperature range. Time the exposure only when the thermometer shows the correct temperature. Avoid opening the door during the exposure period because the chamber will cool rapidly. If the methods of preparation for the various supplies deviate greatly from those summarized in Table 12-2, it is incumbent upon the operator to determine experimentally the time required for the material to reach sterilizing temperature.

TABLE 12-2

SUMMARY OF REQUIREMENTS FOR HOT AIR STERILIZATION OF SUPPLIES

Material	Exposure Period From Time Sterilizer Shows Temperature of—			Quantity and Preparation
	340°F (170°C)	320°F (160°C)	285°F (140°C)	
Glassware		60 minutes		Items must be clean and free from oil or grease.
Instruments (cutting edge)		60 minutes		Instruments must be clean, free from oil or grease and placed on metal tray in sterilizer.
Needles (hypodermic)		120 minutes		Needles may be placed in tubes having restricted sides, with cotton stoppers. Wire mesh baskets serve well as containers for tubes. Remove stylets.
Needles (suture)		60 minutes		Sew needles into gauze pack, wrap in muslin.
Oils	60 minutes	120 minutes		Quantity should be limited to ¼" layer (approx. 1 oz).
Petrolatum—liquid	60 minutes	120 minutes		Same as for Oils.
Petroleum jelly (Vaseline)	60 minutes	120 minutes		Quantity should be limited to ¼" layer (approx. 1 oz) in ointment jar or other similar container.
Petrolatum gauze		150 minutes		Quantity should be limited to 20 strips of 2"×8" gauze and no more than 4-oz white petrolatum in catheter tray with dimensions of 2½"×8"×1¼".
Powders	60 minutes	120 minutes		Quantity should be limited to ¼" layer (approx. 1 oz) in container.
Sulfonamide powders			3 hours	Quantity should be limited to 4 to 5 gm in double envelopes or cotton-plugged test tube.
Syringes (in test tubes)		75 minutes		Place assembled syringe with needle attached in test tube of suitable size. Cover top of tube with foil.
Syringes (Wrapped)		60 minutes		Remove plunger from barrel and wrap in muslin. The needle embedded in gauze may be included in pack.
Zinc peroxide			4 hours	For clinical application, quantity should be limited to 15 to 20 gm in suitable container.

STERILIZATION OF AIR

Bourdillon, Lidwell and Raymond[27] investigated the sterilization of air by passing *B. subtilis* spores through an electrically heated furnace. They concluded that an exit air temperature of 445°F (225°C) was sufficient to kill all spores with an exposure time of 0.4 to 0.6 seconds. Decker *et al.*[28] reported time-temperature studies on the penetration of bacterial spores through an electric air sterilizer. They found 99.9999 per cent of spores were killed by exposure to a temperature of 425°F for 24 seconds. For every 50°F (28°C) rise in temperature, the time of exposure was roughly halved, up to a temperature of 575°F (303°C) which required an exposure of only 3 seconds to achieve this efficiency of kill.

PREPARATION OF SYRINGES

The Supposedly Sterile Syringe

During the past twenty years much has been written about the supposedly sterile syringe and its implications in a variety of conditions attributable to faulty injection technique. Mild inflammations and infections not uncommonly follow the inoculations and injections which play such an important part in modern treatment. Accidents following injections are especially serious when they occur in hospital practice or in the course of mass inoculations and, on more than one occasion, severe and even fatal results have occurred as the result of a contaminated syringe and needle—supposedly sterile. Viral hepatitis may readily be transmitted by contaminated syringes, needles, and other equipment employed for taking venous blood or for capillary puncture.[30,31] Multiple injections with a single syringe and, venipuncture using inadequately sterilized syringes may spread the causative agent of serum hepatitis.[32,33,34]

In a review of this subject by the Medical Research Council[35] in 1945, it was reported that alcohol is used more than any other chemical disinfectant for sterilizing syringes, although the practice is not recommended. With the passage of time this widespread use of alcohol has diminished greatly, and it is no longer the perpetual cause of disquiet to those familiar with its germicidal properties. For the record, however, it must be repeated that alcohol is totally incapable of destroying bacterial spores. The literature records several cases of postoperative gas gangrene conclusively traced to instruments supposedly sterilized by alcohol.[36,37] Complete bacteriological sterility can be achieved only by sterilization in the autoclave, the hot air sterilizer or by means of ethylene oxide gas. Boiling in water will destroy pathogenic organisms, but it cannot be relied upon to destroy resistant spores or the virus of serum hepatitis. A boiled syringe may, if thoroughly cleaned beforehand, be accepted as reasonably safe where sterilization in the hot air oven or autoclave is not possible, but a boiled syringe is not necessarily sterile, and its safety cannot be guaranteed. The cursory treatment of boiling syringes and needles in many physician's offices prior to inoculations is a discredit to the profession.

Of the later recommendations made by the Medical Research Council,[38] those deserving of special emphasis are the following:

A fresh sterile syringe and needle must be used for each injection or aspiration.

The safest and most satisfactory technique for mass inoculations at present is to use a fresh sterile syringe and needle for each subject.

A syringe that has been used for aspiration, e.g. of blood from a vein, or pus from an abscess, or for intravenous injection, which always entails aspiration of blood, must be cleaned and sterilized before it is used again.

It is essential to keep syringes for injection separate from those used for aspiration.

Syringes and needles require thorough cleaning after use, before resterilization.

Contamination of syringes and needles may occur during assembly after sterilization as the result of contact with fingers, dust, or droplets of saliva from either the doctor or the subject, or to contact of the needle with a nonsterile surface.

Handle needles with sterile forceps only, syringes with dry, washed hands, taking care to touch only the outside of the barrel and the handle of the piston.

Do not talk, cough, or sneeze over a sterile syringe. Persons with known or suspected upper respiratory infections must wear masks while carrying out injections.

The practice of "dishing up" a sterile syringe and needle in an open bowl, especially one which contains any liquid, is condemned.

Sterile syringes and needles must be placed in sterile covered containers.

Cleaning

For the busy hospital a centralized syringe and needle service is considered essential. For maximum efficiency the service should be delegated to the central service department, where the procedures of cleaning and sterilizing for all syringes are under one control. If syringes are not thoroughly cleaned after use, sterilization may be ineffective, particularly if the syringe contains traces of oil, grease, or coagulable protein. The following procedure is recommended for the manual cleaning of syringes:

Immediately after use, separate barrel and plunger and rinse thoroughly with cold tap water. This is particularly necessary when the syringe has been used for aspiration of blood or body fluids.

Wash barrel and plunger in warm water to which has been added a safe and effective detergent. Srub outside surfaces with a good grade fibre brush and use a test-tube brush for cleaning inside of barrel. *Avoid scratching*. Be sure and force detergent solution through tip of syringe. (Care should be exercised in selecting a detergent for this application because alkalies, soaps, and many detergents erode the ground-glass surfaces, thereby causing the syringe to leak or bind.) A nonetching and low-sudsing detergent buffered to maintain neutral pH in use solution is best suited for cleaning of syringes. Care should be exercised in selecting a detergent to make sure that it can be easily and completely removed in the rinsing process and that traces as may occur are nontoxic and nonhemolytic.

Rinse in three changes of water. A brush should be used with the first rinse to make sure that all traces of detergent are removed from ground surfaces and graduation marks. The third or final rinse should be made with freshly distilled water.

After final rinsing, permit parts to air-dry and then assemble, taking care to match the serial numbers of barrel and plunger.

Failure to clean syringes immediately after use may result in the plunger sticking in the barrel or the needle sticking on the tip of the syringe. Various methods may be used to separate the "frozen" parts but probably the most successful technic is to use the B-D Syringe Opener. This is an all-metal syringe for loosening any frozen Luer slip or Luer-Lok® syringe. The procedure is to first fill the syringe opener with warm water. Attach it firmly to the tip of the frozen syringe by holding at the base of the barrel. Then apply firm, steady pressure, gradually increasing the pressure until water infiltrates around the plunger and reaches the top of the barrel. Do not grasp the frozen syringe, but rather let it hang free. Keep the pressure steady, and the plunger will gradually be expelled from the barrel. A towel spread beneath the syringe will prevent breakage in the event that it separates with expulsive force. Other methods are sometimes used in an attempt to separate a frozen syringe but their success has not been altogether uniform.

Mechanical Syringe Cleaner

The ever-increasing use of syringes for immunization, antibiotic therapy and hematologic studies has created a major problem of supply for hospitals. The average general acute hospital of two hundred beds may use anywhere from two hundred to three hundred syringes daily. To hand wash this number of syringes is unquestionably an arduous task which consumes a great amount of time and introduces the costly factor of breakage. The most feasible solution to this problem is the use of an efficient, automatic syringe cleaner or washer. Experience in many hospitals justifies the claim that the daily complement of syringes can be thoroughly cleaned, with less handling and less breakage, in approximately one-quarter of the time required by the manual cleaning process. An ultrasonic bath offers an ideal means for the cleaning of syringes and other glassware items.

Sterilization

Dry heat is considered the most satisfactory agent for the sterilization of syringes, principally because all moisture is eliminated, thereby minimizing erosion of the ground-glass surfaces. A common method of preparation is to remove the plunger from the barrel and wrap the parts together in one muslin cover. If desired, the needle can be embedded in gauze and included in the same package. With this method of preparation the exposure period should be not less than 1 hour, preferably 2 hours, from the time that the hot air sterilizer shows 320°F (160°C). Care must be taken to insure that the chamber is not overloaded and that some space is allowed between the wrapped syringes for free air circulation. In an efficient hot air sterilizer, moderately loaded, the rise of temperature in the load should closely follow that of the chamber.

Another method which has certain advantages, especially for the larger syringes, is to place the plunger in the barrel with the needle attached. The assembled syringe is then placed in a Pyrex glass tube or metal container of such diameter that the barrel of the syringe fits loosely in the tube with the flange resting on the top rim. The tube should be of sufficient length to accommodate the syringe with needle attached, without the point of the needle touching the bottom of the tube. (A 10-ml syringe requires a test tube 200 mm in length and 25 mm outside diameter; whereas a 5-ml syringe requires a tube 150 mm in length and 20 mm outside diameter.) With this method the cotton stopper is eliminated because a portion of the syringe extends above the rim of the tube. The upper portion of the tube should, however, be covered with a muslin or paper wrapper.

A technic described by Walter[39] for preparing syringes for dry heat sterilization is worthy of note. After washing the syringes in a mechanical cleaner, they are dried, assembled, and a disposable plastic shield* placed over the syringe tip, as in Figure 12-8. The syringes are then sorted into baskets by size, loaded into the autoclave (at the end of the day's schedule), and with steam admitted to the jacket only, they are dry heat sterilized in an overnight exposure. Upon removal from the sterilizer the syringes are available for immediate use. "The plastic shield seals off the tip of the syringe so that the plunger cannot be removed until the seal is broken between the shield and syringe. This is accomplished by gently twisting the shield and pushing it against the tip. Added advantages of this technic are quick identification of syringe size and storage requiring less space."

The principal disadvantage in the use of dry heat for the sterilization of syringes is the time required to do the job. Even with the most efficient of hot air sterilizers, the time required to process a heavy load of syringes averages 3 to 4 hours. The autoclave with steam to jacket only, serving as a hot air sterilizer, requires a minimum of 6 hours' exposure. It cannot conveniently be used for this purpose during the day because of the demands placed on it for steam sterilization of other supplies. This leaves the hospital with the alternative of either using the autoclave as a hot air sterilizer with an overnight exposure or, during the day, using the more rapid process of sterilizing the syringes with saturated steam under pressure. In the interest of expediency, many institutions favor the steam sterilization process.

When preparing syringes for steam sterilization, they should always be disassembled—the plunger separated from the barrel. If this is not done, direct steam contact to all surfaces cannot be assured and the sterilizing process may be ineffective. The attempted steam sterilization of a dry assembled

---

* Plastic tips for syringes are available from Macbick Co., Wilmington, Mass.

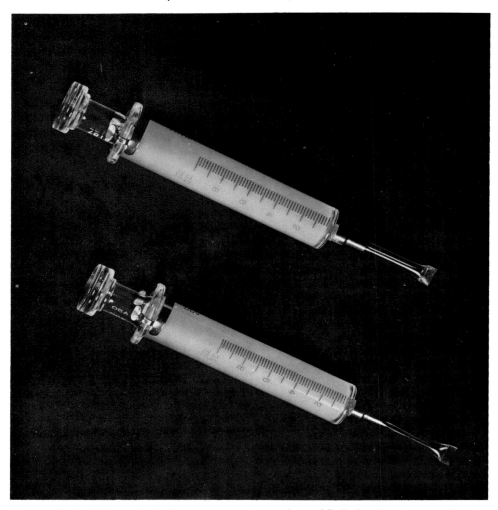

FIGURE 12-8. This method of preparing syringes (assembled) for dry heat sterilization is rapid, efficient, and economical. Plastic shield is placed over syringe tip as shown. Plunger cannot be removed until seal is broken between shield and syringe.

syringe is contrary to established principles. If assembled syringes are to be sterilized by steam, it is necessary to rinse the parts with distilled water, leaving them distinctly moist, just before assembling, packaging, and placing in the sterilizer. The residual film of moisture will then provide steam contact to the inside-surfaces. Unfortunately this method is also objectionable, because the residual water in the assembled syringe during sterilization will attack the ground glass and leach out alkali, which later will destroy certain drugs admitted into the syringe.

Special muslin wrappers facilitate preparation of syringes for steam sterilization. There are two pockets in the wrapper, one for the barrel and one for the plunger. The tie strings sewed to the outside of the wrapper assist in rapid packaging. Syringes packaged in this manner can conveniently be sterilized with bulk loads of dry supplies at 250°F for 30 minutes.

The use of specially fabricated paper bags for packaging of syringes has become very popular in the past few years. When properly carried out, the method is safe, efficient and economical, especially for the hospital where large numbers of syringes must be processed daily. To realize the maximum from this technique the first requirement is to select a paper bag of the right characteristics. It should be made preferably from a white sulfite bond paper of high bursting strength, with controlled porosity to permit adequate steam permeability during sterilization and limited air permeability following sterilization. In addition, all seams and folds of the bag should be uniformly sealed with heat-resistant adhesive to prevent opening up during sterilization.

PREPARATION OF NEEDLES

Cleaning

Like syringes, needles require thorough cleaning as soon as possible after use. Particular attention must be given to the inside of the hub where blood or dirt may have accumulated. The following procedure should be observed in the manual cleaning of needles.

All used needles must be sterilized (decontaminated) prior to processing. This is essential for the protection of personnel. Needles may be placed in a deep tray containing 2% trisodium phosphate solution and sterilized in the autoclave for 30 minutes at 250°F. Remove from sterilizer and rinse under running water.

Insert stylet or needle wire through needle to make sure there is no clogging or obstruction in the cannula. (Always insert stylet through the hub—not from the point.)

Place needles in basin of hot water to which an alkaline detergent capable of dissolving blood has been added. Wash thoroughly inside and out. Use syringe to flush the cannula. Carefully clean inside of hub with a tightly wound cotton applicator.

Rinse well with freshly distilled water and inspect for cleanliness and sharpness. The use of ether, acetone, or alcohol as a final rinse contributes little to the cleaning process. To hasten drying the needles may be placed over a warm radiator or on top of the sterilizer. *If the needles are to be sterilized by steam, some moisture must be present in the cannula at the time of placing in the sterilizer.*

As with syringes, the manual cleaning of large numbers of hollow needles is a difficult and time-consuming task. Human fatigue must eventually take its toll, and when this occurs a percentage of the needles will be poorly cleaned, especially on the inside of the hub and some, perhaps, not at all. The mechanical needle cleaner, now employed in many hospitals, will do much to safeguard cleaning efficiency and to standardize technique. Time study measurement figures show that 2 minutes (average) is required to properly clean one needle. At the top rate of 30 per hour, only 240 needles can be cleaned per day per person by the manual process. In this same period of time, 1 person operating the mechanical needle cleaner can wash 100 needles every 10 minutes or 600 per hour. Obviously the mechanical cleaner effects a tremendous savings in personnel time, insofar as the actual process of washing is concerned. The sequence of operation comprises 1) cleaning out the hub of the needle with a power-driven swab, 2) forcing under pressure three separate cleaning liquids through the cannula, and 3) forcing compressed air through the cannula, leaving it dry and ready for sterilization. The needles are placed in the machine in units of twelve by means of specially designed holders or racks which accommodate all lengths and sizes.

Sharpening

Before sterilization, the point of each needle should be carefully inspected with the aid of a hand lens or magnifying glass to determine if it is damaged and in need of sharpening. Particular attention must be given to the detection and removal of burrs, "fish-hooks," and dull, broken, or misshapen points. The use of a fine Arkansas oil stone is essential for sharpening, also a needle adapter fitted with a handle to hold the needle. A light mineral oil on the stone hastens sharpening, prevents clogging of the grinding surface, and gives a smoother finish. The first step is to grind off any hook on the tip of the needle. Then the bevel must be restored and sharpened. This may be accomplished by placing the bevel flush on the stone at the proper angle, followed by movement of the needle in an elliptical pattern, until it is smooth and shiny. The sides of the bevelled point should then be lightly rubbed on the stone so that it will penetrate skin easily and smoothly. In sharpening a needle with a fitted stylet, care must be taken to keep the stylet in place so that perfectly matched bevels are maintained.

Sterilization

The preferred method for the sterilization of hollow needles is dry heat in the hot air sterilizer. They may also be sterilized in the autoclave with steam in jacket only at 250° to 254°F (15 to 17 pounds pressure) and an overnight exposure period. The dry heat process leaves the needles absolutely dry and assures sterility of the cannula, even when the stylet is left in place. Routinely, needles should not be sterilized with stylets in place because of the possibility of corrosion due to electrolytic action between stylet and needle.

Special tubes of the hour-glass type serve ideally as containers for needles. The restricted sides suspend the needle in the tube and thereby protect

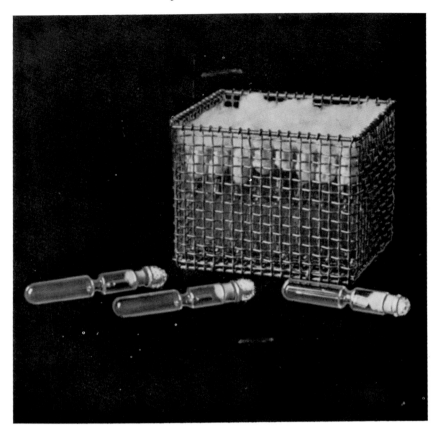

FIGURE 12-9. Needles in special tubes of hour-glass type with constricted sides, stoppered with cotton plugs, may be sterilized by dry heat or by steam under pressure. Constriction supports needle by hub and prevents damage to point.

the point (Fig. 12-9). The open end of the tube is stoppered with a cotton plug. Needles prepared in this manner may then be placed in wire-mesh metal baskets for loading in the sterilizer. It is important to note that the tubes and needles in the middle of the basket will not attain sterilizing temperature as rapidly as those near the sides. In fact, when the sterilizer shows 320°F (160°C), the temperature of the needle in the most centrally located tube is only 277°F (136°C). This needle requires 55 minutes longer heating time to reach 320°F. Therefore, when needles are prepared as in Figure 12-9, the absolute minimum exposure time is 2 hours after the sterilizer shows 320°F.

Needles prepared in this manner can also be sterilized with steam under pressure in the autoclave. If this procedure is followed, each needle should be flushed with freshly distilled water and left distinctly moist, just before placing in the sterilizer. Also the tubes containing the needles should rest on their sides in the sterilizer to facilitate air removal and steam intake to each tube and needle. Under these conditions the exposure period is 30 minutes at 250°F, followed by drying for not less than 15 minutes.

REFERENCES

1. LEWITH, S.: Ueber die Ursache der Widerstandsfähigkeit der Sporen gegen hohe Temperaturen. Ein Beitrag zur Theorie der Desinfektion. *Arch Exp Path Pharmakol, 26*: 341-354, 1890.

2. BARKER, H. A.: The effect of water content upon the rate of heat denaturation of crystallizable egg albumin. *J Gen Physiol, 17*:21-34, 1933-34.

3. KOCH, R., and WOLFFHÜGEL, G.: Untersuchungen über die Desinfection mit heisser Luft. *Mitt Gesundheitsamt, 1*:1-21, 1881.

4. WILSON, G. S. and MILES, A. A.: Topley and Wilson: *Principles of Bacteriology and Immunity.* Baltimore, Williams & Wilkins, 1946, p. 113.

5. MURRAY, T. J.: Thermal death point. II. Spores of *Bacillus anthracis. J Infect Dis, 48*:457-467, 1931.

6. KOCH, R.; GAFFKY, G., and LOEFFLER, F.: Versuche ueber die Verwerthbarkeit heisser Wasserdampfe zu Desinfectionszwecken. *Mitt Gesundheitsamt, 1*:322, 1881.

7. STEIN, C. D., and ROGERS, H.: Observations on the resistance of anthrax spores to heat. *Vet Med, XL*:406-410, 1945.

8. PARK, W. H., and WILLIAMS, A. W.: *Pathogenic Microorganisms,* 10th ed. Philadelphia, Lea & F., 1933, p. 555.

9. OAG, R .K.: Resistance of bacterial spores to dry heat. *J Path Bact, 51*:137-141, 1940.

10. PERKINS, J. J., and UNDERWOOD, W. B.: Unpublished data, 1945.

11. TANNER, F. W., and DACK, G. M.: *Clostridium botulinum. J Infect Dis, 31*:92-100, 1922.

12. MURRAY, T. J., and HEADLEE, M. R.: Thermal death point, I. Spores of *Clostridium tetani. J Infect Dis, 48*:436-456, 1931.

13. DARMADY, E. M.; HUGHES, K. E. A., and JONES, J. D.: Thermal death-time of spores in dry heat. *Lancet, 2*:766-769, 1958.

14. HEADLEE, M. R.: Thermal death point, III. Spores of *Clostridium welchii. J Infect Dis, 48*:468-483, 1931.

15. ECKER, E. E., and SMITH, R.: Sterilizing surgical instruments and utensils. *Mod Hosp, 48*:92-98, 1937.

16. WALTER, C. W.: *Aseptic Treatment of Wounds.* New York, Macmillan, 1948, p. 93.

17. RODENBECK, H.: Ueber die thermische Sterilisation wasserfreier Stoffe und die Resistenz einiger Bakterien bei Erhitzung in solchen Stoffen. *Arch Hyg Bakt, 109*:(2), 67-84, 1932.

18. DARMADY, E. M.; HUGHES, K. E. A., and TUKE, W.: Sterilization of syringes by infrared radiation. *J Clin Path, 10*:291-298, 1957. ·

19. WALTER, C. W.: Sterilization. *Surg Clin N Amer,* New York Number, Philadelphia, Saunders, April, 1942, p. 353.

20. HAWN, C. V. Z., and WALTER, C. W.: The sterile scalpel, *Surg, Gynec Obstet, 99*:118-119, July, 1954.

21. MELENEY, F. L.: *Treatise on Surgical Infections.* New York, Oxford, 1948, p. 591.

22. FLURY, F.: Thesis. Swiss Federal Institute of Technology, Zurich, No. 3202, 1962.

23. GEIST, G.: Explosion bei Glycerinsterilisation. *Deutsch Apoth Zeitung, 101*:110, 1961.

24. GERSHENFELD, L.: Petrolatum gauze. *Amer J Pharm, 126*:112-130, April, 1954.

25. YARLETT, M. A.; GERSHENFELD, L., and McCLENAHAN, W. S.: Petrolatum gauze I. Methods for sterility testing. II. Its preparation and sterilization. *Drug Standards, 22*:205-215, (Nov-Dec), 1954.

26. COMMUNICATION FROM EATON LABORATORIES, Norwich Pharmacal Co., July, 1967.

27. BOURDILLON, R. B.; LIDWELL, O. M., and LOVELOCK, J. E.: Studies in Air Hygiene. Spec Rep Ser Med Res Council, London, No. 262, 1948, pp. 190-207.

28. Decker, H. M.; Citek, F. J.; Harstad, J. B.; Gross, N. H., and Piper, F. J.: Time-temperature studies of spore penetration through an electric air sterilizer. *Appl Microbiol.*, 2:33-36, 1954.

29. Perkins, J. J.: Dry heat sterilization. *Manual of Sterilization and Disinfection, 11*:3-22, 1951.

30. Capps, R. B.; Sborov, V., and Scheifley, C. H.: A syringe transmitted epidemic of infectious hepatitis. *JAMA, 136*:819, 1948.

31. Dull, H. B.: Syringe-transmitted hepatitis: a recent epidemic in historical perspective. *JAMA, 176*:413, 1961.

32. Malmros, H.; Wilander, O., and Herner, B.: Inoculation hepatitis. *Brit med J, 2*:936, 1948.

33. Eichenwald, H. F., and Mosley, J. W.: *Viral Hepatitis, Clinical and Public Health Aspects.* Public Health Service Pub. No. 435. Washington, D.C., Government Printing Office, 1959.

34. Knighton, H. T.: Viral hepatitis in relation to dentistry. *J Amer Dent Ass., 63*:37/21-41/25, 1961.

35. Medical Research Council: *The Sterilization, Use and Care of Syringes.* Kingsway, London, York House, 1945.

36. Nye, R. N., and Mallory, T. B.: Fallacy of using alcohol for sterilization of surgical instruments. *Boston Med Surg J, 189*:561-563, 1923.

37. Medicine and the Law. *Lancet, 2*:941, 1956.

38. Medical Research Council Memorandum, No. 41: *The Sterilization, Use and Care of Syringes.* London, Her Majesty's Stationery Office, 1962.

39. Walter, C. W.: Severe dermatitis is eliminated by complete removal of residual drugs from syringes. *Hosp Topics*, Feb: 81-82, 1954.

Chapter 13

SANITIZATION AND DISINFECTION BY
BOILING WATER

T HE USE of the word *sterilization* is incorrect when applied to boiling water as an agent for rendering instruments and utensils free from all microbial life. Several investigators have shown that boiling water or moist heat at a temperature of 212°F (100°C) is inadequate for the destruction of resistant bacterial spores (see Table 4-4). There is also some question as to the efficacy of boiling water for the inactivation of certain viruses[1,2,3] under ordinary methods of use. Information on the heat resistance of the hepatitis virus is quite inadequate. For these reasons boiling cannot be relied upon for the sterilization of surgical instruments and supplies. It is considered more appropriate to designate the process as one of sanitization or, at best, disinfection.

The official definition of the word "disinfection" adopted by the American Public Health Association is "killing of infectious agents outside the body by chemical or physical means directly applied."[4] Sanitization signifies a process whereby the number of microbial contaminants on utensils is reduced to a safe or relatively safe level as judged by public health requirements. The safe or relatively safe level usually refers to a count of less than one hundred organisms per 4 square inches of a sanitized utensil. Sanitization is a less precise term than disinfection, and it is more appropriately applied to a cleaning process.

THE STATE OF BOILING

The highest temperature that can be attained in boiling water in any open or nonpressure vessel is 212°F (100°C) at sea level. At higher altitudes, the atmospheric pressure is reduced and water will boil at lower temperatures, for example, in Denver boiling occurs at 202°F (94.4°C), and in La Paz, Bolivia at 188°F (86.6°C). It makes no difference how much heat is applied to the vessel—when ebullition occurs, the temperature will have reached the maximum. The application of more heat will simply increase the rate of evaporation and produce more violent boiling. When water boils slowly with the formation of only a few bubbles, liberating very little steam, the condition may be described as "mild boiling." When water boils so rapidly that bubbles form all over the surface, continuously but not violently, the condition may be described as "vigorous boiling." There is no advantage gained in applying so much heat that the water boils violently, giving off clouds of steam. Also, too vigorous boiling will rapidly deplete the water in the vessel and require frequent refilling which is objectionable. The heat should be regulated to maintain a moderate boiling condition.

Instrument and utensil boilers may be vented to the atmosphere to dispose of excess steam, or they may be equipped with condenser vents in which cold water is permitted to flow through a condensing device at the rear of the chamber in such manner as to condense excess steam as fast as it forms. Neither of these methods makes any attempt to conserve heat, they merely dispose of the excess steam created by too vigorous boiling. Regardless of the venting system employed on the boiler, some steam should escape from under the cover to inform the operator that the chamber is filled with free-flowing steam. Not infrequently, in the attempt to keep all steam out of the room or perhaps to conserve heat, the apparatus is regulated for the production of steam at so slow a rate that the temperature above the water may drop below the range at which disinfection should be conducted. Under this condition the water just simmers, very little steam is formed, and the temperature above the water may never get higher than 170°F (76°C). This is hazardous for any article that may extend above the surface of the water or when the apparatus is being used as a steamer only for sanitization.

With the usual simple boiler, the rate of heating can be controlled only by manual regulation of the valve or switch. The operator will turn on the heat to the highest range until the water boils, then the heat is turned down until the desired range is maintained. This requires close attention and some acquired skill. Within recent years automatic devices have been made available for all hospital types of boilers which control the rate of heating. They are known as excess vapor regulators. In service, they utilize the full amount of heat to bring the water to a boil quickly, then automatically reduce the heat to maintain the proper rate of boiling without creating an excess of steam. Figure 13-1 shows application of this type of control to a steam-heated instrument boiler.

BOILING OF INSTRUMENTS FOR DISINFECTION

The preoperative boiling of surgical instruments for disinfection is not recommended except in an emergency and where steam under pressure is unavailable. Some hospitals and clinics continue to routinely boil their instruments in ordinary tap water—with apparently good results. One wonders just how safe this practice is when personal observations show that the exposure times range anywhere from 5 to 30 minutes. In comparison with established standards for surgical sterilization the technic is open to question, and its use should be discouraged in hospitals, clinics, and in professional offices. If the boiling process must be used, it is imperative that the instru-

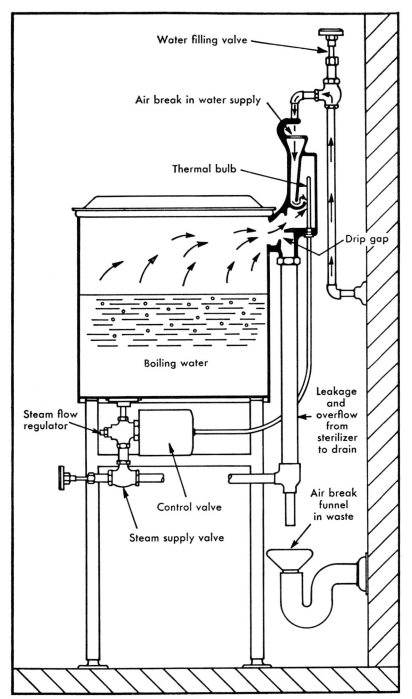

FIGURE 13-1. Steam heated instrument boiler with excess vapor regulator and heat control. This device is neither vent nor temperature regulator. Instead, it automatically controls the rate of heating, to keep water boiling without creating excess vapor or needless waste of fuel.

ments be thoroughly cleaned beforehand to remove traces of dried blood, oil, and grease. Jointed instruments must be opened or unlocked before placing in the boiler. With water boiling at 212°F (100°C) the minimum exposure period should be 30 minutes. At high altitudes the exposure period should be increased about 5 minutes for each 1000 feet elevation above sea level. It is necessary that the boiler contain sufficient water so that all parts of the instruments are well covered. The water level should be adjusted before boiling with at least an inch of water above the instruments.

The bactericidal efficiency of boiling water may be increased by the addition of sufficient sodium carbonate (sal soda) to make a 2% solution or by the addition of sodium hydroxide (caustic soda) so as to make a 0.1% solution in the boiler. Mundel[5] and others [6] reported that the addition of this amount of washing soda markedly increases the disinfecting power of boiling water and also decreases its corrosive action on metal instruments. Bacterial spores in water resisted boiling for about 10 hours, but they were destroyed in a 2% soda solution at 208°F (98°C) in 10 to 30 minutes. Other workers,[7,8] employing a similar technic, demonstrated that when contaminated and oiled instruments were boiled in a 2% soda solution, a period of 10 minutes' boiling was necessary to produce sterilization. Boiling water to which alkali has been added in the above-mentioned concentrations is adequate for the destruction of most spores in an exposure period of 15 minutes.

Scale formation resulting from deposition of lime salts on instruments and utensils routinely boiled is difficult to control, especially in hard water areas. The scale formation can be reduced appreciably by boiling the water for 10 minutes before placing the instruments in it. During this interval, a part of the lime salts in the water will deposit on the heating coils, leaving less to accumulate on the instruments. Frequent draining of the boiler as well as too vigorous boiling contribute to scale formation. The addition of fresh water means the presence of more lime salts. The desirable procedure is to use the water in the boiler throughout the day, then drain and carefully clean the boiler at the close of the day. Water softeners are also of some advantage, but they do not entirely overcome the difficulty. Oil or grease should never be permitted in any instrument boiler. These substances provide a protective barrier for bacteria through which the moist heat cannot penetrate. The use of boiling type "sterilizers" for surgical sterilization of instruments and utensils has become outmoded because the margin of safety with steam under pressure is greater, the time required is less, and the instruments are maintained in better condition.

Dineen[9] has proposed a new method for "disinfection" of endoscopic instruments. It involves immersing the contaminated instrument in a water bath at 185°F (85°C) for 1 hour. The cement used in the lens system of the instrument must, of course, be able to withstand this degree of heat. The method is effective for the destruction of most pathogenic organisms, including *M. tuberculosis, Staphylococcus aureus, E. coli, P. vulgaris,* and *Ps. pyocyaneus.* Enterococci are not uniformly eliminated. Most authorities recommend ethylene oxide gas as a superior process for sterilization of endoscopic instruments.

BOILING OF UTENSILS

The procedure given above for the disinfection of instruments by boiling also applies to utensils. It is a hazardous practice to attempt disinfection if parts of the utensils extend above the surface of the water. If the utensils are nested with parts exposed above the water it will be difficult for steam to contact all surfaces. Even when the utensils are turned bottom side up, air will be pocketed in them, thereby preventing steam contact to all surfaces. The requirement should be strictly enforced that all utensils be completedly submerged during the boiling process. The exposure period should be 30 minutes from the time boiling temperature had been reached. As with instruments, dependable technique demands that the utensils undergoing disinfection be thoroughly cleaned beforehand. Do not permit the utensils to remain in the boiler for any considerable period of time after boiling. As the steam condenses and the water cools upon standing, air containing dust particles will be drawn into the chamber with the possibility of the utensils becoming contaminated.

TERMINAL DISINFECTION OF INSTRUMENTS BY BOILING

The immediate care of instruments and utensils used on "septic" cases is of serious concern, especially where facilities are not available for use with steam under pressure, such as the pressure instrument washer-sterilizer. At best, boiling water is a poor substitute for steam under pressure, but when an emergency occurs and the only equipment available is an instrument boiler, the most practicable procedure yielding reasonable precautionary measures must be followed. This means that some method must be used whereby the microbicidal efficiency of boiling water can be depended upon to decontaminate the instruments and to protect the employee against the infectious hazard in later cleaning of the instruments. Immediately following the operation, the instruments (unlocked and open) should be transferred to the boiler and sufficient trisodium phosphate added to the water so as to make a 2% solution. With the instruments completely submerged, the water should then be brought to a brisk boil and the boiling continued for not less than 15 minutes. The instruments may then be cleaned in the usual manner. The alkalinity due to the trisodium phosphate will assist in solubilizing the organic matter on the instruments and it will also enhance the microbicidal efficiency of the boiling water.

CLEANING AND SANITIZING AGENTS

Water is the universal cleaning and sanitizing agent, and an adequate supply of hot water is the strongest weapon against dirt. Although water alone possesses some detergent value, it is largely ineffective for the removal of proteinaceous soil, oil, and grease from the surfaces of instruments and utensils. The addition of a suitable detergent to water is, therefore, of the greatest importance for effective cleaning. The purpose of the detergent is to facilitate the exchange of a soiled-surface condition for a clean surface plus a soiled detergent. This exchange process, which, in effect, constitutes the cleaning operation, is dependent upon the kind of surface being cleaned, the nature and amount of soil, the composition and concentration of the detergent, time of exposure to the cleaning agent, hardness of the water, pH of the cleaning solution, and the mechanical factor of agitation or scrubbing. Heat is also a component of the detergent system. It enhances the separation of soil from articles by increasing the reaction rate between detergent and soil.

Most detergents may be classified as either highly alkaline, moderately alkaline, neutral, and acid cleaners. The highly alkaline detergents usually contain sodium hydroxide or caustic soda as the primary active ingredient, for dissolving power, to which is added sodium metasilicate as a corrosion inhibitor and water softener. Usually trisodium phosphate or a pyrophosphate is added to the formulation to prevent calcium and magnesium salts from precipitating out when the detergent is used in hard water. One or more wetting (surface active) agents is also added to increase the wetting, penetrating, spreading, and rinsing properties of the formulation. As a rule, the highly alkaline detergents possess rapid dissolving power for dried blood or protein and for emulsifying fats and oils. They are corrosive to aluminum and will readily attack ground-glass surfaces such as syringes. They are not harmful to rubber.

The moderately alkaline cleaners, of which there are many commercially available, are of variable composition. They usually contain sodium carbonate or soda ash, sodium metasilicate, and one or more phosphate compounds as the basic ingredients. A surface-active or wetting agent is also added to enhance the detergent properties. The moderately alkaline detergents are the most satisfactory for general purpose use. They are less corrosive than the highly alkaline cleaners, but they may attack aluminum and ground glass surfaces, including syringes. Representative of this class are products such as Calgonite, Haemosol, and Alconox®.

The neutral cleaners are those products which in use solution develop a pH close to neutrality. They are mixtures of strong wetting agents to which are added neutral phosphate compounds or other fairly neutral builders to give the solution detergent properties in addition to the surface-active effects of the wetting agents. The synthetic (household) detergents offer many examples in this classification. Acid detergents operate in the pH range substantially below 7.0. The acid properties are usually obtained through the incorporation of a mild organic acid or phosphoric acid in the formulation to which is added an effective wetting agent. The acid detergents exhibit low-sudsing properties. They are useful for the removal of certain types of soil such as "milkstone" from dairy equipment. The traditional product known as green soap is still widely used in hospitals. It is not an effective detergent, much less a sanitizer or disinfectant.

Many detergents sold today for home and institutional applications contain an active chlorine releasing compound. Combined with the power to destroy organic matter, the available chlorine also exerts bleaching and sanitizing action. If to these properties are added those of the phosphates, silicates, the nonionic wetting agents, and high alkalinity, the result is a potent, heavy-duty cleaning compound. Such a detergent should be especially well suited to the removal of greasy and proteinaceous soils.

Knowledge of the forces involved in the deposition and binding of soils on hard surfaces and how best to clean these surfaces is highly empirical.[10] This is one reason why frequent conflict occurs in the cleaning recommendations of public health agencies, equipment manufacturers, and detergent suppliers. With the tremendous increase in synthetic detergent chemicals, it has become a most difficult task for the average hospital departmental supervisor or the purchasing department to decide what detergent is best suited to his needs. The general term *detergent* covers a multitude of variations.

SANITIZATION OF DISHES

Wherever possible, equipment designed specifically for the washing of dishes should be used. When an efficient detergent is employed in an approved type dishwashing machine,* followed by a hot water rinse, the dishes and utensils are rendered clean and the bacterial count is reduced to a safe level. In addition to approved equipment properly installed, the following conditions must be observed:

- Individuals responsible for operating dishwasher must be thoroughly trained.
- Adequate volume of hot water with temperature maintained at 160° to 165°F (71° to 74°C). Rinse water at 180° to 190°F (82° to 88°C).
- Adequate wash spray pressure and volume. Spray openings and wash arms must be kept clean and in proper working order.
- Approved type and use dilution of detergent.
- Proper flow pressure in rinse line—15 to 30 pounds per square inch as it enters the machine.

* National Sanitation Foundation, Standards No. 3.

After washing, the dishes should be dried in the air. Hand wiping should not be permitted. The clean dry dishes should be stored in a clean environment, protected from all sources of contamination such as dust, insects, water droplets, and condensation. Personnel should be instructed in the correct way of handling sanitized dishes so that surfaces which come in contact with food or lips are not touched by hands. Glasses should be picked up by the bottom, cups and silverware by handles. Any cracked or chipped dishes are difficult to effectively sanitize and they should be discarded.

In the event that proper equipment is not available, a utensil boiler may be used for sanitization or terminal disinfection of dishes. Residual particles of food must be removed from the dishes before placing them in the boiler. Plates and saucers should be stacked on edge in the tray or basket, and cups or other deep dishes should rest on their sides so that water will drain from them. All articles must be submerged in the water. A sufficient amount of low-foaming detergent is then added and the dishes are boiled for 15 minutes.

THE INDIVIDUAL PATIENT'S UTENSILS

Separate bedside utensils (wash basin, emesis basin, bedpan, urinal) must be provided for each patient during his hospitalization. The use of communal equipment in hospitals should not be permitted. There are various procedures in use today for the cleaning and disinfection of these utensils. Some are effective, others are little more than a gesture, e.g. wiping out the basin with a disinfectant solution. In many hospitals the utensils are delivered to the central service department, via conveyor, dumbwaiter or elevator, for washing, wrapping, and sterilization by steam under pressure. This is a particularly desirable procedure to follow for terminal treatment of the utensils upon discharge of the patient. It has been criticized on the grounds that supplies of this type used by the general hospital patient do not require sterilization for safety. Also, it has been said that it is difficult to maintain control over the procedure because of failures on the part of the floor personnel to arrange for delivery of the utensils to central service.

In other institutions adequate facilities are available for sanitization and/or sterilization of the utensils in nursing-unit utility rooms. In more than a few hospitals, it is common practice to subject the utensils to routine washing, however cursory it may be, with no further attempt at sanitization or sterilization. It would seem that in all fairness to the patient the minimum daily treatment given to utensils should be the equal of the dishes and eating utensils furnished on the food tray. This requirement can be met through the use of a utensil washer-sanitizer designed specifically for the application. A typical unit is shown in Figure 13-2. The total process cycle time is twenty-two-and-one-half minutes, of which 6 minutes will be consumed in the detergent wash and 8 minutes for sanitization with water

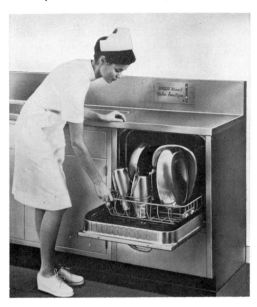

FIGURE 13-2. Utensil washer-sanitizer for mechanical cleaning and sanitizing of patient's utensils. Total cycle time is 22½ minutes, of which 6 minutes will be consumed in detergent wash and 8 minutes for sanitization at water temperature of 200°F (93°C). This is not a sterilizer.

maintained at a minimum of 200°F (93°C). An impeller forces the heated water over, into, and around the utensils. *It is not a sterilizer.*

The utensil washer-sterilizer furnishes another mechanical means of processing soiled patient utensils without the risk of releasing contaminants to the environment as so often occurs in the manual washing process. It also permits utensils to be kept on the nursing floor for sanitization and rapid return to the bedside. It is necessary to position the utensils correctly in the chamber for most effective cleaning (Fig. 13-3). The inside surfaces of bedpans may present a problem. All washer-sanitizers should be equipped with a thermometer or time-temperature recorder to show if proper temperatures are developed during each phase of the cycle. The interior of the unit must be cleaned frequently to keep it free of soil and scale which may contain bacteria and protect them against the sanitizing action of the hot water. Failure to clean the equipment regularly may result in cross-contamination of utensils.

It must be acknowledged that each new patient admitted to the hospital is entitled to a freshly sterilized kit of utensils. The recommended procedure is as follows:

When the patient leaves the hospital room, the various utensils are collected and washed with hot water and detergent (mechanically) in the

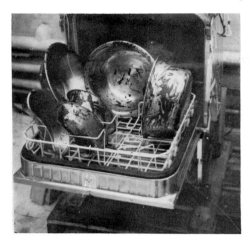 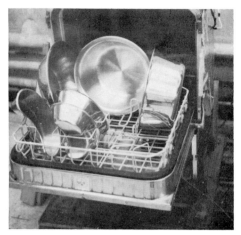

FIGURE 13-3. This illustrates method used to determine cleaning efficiency of utensil washer-sanitizer. Utensils were smeared with excessive amounts of artificial soil, then processed in the unit, and finally examined for residual traces of soil by wiping all surfaces with clean white towel. Soil was made from mineral oil, peanut butter, corn meal, and India ink. Areas found most difficult to clean are the undersurface of curled edge of wash basin and the undersurface of seat bedpan.

cleanup area of the utility room or the Central Service Department. After drying and inspection the utensils are wrapped in a double-thickness muslin cover. Washbasins, emesis basins, and cups should be packaged as a unit. The packaged kit is then sterilized in the autoclave at 250°F for 20 minutes, followed by 15 minutes drying. The kit is then removed from the sterilizer, placed in clean storage, or transferred to the bedside table in the patient's room.

Utensils used in the care of infectious patients must be *sterilized* (decontaminated) before placing into general circulation or for use by the next patient. The bedpan should be assigned solely to the individual patient with infectious hepatitis and thoroughly cleaned and carefully handled between uses until it can be sterilized. Wherever facilities permit, it is preferable to wash and sterilize mechanically after each use of the bedpan. If there is no established isolation unit on the floor, the utensils from the infected patient must be sent to the most conveniently located washer-decontaminator, such as one in the Central Service Department. The contaminated utensils should be placed in a protective covering (waterproof plastic bag), sealed, appropriately identified, and transferred from the patient's room to the department for processing.

Sanitization of Bedpans and Urinals

The objective in the handling of bedpans and urinals is to dispose of the excreta under the most sanitary and least offensive conditions, and at the same time to disinfect the utensils insofar as the communicable disease organisms are concerned. Hospital personnel are well acquainted with apparatus known to the trade as bedpan washers and sterilizers. To designate such equipment as a "sterilizer" is incorrect because in normal usage no attempt is made to sterilize the utensil nor is the process capable of sterilization in the strict sense of the word. In certain instances the equipment does nothing more than flush out the contents of the bedpan. Unfortunately the term has been firmly established in the minds of hospital people as well as the manufacturers of the equipment and that name will undoubtedly continue to be used.

In recent years very few improvements have been made on apparatus designed for the washing and disinfecting of bedpans and urinals. With the automatic unit shown in Figure 13-4, the operator brings the soiled pan or urinal to the fixture, presses the foot pedal to open the cover, inserts the

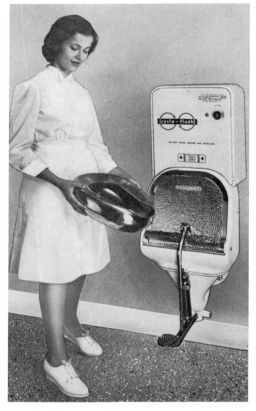

FIGURE 13-4. Automatic bedpan washer-sanitizer. When foot pedal is depressed, door opens and spreads locking clamps to receive bedpan or urinal. Cycle is started by pressing push button. Pilot light comes on, attendant is then free to leave unit, returning later to remove utensil.

utensil within the flexible arms and removes her foot from the pedal. The cover closes automatically and at the same time the utensil is emptied. She then touches the push-button with her forearm and this starts an uninterrupted cycle of washing and steaming. The first action is that of a cold-water wash with inside and outside flushing of the utensil as well as complete flushing of the chamber. The scrubbing action of the jet stream of water is enhanced through air entrainment. After washing with cold water for ½ minute, the unit automatically shuts off the water supply and instantly admits live steam to the chamber for 1 minute (a steaming period of less than 1 minute is considered unreliable). A bleeder trap is connected to the steam supply line which constantly bleeds condensate from the line, thereby assuring exposure to live steam throughout the sanitization period. The pilot light remains on during the entire cycle, warning a second operator that the fixture is in use and the door should not be opened until the cycle is completed. In a fixture of this type, steam is liberated direct from the supply line at close range against the surfaces of the utensils. The utensil heats rapidly because of its fixed proximity to the source of steam. Under these conditions short exposure periods are permissible for disinfection. The efficiency of the process is dependent largely on the removal of soil during the flushing phase.

Bedpans Containing Oil

Pans containing stools from oil enema patients cannot be properly cleansed by this or any other similar washing and steaming process. The excreta will be flushed out but residual oil globules will remain in the pan. Placing paper in the bottom of the pan before use will reduce the difficulty of cleaning, but personnel are prone to forget this detail. Oily pans can only be rendered clean by use of a toilet brush and detergent. In some hospitals the brush is suspended close to the bedpan cleaning fixture and the detergent is kept on a shelf nearby. The operator can hold the cover open with the foot pedal in position to cleanse the pan and so apply the brush and detergent. But this is an awkward procedure and proper cleaning occurs only now and then with unusually painstaking personnel. It is considered better practice to provide a clinical sink close to the bedpan washer that is used largely for this one purpose. Then when an oily pan is encountered, it is taken immediately from the bedpan washer to the sink, scoured with brush and detergent, and returned to the fixture for a second cycle which renders it clean and sanitized. Mechanical cleaning with hot water and detergent is a far superior process because it guards against dispersal of organisms and prevents contamination of the environment.

Flushing a washdown type of water closet can produce a bacterial aerosol.[11] In fact, any process conducive to splashing or frothing produces droplets which remain suspended in the air. These droplets or their droplet nuclei may be infective.

Disposal of Body Discharges

In communities where the sewage disposal system provides adequate control for enteric diseases, the excreta may be emptied directly into the flushing utility hopper or toilet bowl. This should be done as carefully as possible so as to avoid splattering and contamination of the surrounding area. Where the sewage disposal system does not provide adequate control over enteric diseases such as typhoid, infectious diarrheas, or infectious hepatitis, it is necessary to disinfect stools, urine, and liquid wastes before disposal into the sewage system. The stools should be broken up with a tongue depressor and emptied into a container (covered) of 5% phenol solution. Add one and-one-half ounces of phenol to 1 quart of water. After thorough mixing of feces or urine with the disinfecting solution, the mixture should be allowed to stand for at least 2 hours before being emptied into the hopper or toilet. NOTE: The ability of chemical disinfectants to inactivate the virus of infectious hepatitis is not well established.

Alternate Method of Handling Bedpans

Modern planning does not make provision for the installation of bedpan washing and disinfecting equipment within the utility room, unless the room is divided into soiled and clean work areas. With this arrangement, experience has shown that one bedpan washer-sanitizer will serve about 15 patients adequately. This figure is used as a guide for hospitals desiring to install such equipment. In private or semiprivate rooms where toilet facilities are available, the toilet is usually equipped with a bedpan flushing attachment, as shown in Figure 13-5. The bedpan is cleaned here and retained until the patient leaves. Then it is taken to the washer-sanitizer located on the nursing unit or central service, cleaned, packaged, sterilized, and returned for use by the next patient. This method saves time and undesirable traffic through corridors.

Routine Care of Bedpan Washer

The type of bedpan washer shown in Figure 13-4 incorporates certain features of design which have done much to eliminate the serious objections inherent in earlier designs. One highly important feature is the loose-fitting cover which serves a twofold purpose. The cover is baffled on the inside so that in normal usage there is no leakage of water. The loose-fitting design of cover also serves as an overflow so that pollution can rise in the chamber, under adverse conditions, not appreciably higher than the bottom of the cover. Similarly the loose-fitting cover serves to admit room air to the chamber for continuous aeration. The effect is that of a chimney on any fuel-consuming stove or furnace. Room air enters, entrains with odors or vapor, and passes up the vent stack. Lacking the loose-fitting cover or its equivalent opening for air intake, odors are trapped in the chamber offensively.

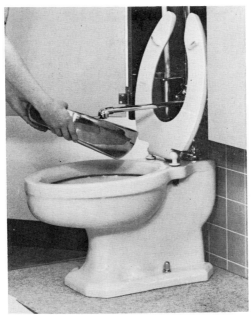

FIGURE 13-5. A diverter valve for flushing of bedpans. It operates by simply lowering spray arm and tripping regular flush valve. One third of normal water flow to toilet is diverted to spray arm for rinsing bedpan.

The bedpan washer-sanitizer needs occasional cleaning with a toilet brush just as ordinary toilet bowls are cleaned. The white porcelain enamel finish of the hopper serves a useful purpose in making immediately apparent any soiled surfaces. Obviously the soiled surfaces can only be seen when the cover is opened, but it is a matter of good housekeeping as well as sanitation, to frequently scrub the interior of the washer. It is no mark of commendation, for the otherwise well-managed hospital, to find bedpan washers that have never been cleaned out since installation. Strict floor supervision can surely govern the cleaning of this equipment as frequently and as thoroughly as toilets are cleaned.

In former years attempts were made to build apparatus in which the contents of bedpans and urinals could be disinfected before releasing into the sewage system. Needless to say, the equipment never proved satisfactory and sanitary protective features were largely ignored. Today the need for such equipment has been largely done away with as the result of the modern city sewage disposal plant. There is considerable room for product improvement in bedpan handling equipment. Generally speaking, it is in the interest of better patient care and environmental sanitation to wash and sanitize a bedpan in a mechanically operated unit. The initial emptying of the pan must, of course, take place in an open area such as the toilet or in an enclosed bedpan flusher. The latter method is superior. Perhaps the answer lies in the use of the disposable bedpan, provided a safe and efficient means is available for its disposal.

REFERENCES

1. EDITORIAL: *Med Times,* 79:443, 1951.
2. LENARD, A.: Poliomyelitis—the possibility of syringe transmission. *Med Times,* 79:395-399, 1951.
3. KNIGHTON, H. T.: Viral hepatitis in relation to dentistry. *J Amer Dent Ass,* 63:37/21; 41/25, 1961.
4. GORDON, J. E. (Ed.): *Control of Communicable Diseases in Man,* 10th ed. New York, Am. Public Health, 1965, p. 14.
5. MUNDEL, O.: Über das Sterilisiervermögen von siedender Sodalösung bei vermindertem Atmosphärendruck. *Z Hyg Infektionskr. 120:*267, 1937.
6. VON JETTMAR, H. M.: Über die Sporozide Wirkung heisser Sodalösung. *Arch Hyg Bakt, 119:*223, 1938.
7. ECKER, E. E., and SMITH, R.: Sterilizing surgical instruments and utensils. *Mod Hosp,* 48:92 (March), 1937.
8. SOBERNHEIM, G.: Ueber Instrumentensterilisierung. *Schweiz Med Wschr,* 62:1034, 1932.
9. DINEEN, P.: The "sterilization" of endoscopic instruments. *JAMA, 176:*100-103, 1961.
10. JENNINGS, W. G.: An interpretive review of detergency. *Food Tech,* 17:53-61, 1963.
11. DARLOW, H. M., and BALE, W. R.: Infective hazards of water closets. *Lancet, 1:*1196-1200, 1959.

CHEMICAL DISINFECTION

T HE NEED for safe and effective chemical disinfectants is of great practical importance to the hospital. They are required for the destruction
of organisms present on delicate instruments and supplies which cannot be
rendered sterile by other means due to their heat-sensitive characteristics.
Efficient surgical antiseptics are also required to assist in the degermation of
the hands and arms of the surgeon as well as the skin of the patient at the
operative site. General utility disinfectants are likewise essential for institutional use in order to minimize the infection hazards from enteric, respiratory, and other pathogens present on floors, walls, and furniture.

DEFINITIONS

Disinfection: By definition this is any process, chemical or physical, by
means of which pathogenic agents or disease-producing microbes are destroyed. It is essentially a process which will destroy the infectious agents,
usually the communicable disease organisms, but not necessarily exacting to
kill resistant bacterial spores. The more common disinfecting agents are
chemicals, boiling water, flowing steam, and ultraviolet radiation. As ordinarily employed, the disinfection process may or may not be adequate for
the destruction of tubercle bacilli, and for the inactivation of enteroviruses
or hepatitis viruses. Disinfectants should be used on inanimate objects only.
They should not be confused with the use of antiseptics as applied to the
body.[1]

Sterilization: Sterilization may be defined as any process by means of
which all forms of microbial life (bacteria, spores, fungi, and viruses), contained in liquids, on instruments and utensils, or within various substances,
are completely destroyed. The word "sterile" denotes the complete freedom
from, or absence of all living microbes and other forms of life. In the strict
sense of definition, sterile is an absolute term, but the word is subject to
common misusage and misinterpretation by both laymen and professional
people. The Council on Pharmacy and Chemistry of the American Medical
Association[2] has reported on this subject as follows:

> The Council on Pharmacy and Chemistry has formally gone on record as
> disapproving of the use of the terms 'sterile,' 'sterilize' and 'sterilization' in
> a bacteriologic sense other than in their correct scientific significance; i.e.,

meaning the absence or destruction of all microorganisms. These terms are not relative and to permit their use in a relative sense not only is incorrect but opens the way to abuse and misunderstanding.

Germicide: A germicide is anything that will destroy germs or microbes. Common usage involves the application of chemical agents to kill disease-producing germs, but not necessarily resistant bacterial spores. Germicides are usually employed in solution form for application to living tissue as well as inanimate objects. Other commonly used terms with similar definitions are bactericide, fungicide, virucide, and sporicide.

Antiseptic: Antiseptics are substances which, when applied to microorganisms, will render them innocuous either by killing them or preventing their growth, according to the character of the preparation or the method of application. They are preparations made especially for application to living tissue. If the substance is of such a nature or is used in such a way as to only prevent the growth of bacteria, it may be classed as a bacteriostatic agent.

Bacteriostat: A chemical agent that has the property of inhibiting bacterial growth. Bacteriostatic action is reversible; when the agent is removed, the cells will resume normal multiplication.

THE NATURE OF CHEMICAL DISINFECTION IN THE HOSPITAL

Disinfection is most often practiced with chemicals, usually in solution, and use of the terms *disinfection* and *chemical disinfection* are interchangeable. Under certain conditions actual sterility can be achieved, but, as it is practiced most of the time, chemical disinfection does not do this. How much it does, or can do, especially in the hospital environment, is the purpose of this discussion.

Hospital disinfection consists of two major types of applications. The first is the disinfection of inanimate materials such as floors, furniture, equipment, and instruments. Regardless of whether the chemicals are used as liquids, gases or aerosol mists, they should be referred to as *disinfectants*. The second application is the disinfection of body surfaces, a practice called *antisepsis* to distinguish this special application from disinfection in general. When used this way, chemicals become *antiseptics*. It is important for an understanding of chemical disinfection as a whole, and certainly for the purposes of this discussion, that the reader be aware of the fact that the same chemical compound (alcohol, for example) may be used both as a disinfectant and as an antiseptic.

It is desirable to think of the disinfection of inanimate materials as consisting also of two types of applications: 1) housekeeping disinfection which deals with floors, walls, furniture, and 2) instrument-equipment disinfection. Furthermore, instrument-equipment disinfection is, in turn, made up of two different categories based on the risk of infection involved in the use of the disinfected materials. One of these involves *critical items* that are introduced beneath the surface of the body or attached to objects which may be so used, e.g. forceps, scalpel blades, and plastic components of the heart-lung oxygenator. Consequently, any contamination whatsoever must be destroyed; in other words, one must approach or achieve actual sterility. The problem here is very different from that encountered with pieces of equipment such as anesthesia apparatus and telescopic instruments which may be called *semicritical* because they only come in contact with unbroken skin or mucous membrane. The divisions of chemical disinfection just described appear in Table 14-1. It may seem at this point that the subject is unnecessarily complicated by creating artificial and inconsequential categories. But this is not so, because these divisions are based on the fact that each one presents a different set of requirements for acceptable disinfection, and failure to recognize these differences has confused and seriously hindered progress in this field.

TABLE 14-1

HOSPITAL GERMICIDES

APPLICATION VERSUS CIDAL ACTION EXPECTED

	Bacteria			Viruses	
	Veg.*	Tbc.**	Spores	Lipid	Nonlipid
Disinfection					
Instruments and equipment					
Critical	+	+	+	+	+
Semi-critical	+	+	−	+	+
Housekeeping	+	+	−	+	+ or −
Antisepsis	+	+ or −	−	+	+ or −

* Veg.—vegetative (nonsporulating) bacteria
** Tbc.—tubercle bacillus

The most pronounced difference in requirements is between antisepsis and the disinfection of inanimate objects. Bacteria and fungi have cell walls that are more resistant to chemical injury than our own tissue cells. Therefore, only the special keratinized cells of the skin and the epithelial lining of mucous membranes can tolerate the irritating action of germicides. Since antiseptics are applied directly to skin and mucous membranes, the maximum concentration of a germicidal chemical which can be used this way is limited by its toxicity for these tissues. Thus there are not nearly so many useful antiseptics as there are disinfectants. Strong disinfectants like formaldehyde and glutaraldehyde, in the concentrations used for inanimate objects, are entirely too toxic for tissue, and they will lose much of their germicidal power if they are diluted to the point where they are nontoxic. The phenolic germicides are also examples of good disinfectants that do not qualify as good antiseptics, irrespective of concentration, and for the same reason. An exception is hexachlorophene, a phenolic compound heavily modified by the addition of chlorine to the molecule, which is a relatively nontoxic compound with a useful level of bactericidal activity. A few other germicides can also be tolerated on our skin in concentrations that effect significant reduction in the microbial population, and this select group constitutes the useful antiseptics (Table 14-2).

The best housekeeping disinfectants are not the best instrument disinfectants. The phenolics, for example, deserve their widespread use on floors, walls, and furniture, but they are not good choices for instruments. Conversely, formaldehyde-alcohol, an excellent instrument solution, is completely inappropriate for floors. And finally, some instrument-equipment germicides are satisfactory for semicritical items but do not have sufficient tuberculocidal, virucidal, or sporicidal activity to qualify them for critical items.

It must be clear by now that there is no such thing as an "all purpose" germicide. If the same germicidal solution is used for all the different applications needed for good hospital asepsis, it will fall short in one or more of

TABLE 14-2

CLASSES OF CHEMICAL
COMPOUNDS USEFUL AS DISINFECTANTS AND ANTISEPTICS

	Disinfectants	*Antiseptics*
Vegetative bacteria	Many	Few
Lipid viruses	Many	Few
Nonlipid viruses	Mod. no.	Very few
Tubercle bacillus	Few	Very few
Bacterial spores	Very few	None

these applications of the performance available with some other germicide. And this is still true even though appropriate adjustments are made in the concentration of that germicide to suit each application. The proper practice of chemical disinfection, therefore, is based on the selection of the best available germicide for each type of application and its use in the most effective way. To do this one must know the nature of microbial contamination, the major principles of chemical disinfection and the properties of the available germicides.

NATURE OF MICROBIAL CONTAMINATION

The four major classes of microorganisms are bacteria, viruses, fungi, and animal parasites. For the practical purposes of this chapter the last two classes may be disregarded; thus the problem of hospital disinfection is how to destroy bacteria and viruses.

The nature of bacteria and viruses, with special reference to germicidal resistance, has been described by Spaulding.[3] Bacteria usually occur as vegetative (growing) cells, but a few species also produce spores. Bacterial spores are the most resistant form of microbial life, and their resistance to germicides is enormously greater than that of vegetative cells. The tetanus bacillus in its vegetative form, for example, is no more resistant to a disinfectant than the staphylococcus, but the tetanus spore survives exposure to many of the commonly used germicides for days, or weeks, or even months. Consequently, the statement that a certain germicide "kills spore-formers" is meaningless and misleading.

Once formed within the bacterial cell, the spore remains dormant until the proper growth conditions cause it to germinate into a vegetative cell. Since this dormant period may last for years, viable spores are disseminated so widely in nature that we must assume they are present in most situations involving hospital disinfection. And because it takes a relatively long exposure to very strong germicides to destroy them, spores constitute the principal obstacle to chemical sterilization.

In contrast, the differences among the various kinds of vegetative bacteria are relatively minor, with one exception. This is the tubercle bacillus which, because of its waxy envelope, is comparatively resistant to aqueous germicides, and almost completely so to quaternary ammonium ("quats") compounds and hexachlorophene. Among the other vegetative bacteria the staphylococci and enterococci (intestinal streptococci), which are gram-positive; and *Salmonella* and *Pseudomonas* species, which are gram-negative, are somewhat more resistant than the rest.

The gram-positives as a whole are more resistant to some classes of germicides, whereas the gram-negatives are more resistant to others. These differences assume practical significance only when marginal concentrations of germicide are being used. *One of the most important improvements in hospital disinfection that could be made at the present time would be widespread adoption of concentrations of proprietary disinfectants (not antiseptics) twice as strong as those currently recommended by their manufacturers.* Incidentally, antibiotic-resistant "hospital" strains of staphylococci are no more resistant to germicides than any of the other staphylococci.

Viruses also differ in germicidal resistance, and these differences are very important. Furthermore, the number of human pathogenic viruses is at least as large as the number of pathogenic bacteria, and since they are frequently present on and in our bodies, we must assume that pathogenic viruses are regularly contaminating our hospital environment.

The major concern about viral resistance has to do with the hepatitis viruses, infectious (IH) and serum (SH). Because man is the only animal species known to be susceptible to them, the proper tests to determine germicidal resistance have never been performed. Until this is done, the correct statement to make about their resistance to chemicals is that we do not yet know the answer. On the other hand, we have reason to believe they are more resistant than most—and perhaps all—other viruses. Consequently, it is necessary to use a *sterilization* procedure whenever destruction of IH or SH virus is required.

The other viruses also differ significantly in resistance to antimicrobial chemicals. One of these differences is based on the composition of the protein coat of viruses. Klein and Deforest[4] have found that the presence of lipid in that coat makes the viruses so constituted (lipid viruses) susceptible to certain germicidal solutions that are nonlethal for viruses free of lipid (nonlipid viruses). And among the resistant, lipid-free viruses are found the very important enteroviruses containing the poliomyelitis, Coxsackie, and Echo groups, many of which are human pathogens. Therefore, we now recognize the existence of two distinct classes of viruses with respect to chemical disinfection (see Tables 14-1 and 14-2).

PRINCIPLES OF CHEMICAL DISINFECTION

How Germicides Kill Microorganisms

A good germicide must be rapidly lethal for microorganisms in its use concentration. Some strong disinfectants do this the same way heat does, by coagulating the protein of microbial cells. This is exactly the same process as the clotting of milk casein or the hardening of egg white. The change is irreversible. Thus, formalin (solution of formaldehyde in water) in high concentrations kills most vegetative bacteria on contact, but it also does the same thing to tissue cells. This is the reason strong (high-level) disinfectants cannot be used as antiseptics. More often, however, the germicidal effect is based not upon actual coagulation but upon a less obvious denaturation of protein. Much of the microbial cell is made up of proteins some of which are enzymes. Being complex molecules, they are subject to alteration or denaturation by heat or by chemicals. Although this process is slower than gross coagulation, denaturation kills the cell if essential enzymes or vital structures are affected.

There are other bactericidal mechanisms, and a single disinfectant may work through several of them. Phenolic compounds in disinfectant concentrations, for example, cause rapid lysis of the bacterial cell, leakage of cell constituents without lysis, or death by denaturing enzymes, depending upon the strength of the germicide and the species of bacterium.

A third level of germicidal action is represented by some of the antiseptics. Germicides are protoplasmic poisons, meaning that they kill all kinds of cells, microbial and tissue. Consequently, as pointed out earlier, body application of germicidal solutions is limited to intact and relatively tough tissues, namely skin and mucous membrane. But even then, the maximum concentrations that can be tolerated are still relatively weak (low-level) germicides which bring about their "cidal" effects in subtle ways, such as oxidation of essential enzymes (iodine), gradual alteration of the cell membrane to produce leakage of protoplasm ("quats"), binding of enzymes (mercurials), or by some unknown mechanism (hexachlorophene). Germicidal effects of these types take place slowly (hexachlorophene), and they can often be reversed by adding a neutralizer, e.g. soap, to a "quat."

The mechanisms just described pertain to vegetative bacterial cells. Sporicidal action is not well understood, but it is apparent that the thick wall and low water content of spores are important. The mechanism of virucidal action is probably based on denaturation and coagulation of protein, but there is more to it than that.[4]

Influence of Numbers

The larger the number of bacteria contaminating skin or inanimate objects, the longer it takes for a germicide to destroy them all. The reason is that all bacterial populations are heterogeneous, even if all the contamination is a single type of microorganism. In other words, genetic mechanisms produce mutations among bacteria which make them different from each other in many ways, including resistance to germicides; and extensive multiplication of a bacterial population produces a corresponding increase in the number of resistant mutants. A practical illustration of this point is shown in Table 14-3.

TABLE 14-3

EFFECT OF NUMBERS ON SPORICIDAL TIME

B. subtilis Spores. Germicide: 8% Formaldehyde-isopropanol, 0.5% G-11

Spore Count *(per blade)*	*Test Procedure*	*Results*	
		Positive	*Negative*
100,000	Dried blood blade	2 hrs.	3 hrs.
1,000	Dried blood blade	1 hr.	2 hrs.
10	Dried blood blade	—	30 min.

(Data from Spaulding)[3]

The application of this principle to instrument disinfection is the necessity for good physical cleansing prior to disinfection. By reducing the number of microorganisms which must be destroyed, one correspondingly shortens the time required to bring about complete destruction ("disinfection time"). This principle also applies to all other types of disinfection, including housekeeping and antisepsis.

Influence of "Soil"

Organic dirt such as blood, plasma, feces, and tissue absorbs germicidal molecules and inactivates them. Thus, only the excess free chemical is left to act. This is, of course, a second—and the major—reason for thorough cleansing of instruments and certain other items prior to application of chemical disinfection.

Strong concentrations of some germicides usually retain a safe level of activity in the presence of heavy organic soil, e.g. phenolic disinfectants. Iodophors (iodine-detergent complexes), on the other hand, are much more subject to inactivation by organic soil, and so are the "quats" and chlorine compounds. The adverse effect of organic soil is, of course, correspondingly greater with weak concentrations and with low-level germicides than it is with strong ones and with high-level germicides.

Influence of Germicide Concentration

The point has already been made that the disinfection time can be shortened by first reducing the amount of the contamination, both in the form of numbers of microorganisms and in the quantity of organic soil. The disinfection time can also be shortened by increasing the concentration of germicide, as illsutrated in Table 14-4 where the number of bacteria and other test conditions remain the same, the only variable being alcohol concentration. In the presence of more chemical, additional "cidal" mechanisms come into play, and those already in effect are increased in intensity.

TABLE 14-4

ETHYL ALCOHOL: CONCENTRATION VERSUS "CIDAL" ACTION

(From Morton)[5]

(Free Suspension—Room Temperature)

%/Vol.	Staph. Aureus		Pseudo. Aeruginosa	
	Pos.	Neg.	Pos.	Neg.
100	40 sec.	50 sec.	—	10 sec.
95–60	—	10 sec.	—	10 sec.
50	10 sec.	20 sec.	—	10 sec.
40	45 sec.	60 sec.	—	10 sec.
30	45 min.	60 min.	—	10 sec.
20	2 hrs.	3 hrs.	25 min.	30 min.

Some germicides are appropriately used only as strong (high-level) concentrations. This is the case with 8% formaldehyde, 2% glutaraldehyde and 12% ethylene oxide which are actually sporicides and therefore sterilizing agents when adequate exposure times are used.

Most low-level germicides become high-level ones when the usable concentration is increased sufficiently. Thus, iodophors and certain phenolics are tuberculocides of practical value at 450 ppm and 3% respectively.

Influence of Temperature

The rate of disinfection is accelerated with an increase in temperature. This is important when considering the application of disinfectants to various tempered surfaces within an institution. One should not expect that a cold surface such as the interior of a refrigerator can be disinfected as rapidly as a warm surface.

Even more important, other vegetative bacteria—and probably viruses as well—are destroyed more rapidly by a modest increase in the concentration of many germicides. Bactericidal tests in the writer's laboratory showed this to be so with "quats," iodophors and phenolics. To repeat a suggestion made earlier in this discussion, the rapidity of disinfection can be significantly increased by employing twice the recommended use concentrations of many proprietary disinfectants.

PROPERTIES OF GERMICIDES

Most germicides are used as aqueous solutions. The water brings the chemical and microorganism together and constitutes the "water of reaction" without which the disinfection process practically stops. A few germicidal chemicals have vapor pressures low enough to be gases at room temperature, and these compounds can be used as gaseous disinfectants or sterilizing agents. Table 14-5 lists the major classes of germicides in use at the present time and summarizes the salient properties of each class. The notations are based upon experience, published laboratory data, and in-use reports. Some of the evaluations and properties which had to be limited to one or two words in the table, in order to fit the format, need some qualification and discussion. As in the table itself, these comments pertain only to bacteria.

Liquid Germicides

Mercurials (Heavy metal compounds)

Relatively high concentrations are required to achieve significant "cidal" activity. The compounds are slow acting and most are bacteriostatic. The use of mercuric oxycyanide for the soaking of cystoscopes and catheters

TABLE 14-5

EVALUATION OF GERMICIDES

	General Usefulness as		(Bacteria only) Effectiveness Against		Other Properties
	Disinfectants	Antiseptics	TBC	Spores	
Liquid					
Mercurial compounds	None	Poor	None	None	Static only; inact. by org. matter; bland.
Phenolic compounds	Good	Poor	Good	Poor	Bad odor; irritating; not inact. by org. matter or soap; stable.
Quaternary ammonium compounds ("quats")	Good	Good	None	None	Neutr. by soap; rel. nontoxic; odorless, absorbed by gauze and fabrics.
Chlorine compounds	Good*	Fair	Fair*	Fair*	Inact. by org. matter; corrosive.
Iodine and iodophors	Good	Good	Good§	Poor§	Staining temporary; rel. nontoxic; corrosive.
Alcohols	Good†	Very good†	Very good†	None	Volatile; strong conc. required; rapidly cidal; inact. by org. matter.
Formaldehyde	Fair	None	Good‡	Fair†	Toxic; irritating fumes.
Glutaraldehyde	Good	None	Good	Good	Low protein coagulability; aqueous sol. useful for lens instruments and rubber articles. Limited stability. Corrodes carbon steel objects after 24 hours exposure.
Hexachlorophene	Fair	Good	None	None	Slow acting; not neutr. by soap; H₂O insol.; alc. sol.; inact. by organic matter.
Combinations:					
Iodine-alcohol	Fair	Very good	Very good	None	Stains fabrics.
Formaldehyde-alcohol	Good‡	None	Very good‡	Good‡	Toxic; irritating fumes; volatile.
Gas					
Ethylene oxide	Special	None	Good	Good	Poisonous; expensive; penetrating.
Beta-propiolactone	Special	None	Good	Very good	Vesicant; carcinogenic; expensive; unstable.

(*) 4–5% conc. (†) 70–90% conc. (‡) 5–8% formaldehyde (12–20% formalin) (§) 450 or more ppm available iodine.

should be discontinued. It is not a reliable disinfectant. For these reasons the mercurials have little value in modern disinfection.

Phenolic Compounds

Phenol or carbolic acid is the oldest of the germicides. Although the parent chemical is no longer used, some of the hundreds of compounds derived from it constitute the phenolic substitutes (or simply the phenolics). This class is the most popular one for housekeeping disinfection, and properly so. Not only are the phenolics good bactericides, but they also have the desirable property of stability, meaning that they remain active after mild heating and prolonged drying. Thus, subsequent application of moisture to a dry surface previously treated with a phenolic can redissolve the chemical so that it again becomes bactericidal. In addition, concentrations of the order of 2 to 3 per cent remain quite active when in contact with organic soil; for this reason phenolics are also the disinfectants of choice for dealing with fecal contamination. On the other hand, unpleasant odor and tissue irritation preclude their useful application on the skin and on objects which come in intimate contact with mucous membranes, e.g. anesthesia equipment.

Quaternary Ammonium Compounds

The synthetic chemists have created hundreds of chemical compounds with detergent properties, many of which are universally used for cleansing. One group, known as the cationic detergents, contains quarternary ammonium compounds with good germicidal activity. Zephiran® is the prototype.

The "quats" have enjoyed wide usage both as disinfectants and antiseptics. They have the important property of being bland and, therefore, popular with the user. On the other hand, certain limitations have become apparent in recent years. They are selectively absorbed by fabrics so that a 1:1000 solution becomes a 1:1500 or 1:2000 if gauze is immersed in such a solution.[6,7] This situation has apparently resulted in severe, and even fatal, infections.[8] Hospital infections from other uses—or misuses—of "quats" were reported and reviewed by Lee and Fialkow.[9] Even the use of hard water for dilution reduces the active concentration of Zephiran.[10] If it is desired to soften water for use with "quats," sodium carbonate (washing soda), trisodium phosphate, borax, or the sodium salt of ethylene diamine tetra-acetic acid should be used.[11] Sodium hexametaphosphate (Calgon®) has an inactivating effect and it should be used with caution.

In general recognition of the fact that the traditional 1:1000 concentration was not enough, it has become common practice in recent years to use 1:750; and in the writer's opinion it should be further increased to 1:500. The "quats" are devoid of tuberculocidal activity.[12]

Their value as antiseptics is limited by the fact that, being cationic compounds, they are neutralized by anionic chemicals such as soap. Nevertheless, their blandness for tissue is a favorable property, and it makes them particularly suitable for vaginal "preps" and other mucous membrane applications.

Chlorine Compounds

Inorganic chlorine is valuable for the disinfection of water. However, normal chlorine dosages usually employed in the simple chlorination of a water supply may not inactivate the infectious hepatitis virus (IH).[13] Cysts of *Endamoeba histolytica* resist chlorine concentrations greater than can be tolerated in potable water. The hypochlorites (sodium and calcium) are the most useful of chlorine containing compounds for practical disinfection in the hospital. Their germicidal power is dependent upon the release of free hypochlorous acid. Chlorinated lime contains 30 to 35 per cent calcium hypochlorite. Commercial laundry bleaches such as Clorox® are solutions of sodium hypochlorite. The equivalent U.S.P. solution contains about 5% sodium hypochlorite. These solutions are useful for disinfection of bedpans, urinals, toilets, and floors. They should not be used for disinfection of metal instruments.

All hypochlorites deteriorate upon aging, either in solution or powder form. Their germicidal efficiency is reduced in the presence of organic matter. Also, acid-fast organisms, including *M. tuberculosis,* are resistant to hypochlorites.

Iodine and Iodophors

Iodine is a good bactericide, but it stains fabrics and tissue. The staining can be reduced and made temporary by complexing iodine with a detergent. Such complexes are known as iodophors, and many of them have been placed on the market as disinfectants and antiseptics. Some of them are unstable in the presence of hard water, heat, and organic soil; yet they are reliable general purpose disinfectants if employed in adequate concentration. Instruments are likely to be corroded.

They are good antiseptics because they are relatively nontoxic and produce rapid degerming. The old problem of iodine burns was the result of careless contact with excessively high concentrations and need not be considered any longer. The germicidal action is due mostly or entirely to the release of free iodine and not to the complex itself.

The Alcohols

This subject was recently reviewed by Spaulding in some detail.[14] Therefore, the present discussion is confined to summary comments. Ethyl and isopropyl alcohol are much more useful as antiseptics than as disinfectants. Disinfectants can act only as long as they are in solution, and this means that the alcohols become ineffectual as soon as they evaporate. Although this property has the advantage of leaving no residue on treated surfaces, it often makes repeated applications desirable in order to get adequate exposure.

Nevertheless, the alcohols are rapidly bactericidal and, in the writer's experience, they are the most active germicides against the tubercle bacillus. They can be relied upon to destroy other vegetative bacteria promptly, provided little or no organic soil is present and they have not been diluted too much. Since it is convenient to use a single concentration throughout the hospital, one can select 85 per cent by volume as suitable for general use. Because the alcohols rapidly lose their "cidal" activity when diluted below 50 per cent concentration (see Table 14-4), solutions should be watched closely with this in mind and discarded at frequent intervals. The alcohols dissolve cement mountings of lensed instruments and they blanch the asphalt tiles of floors. On long exposure they harden and swell plastic tubing, including polyethylene.

Formaldehyde

Aqueous solutions are known as formalin. When purchased commercially formalin is a solution of approximately 40% formaldehyde in water. Therefore, 8% formaldehyde is 20% formalin. This strong concentration is a high-level germicide, and its activity is further increased by adding alcohol. A combination of 8% formaldehyde and 70% isopropyl alcohol is rapidly bactericidal and even a sporicide. Sterility can be expected within 3 hours exposure. Its tuberculocidal action is extremely rapid. Formaldehyde and cresol solutions appear to be effective for destroying *Histoplasma capsulatum* in soil.[15] The irritating fumes of formaldehyde limit its usefulness; and its toxicity for tissue requires that materials treated with it be thoroughly rinsed before use.

Glutaraldehyde

This chemical relative of formaldehyde appears to be somewhat more active than formaldehyde in that a 2% aqueous alkaline concentration has been reported as the approximate equivalent of 8% formaldehyde in alcohol.[16] It is a high-level disinfectant. Spores are destroyed within 3 hours, and it is tuberculocidal within a few minutes. It is the liquid disinfectant of choice for lensed instruments and certain critical items which should be sterile when used.[17]

Gaseous Disinfectants

These include formaldehyde and two chemicals used for "gas sterilization," ethylene oxide and beta-propiolactone. All are highly toxic and, therefore, not involved at all with antisepsis. Since these chemicals are limited in

application to inanimate objects and since their "cidal" activity is subject to the same kinds of limitations as germicides in general, they should be designated as disinfectants rather than sterilizing agents. When used appropriately one of them, ethylene oxide, is a practical agent for producing sterility, and under such conditions—and only then—should the process be termed "gas sterilization."

Formaldehyde

This preparation has been employed as a fumigant for many years, as has the formaldehyde chamber in operating rooms. The bactericidal effect is disappointing unless much moisture (70% relative humidity, or higher) is present. This much moisture promotes corrosion of metal, and the fumes are irritating. The vapor penetrates articles poorly. Studies have shown that formaldehyde cannot be recommended for disinfection of fabrics contaminated with smallpox virus or with anthrax spores. Unless special care is exercised it is not suitable for the destruction of tubercle bacilli on woolen garments and toys.[18]

Ethylene Oxide

Ethylene oxide has a much more rapid sporicidal action than formaldehyde.[19] This property has led to the development of "gas sterilization" as a very useful commercial process for medical and surgical items. The conditions of application, equipment and controls recommended by manufacturers are such as to ensure sterility. Thus, the designation of chemical sterilization is entirely appropriate. The general subject of ethylene oxide sterilization is discussed in detail in Chapter 19.

Beta-propiolactone (BPL)

Beta-propiolactone is the most rapidly sporicidal of the three gases, but it has too many detrimental properties to be suitable for hospital disinfection (see Table 14-5). Recent investigations have supported the earlier findings relating to the carcinogenic properties of this compound.[20,21]

PROBLEMS IN THE EVALUATION OF GERMICIDES

Commercialism

The first problem is commercialism. Hospitals, the users, are faced with a plethora of proprietary solutions, hundreds of which are insignificant modifications—if, indeed, they are modifications at all—of well-known products. Many of them are promoted vigorously and backed by claims that do not stand up. As early as 1959, there were registered with the United States Department of Agriculture about 450 products specifically recommended for hospital application.[22] There are presently over 8000 registered disinfectants. Fortunately, this Federal agency is doing much to curb the sale of poor germicides. Dr. Stuart and his associates at the U.S.D.A. have established minimum criteria which must be met if the product enters interstate commerce, and these "official" standards provide a practical device for the elimination of products which do not fulfill the claims made for them.

The second problem is how to evaluate germicides. This is a complex technical subject which belongs to the microbiologist, and it is not appropriate to this discussion. However, a few comments of a general nature may be helpful to the reader.

Testing Methods

These consist of laboratory tests and in-use tests. The former may be dismissed with the remark that the emphasis in the "official" tests seems to be on minimum standards; whereas it might better be spent on ways to select the best germicide for a specific application, i.e. by practical or *in-use testing.*

In-use tests with critical and semicritical articles involve nurses and Central Service personnel who assist the microbiologist in determining whether the results of laboratory tests hold up in actual practice. With floor decontamination this means a series of cleaning-disinfection tests which, if properly designed and carried out, will answer the question, How can we get the most efficient decontamination? Good examples of in-use testing of operating rooms and of the floors in hospital wards are those of Kundsin and Walter,[23] Adams and Fahlman,[24] Finegold *et al.*[25] and Ostrander and Griffith.[26] One investigator reported that under actual hospital conditions plain water reduced the bacterial count more than did a detergent-disinfectant combination.

Similarly, in-use testing of anesthesia equipment can be a comparative study of several disinfectants to determine which one, under controlled conditions, shows the fewest viable microorganisms. Smith and Howland[27] did such a study in 1959.

The evaluation of antiseptics *must* be done by in-use testing because *in vitro* laboratory tests mean very little. The best method for doing this is the serial basin procedure of Price[28] which, unfortunately, is a tedious, inconvenient and time-consuming one. Consequently, short-cut methods are generally resorted to, and with corresponding reductions in the value of the results.

FOGGING AND SPRAY DISINFECTION

Fogging

Considerable interest has developed in this convenient and labor-saving application of room disinfection. The dispensers currently available do not produce thorough and even distribution of germicidal solution throughout the room. Until they do, it appears that fogging should be considered, as suggested recently,[29] a "supplementing technique to an overall contamination control program." Hackett and Macpherson[30] found that fogging does not provide effective decontamination, and it does not reduce the time required for terminal care of rooms housing contagious disease patients. The writer must add his own concern at the potential harm that may result from inhaling protoplasmic poisons over a long period of time.

Spray Disinfection

The direct spraying of a surface for a sufficiently long time to produce a film of disinfectant solution should be the equivalent of the usual method of application, although a long hose attachment may be required so as to bring the nozzle close to the surface. A spray seems to be the only convenient way to get disinfectant through ventilator gratings and into crevices. It is important to remember, however, that a light spray which fails to blanket a surface is not the equivalent of direct application.

SELECTION OF DISINFECTANTS

Even though the user has a good working knowledge of the nature of microbial contamination, the principles of disinfection and the comparative value of available germicides, some practical suggestions may be helpful in selecting the best one for a particular purpose.

The user should first determine the level of disinfection required. If the application is the disinfection of a critical item such as transfer forceps, select a high-level solution that is capable of producing sterility if resistant forms are present. When there is a risk of exposure to tubercle bacilli, but not to spores, a good tuberculocide is adequate. Thus it is necessary to consider both the types of microorganisms likely to be present and the nature of the application.

There are many proprietary germicidal solutions which have not been subjected to in-use testing. Thus, it seems advisable for users who are unable to get a good bacteriological opinion to choose "brand name" products which are sold in interstate commerce since these come under Federal jurisdiction and have probably been approved as meeting acceptable standards.

When considering an unfamiliar disinfectant ask for comparative data with a standard germicide of the same type, for example, Zephiran, if it is a "quat," or Wescodyne® if it is an iodophor. Ask a microbiologist to evaluate the data.

The recommendation outline given below should be consulted.

Recommendations for Chemical Disinfection of Medical and Surgical Materials[†]

Comment: We have been able to evaluate only a small proportion of the total number of proprietary and nonproprietary germicides. The ones named

[†] From: Chemical disinfection in the hospital, by E. H. Spaulding. *J Hosp Research,* 3:5-25, 1965.

here gave the best results in laboratory and/or hospital tests. Many others may be satisfactory.

Bacteria: For the purposes of disinfection, bacteria fall into three types: ordinary vegetative bacteria such as staphylococci, tubercle bacilli, and spores. *Provided prior cleaning is thorough,* satisfactory disinfection can be obtained as follows:

A. VEGETATIVE BACTERIA AND FUNGI.

    1. *General comment*—Many germicides fulfill these easy requirements.

        (a) 80 to 90% ethyl or isopropyl alcohol*;

        (b) strong formaldehyde-alcohol solutions* of the Bard-Parker Germicide type;

        (c) cationic quaternary ammonium solutions such as Zephiran*, 1:750 aqueous;

        (d) 1% phenolic germicides such as Amphyl**, O-syl**, San Pheno X, and Staphene;

        (e) 2% phenolic germicide-cleansers such as Di-crobe, Tergisyl, and Vesphene;

        (f) iodophors such as Hi-Sine*, Ioclide*, and Wescodyne*, 75 ppm available iodine;

        (g) 2% activated glutaraldehyde, aqueous (Cidex).

    2. *Smooth, hard surfaced objects*—5 minutes exposure to any of the solutions in A.1. If the object is metal, add 0.2% sodium nitrite to solutions marked*, and 0.5% sodium bicarbonate to solutions marked ** to prevent rusting.

    3. *Rubber tubing, "Shellac" and "Web" catheters*—Flush by syringing with solution A.1. (c), (d), (f), or (g), and immerse in the same solution for 10 minutes. Follow by a sterile water flush and rinse.

    4. *Polyethylene tubing*—Same as A.3. Solutions A.1 (a) and (b) are very satisfactory if tubing is clean.

    5. *Lensed instruments*—Cleanse and immerse for 5 minutes in A.1. (g). Rinse with sterile water.

    6. *Hypodermic needles and syringes*—until more is known about the chemical resistance of the hepatitis viruses the only safe method is heat sterilization.

    7. *Hinged instruments*—cleansing must be particularly thorough. Then immerse for 20 minutes in any of the solutions in A.1. except (e). See A.2. for comment on rust prevention.

    8. *Floors and walls*—A disinfectant is no substitute for soap and water. Use one of the phenolic germicide-cleansers in A.1. (e), or a good detergent scrub followed by an A.1. (d) solution.

    9. *Furniture and plastic bedding covers*—use one of the solutions in A.1. (d) or (f).

B. ORGANISMS IN A. (Vegetative Bacteria and Fungi) PLUS TUBERCLE BACILLUS.

    1. *General comment*—The "quats" should not be used; and the concentration of phenolic or iodophor is increased.

(a) 80 to 90% ethyl or isopropyl alcohol;

(b) strong formaldehyde-alcohol solutions of the Bard-Parker Germicide type;

(c) the phenolic germicides in A.1. (d) in 2% final concentration;

(d) the phenolic germicide-cleansers in A.1. (e) but in 4% final concentration;

(e) a strong concentration (450 ppm of available iodine) of one of the iodophors in A.1. (f);

(f) 2% activated glutaraldehyde.

2. *Smooth, hard surfaced objects*—2 minutes exposure to (a) or (b); 5 minutes to (f); 10 minutes for the other solutions in B.1.

3. *Rubber tubing, "Shellac" and "Web" catheters*—flush by syringing with B.1. (c), (e) or (f). Then immerse in same solution for 5 minutes (f) or for 10 minutes (c) or (e). Rinse and flush thoroughly with sterile water.

4. *Polyethylene tubing*—use B.1. (f) as in B.3. OR flush by syringing with B.1. (c) or (e) and then with water; follow with a B.1. (a) or (b) flush and immerse for 2 minutes.

5. *Lensed instruments*—cleanse and immerse in B.1. (f).

6. *Hypodermic needles and syringes*—see A.6.

7. *Hinged instruments*—cleansing must be particularly thorough. Then immerse for 20 minutes in B.1. (a), (b), (c), (e) or (f.) See A.2. for comment on rust prevention.

8. *Floors and Walls*—thorough cleansing with B.1. (d).

9. *Furniture and plastic bedding covers*—Use B.1. (c) or (e).

C. ORGANISMS IN A. AND B. PLUS SPORES.

1. *General comment*—the only solutions that qualify as acceptable sporicides are as follows:

(a) strong formalin-alcohol solutions of the Bard-Parker Germicide type;

(b) 2% activated glutaraldehyde (Cidex).

2. *Smooth, hard surfaced objects*—at least 3 hours exposure to C.1. (a) or (b).

3. *Rubber tubing, "Shellac" and "Web" catheters*—flush with and immerse in solution C.1. (b) for at least 3 hours.

4. *Polyethylene tubing*—same as B.4. except for immersion of at least 3 hours.

5. *Lensed instruments*—use C.1. (b) for 3 hours.

6. *Hypodermic needles and syringes*—See A.6.

7. *Hinged instruments*—cleansing must be particularly thorough. Then immerse in C.1. (a) or (b). See A.2. for comment on rust prevention.

8. *Floors, walls, furniture*—the sporicides in C.1. are not applicable. Therefore spores must be removed mechanically by thorough cleansing.

Viruses[*]

Use 10 minutes exposure in 80 to 90% by volume *ethyl* alcohol, formaldehyde-alcohol solution of the Bard-Parker Germicide type, 2% glutaraldehyde (Cidex), or an iodophor at 150 ppm or more available iodine.

NOTE: all articles which may carry hepatitis virus should be heat sterilized.

[*] Based upon the tests and opinions of Dr. Morton Klein, Department of Microbiology, Temple University Medical School.

Supplementary Recommendations

Transfer forceps—Solution A.1. (b) or (g).

Contaminated cases:

    Instruments—soak in a solution in A.1. (c), (d), (e), (f) or (g) for 10 minutes. Cleanse sharps and follow procedure in C.2. Autoclave everything else that can be sterilized this way.

    Furniture, floors—See A.8.

Oral thermometers—wash with soap and water; wipe dry and store in 80 to 90% ethyl alcohol containing 0.2% iodine.

Anesthesia apparatus—immerse in or wipe with solution A.1. (a) or (g).

Complex heat-labile items (e.g. heart-lung oxygenator parts)—ethylene oxide, 850 mg/liter, for at least 3 hours (see Chapter 19).

SURGICAL SCRUBS AND PREOPERATIVE SKIN DISINFECTION[*]

PHILIP B. PRICE, M.D.

PREOPERATIVE SCRUBBING and surgical antisepsis are matters not only of scientific interest but of great practical importance as well.

A weak link in the chain of surgical technique is inability to sterilize skin without destroying it. The surgeon is compelled to operate with hands that cannot be fully disinfected and make incisions through skin that cannot be made entirely germ-free.

Historically, skin disinfection has always been a controversial subject in both theory and practice; it remains to this day in a state of considerable uncertainty and confusion.[31]

One reason for disagreement is that many students of the problem have been concerned primarily with the numbers of culturable organisms that can be washed off the skin, not realizing that the more important consideration is the numbers and sorts of germs left on the skin after mechanical cleansing and chemical disinfection.

Furthermore, antibacterial agents behave differently *in vitro* and on living tissues. It is now generally recognized that the action and value of antibacterial agents on skin or in wounds can be measured reliably only when those substances are tested under conditions of actual use. It is possible for a given agent to be strongly bactericidal or highly bacteriostatic in test tubes and Petri dishes and yet be relatively ineffectual in surgical practice.

Another source of disagreement is that many studies have been made and published wherein investigators have failed to distinguish between bacteriostatic and bactericidal effects, have not employed suitable antidotes in their tests, and have not fully appreciated the inhibiting influences of minute traces of certain chemicals on the growth of bacteria in cultures.

THE SKIN

The irregularly ridged and pitted epidermal surface, upon suitable magnification, is seen to be composed of innumerable flat translucent cells. They lie many thick, are stuck to each other and to underlying cells, and form a watertight covering for the body. The most superficial cells become desic-

[*] Permission granted by *Journal of Hospital Research* to reproduce this material.

cated, lose their attachments, and are easily rubbed off. The numbers of such cells insensibly lost from the surface of the body every day is incredibly large. Bernstein[32] counted millions of them in handwashings. Their place is taken by underlying epidermal cells which have been pushed slowly to the surface, losing their nuclei in the process, and suffering transformation from living protein-filled cells to flat masses of inert keratin. Bacteria are present on and under the superficial, loosely attached, lifeless cells, but few if any are found in or between living cells beneath.

Sweat is normally a weak solution of sodium chloride with small amounts of urea, potassium salts, and lactic acid, and traces of compounds of calcium, magnesium, sulfur, and phosphorus. The amounts of these ingredients depend upon the health of the body and the profuseness of secretion. With active perspiration, the salt content rises and the nitrogen content falls. According to Mosher,[33] the pH may range from 4.2 to 7.5, although ordinary variations are much narrower, from 5.02 to 5.71. Since normal sweat is slightly acid and mildly bactericidal, and the flow is continually outward, bacterial invasion of these ducts is relatively uncommon. Sweat is usually sterile as it emerges from pores onto the skin surface, but there it picks up surface bacteria and quickly becomes highly contaminated.

The fatty secretion of sebaceous glands is a very different substance. Its exact composition is not known, but it contains fats, soaps, cholesterol, albuminous material, epithelial cells, organic detritus, and inorganic salts. Within the glands and ducts the secretion is semifluid, but in the open hair pits and on the exposed epidermal surface it tends to "set" into firmer consistency, coating the entire surface of the body. This coat serves a useful purpose in protecting the skin and making it water-repellent. Ordinary washing with soap and water does not remove it fully. Sebum has very little antibacterial action; consequently, infection of hair follicles is common. Bacteria can be demonstrated occasionally in normal sebaceous ducts and glands.

The Bacteriology of Healthy Skin

The cutaneous bacterial flora is composed of transient and resident organisms.[34] Transients vary tremendously in number and kind. Virulent germs may be present as well as saprophytes. Test bacteria placed on skin are transients. Fortunately for our health, most of the extraneous microorganisms that get on the skin soon disappear from its surface. Some die; others fall off, are rubbed off on clothes, or are washed off. In general, transient bacteria are more abundant on the exposed skin of the hands and face. Enormous numbers of them may be collecting under nails, on the scalp and feet, in the umbilicus and perineal area, and in major folds and creases where microorganisms are protected and conditions are favorable for growth. Depending on the condition of the skin and the numbers of bacteria present, it takes from 5 to 10 minutes of washing with soap and water to remove all transients (contaminants) from the hands. They can be killed with relative ease by suitable antiseptics.

Residents form the stable bacteria population of the skin. They live and multiply there. Some of them die there; many are rubbed off or are washed off. Under ordinary conditions of life, increases tend to balance losses, so that on the same person the total number of resident microorganisms remains fairly constant. Inasmuch as the resident bacteria are firmly attached to the cutaneous surface, washing removes them slowly. They are less susceptible than transients to the action of antiseptics. Residents are composed largely of staphylococci of low pathogenicity, but some pathogens are almost always present. Prolonged or frequent exposure of the skin to large numbers of bacteria, particularly to pathogenic bacteria, may alter the usual composition of the resident flora and increase its potential infectiousness.[35]

Some persons habitually carry a much larger flora than others, but it is not possible simply by looking at skin to say whether its flora is large or small. The rate at which the cutaneous flora is reduced by scrubbing varies with different individuals. These variables add unavoidable uncertainties to any arbitrary rigid schedule of preoperative scrubbing.

In addition to the resident flora just described, there is a reservoir of bacteria hidden deeply in the skin.[36] The superficial resident flora comes off in washings at a regular rate, whereas the deep bacteria begin to appear in washings in appreciable numbers only after many minutes of scrubbing. *This observation strengthens a time-honored belief that it is not possible to sterilize skin without destroying it.* The deep resident flora appears to have about the same composition as the superficial resident flora; that is to say, it contains approximately the same proportion of pathogens. Little is known as yet about the size or precise location of the deep flora. It is probable that many of these bacteria are harbored in sebaceous ducts and glands.[37]

The cutaneous bacterial populations in various parts of the body tend to vary in size according to a definite pattern.[38] The forehead, for example, appears to have an extraordinarily large flora, whereas the back has a surprisingly small one. Some of the areas frequently operated on (abdomen, chest and legs) have floras roughly similar in size to those found on hands and forearms.

Conventional scrubbing decreases the resident flora slowly, at roughly logarithmic rates, about half the bacterial population present being removed with each 6 minutes of scrubbing. In general, the larger the initial flora the slower the rate of reduction by scrubbing. When the skin has been effectively degermed by scrubbing or by application of antiseptics, regeneration starts promptly. Richards[39] found that regrowth was approximately 25 per cent complete in 24 hours, 73 per cent in 3 days, and 100 per cent in about a week. The rate of regrowth on hands and arms is found to be greatly accelerated whenever surgical gloves and gown are worn.

The basic problem of skin disinfection, therefore, is simple and rational, however difficult it may be in actual practice to achieve fully the desired results. The potentially infectious bacteria are virtually all on the cutaneous surface. Most of the transients, pathogenic and nonpathogenic, are readily removed by soap and water. The remaining flora is best attacked by means of suitable chemical antiseptic agents. These antiseptics should be capable of destroying bacteria of the skin without damaging the skin itself. For maximal effect, all dirt, grease, and other extraneous material should be removed first (with soap and water) so as to permit optimal contact between the chemical agent and the bacteria. That contact will be augmented and the antiseptic effect increased if the antiseptic is applied to the skin with friction.

In preparation of the hands and arms for operation, therefore, the surgeon should place reliance on adequate scrubbing to remove dirt and grease, transient bacteria, and, incidently, a portion of the resident flora. Further disinfection is best accomplished by washing in one or more suitable antiseptic solutions. Those solutions should be effective bacteriologically yet entirely innocuous on skin, even with repeated and frequent use.

Preoperative preparation of the patient's skin presents a somewhat different problem since prolonged scrubbing is not usually feasible. Instead, the site of operation receives an ordinary bath, may be shaved, and is treated principally by application of antiseptics with gauze sponges. Use of relatively strong antiseptic preparations for this purpose is permissible since repeated applications are not ordinarily required.

In the case of hands and arms, additional protection from infection is provided by wearing sterile gown and rubber gloves at operation. Even so, complicating problems may arise. Should the sleeve or any other portion of the gown get wet, underlying bacteria are able to pass readily through the fabric and contaminate its sterile surface. As mentioned already, rapid multiplication of remaining skin bacteria occurs under rubber gloves, so that punctures and tears in the glove, which occur more frequently than many operators realize, may result in leakage of large numbers of microorganisms into the wound. There have been many attempts, mostly unsuccessful, to find methods of preventing the multiplication of bacteria under gloves. There have also been efforts to provide analogous protective coverings for the patient's skin at the operative site by means of adherent impervious plastic sheets.

EVALUATION AND USE OF SPECIFIC SURGICAL ANTISEPTICS

Soap

Soap is a feeble antiseptic. A cake of nonmedicated soap will disinfect itself quickly after it has been used, but, per se, it is relatively ineffective in disinfecting the skin. Its great value lies in its nonirritating detergent action, especially when washing is combined with mechanical friction.

For preoperative scrubs a preliminary toilet of the nails is recommended, followed by a 7-minute wash, using soap, a good nylon-bristle brush, and running warm water, not neglecting any area between the finger tips and a level well above the elbows. That procedure can be depended upon to remove all grease and dirt, all contaminating bacteria, and about half the resident flora.[34,35] Then the hands and arms should be dried with a sterile towel so that the following antiseptic solution will not be diluted and weakened by water left on the skin.

Soap is useful in preparation of the patient's skin for operation but, generally speaking, it does not have as large a role as in hand disinfection. Washing the field of operation in the operating room prior to surgery is sloppy and may be dangerous if sterile drapes and gowns become wet as a result. It is better to wash the area ahead of time and have it reach the operating table grossly clean and dry.

Tests[34,35] have shown that it makes little difference whether the detergent used is cake soap, liquid soap, or tincture of green soap. If the tap water employed is very hard, a synthetic detergent may be preferable, but its degerming action will not be greater than that of ordinary soap used with soft water.[60] Medicated soaps (except those containing hexachlorophene) possess no advantage over nonmedicated,[35] they are more expensive, and occasionally are found to be irritating. Pure soap is rarely irritating to the skin if it is not used in a too-concentrated liquid form.

Hexachlorophene

Hexachlorophene, a bis-phenol, is one of the few known antiseptics that do not lose most of their antibacterial potency in the presence of soap. Consequently, hexachlorophene has been combined with soap and other detergents, and has been recommended for surgical preparation of hands and the field of operation.

Many highly favorable reports were published, particularly during the years immediately following discovery and introduction of the agent.[40,43] Walter and associates[44] proposed the use of a synthetic detergent vehicle with 3% hexachlorophene (originally termed pHisoderm, now usually called pHisoHex,®) which is thought to be even more effective than the soap preparations. It has been asserted that persons who operate regularly no longer need to scrub in the old-fashioned manner, nor soak their hands in irritating solutions; instead it is necessary only to lather the hands and arms for 2 or 3 minutes with hexachlorophene soap. It is alleged that washing with this antiseptic soap daily will not only reduce the cutaneous flora to a low level but keep it persistently low. These glowing recommendations, together with the desire of many operators for a quick easy method of preparing for operation, have resulted in an extraordinarily rapid adoption of hexachlorophene preparations in the hospitals in this country.

In a great many operating rooms at the present time[31] hexachlorophene soap and pHisoHex have replaced the conventional scrub and alcohol wash. And in some hospitals, the field of operation is prepared by a brief wash with hexachlorophene or pHisoHex, followed by application of Zephiran. It is only natural that the initial enthusiastic reports about hexachlorophene should have been followed by more critical reevaluations.[45,48]

Correct evaluation of the antibacterial effectiveness of hexachlorophene preparations on skin is fraught with peculiar difficulties because of insolubility of the chemical in water, the bacteriostatic effects of even minute traces of the substance in cultures, and the lack of a fully effective neutralizing agent. Extreme care must be taken, therefore, in making tests and in interpreting the results.

The author, after two years of intensive experimental and clinical study of hexachlorophene, came to the following conclusions:[48]

> Quantitative and qualitative tests of skin disinfection, using the serial basin handwashing method and a new spot-testing technic, with control of bacteriostatic effects in cultures, demonstrate that the presently popular brief period of handwashing with soap or a synthetic detergent containing hexachlorophene (G-11) is not as efficacious as has been so enthusiastically claimed.
>
> Hexachlorophene does not disinfect the skin quickly, as alcohol does, but much more slowly . . . This slow degerming action is attributed to a film of the agent left on the hands after washing with the medicated soap. In order to achieve this desired effect, it is necessary to use G-11 soap exclusively and frequently, (i.e. many times a day) . . .
>
> It appears that the bacterial populations of the hands of different people vary in susceptibility to the agent. The fact that some individuals harbor a bacterial flora that is resistant to the action of hexachlorophene injects a disturbing element of uncertainty into its exclusive use in preparing the hands for operation. Even in those persons whose cutaneous bacterial flora has been shown by appropriate tests to be sensitive to hexachlorophene, an occasional brief wash with G-11 soap cannot be relied on to keep the hands relatively free from infectious germs.
>
> Comparative studies show that the conventional scrub followed by a 3-minute wash in 70% alcohol is much more effective bacteriologically, and more consistently so, than a brief lathering with G-11 soap or pHisoderm.

Further studies and experience on the part of myself and others have not led me to change those views. Furthermore, hexachlorophene is one of the antiseptics that shows a "rebound" effect; that is to say, ordinary scrubbing with hexachlorophene soap is followed (during succeeding days of nonuse) by temporary excessive regeneration of the cutaneous flora of the hands and arms.[45,49] Thus the occasional operator may unwittingly complicate the problem of his preoperative hand preparation.

On the other hand, Richards[39] states that the only way to slow down the otherwise seemingly unavoidable, rapid, potentially dangerous regeneration of residual cutaneous bacteria under sterile rubber gloves is to rinse the hands in a pHisoHex solution immediately prior to putting on the gloves.

The slowly acting hexachlorophene preparations have little value in preparation of the patient's skin for operation when they are used, as most antiseptics are, in a single brief application. There is an important place for them, however, in operations of election where the site of operation can be washed with hexachlorophene soap three or four times a day for several days preoperatively. This procedure will enable the patient to come to operation with that skin area fairly well degermed. It is not necessary for the part to be covered with sterile wrappings during that period or preparation; indeed, that is apt to be a disadvantage. This method of using hexachlorophene preoperatively is especially valuable in preparation of such areas as hands, feet, face, ears, and external genitalia.

Ethyl Alcohol

Although ethyl alcohol has had a long and honorable history as a skin disinfectant, and is still considered by the author to be on the whole the most effective and satisfactory hand disinfectant available, it is currently used significantly less frequently in operating rooms in the United States and Canada than formerly was the case.[31] Reasons for this loss of popularity are not clear.

Concentration is important. Strengths between 70% by weight (approximately 80% by volume when prepared at room temperature) and 92% by weight (commercial alcohol, 95% by volume) are all about equally effective in reducing the bacterial flora of the skin. For routine use, 70% by weight is recommended.[50,51] It spreads evenly, wets efficiently, and dries slowly (a desirable characteristic), and because it is almost completely innocuous, unless it happens to contain some irritating denaturing substance. Solutions of alcohol (the 70% solution, for example) exposed in an open vessel for periods of time tend to lose strength slowly because the alcohol fraction evaporates more rapidly than the water fraction.

Timing is also important. Washing the hands and arms for 1 minute in 70% by weight alcohol has a degerming effect equivalent to 6 to 7 minutes of scrubbing, and washing for 3 minutes will be as effective as approximately 20 minutes of scrubbing. If in addition one rubs the skin with sterile gauze or washcloth while using the alcohol, that degerming rate will be enhanced. The same basin of alcohol solution may be used by a succession of operators. At the day's end the used alcohol can be salvaged by filtering it through filter paper and bringing it back to its original strength with the aid of an alcoholometer and appropriate tables.[51]

Isopropyl Alcohol

Isopropyl alcohol degerms the skin fully as well, or even a little better, than ethyl alcohol. Solutions 70% or stronger are recommended. In contradistinction to ethyl alcohol, the bactericidal action increases with concentration, so that full strength (99%) is more effective than 70%.[49]

Since isopropyl alcohol is nonpotable, it may be obtained in unadulterated form and without the restrictions and taxes commonly associated with ethyl alcohol. Isopropyl alcohol is a more efficient fat solvent, however, than ethyl alcohol; consequently, it tends to defat the skin when used repeatedly in concentrated solution, leaving the hands rough and scaly with an uncomfortable feeling of dryness. For this reason it is not recommended for routine use as a hand antiseptic, however useful it may be in preparation of the patient's skin for operation.

Mercurials

Evaluation of mercurials as skin antiseptics is peculiarly difficult. No group of antiseptics has in its day received more enthusiastic acclaim but in the long run has proved to be more disappointing.

Mercurials are highly bacteriostatic. Small quantities carried over into cultures may inhibit growth. Moreover, both inorganic and organic mercurial compounds tend to combine with bacterial cells in some sort of union or complex that is not broken by washing in water or excessive dilution. As a result, suitable antidotes are necessary to avoid deceptive bacteriostatic effects in cultures. In addition, there is some evidence that mercurials react with the epidermis to form "films" which cover the underlying bacteria without destroying them or preventing their multiplication. A false illusion of a sterile skin surface may thus be created. To complicate the matter further, alkaline sulfides (used as antidotes) and other reducing agents seem to increase the size of the cutaneous flora. These confusing problems have been studied[52,53,54] but have never been satisfactorily resolved.

Solutions of mercuric chloride and potassium mercuric iodide, once universally used for hand disinfection, have now been almost completely discarded,[31] and rightly so, for they tend to irritate or injure the skin without degerming it effectively.

Organic mercurials (Merthiolate,® Mercurochrome,® Mercresin,® Metaphen®) are also far less popular than they were a generation ago. Tinctures of these compounds are bacteriologically more effective than aqueous preparations in preparing the skin for operation, but they are not as efficacious in that respect as simple 70% ethyl alcohol.[36]

Benzalkonium Chloride—Zephiran

Quaternary ammonium compounds have come into wide usage since their introduction as medicinal disinfectants by Domagk in 1935. Cationic forms are efficacious against both gram-positive and gram-negative bacteria, whereas anionic preparations are active chiefly against gram-positive organisms, and nonionics bacteriologically are virtually powerless. The preferred cationic compounds are incompatible with many chemicals,[55] and their antibacterial activity may be largely or completely neutralized by alkaline soap.[56]

Benzalkonium chloride—Zephiran, the cationic preparation of choice in this country, is a powerful, rapidly acting germicide against test bacteria *in vitro*, but on skin, under conditions of ordinary use, its antiseptic action is not as great as many investigators believed originally. This loss of power is due in part, especially in the case of aqueous solutions, to the traces of soap regularly left on skin after ordinary washing.[56] When Zephiran is to be used, therefore, it is advantageous to make sure that all soap has been removed from the epidermal surface. Simply rinsing off the suds will not do; even prolonged rinsing in running tap water is not entirely effective; but a brief wash with 40 to 70% ethyl alcohol will remove all the soap.

Tincture of benzalkonium is a more effective skin antiseptic than aqueous solutions, though no better than plain 70% alcohol. Indeed, there is evidence[56] that a considerable portion of the degerming effect of tincture of benzalkonium is attributable to the alcohol-acetone solvent.

From what has been said, it should be clear that it is illogical to wash with Zephiran immediately after using hexachlorophene soap. Washing the hands in Zephiran just before putting on sterile rubber gloves does not appear to inhibit the rapid regeneration of skin bacteria under the gloves.[39]

Iodine

Iodine has long been considered a superior skin antiseptic. It is a broad-spectrum germicide, effective against ordinary aerobic cutaneous bacteria as well as against pathogenic strains resistant to antibiotics. It also kills anaerobes, sporulating bacteria, and many fungi. The main reason it has fallen into disuse as a preoperative skin antiseptic is that the old standard preparations so often caused burns or irritations, and some persons were found to be hypersensitive to the halogen. These defects can be largely avoided, however, if less concentrated preparations are employed.

Aqueous solutions of iodine should be used with caution, if at all. Lugol's solution (iodine 5, potassium iodide 10, distilled water q.s. ad 100) may be dangerous if applied to large areas of skin. Three subjects in the author's laboratory, one after the other, who washed their hands and arms in the solution to test its antiseptic effects, were all badly burned, and one of them had to be hospitalized for systemic symptoms of iodism. A 2% water solution of iodine-iodide (iodine solution) has been recommended as a superior skin antiseptic,[57] but the author has found it less effective bacteriologically and more irritating than 2% alcoholic solution.[49] Old-fashioned "tincture of iodine" (7% iodine and 5% potassium iodide in 83 to 88% alcohol) was much too strong. The former "half-strength tincture of iodine" was even more prone to cause burns because rapid evaporation left rims of highly concentrated iodine on the skin. Modern iodine tincture (2% iodine, 2.4% potassium iodide, 44 to 50% alcohol) is a very effective, reasonably safe skin antiseptic. Superior to that, however, in my opinion, is a preparation of a 1 or 2% iodine and an equal amount of potassium iodide in 70% (by weight) ethyl alcohol. This solution spreads evenly, dries slowly (a desirable characteristic), does not burn the skin, and rarely causes the patient discomfort of any sort. Quantitative bacteriologic tests in my laboratory show these preparations of iodine to be extremely effective in reducing the cutaneous flora.[49,60] These newer preparations of iodine merit a larger place of usefulness in present-day operating rooms.

Iodophors

Iodophors are combinations of iodine with detergents, solubilizers, or other "carriers." A large number of them have been produced and recommended which have in common iodine bound in a chemical complex in solution in an aqueous medium. They differ from each other in type of carrier used, degree of acidity, color, and odor. Most of them are said to have about 1% "available" iodine which theoretically is slowly released to become effective against bacteria.

As mentioned previously, iodine is known to be extremely effective as a wide-spectrum local antiseptic when applied to healthy skin, but in traditional preparations these merits are counterbalanced by proneness to local skin damage, to allergic or toxic effects in sensitive persons, and to reactivity with metals. Iodophors, in contrast, are free from those defects and yet (it is said) retain the advantages of iodine as an antiseptic. An added virtue claimed for iodophors is that the detergent present serves to cleanse the skin at the same time that the iodine is acting.

It is easy to demonstrate that iodophors are good cleansing agents; that they are not unpleasant to use, do not irritate the skin or produce allergic reactions; that they are free from irritating fumes or odors; that the light-yellow stains produced by them are readily washed off with water; and that they do not react with metals. Reports also indicate that iodophors are effective sanitizers for floors, eating utensils, and other similar items. It is not so certain, however, that iodophors are nearly so effective as skin antiseptics. Indeed, when tested critically under conditions of actual use, iodophors are found to be only moderately effective degerming agents.[49,58] None of them appears to be nearly as potent as simple alcoholic solutions of iodine, or as good as ethyl alcohol itself. It would seem that in producing preparations that are comparatively harmless to skin, manufacturers have provided solutions that are relatively weak degermers of skin. The attractive hypothesis of slow release of free iodine to act upon the resident cutaneous flora does not stand up under tests which reproduce conditions of actual use.[60]

A possible exception to these general observations regarding iodophors is provided by a new preparation called Surgidine,® which the author has had opportunity to study thoroughly in his laboratory. That is the trade name given to a combination of nonylphenoxypolyethanol-iodine with selected wetting agents, solvents, and emollients. It is supplied* in both aqueous and alcoholic forms. The aqueous preparation, which is completely harmless on skin, was found to be a fairly good antiseptic, reducing the resident flora by about one-third with each minute of application with gauze friction.[60] That is a slightly better result than was obtained in similar tests with any of the other iodophors studied.[58] The alcoholic (80% ethyl alcohol) solution, said to contain 10,000 ppm "available" iodine, also harmless on skin, is more efficacious, comparing favorably with 70% ethyl alcohol, tincture of Zephiran, and simple 1% tincture of iodine.[60]

RECOMMENDATIONS

Preoperative Preparation of the Operator's Hands

Schedule of Choice for the Initial Scrub of the Day

—Come to the scrub sink with grossly immaculate hands.

—Examine the nails critically; if need be, trim them with scissors and clean them with a nail file.

—Scrub vigorously and steadily for at least 7 minutes by the clock, using a good surgical handbrush, soap, and warm running water. Nylon-bristle brushes, which can be heat-sterilized without becoming flabby, are most satisfactory. The type of soap used does not matter very much. Hexachlorophene soap or pHisoHex may be used if desired, but the scrubbing time should not be lessened for that reason. After several decades of clinical experience and laboratory studies, the author's personal preference is for pure, nonmedicated soap in cake form. Every part of each hand and arm should receive its full share of scrubbing, from the finger tips to a level well above the elbows, with special attention to brushing the nails. During the scrub, at intervals of about 1 minute, the accumulated lather should be washed off, fresh soap applied, and brushing resumed.

—After the final rinse, dry the hands and arms with a sterile towel. Failure to include this step will result in dilution and weakening of the antiseptic alcohol solutions.

—Wash the hands and arms briefly in a basin of 95% ethyl alcohol. This step will in itself have some degerming effect, but its main purpose is to remove all remaining water from the skin.

—Pass immediately to a basin half full of 70% (by weight) ethyl alcohol. Wash for 3 minutes by the clock, using a sterile washcloth to rub, gently but firmly, every part of the scrubbed area repeatedly. The small amount of

---

* Ingram & Bell, Ltd., Toronto, Ontario. Also Wallace Pharmaceuticals, Cranbury, New Jersey.

95% alcohol carried over into this basin will help to counteract the inevitable gradual weakening of the 70% alcohol solution by evaporation.

—Lather the hands and arms with a few milliliters of pHisoHex and rinse off the suds, or wash briefly in a sterile pHisoHex solution; dry with a second sterile towel.

—Put on sterile gown and gloves.

This schedule, properly and conscientiously carried out, requires 12 to 15 minutes, but it is time well spent. It is actually not laborious; it does not injure or irritate the skin, even after countless repetitions; it can be depended on to remove all dirt, grease, and transient microorganisms, and about 98 per cent of the resident cutaneous flora; and multiplication of the remaining bacteria under the gloves will be inhibited to some degree. As a result, the danger of infecting operative wounds by punctures or tears in gloves is reduced to a minimum.

Schedule for Succeeding Operations

—Strip off the used gown and gloves.

—Wash the hands and arms with soap but without brush in warm running tap water to remove powder, sweat, and possible blood stains.

—Dry with a sterile towel.

—Wash briefly in 95% alcohol.

—Wash for 1 minute in 70% alcohol, rubbing the skin with the washcloth.

—Lather with pHisoHex; rinse off; dry with a second sterile towel.

—Gown and glove.

This entire procedure will require only 6 to 7 minutes, but the hands and arms will, under these conditions, be disinfected as thoroughly as they were initially following the use of the first schedule described.

NOTE: If the operator should have come in contact with pus or other infected material during an operation, it is recommended that he observe the initial schedule in its entirety before going on to the next operation.

A "Short Scrub" for Minor Operative Procedures.[48,60]

—Scrub for 3 minutes with either ordinary or hexachlorophene soap.

—Dry the hands with a sterile towel.

—Wash for 1 full minute in 70% ethyl alcohol, rubbing with the washcloth.

This routine was adopted by the author's surgical service for such minor operations as biopsies, cystoscopies, and spinal punctures. Frankly, it was a concession to operators who were unwilling to go through the long scrub schedules for such minor surgical procedures. Even so, it was found upon careful measurement to be superior in degerming effect to the prevalent 3-minute scrub with hexachlorophene soap. It is easier to defend this technique on pragmatic than on philosophical and idealistic grounds.

Preoperative Preparation of the Patient's Skin
"Ward Prep"

Wash the area with soap and water, making sure that it is grossly quite clean. An ordinary shower or tub bath can be used satisfactorily for that purpose.

Shaving is not mandatory in all cases; indeed, it may be more disadvantageous than beneficial in many cases, but where coarse long hairs are present, it is clearly indicated. The almost invisible fine hairs, on the abdomens of children and most women, for example, do not in any way hinder application or action of surface antiseptics, nor, in the author's opinion, do their presence increase the chances of postoperative infections.

If the operative site is to be shaved, a clean safety razor should be used with a new blade and adequate soap lather, and great care should be taken to avoid scratching or nicking the skin. It has been found[60] that even skillfully performed shaving of the abdomen may be followed, after a few hours, by abnormal increases of the cutaneous bacterial flora, and that slight scratches, nicks, and excoriations may result in surprisingly large bacterial counts with many pathogens present.

The old custom of applying antiseptics as part of the "ward prep" and then wrapping the part in sterile dressings has been found to be bacteriologically useless[60] as well as psychologically harmful. Washing the field of operation in the operating room prior to surgery is sloppy, and may be dangerous if sterile drapes become wet as a result. It is better to wash the area ahead of time and have it reach the operating table grossly clean and dry.

Chemical Disinfection

The problem of disinfecting the patient's skin for surgery differs in several important respects from that of hand disinfection. The site of operation is not subjected to prolonged scrubbing with a brush. Although it may appear grossly clean, it still harbors a large bacterial flora, both transcients and residents (including some pathogens), which are protected to some extent by remaining extraneous oils and natural fats. This flora may be unusually large and potentially infectious, as already mentioned, if the "ward prep" has scratched or excoriated the surface. That may also be the case if there is a nearby infection, or a draining sinus, or a colostomy, seeding the operative site with contaminating organisms. Even a distant infection, such as a sore throat, may contribute an abnormally large number of pathogenic bacteria to the existing flora. Yet the person preparing the field of operation is expected to disinfect the skin surface quickly and thoroughly—quickly because the surgical team is in a hurry and the crowded operating room schedule demands it, thoroughly because a considerable area of skin is, as a rule, exposed during operation and remains a potential source of infection.

Although the patient's skin will usually tolerate stronger and harsher antiseptic solutions in a single application than are permissible on hands which must be disinfected repeatedly day after day, one is limited nevertheless to preparations which are not injurious. Even with these stronger antiseptics, reaction time between the chemical and the bacterial flora cannot be ignored. *There is no such thing as instantaneous skin disinfection by means of an antiseptic.* Generally speaking, the longer an antiseptic has to act, the more effective it will be. However, the contact between bacteria and the bactericidal agent can be augmented and the rate of disinfection of skin increased in consequence if gauze friction is used to apply the antiseptic. Spraying the antiseptic solution on the skin is a significantly less effective technique bacteriologically.[60]

Methods used to prepare the operative field vary not only from hospital to hospital but from time to time. Reasons for adoption of the routines employed are not always clear or logical. King and Zimmerman[31] properly ask, "Does the wide variety of procedures now in use mean that all technics are good, that they are all equally bad, or just that it does not make any difference?" There is a clear need for more uniformity in this regard in operating rooms generally—uniformity based on "specific and authoritative recommendations" which in turn are scientifically founded on acceptable standardized laboratory tests and critical clinical evaluations.

The following procedures are those which have received highest rating in the author's laboratory on the basis of tests which reproduce, as nearly as possible, conditions of actual use in surgical practice:

A. Apply alcohol
   Apply benzalkonium
   Apply alcohol
   Apply benzalkonium
   Apply alcohol
   Drape

The antiseptics are applied with gauze sponges. Alcohol used, 70% ethyl (by weight) or 70% isopropyl alcohol. Benzalkonium, 1:1000 tincture of Zephiran, tinted

B. Apply alcohol
   Apply iodine
   Apply alcohol
   Apply iodine
   Apply alcohol
   Drape

Antiseptics are applied with gauze sponges. Alcohol used, 70% ethyl or 70% isopropyl. Iodine preparation, 1 or 2% iodine in 70% (by weight) ethyl alcohol.

C. Apply alcohol
   Apply iodophor
   Apply alcohol

Apply iodophor

Apply alcohol

Drape

Antiseptics are applied with gauze sponges. Alcohol used, 70% ethyl or 70% isopropyl. Iodophor preparation, tincture of Surgidine.

D. For especially sensitive or delicate areas (perineum, around the eyes):

Apply aqueous iodophor solution repeatedly; or

Apply aqueous Zephiran solution repeatedly (first washing the skin thoroughly to remove any residual soap); or have the patient wash the area with hexachlorophene soap or pHisoHex for 3 to 5 days, several times each day, before coming to the operating table.

E. For operations of election involving areas (hands, feet, ears, face, male genitalia) where ordinary "painting" with antiseptics is difficult and possibly imperfect.

Have the patient wash the area with hexachlorophene soap or pHisoHex for 3 to 5 days, several times each day, prior to operation; then at the operating table follow with Schedule A, B, or C, modified as may be required to meet the special situation.

REFERENCES

1. Reddish, G. F.: *Antiseptics, Disinfectants, Fungicides and Sterilization.* Philadelphia, Lea & F., 1954, p. 25.
2. American Medical Association: Report of the council on pharmacy and chemistry. Use of the terms "sterile," "sterilize," and "sterilization." *JAMA, 107*:38, 1936.
3. Spaulding, E. H.: Principles of microbiology as applied to operating room nursing. *AORN, 1*:49-57, 1963.
4. Klein, M., and Deforest, A.: Antiviral action of germicides. *Soap and Chemical Specialties, 39*:70-72, 95-97, 1963.
5. Morton, H. E.: The relationship of concentration and germicidal efficiency of ethyl alcohol. *Ann NY Acad Sci, 53*:191-196, 1950.
6. Kundsin, R. B., and Walter, C. W.: Investigations on adsorption of benzalkonium chloride USP by skin, gloves and sponges. *Hosp Topics, 36*:108-113, 1958.
7. Myers, G. E., and Lefebvre, C.: Antibacterial activity of benzalkonium chloride in the presence of cotton and nylon fibers. *Canad Pharmaceut J, 94*:55-57, 1961.
8. Plotkin, S. A., and Austrian, R.: Bacteremia caused by *Pseudomonas sp.* following use of materials stored in solutions of a cationic surface-active agent. *Amer J Med Sci, 235*:621-627, 1958.
9. Lee, J. C., and Fialkow, P. J.: Benzalkonium chloride—source of hospital infection with gram-negative bacteria. *JAMA, 177*:708-710, 1961.
10. Babcock, K. B.: Maintaining standards and quality care in the operating room. *OR Nursing, 2*:44-86, 1961.
11. Finch, W. E.: *Disinfectants.* London, Chapman and Hall, Ltd., 1958, p. 90.
12. Hirsch, J. G.: The resistance of tubercle bacilli to the bactericidal action of benzalkonium chloride (Zephiran). *Amer Rev Tuberc, 70*:312-319, 1954.
13. Safety Committee (Calif Water Pollution Control Assoc): Report on hepatitis. *J Water Pollut Contr Fed, 37*:1629-1634, 1965.
14. Spaulding, E. H.: Alcohol as a surgical disinfectant. *AORN J, 2*:(5)67-71, 1964.
15. Tosh, F. E.; Weeks, R. J.; Pfeiffer, F. R.; Hendricks, S. L., and Chin, T. D. Y.: Chemical decontamination of soil containing *Histoplasma capsulatum. Amer J Epidemiol, 83*:262-270, 1966.
16. Stonehill, A. A.; Krop, S., and Bobick, P. M.: Buffered glutaraldehyde, a new chemical sterilizing solution. *Amer J Hosp Pharm, 20*:458-465, 1963.

17. O'Brien, H. A.; Mitchell, J. D., Jr.; Haberman, S.; Rowan, D. F.; Winford, T. E., and Pellet, J.: The use of activated glutaraldehyde as a cold sterilizing agent for urological instruments. *J Urol*, 95:429-435, 1966.

18. Committee on Formaldehyde Disinfection, (Publ Health Lab Service): Disinfection of fabrics with gaseous formaldehyde. *J Hygiene*, 56:488-515, 1958.

19. Phillips, C. R.: Gaseous sterilization. In *Becton, Dickinson Lectures on Sterilization.* Rutherford, New Jersey, Becton, Dickinson and Company, 1957-59, pp. 33-50.

20. Dickens, F., and Jones, H. E.: Carcinogenic activity of a series of reactive lactones and related substances. *Brit J Cancer*, 15:85, 1961.

21. Dickens, F., and Jones, H. E.: Further studies on the carcinogenic and growth inhibitory activity of lactones and related substances. *Brit J Cancer*, 17:100, 1963.

22. Stuart, L. S.: How effective are chemical germicides in maintaining hospital asepsis? *Hospitals, 33*:46-47, 59, 62, 66, 1959.

23. Kundsin, R. B., and Walter, C. W.: In-use testing of bactericidal agents in hospitals. *Appl Microbiol, 9*:167-171, 1961.

24. Adams, R., and Fahlman, B.: Prevention of infections in the operating room. *Trans Amer Acad Ophthal Otolaryng, 65*:16-32, 1961.

25. Finegold, S. M.; Sweeney, E. E.; Gaylor, D. W.; Brady, D., and Miller, L. G.: Hospital floor contamination: controlled blind studies in evaluation of germicides. *Antimicrob Agents Chemother* Amer. Soc. Microbiol., Ann Arbor, Mich. 1962, pp. 250-258.

26. Ostrander, W. E., and Griffith, L. J.: Evaluation of disinfectants for hospital housekeeping use. *Appl Microbiol, 12*:460-463, 1964.

27. Smith, J. R., and Howland, W. S.: Endotracheal tube as a source of infection. *JAMA, 169*:343-345, 1959.

28. Price, P. B.: Skin antisepsis. In *Becton, Dickinson Lectures on Sterilization.* Rutherford, New Jersey, Becton, Dickinson and Company, 1957-1959, pp. 79-98.

29. McGray, R. J.; Dineen, P., and Kitske, E. D.: Disinfectant fogging techniques. *Soap and Sanitary Chemicals, 40*:75-78, 112-114, 1964.

30. Hackett, J., and Macpherson, C. R.: Studies on "Fogging" as applied to hospital room disinfection. *Ohio Med J, 59*:263-265, 1963.

31. King, T. C., and Zimmerman, J. M.: Skin degerming practices: chaos and confusion. *Amer J Surg, 109*:695-698, 1965.

32. Bernstein, L. H. T.: Technic for studying the epithelial cells of the skin in relation to disinfection. *J Invest Derm, 11*:49-61, 1948.

33. Mosher, H. H.: Simultaneous study of constituents of urine and perspiration. *J Biol Chem, 99*:781-790, 1933.

34. Price, P. B.: The bacteriology of normal skin; a new quantitative test applied to a study of the bacterial flora and the disinfectant action of mechanical cleansing. *J Infect Dis, 63*:301-318, 1938.

35. Price, P. B.: New studies in surgical bacteriology and surgical technic. *JAMA, 111*:1993-1996, 1938.

36. Price, P. B.: Disinfection of the skin. *Drug Standards, 19*:161-173, 1951.

37. Lovell, D. L.: Skin bacteria; their location with reference to skin sterilization. *Surg Gynec Obstet, 80*:174-177, 1945.

38. Richards, R. C., and Price, P. B.: Regeneration of skin flora under normal conditions. *Surg Forum, 12*:34, 1961.

39. Richards, R. C.: Some practical aspects of surgical skin preparation. *Amer J Surg, 106*: 575-580, 1963.

40. Traub, E. F.; Newhall, C. A., and Fuller, J. R.: Value of a new compound (dihydroxyhexachlorodiphenyl methane) used in soap to reduce the bacterial flora of human skin. *Surg Gynec and Obstet, 79*:205, 1944.

41. Udinski, H. J.; Reduction in total skin flora by the daily use of a soap containing dihydroxyhexachlorodiphenyl methane. *J Med Soc New Jersey, 42*:15-17, 1945.

42. Seastone, C. V.: Observations of the use of G-11 in the surgical scrub. *Surg Gynec Obstet, 84*:355, 1947.

43. DISCUSSION: *Ann Surg, 134*:482-485, 1951.

44. WALTER, C. W.: *The Aseptic Treatment of Wounds.* New York, Macmillan, 1948, p. 185.

45. PRICE, P. B., and BONNETT, A.: The antibacterial effects of G-5, G-11, and A-151, with special reference to their use in the production of a germicidal soap. *Surgery, 24*:542-554, 1948.

46. BLANK, I. H., and COOLIDGE, M. H.: Degerming the cutaneous surface. II. Hexachlorophene (G-11). *J Invest Dermatol, 15*:257-263, 1950.

47. BLANK, I. H.; COOLIDGE, M. H.; SOUTTER, L., and RODKEY, G. V.: A study of the surgical scrub. *Surg Gynec Obstet, 91*:577-584, 1950.

48. PRICE, P. B.: Fallacy of a current fad—the 3-minute scrub with hexachlorophene soap. *Ann Surg, 134*:476-482, 1951.

49. PRICE, P. B.: Local antiseptics. In *Drugs of Choice.* Walter Modell (Ed.) Saint Louis, Mosby, 1966, pp. 133-144.

50. PRICE, P. B.: Reevaluation of ethyl alcohol as a germicide. *Arch surg, 60*:492-502, 1950.

51. PRICE, P. B.: Ethyl alcohol as a germicide. *Arch surg, 38*:528-542, 1939.

52. PRICE, P. B.: Mercuric chloride, potassium mercuric iodide, and Harrington's solution in skin disinfection. *Surg Gynec Obstet, 69*:594-601, 1939.

53. CROMWELL, H. W., and LEFFLER, R.: Evaluation of "skin degerming" agents by a modification of the price method. *J Bacteriol, 43*:51-52, 1942.

54. POWELL, H. M., and CULBERTSON, C. G.: Assay of antiseptics at different times after application to human skin. *Ann NY Acad Sci, 53*:207-210, 1950.

55. LAWRENCE, C. A.: Quaternary ammonium compounds. In *Antiseptics, Disinfectants, Fungicides, and Chemical and Physical Sterilization.* George F. Reddish (Ed.) Philadelphia, Lea & F., 1957, pp. 586-587.

56. PRICE, P. B.: Benzalkonium chloride (Zephiran chloride) as a skin disinfectant. *Arch Surg, 61*:22-23, 1950.

57. GERSHENFELD, L., and WITLIN, B.: Iodine as an antiseptic. *Ann NY Acad Sci, 53*:172-182, 1950.

58. KING, T. C., and PRICE, P. B.: An evaluation of iodophors as skin antiseptics. *Surg Gynec Obstet, 116*:361-365, 1963.

59. PRICE, P. B.: Hand scrubs and skin preparations. *Hosp Topics, 38*:61-68, 1960.

60. UNPUBLISHED DATA, Author's Experimental Laboratory.

Chapter 15

THE CENTRAL SERVICE DEPARTMENT

EVOLUTION OF THE CENTRAL SERVICE DEPARTMENT

I N TODAY'S Hospitals, the presence of a department whose main responsibility is focused on preparing and maintaining the many life preserving articles and pieces of equipment is becoming commonplace and mandatory. This is the Central Service Department as we know it today. The American College of Surgeons[1] gave impetus to the development of this department when it instituted a movement some years ago to standardize surgical dressings and centralize the preparation and handling of all surgical supplies into one unit. For a long time, in many hospitals, this department was referred to as Central Supply or Sterile Supply and is still known by that name in some institutions. Many of the dressings dispensed from this source were prepared by volunteer workers or the hospital ladies auxiliary. By definition, the Central Service Department comprises that service within the hospital which processes, issues, and controls professional supplies and equipment, both sterile and unsterile, to all departments and units of the hospital for the care and safety of the patients.

Many workers associated directly with hospitals, and others connected with government agencies and industry helped to develop the present concept of sterile supply centralization. The early contributions of the late W. B. Underwood[2,3] are particularly noteworthy. His extensive studies relating to the planning and organization of work in the Central Service Department, from the administrative and technical viewpoints, led to a number of significant and important findings. In brief, his pioneering efforts did much to establish the basic philosophy of centralization which, when put into practice later by many hospitals, was proved invaluable.

During the early era, centralized sterilization of all supplies required for the entire hospital took place in surgery. There were fewer operations to prepare for, operating room personnel had the time to carry out the task, and the department was considered the most knowledgeable on the subject of sterilization. When surgeries became busier and it was no longer practical to have the sterilizers in the operating room, they were relocated into a surgery work room and the operating room supervisor still monitored their use. The usual surgical dressings, needles, syringes were prepared and sterilized in this room, then distributed to the various wards, units, or departments of the hospital. Even today in many hospitals, this is still the procedure and the source of all sterile supplies for the operating rooms and patient care units. Inappropriately this work room is often referred to as central supply. This is by no means what is implied by the term Central Service as used at present.

The purpose of Central Service is often misconstrued. In this department it is practical to prepare, sterilize, and issue all professional supplies for the hospital except, in some instances, instruments used in the operating and delivery rooms, supplies for the infant formula, and laboratory services. For many years, processing activities were carried out in the department or area where they were to be used. In some hospitals with facilities for steam sterilization in the operating rooms and water, instrument and utensil sterilization in the patient care units, it was assumed that a perfectly satisfactory supply processing system had been achieved. With this arrangement, it cannot be denied that many sterilization facilities had been provided, but who operated these numerous sterilizers? Under such conditions it was difficult to establish and maintain anything approaching standardization of sterilizing techniques throughout the institution. Thus, the situation where the operation of the sterilizers was everyone's business but no one's responsibility constituted one of the valid reasons for establishment of the comprehensive Central Service Department. The Department continues to assume a greater role in the function of the hospital. The services rendered have expanded in scope since the days of the Central Sterile Supply Room and Central Dressing Room.

The gradual introduction and acceptance of disposable items for patient care has had definite bearing on the layout and facilities needed to operate the department. While processing activities in some instances are diminishing due to the use of disposable needles, syringes, gloves, and many routine treatment sets, the overall responsibilities of Central Service are not. As the need for certain items or services is reduced, Central Service is taking on new assignments, often related to direct patient contact. The departmental role is becoming more complex because the hospital health team has grasped a new meaning of Central Service relating to a high degree of specialization in patient care. Teams for intravenous therapy, inhalation therapy, surgical preparation, and patient transport are functioning out of Central Service.[4,5,6,7] There has also been a change in hospital organizational concept and the Department may soon become part of a Materials Management[8] or Central Stores and Dispatch Department. On the other hand, there are hospital management authorities who believe that with the adoption of substantial quantities of disposables, decentralized processing of re-usable articles should be resumed. Emphasis is presently being placed on the combined operation of stores, inventory, processing, distributing, and accounting of supplies and material used in patient care. Apparently Central Service operations will continue to be in flux[9,10] as methods, standards, and customs of medical practice change the hospital.

OTHER CONCEPTS OF CENTRAL SERVICE

Two different concepts of Central Service operation have been instituted in Great Britain.[11,12,13,14,15] One is the regional central supply service for a group of hospitals and the other a central supply service located and operated within the individual hospital which is similar to the Central Service Department in hospitals in North America. A standard kind and limited variety of supplies such as ward instruments, theatre and labor-room linen packs, ward packs (treatment trays, dressings), and theatre supplements are provided by the regional central service. Hospitals participating in the regional supply program must provide supporting services and material for use with those purchased. The individual hospital central supply department provides both standard and special needs.

The physical facilities used by both types of departments are similar, except that the regional Central Sterile Supply is larger and many factory-type production operations are used. Very few pieces of small apparatus are handled. All items to be reprocessed are considered contaminated; however, the decontamination procedure includes mainly washing and drying. Workers assigned to this area wear protective clothing, and the decontamination section is segregated from all other aspects of processing. Disposable needles and syringes are used to considerable extent. Parts of treatment sets are made up of disposable articles such as aluminum foil, solution cups, and towels in the dressing sets.

Paper, aluminum foil, and nylon[11,16] are used more commonly as wrapping materials than cloth is. Containers used for irrigating solutions are made of borosilicate glass, soda lime glass, and aluminum. The sterilizing equipment in these departments consists of high vacuum and gravity steam sterilizers, ethylene oxide sterilizers, infrared (dry heat) sterilizers, hot air, formaldehyde and steam disinfectors. There is a difference in the manner in which supplies are offered for use in the regional supply system. Supplies are packed in foot lockers or corrugated cartons at the regional Central Sterile Supply, transported via truck to the participating hospital, and placed in the ward storage units for use in the same containers.

In hospitals with a separate Central Sterile Supply Department, the required individual articles or units of supplies are placed in the ward storage cupboards. Soiled supplies are collected and returned for reprocessing in metal containers, polyethylene bags, or plastic buckets under the regional system. The hospitals that maintain their own Central Sterile Supply have special collection containers in the soiled utility rooms where articles are grouped according to category, i.e. syringes, small glassware, needles, instruments utensils, and rubber goods. Work studies and mechanical devices are being used to improve operation of both types of Central Sterile Supply services. The operation and management of the departments is influenced to great extent by the hospital infection control officer and pathologist. The concept as practiced in Britain is designed to fit the British Hospital Service.

ADVANTAGES OF A CENTRAL SERVICE DEPARTMENT

The recognized advantages of centralization are efficiency, economy, and safety. When properly organized, the system promotes efficiency through good supervision of cleaning, maintenance, and sterilization of materials. The problem of standardization, uniformity, and coordination of materials and procedures are more easily controlled because the work is under constant supervision by an individual who devotes his entire time to this activity. A central service department is also economical because it avoids duplication of equipment infrequently used. The life of materials is prolonged through more efficient handling and better methods of preparation and sterilization. Procedures do not vary from day to day with changing personnel. The use of nonprofessional personnel, working under competent supervision, with assembly-line methods and mechanical equipment, results in marked savings for the hospital. One group of nonprofessional workers whose primary function is the preparation of supplies can be trained to perform correct technics when the system is highly standardized and adequately supervised. This relieves professional personnel for other duties, not the least of which are patient care activities.

A summary of the advantages of centralization of sterile supplies would be incomplete without the recognition that it contributes to safer and more exacting processing procedures. The old decentralized system of sterilization on several floors and in several departments by many people was not conducive to monitoring of personnel activity to prevent sterilization failures. Cases have been recorded where loads of supplies were inadequately exposed to sterilizing conditions, some where steam was never admitted to the chamber of the sterilizer, and in more than a few instances, the entire process of sterilization had been omitted. The evidence against oversterilization of supplies is equally as bad from the standpoint of destructive effect on materials. Here no hazard is involved insofar as unsterile supplies are concerned but the destruction of materials has incurred unnecessary costs for the hospitals. These unsatisfactory practices do not always occur through the fault of the individual but rather because of interference with other, and perhaps, imperative duties. Centralization has taken the operation of sterilizers out of the class of "everybody's business and no one person's individual responsibility," and placed it in a highly specialized class with both supervision and responsibility centered on the shoulders of one person, the central service supervisor.

PHYSICAL FACILITIES AND EQUIPMENT

Before a drawing of Central Service is prepared for a hospital, preliminary planning sessions should be conducted by a hospital building committee. Planning for the department is usually best accomplished with a committee consisting of the administrator, the architect, director of nurses, systems consultant, technique consultant, the person who will be responsible for the management of the department, and representatives from the various departments planning to use the services. The responsibilities of the planning committee include definition[17] of the objectives for the department as they relate to the total operation of the hospital, and a concise delineation of functions of the department.

Location of the Department in the Physical Plant

In recent years the department has been situated in various areas influenced by the following: 1) availability of vertical transportation systems, 2) degree of service to be provided to the special areas such as operating and obstetrical suites, emergency and outpatient departments, and 3) proximity of other departments which provide materials for processing such as laundry and general stores.

The present trend in Central Service planning is for greater centralization of services and a total logistics system.[18] All inclusive Material Management Departments which encompass the elements of receiving, processing, distribution, recovery, disposition, and inventory control of supplies used in operation of the hospital and for all phases of patient care are being created in some institutions. These departments are being located on the same level as supply-receiving platforms and where the material for distribution from the central linen room, pharmacy, central stores, flower and mail room, sanitation services (housekeeping), and medical records is situated so that supplies and equipment can be moved by an automated vertical transportation system. In the small hospital, Central Service may be located near to or on the same floor as the operating and obstetrical suites.

Irrespective of the size of the hospital, the location selected for the department should be in a dust-free area, well ventilated, separated from the general storeroom by an impervious wall to preclude the contamination of supplies by vermin or insects, easy to maintain and have direct access to the vertical transportation system. The placement of the department should allow for some expansion and not be too remote from the hub of hospital operation so that personnel will not feel isolated or be reluctant to go to the department at a time other than the normal work day.

Factors Which Affect the Plan

It is no longer practical to use a predetermined figure for space allocation in the planning of Central Service because of the great number of variables in departmental functions. The space requirements for each department will be determined after the following have been made known:

—The material transportation systems to be installed—dumbwaiters, cart/elevator, vertical and horizontal conveyor, monorail conveyor, service elevators, pneumatic tube.

—The degree of centralization for materials handling—will some articles be reprocessed for use at the using area; will purchased ready-to-use articles be distributed from Central Service; will general linen supply, pharmacy supply, records be dispatched through Central Service?

—Concept of supply processing to be followed—total decontamination of all reusable articles on a centralized basis. Will some processing be done automatically or manually?

—Articles and quantity of each to be reprocessed—if the volume of material to be reprocessed is large and includes utensils and instruments from the operating and obstetrical suites, rubber gloves, patient's bedside utensils, then facilities must be proportionately greater and more work stations will be needed.

—Equipment to be located in the department—how many units and what kind, such as mechanical washers, washer sterilizers, dry heat sterilizers, gas sterilizers, steam sterilizers, conveyors, wheeled equipment washer, water stills, and sonic energy cleaners?

—Structural form of the building—the position of support columns, column patterns, pipe chases, stair wells, windows, drop ceilings, materials of construction, number of floors above and/or below the level where Central Service is to be located; whether it will be a high rise building of one or two stories or a low rise building attached to a multistoried structure, all have bearing on the space requirements and kind of department which can be planned.

Automated Material Processing and Distribution System

The rising cost of patient care, increasing demands for personal time and attention, coupled with greater patient loads and need for improved processing methods, have been largely responsible for the development of an *automated material processing and distribution system*. This system is a comprehensive method of hospital material handling, incorporating the elements of receiving, processing, storage, distribution, recovery, horizontal and vertical transportation, waste disposition, reprocessing and inventory control. The scope of the system includes, but is not limited to, the following hospital areas: general stores, central processing, pharmacy, laundry and dietary, medical records, housekeeping, patient care units, utility areas, patient rooms, surgical suite, obstetrical suite, emergency department, outpatient department, pathology and laboratories, x-ray department, intensive and other special diagnostic and care units, morgue autopsy unit, and central dispatch. With an automated distribution system, material can be moved throughout the hospital complex without personnel.

The system is comprised of two parts: *primary transportation system* to distribute bulk loads and a *supplementary transportation system* to handle small unit loads such as an extra food tray, pharmacy item, treatment tray, blood bottle, or medical records. A series of horizontal and/or vertical passageways are employed to move the loads through single and multiple structured buildings. A schematic diagram to illustrate this movement is shown in Figure 15-1. The same passageway is used for movement of clean and soiled materials.

Unmanned portable carts are used to convey articles in the primary system. The cart guidance base may be self-propelled and electronically guided or mechanically propelled and electromechanically guided. The material-holding cart is a closed container which encases clean loads and guards against environmental contamination. The interior of the cart is designed for dietary service in accordance with individual hospital requirements or for general purpose use. The general purpose cart has a fixed central divider and nonremovable shelving which can be folded back to form bins or a combination of bins and shelves. When a self-propelled electronically guided propulsion and guidance system is employed, the material-holding section is removable and may be left at an appointed location to hold contents until they have been used or for receipt of soiled articles following use. The propulsion and guidance base may then be used as a separate section to move additional supply loads. Horizontal travel by the cart is limited to utility or nontraffic passageways. The self-propelled electronically guided system employs an elevator-type lift whose height is only limited by local safety codes. Carts are automatically accepted and ejected from a shaft of one or two car capacity. The cart lift will travel twelve floors, eject the cart, and return to its place of origin within two minutes.

The mechanically propelled electromechanically guided cart is moved on a dual support, multiple-flight-type lift to a ten floor height limitation. The shaft will accommodate a single cart module and continuously accept and eject the portable carts automatically. It takes two minutes for the support to travel ten floors and eject the cart. For a multiple flight system the time required for return is not significant. The supplementary system carries unit loads in a specially designed, enclosed module to destination and return through the same horizontal and vertical passageway as the cart travels in the primary system. The module will deliver items such as supplementary or delayed meals, medical records, or any article of limited dimensions required on an emergency basis.

Operation of the automated material-processing and distribution system originates in the central processing department. This department, Figure 15-2, is divided into several areas according to function.

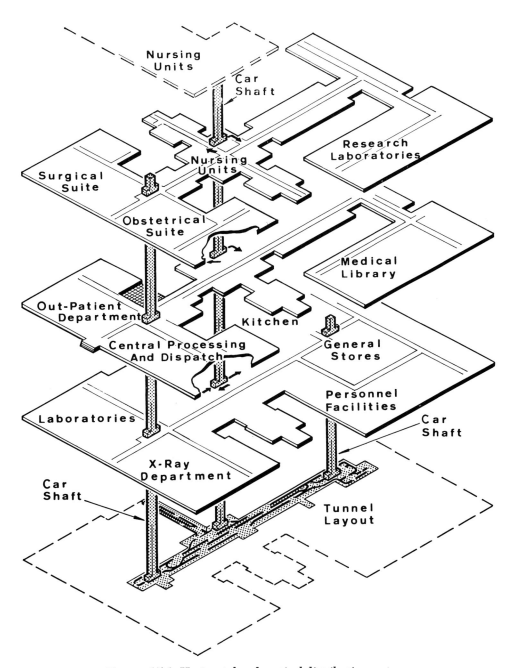

FIGURE 15-1. Horizontal and vertical distribution system.

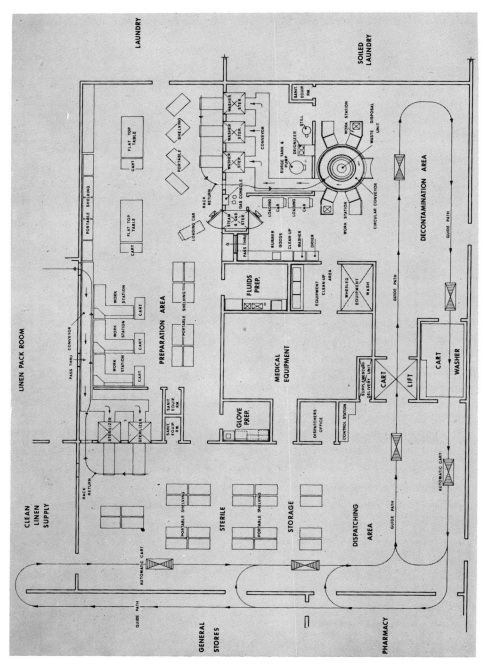

Figure 15-2. Schematic plan for automated material processing and distribution department.

DECONTAMINATION AREA. This is the area where soiled articles to be reprocessed are received, sorted, prepared for washing and decontamination, and disposition of waste takes place. It is separated by physical barriers from other sections of the department because contamination from all used items is concentrated here. The equipment and facilities are designed to allow materials to be decontaminated effectively and according to the needs of each article.

Material is returned from the using departments via the guided cart, separate tote-box system, or by any other transportation means and received at the circular conveyor station. Reprocessable articles are removed from protective coverings and placed upon the general purpose circular conveyor as shown in Figure 15-2. The items are then selected according to type by the worker, placed into an appropriate rack which is automatically moved onto a conveyor and transported to the washer-sterilizer. All operations of the washer-sterilizer are automatically programmed to accept filled racks or maintain them on the loading ramp if a washer-sterilizer is not available. Upon completion of the cleaning and decontamination cycle, the rack is ejected into the preparation and packaging areas.

Articles which are heat and moisture sensitive are cleaned manually at one of the work stations adjacent to the conveyor station and decontaminated in the double door steam and gas sterilizer or by chemical disinfection. The articles treated by chemical disinfection or washed in a mechanical washer-sanitizer are transferred to the preparation area via a pass-through window. The inclusion of a household type washing machine for cleaning of gloves in the decontamination area is optional. When required, a glove dryer can be located here.

Disposable material and refuse is placed in the center of the circular conveyor leading to a waste disposal unit in the space beneath. If a waste disposal unit is not available in the circular conveyor, provisions for moving waste to an incinerator or trash-holding receptacle must be made. Soiled linen is placed in a laundry-holding receptacle or transported directly to the laundry.

Certain pieces of inhalation-therapy equipment and other therapeutic and orthopedic apparatus of dimensions which permit them to be accommodated in one section of the enclosed cart can be returned from the area of use in the guided cart and received at the equipment-processing station in the decontamination area. Large or wheeled equipment which will not fit into the guided cart is returned via the service elevator for reprocessing in the decontamination room.

In certain instances it has been recommended that dish scraping and processing of dinnerware, glasses, and eating utensils be part of a centralized material-handling program. Soiled dishes and utensils are placed on a separate conveyor turntable located in the receiving area and designated solely for dietary use. They are racked at the work station, conveyed to a standard conveyorized continuous-process dishwashing machine and automatically ejected into the clean-dish room.

After all articles have been removed, the transportation cart enters a mechanical washer which employs a detergent-sanitizer to clean the interior and exterior. Following the wash and rinse cycle, the cart is dried with circulating hot air for approximately 2 minutes and exits with only residual moisture which dries rapidly as it is moved into position for use in the processed storage and dispatch area.

PREPARATION AREA. Clean supplies from the decontamination area, laundry, or general stores are temporarily stored in this area prior to packaging. Some items which have been decontaminated and which are not necessarily to be maintained in a sterile state for patient use, can be confined in a protective cover prior to placement in storage. Flat-top work tables are shown for this purpose on the plan Figure 15-2. Articles ejected from the washer-sterilizer are removed from their racks and placed on portable shelving labeled to receive the specific articles. The empty racks are returned to the decontamination area on an overhead conveyor.

Articles which require wrapping prior to sterilization and wrappers are brought to the work stations on portable shelves. The stations may be designated for packaging certain articles, e.g. instrument kit make-up, utensil kit make-up, tray preparation, special supply make-up station, and others as required. After the necessary assembling and wrapping process has been completed, the packages are placed in a basket designed to hold supplies during sterilization and moved by conveyor to a position to be accepted in the sterilizer. Following the sterilization process, the items automatically exit into the processed storage area.

SEGREGATED PROCESSING FACILITIES (GLOVES, SOLUTIONS, AND LINENS). Gloves require conditioning with powder before packaging. It is necessary to isolate this activity to restrict dissemination of the powder throughout the institution.

NOTE: *The use of glove powder is a hazard* (see page 224). The glove preparation area on the plan Figure 15-2 shows a counter for sorting of cleaned gloves, a cabinet for holding prior to testing, a glove tester, powderer, counter for wrapping, storage facilities for wrappers and packaging accessories such as wicks and tape labels.

In order that all the requirements for preparation of surgical and external fluids can be met, as well as to avoid dust and particulate matter from gaining access to the fluids, a separate room is essential for the process. The fluids-preparation facility is equipped with a rinsing device for the final distilled water rinse of flasks. A place to rinse and hold collars and caps, a flask filling unit, and a work counter for labels and ingredients are also required. The filled and capped solution bottles are placed directly on a sterilizer loading car for transfer to the sterilizer.

Linen used in packs for special-care areas requires careful inspection for holes, tears, worn spots, and folding to allow ease of handling at point of use. Dust and lint are by-products of the handling involved to fulfill the special requirements. Therefore, linen processing should be a segregated activity. Although this facility is not shown in Figure 15-2, the work flow in the room is from laundry truck to the table for inspection and folding, then to portable shelf for temporary holding, to work table for pack make-up and wrapping, to basket and conveyor, and finally to the sterilizer.

PROCESSED STORES AREA. As articles are ejected from the sterilizer, they are removed from the sterilizer baskets and placed on a portable storage cart or into a cupboard, dependent on the type of article, frequency of use, and area of use. The empty baskets are returned to the preparation area on an overhead conveyor. Articles which are purchased ready for use, are removed from their shipping cartons in a break-out area and transported to the department for storage on a cart or in a cupboard.

DISPATCH CENTER. The dispatch center is the heart of control for the entire automated processing and distribution system. It encompasses the elements of material management, remote station traffic information and control, and dispatch of material throughout the hospital complex. The specific functions of material management are inventory control, storage, requisitioning, maintenance of stock levels, and distribution scheduling.

The remote station information panel informs the dispatcher of the availability of stations in the clean supply area to receive carts with supplies, destination of carts in the system, carts in position at the soiled recovery stations, and the operational conditions of the horizontal and vertical system. Material is dispatched through the hospital according to a predetermined schedule based on use requirements. Items transferred from other sources such as general linen supply, general stores, housekeeping, pharmacy, and mail room are received at the dispatch point, placed into a cart, and directed to point of use via the automated system. The material dispatched from the control point in Central Service via cart or small supplementary module arrives at the patient care unit or other using unit in a clean supply terminal and it must be moved with manual guidance. The terminal may accommodate one or two carts depending upon the space allotted in the plan and the number of patients to be served at each level.

MEDICAL EQUIPMENT DECONTAMINATION AND STORAGE. A room for maintaining and decontaminating parts of medical equipment is located between the central decontamination area and medical-equipment storage area. The work area includes a triple sink unit with counter on each side and a cubicle for washing wheeled equipment or parts of apparatus which will withstand such treatment. Parts of apparatus which can be washed and decontaminated in the washer-sterilizer or gas sterilizer are processed in that manner. Following decontamination the parts are taken to the storage room, where the units are reassembled, checked for proper working condition, and protected until time of dispatch. Before plans are made for a medical-equipment storage room, the number of pieces of apparatus maintained in storage most of the time and the dimensions of each should be known. Storage facilities which will conserve space, yet permit ready access to the items are desirable. There must be some space allowance for acquisition of new apparatus which will be made available as a result of advances in medical research.

Prior to the planning for an automated material-processing and distribution system for a hospital, a study of material-processing needs and the supply-distribution pattern should be conducted. Figure 15-2 illustrates one physical arrangement in which the functions described in the text may be accomplished.

Conventional Plan for Central Service

Figure 15-3 shows a schematic layout of a conventional Central Service Department. The plan is made up of six specific processing areas.

RECEIVING AND CLEANUP AREA. This area provides space and facilities to clean articles and equipment returned to the department. To the left of the entrance the plan shows one hamper for soiled linen; two refuse containers to receive burnable and nonburnable waste; a clinical sink to receive liquid waste or for prerinsing of some articles, and a triple sink with cleanup counter for manual washing of articles, cleaning and disinfecting of thermometers. The center-island work unit has on one side a work counter for receiving and racking of utensils and other articles to be washed in the utensil washer and on the other side are two work stations, one to receive and preclean instruments, syringes, and other glassware to be processed in the sonic energy cleaner and the other to receive and prepare gloves for washing in the glove washer. A dryer is shown for glove drying.

Space is available in this area for parking of carts used to collect soiled material for reprocessing. A separate cart is often used for the collection of flasks and it is located near the flask cleanup area. The flask washer and drainage cart are used for flask processing. A double sink unit is included for cleaning of reusable flask collars and caps.

Adjacent to the receiving and cleanup area, facilities are shown for cleanup, check, and reassembly of equipment. Parts of apparatus which can be washed mechanically—in utensil washer, sonic cleaner, or household-type

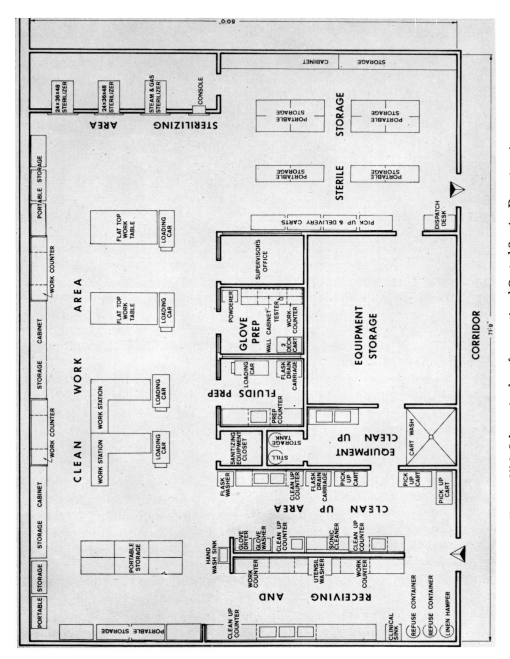

FIGURE 15-3. Schematic plan of conventional Central Service Department.

washer—should be cleaned that way. A double sink unit is provided for manual cleaning of parts of apparatus which cannot be subjected to a mechanical process. A cart-wash cubicle is shown for mobile equipment.

CLEAN WORK AREA. This is where many cleaned and decontaminated articles are inspected, reassembled into special kits, packaged, and labeled in preparation for sterilization. Portable storage is included for temporary holding and transfer of cleaned articles from the receiving area to a work station; also for storage of linen used for wrapping of packages. Storage cabinets are located in this section for reserve supplies from central stores and items not required frequently for processing.

The two work stations of functional design can be assigned to treatment tray assembly and preparation of supplies for clinics, emergency room, or special diagnostic units. The flat-top work tables may be used for packaging articles to be sterilized in the ethylene oxide sterilizer or assembly of instrument kits for delivery and operating rooms. If included as part of the service to be rendered, linen pack assembly may take place on one of the flat-top work tables. The linen should have been inspected and folded in a manner acceptable for pack make-up prior to delivery to Central Service. Inspection and folding of linen is not recommended for this area because of the release of lint and dust particles. When it is necessary to carry out this function in Central Service, a separate enclosed area with effective air-conditioning should be provided.

Two work counters fixed along the wall may be used for thermometer packaging and for preparation of special ointment or medicated gauze. Sterilizer loading cars are located close to production points so that material prepared for autoclaving can be placed directly on them to eliminate rehandling.

SEGREGATED PROCESSING AREAS. *Fluid preparation:* the flask filling, capping, and labeling activity must take place in an area free from dust and particulate matter and, therefore, it should be segregated from other processing areas. Facilities for this activity comprise the flask-drainage cart, flask-filling counter, storage for solution ingredients, and sterilizer-loading car.

Glove Preparation: Glove powder used to condition gloves prior to packaging for sterilization is easily carried on air currents and must be confined so that it will not be dispersed throughout the hospital and become a source of contamination. For this reason glove processing must be done in an enclosed area with controlled ventilation. The facility is equipped with a glove powderer, storage cabinets for wrappers, wicks, tape labels, glove tester, and cart to receive baskets of packaged gloves. Glove powder contributes to hazards in patient care and environmental control, and it should be eliminated if possible.

STERILIZING AREA. Equipment necessary to fulfill sterilizing requirements is located in this area. Two steam sterilizers and one combination ethylene oxide and steam sterilizer are shown on the plan. In some departments a hot air sterilizer is included for articles which require this method of sterilization. There is space to accommodate sterilizer loading cars filled with supplies while they cool prior to transfer to sterile storage.

The supervisor's office is located in the preparation area. In the past it was considered necessary that she be located in this section in order to monitor the operation of the sterilizers so that the procedure would be carried out correctly. Some supervisors feel that their office should be located in the center of the department to permit them to oversee all activities. The location of the supervisor's office has little to contribute to the act of supervision itself. Therefore, it would be desirable to have the supervisor's office located at a point where she would be accessible to personnel in Central Service and to personnel from other departments or outside of the hospital without their having to enter any area of the department.

STERILE STORAGE AREA. The sterile storage area is fairly remote from the soiled receiving and cleanup section so that sterile supplies can be protected from extraneous contamination. Fixed storage is indicated for articles dispensed infrequently and for some items which arrive ready to use from stores. Articles which have a high volume of use or rapid turnover are stored on carts. Carts used to deliver supplies to the hospital departments providing patient care are stocked and parked in this area. A dispatch desk is located at the dispensing door. The dispensing and distribution records, sterilizer recording charts, and sterilization control test reports are stored in the dispatch desk.

EQUIPMENT STORAGE. This room is located adjacent to the dispatch desk to facilitate dispensing and control of apparatus.

Basic Equipment for Centralized Material Processing

Washer-decontaminator

Preventing the release of contaminants from inanimate objects is of major concern to hospitals. The presence of infectious agents on used articles constitutes a hazard to personnel required to handle and clean the article. Aerosols created during the manual cleaning of many objects used in the daily treatment of patients contribute to the buildup in microbial populations in the hospital environment. This hazard can be minimized and a controlled standard for decontamination realized if an automatic washer-sterilizer is located in the hospital. Equipment of this type may be part of an automated material processing and distribution system or it may be an independent unit installed in a pertinent location. Regardless of the way it is acquired for use in the hospital, it is a desirable piece of machinery because it not only washes and sterilizes, but it also fulfills the requirements for the present trend toward centralization of processing of all soiled equipment with de-contamination as the initial step in the process.

The washer-sterilizer shown in Figure 15-4 is designed to automatically accept baskets of articles which are heat and moisture stable, wash and ster-ilize them with saturated steam, and discharge the load at the end of the processing cycle. The basic unit is a double door chamber with dimensions of $18 \times 25 \times 30$ inches. The chamber floor is fitted with tracks for the material-holding basket. Twelve strategically located revolving spray heads, each with multiple nozzles as required, provide washing action in the cham-ber. A water sump with steam jet heats the wash and rinse water while it is pumped to the spray heads. The water sump manifold has a riser valve to admit water to spray heads designed for washing special articles in the material-handling baskets. The features of construction and sanitary fittings prevent backflow of pollutants into the water supply system and unit. The performance cycle of the washer-sterilizer is as follows: The door on the input side of the machine is raised when a loaded material-handling basket

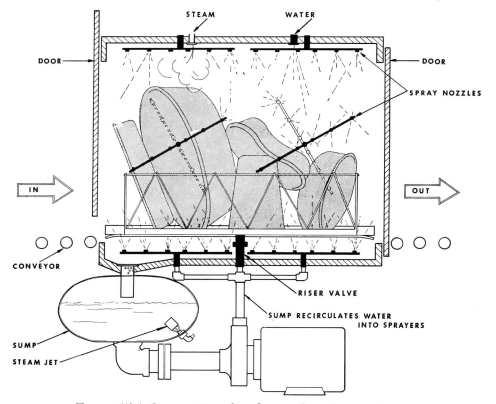

FIGURE 15-4. Cross section of washer-sterilizer-decontaminator.

moves forward on the conveyor. The door lowers and locks automatically when the basket is inside the chamber and the feeding mechanism has been withdrawn from the unit. Each load of material is subjected to a series of events. Upon activation, a measured amount of water enters the sump. The water is then pumped (recirculated) through the spray head and riser valve nozzles to force powerful jets of detergent water onto the load, while the steam jet heats the water. When the wash phase is completed, the detergent water is discharged to the waste. The chamber then fills with cold tap water, which is gradually heated by the steam jet during the rinsing cycle. The rinse water is drained from the chamber and replaced by deionized or distilled water as required for a final rinse. After water from the final rinse is drained from the sump, the chamber is charged with steam for the sterilizing phase. This process is terminated automatically with the evacuation of the chamber to 20 inches mercury and then returned to atmospheric pressure by filtered air. It takes 15 minutes to complete the washing and sterilizing cycle for one full basket of articles.

Upon completion of the cycle, the door on the unloading end will raise, and the basket of material will be automatically moved to a discharge ramp. When the basket has cleared the exit, the door will lower and lock automatically. The automatic opening and closing operation for the doors in conjunction with the processing cycle can be continuous without operator attention. The washer-sterilizer is designed to process an extensive variety of articles. Instruments, surgical brushes, trays, bowls, soap dishes, emesis basins, urinals, bedpans, bath basins, kick buckets, dressing jars and tumblers, flask collars and closures, ice bags, ice collars, hot water bags, assorted glassware, flasks, beakers, and bottles are examples of some of the heat- and moisture-stable articles which can be processed in the unit. The washer-sterilizer fulfills the basic equipment requirement for a centralized decontamination service. In hospitals where a program for total centralized decontamination will not be followed, consideration should be given to locating a washer-sterilizer in areas where all articles are considered infectious such as the operating suite, obstetrical suite, and isolation unit.

Waste Removal

Waste removal is a growing problem in hospitals and other institutions. The volume to be removed per hospital has increased steadily since the early nineteen-sixties. In 1967, the accumulated sum of more than 10 pounds of waste per bed per day has been recorded[19] and an escalation is anticipated due to the increased consumption of disposable medical and surgical supplies, and prepackaged foods which lessen wet garbage but add to the volume of paper and plastic waste. The composition of this growing waste load generates high degrees of latent heat during incineration. Recent studies[20] have shown that this admixture of paper, plastics, and wet garbage raised the

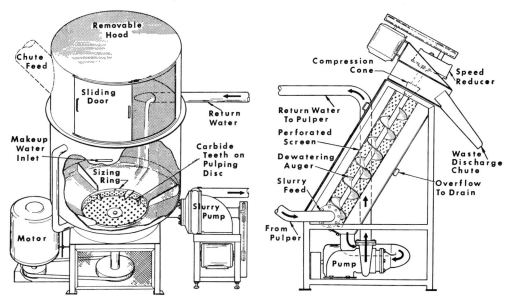

FIGURE 15-5A. (*left*) A Wascon pulping unit, part of a waste disposal system.
FIGURE 15-5B. (*right*) Water press.

latent heat of hospital waste from an average of 3500 BTU per pound in 1960 to a current level of 9000 BTU per pound. The problem of greater volumes of waste and higher latent heat is being further compounded by incinerators of inadequate capacity, grates burning out, and refractory linings spalling (chipping) due to unacceptably high waste latent heat. Overloaded incinerators produce smoke and fly ash in excess of the present stringent ordinances. Unfortunately the latent-heat rise in hospital waste was not anticipated by many engineers, and it is difficult to comply with most low smoke emission regulations even when incinerators installed as recently as one or two years ago are used. The permissible density of smoke from an incinerator, as specified by most of these laws or ordinances, must not exceed a specified Ringlemann Smoke Chart number measured in a manner prescribed by the U. S. Department of Interior (Bureau of Mines) in its Information Circular 7718. Incinerators which can handle high latent heat waste and still comply with smoke abatement ordinances are currently in the research stage.

Some hospitals are facing the waste problem by the installation of compactor-type carts, fireproof trash chutes, and pulping systems. Waste pulpers have minimized waste management problems by reducing the bulk as much as 80 per cent. Since the effluent is usually buried and there are no smoke or incinerator problems, pulping is being extolled as the method of choice for waste handling.

One type of pulping system (Wascon®) functions as a complete, totally closed loop after feed in, operates automatically, and deposits the end products into waste containers. This pulping system is designed to accept virtually any kind of waste, and specifically, such materials as paper, corrugated cartons, plastic items, flasks, glass bottles, rags, leather, plastics, aerosol cans, food waste, milk cartons, and disposable dinnerware. The machine consists of a pulper and water press as shown in Figure 15-5A and 15-5B. Upon pressing a button to activate the unit, the receiving tank is filled with water to a predetermined level. The proper water level is then automatically maintained during operation. The pulping disc, studded with carbide teeth rotates at 3000 rpm creating a vortex to draw the waste down into the water where it is abraded and converted to a slurry. Metal and other hard objects are mutilated, reduced in volume and ejected into an integral trash box where they can be easily removed. The slurry composed of two per cent solids and 98 per cent water is pumped through a perforated sizing ring and transported in closed piping to the water press. The slurry is then conveyed upward in the press by a dewatering auger which forces the water through a perforated screen to be pumped back to the pulper for reuse. The remaining semidry pulp, reduced to 20 percent of its original volume, is discharged into a waste container.

Two main applications of this system in hospitals are the handling of general waste and the handling of waste produced in dietary departments. Pulpers may, however, be placed anywhere in the hospital where waste is generated or accumulated. The general-waste system is used to handle waste from patient care units, store rooms, central service, pharmacy, offices, and other service areas of the hospital. The units may be floor mounted or pit mounted and fed in a variety of ways. Floor-mounted pulpers can be fed by hand, conveyor, hopper dumper, or combined with a trash chute. When installed with a trash chute, waste can be confined in bags and dropped down the chute. As the bag enters the pulper, it passes a sensor which starts the unit. Pit-mounted pulpers will receive carted waste which is dumped into the unit at the floor level, waste raked in from the floor or from chutes.

For special applications where all material is channeled to one point for reprocessing or disposal, the pulper may be mounted under the counter in a Central Service Department receiving area or in a conveyor sorting unit. This kind of installation is shown in Figure 15-2. Where this type of system is used, trash is bagged at the point of use, transported to Central Service at a predetermined time, and dropped in the pulper in the receiving section of the department. After the waste is broken down in the pulper, the slurry is conveyed to a water press located at a near or distant point where the semidry pulp is discharged into waste collection containers or hoppers for removal to a land fill.

Determining Sterilizer Requirements

The kind and number of sterilizers required for a Central Service Department should be determined on the basis of actual productivity needs. It is no longer practical to render a decision on sterilizer requirements based solely on chamber size. A more accurate method, utilizing the concept of unit productivity, has been developed to assist in determining the number, size, and type of sterilizers necessary to process the sterile-supplies quota for any hospital under actual work conditions. Five basic factors must be taken into consideration:

· Cubic capacity of each sterilizer.
· Average output productivity per processing hour, based on full practical loads.
· Methods of loading and accessory equipment.
· Characteristics of each type of sterilizer, including method of air removal, heat-up time, drying efficiency and the average cycle time for each type of load.
· Hours per day that each sterilizer will be used; ratio of processing time to "down" time.

There are many variables which influence the ratio of processing time to "down" time. Among these are such essential time factors as door opening and closing (manual and power operation times are identical), loading and unloading time, personnel efficiency, and flow patterns of both clean and unclean supplies. The newer sterilizers operating under automatic control are so much faster than the conventional gravity displacement units that the Central Service bottleneck has shifted from the sterilizer to the loading or distribution areas.

The productivity concept provides a prototype of measure for the selection of sterilizers based on the output potential of each type of sterilizer in terms of the cubic feet of material processed per hour. This is illustrated graphically in Figure 15-6 for three types of sterilizers in three different sizes for each. The total chamber capacity is never fully utilized and therefore it becomes a theoretical figure. It does, however, provide the starting point from which rates of production per hour of full practical loads can be determined, with consideration for the loading car, shelf, and air space, and approved loading techniques.

The total chamber capacity is shown on the chart by *heavy diagonal bar lines.* The total productive capacity in cubic feet per hour (full loads) during continuous operation is represented by the *light diagonal bar lines.* The hourly productive capacity which can be expected under average conditions for each type and size of sterilizer is designated by the *heavy vertical bar lines.* This line represents the most realistic figure for personnel to use in determining the anticipated productivity of a new sterilizer.

Even though a sterilizer is potentially capable of sterilizing larger volumes of material per hour, recent surveys made in hospitals have demonstrated only the cubic feet of material shown on the chart by *heavy vertical bar lines* can be considered typical of actual situations. In order to use the chart (Fig. 15-6) effectively, one should first prepare an estimate of the cubic feet of material to be processed per hour or per day in the individual

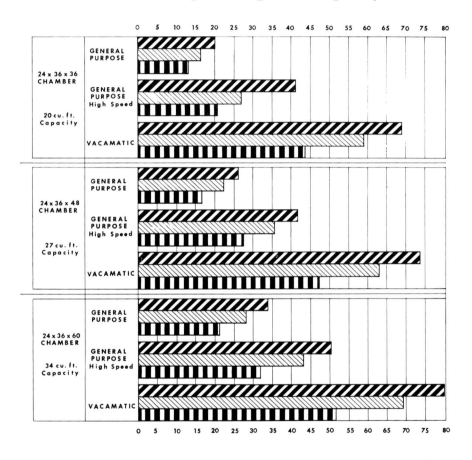

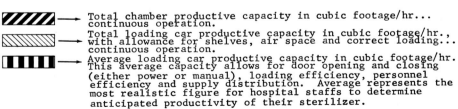

→ Total chamber productive capacity in cubic footage/hr... continuous operation.

→ Total loading car productive capacity in cubic footage/hr., with allowance for shelves, air space and correct loading... continuous operation.

→ Average loading car productive capacity in cubic footage/hr. This average capacity allows for door opening and closing (either power or manual), loading efficiency, personnel efficiency and supply distribution. Average represents the most realistic figure for hospital staffs to determine anticipated productivity of their sterilizer.

FIGURE 15-6. Sterilizer productivity chart.

hospital. With this information available, the output per cycle for each type of sterilizer can be computed as follows:

$$\frac{\text{productivity of sterilizer}}{60} \times \text{total cycle time} =$$

volume of material processed per cycle

The productive capacity of various sterilizers in units of hard goods, fabrics, and liquids and the corresponding total cycle times is given in Table 15-1.

ORGANIZATION AND ACTIVITIES OF THE DEPARTMENT

The primary requisites for good organization of the Central Service Department are a clear understanding of functions and well-defined responsibilities. Activity-wise, the greatest amount of time in Central Service operation is spent in the processing of supplies and apparatus used in patient care. The degree of centralization of processing will vary from hospital to hospital; however, there is a general trend toward more centralization in control and processing of material. The services to be provided by the department should be defined in writing and changed whenever the pattern of hospital operation changes.

Change in Concept of Processing Supplies

In many hospitals there is a pressing need for an upgrading in material-processing techniques in order to effectively combat environmental sepsis and to assist in the control and prevention of hospital-acquired infections. A composite chart, taking into consideration the many problems facing hospital personnel in attempting to select and standardize on reliable, high-quality techniques for processing of supplies, equipment, and furnishings needed for patient care, has been assembled. This chart, shown on pages 388 to 402, deals with the decontamination methods for a large variety of articles along with recommended methods for making articles safe for use on the next patient. The objectives of the processing methods are the following:

—To render contaminated articles safe for handling and subsequent reprocessing by employees.
—To prevent contamination of wounds through well defined pre-use and preoperative treatment of instruments and other articles so as to render them sterile.

It is the goal of the selected process methods to maintain the integrity of the aseptic barrier. All material and equipment should be confined in a protective wrapper or container immediately after its use on the patient has been discontinued. Recommended methods for sanitization, disinfection, or

TABLE 15-1

PRODUCTIVITY OF HOSPITAL STERILIZERS

STEAM-POWERED STERILIZERS

Chamber Size (Inches)	Type Load	Productive Capacity (Units) see note 1	TOTAL CYCLE TIME (MINUTES) see note 3								Vacamatic ® see note 2
			General Purpose		General Purpose High Speed		Laboratory		Laboratory/ Isothermal ®		
			250 F	270 F	250 F	270 F	250 F	270 F	250 F	270 F	
16x26	Hard goods	5	18-25	7-13			18-25	7-13	18-25	6-13	
	Fabrics	1	53-57				53-57				
	Liquids	10	62-71				62-71		56-63		
20x38	Hard goods	8	18-25				18-25		18-25		
	Fabrics	1	50-59				50-59				
	Liquids	16	72-86				72-86		68-76		
16x16x26	Hard goods	6	19-25	8-14	19-25	8-14	19-25	8-14	19-25	8-14	
	Fabrics	1	47-52			36-38	47-52				
	Liquids	15	69-78		69-78		69-78		62-70		
20x20x38	Hard goods	10	19-25	9-15	19-25	9-15	19-25	9-15	19-25	8-14	
	Fabrics	1	56-61			36-38	56-61				
	Liquids	32	86-100		86-100		86-100		80-88		
24x36x36	Hard goods	14	19-25	8-14	19-25	8-14	19-25	8-14	19-25	8-14	21-24
	Fabrics	6	49-55			40-42	49-55				18-22
	Liquids	120	80-95		80-95		80-95		68-76		75-85
24x36x48	Hard goods	16	21-27	9-15	21-27	9-15	21-27	9-15	21-27	9-15	22-26
	Fabrics	8	53-59			42-44	53-59				21-26
	Liquids	165	96-100		96-110		96-100		78-87		83-93
24x36x60	Hard goods	20	22-28	10-16	22-28	10-16	22-28	10-16	22-28	9-15	24-27
	Fabrics	10	56-62			44-46	56-62				25-27
	Liquids	210	112-123		112-123		112-123		87-98		92-100

Notes:

1. Includes allowances for shelves or other loading equipment, space for steam circulation and correct loading; figures shown are based on test loads as follows:
   Hard goods—unwrapped stainless steel utensils, adult bedpans.
   Fabrics—packages (each 12×12×20″) of muslin wrappers, surgical gowns, sheets, or similar linens.
   Liquids—one liter capped and collared borosilicate glass flasks each containing 1050 ml water.
2. Liquids processed with sterilizer operating on the gravity air removal principle at 250°F.
3. Cycle time is based on load at 70 to 76°F atmospheric pressure about 14.7 psia and steam to the sterilizer at 50 to 80 psig.

sterilization of equipment can then be followed to assist in the control of microbial populations within the hospital.

The articles listed on the chart have been categorized according to the intended application or usage. No attempt has been made to list every item used in the care of patients. The examples given comprise articles used most frequently, other articles commonly overlooked and, perhaps, processed inadequately, and finally those articles which by nature do not permit processing by conventional methods of sterilization. The methods shown on the chart include wash and sanitize, disinfect, wash and sterilize, and sterilize only. In order to decontaminate articles, they must be washed and sterilized, sterilized only, or, at least, disinfected before they can be considered safe for handling and before further preparation is undertaken prior to use by the next patient. No distinction in the processing of supplies is made, all articles and furnishings are considered potentially contaminated and therefore they require decontamination. *In using the Materiel Process Chart, the operator should follow the methods indicated in the column headings by reading from left to right to accomplish decontamination and preuse preparation.* In many instances more than one method must be employed. For some articles a choice of methods is indicated by "or" and selection of the process is dependent upon the mechanical equipment available in the hospital. The selection of alternate methods with lower orders of efficiency should not be permitted. Wherever possible, manual washing and sanitizing should be avoided because of the opportunity for release of microorganisms into the surrounding area by means of aerosols and the splashing of water. The preferred method is to wash and sanitize or wash and sterilize in closed mechanical equipment designed for specific application. Mechanical cleaning prevents the release of contaminants to the environment, including personnel, and it provides a controlled process largely free of the human element.

Manual disinfection means that the article is to be immersed in an effective germicide solution for a specific period of time, followed by careful cleaning to render the article safe for further processing and packaging prior to sterilization before reuse. Preliminary soaking is a necessary step in manual disinfection. If any scrubbing is necessary, the article, brush, and hands must be submerged. Manual cleaning and sanitization have been recommended only for those items which do not tolerate high temperature, or for other articles so constructed that they do not permit mechanical washing prior to sterilization.

Positive cleanliness is the primary criterion for articles which require packaging and sterilization prior to their use for treatment of patients. If there is an appreciable delay between the time of decontamination and final processing for reuse, the article should be rewashed before it is packaged for sterilization. Never assume that an article cleaned on some previous date is still clean.

After decontamination, some articles which are not required in a sterile state for patient use may be confined in wrappers or covered to protect them from dust and soil accumulated through handling or during storage. Many articles should be wrapped for the final sterilization step so that sterility will be preserved until the time of use. Some decontaminated articles will be included as part of a set or treatment tray, thereby eliminating the need to specify wrapping. The chart specifies the articles necessary to wrap following decontamination and subject to a resterilization cycle prior to release for use. Use of the chart requires careful attention to Sub-Note references at the end of the chart. These are included to clarify the recommendation of a process method or to caution the operator before implementation. The processing methods can normally be adapted to physical facilities in the individual hospital.

Linen Processing

Centralized linen processing affords many advantages to the hospital. From a personnel standpoint, a decrease in rehandling, transporting, and refolding of linen saves labor; workers become proficient and more productive because they are doing a repetitive task, and staff members in areas which require special packs such as operating suite, obstetrical suite, and nursery can be used for more technical duties. In a centralized linen processing facility, lint can be controlled, thereby decreasing the hazard of contamination and contributing to a better standard of sanitation in the clinical areas. There is better control of linen replacement, as all discarding is done in one place. The decision for mending or replacement is made in the central linen processing room. Through interdepartmental cooperation, pack content, folding methods, and content arrangement can be compared, dissimilarities reduced, and standardization with greater efficiency in the central linen room realized.

Physical facilities for linen processing should contribute to efficient work flow. A holding area should be provided in the room for linen to be inspected and handled for pack make up so that it is not subject to contamination in public corridors or thoroughfares. Self-leveling carts facilitate removal of linen from the carts and decrease awkward bending by the worker. If the activity is to be carried out in the Central Service Department, the area should be segregated or enclosed as a separate unit. Lint and dust are by-products of this operation and will settle on all horizontal surfaces in the department. This point must be remembered when transporting wrapped supplies to critical areas of the hospital. Such soil can be a vehicle for transmission of contamination. Because of the problems cited, many hospital administrators have classed this activity as a laundry function and provided facilities in the laundry for linen processing. In some parts of the country, linen for hospital use is laundered commercially on a contract basis. Some commercial laundries have undertaken the task of preparing linen packs and bundles according to the manner prescribed by the subscribing hospitals.

Linen used in special areas where observance and maintenance of aseptic technique is mandatory requires careful inspection and must be free of worn spots, tears, flaws, holes, or lint. The inspection process is made easier if a table illuminated from beneath is used, and combined with the sorting, folding, and delinting operations. Delinting can be done with a firm-bristle brush, adhesive tape, or commercially available delinting apparatus.

MATERIEL PROCESS CHART

To Render Safe for Employee Handling (Terminal Treatment or Decontamination to Prevent Cross Contamination)
to Render Safe for Next Patient (Pre-Use and Preoperative Treatment to Prevent Contamination)

Order of Processing is from Left to Right

ARTICLE	Wash & Sanitize — Manual: Hot Water & Detergent	Wash & Sanitize — Manual: Water & Detergent Germicide	Wash & Sanitize — Mechanical: Hot Water & Detergent	Disinfection — Manual: Chemical Solution	Wash & Sterilize — Mechanical: Water & Detergent & Steam @ 270°	Sterilize — Mechanical: Steam Autoclave	Sterilize — Mechanical: Ethylene Oxide Gas	Sterilize — Mechanical: Dry Heat Hot Air	Packaging: Wrap (15)	Packaging: Optional (16) Wrap	Packaging: Include With (17) Other Articles	Packaging: No Wrap — Does Not Apply (18)	Packaging: Protect (19)	Sterilize — Mechanical: Steam Autoclave	Sterilize — Mechanical: Ethylene Oxide Gas	Sterilize — Mechanical: Dry Heat Hot Air
A. Instruments and other articles used in body orifices, naso-pharynx, respiratory tract, in wounds, burn cases, and all surgical operations, septic or otherwise. Also articles used on patients in isolation. Anesthesia and inhalation therapy equipment.																
Examples:																
1. Instruments for examining purposes:																
ear specula, nasal specula, metal tongue depressor, laryngoscope blade, broncho-scope made of heat resistant metal, nylon (3)					X				X					X		
laryngoscope handle, light carriers, gastroscope, hypothermia thermometer and other items so constructed making them heat sensitive		X		X					X						X	
2. Dental instruments:																
heat resistant metal: e.g., extracting forceps, probes, suction tips, Carpule® holders					X					X				X		
heat sensitive : nylon or other (3)				X					X						X	
moisture sensitive: e.g., handpieces, drills, contra-angles (3) (4)	X					X	X	X	X					X	X	X

MATERIEL PROCESS CHART

To Render Safe for Employee Handling (Terminal Treatment or Decontamination to Prevent Cross Contamination)
to Render Safe for Next Patient (Pre-Use and Preoperative Treatment to Prevent Contamination)

Order of Processing is from Left to Right — ARTICLE	Wash & Sanitize — Manual — Hot Water & Detergent	Wash & Sanitize — Manual — Water & Detergent Germicide	Wash & Sanitize — Mechanical — Hot Water & Detergent	Disinfection — Manual — Chemical Solution	Wash & Sterilize — Mechanical — Water & Detergent & Steam@270°	Sterilize — Mechanical — Steam Autoclave	Sterilize — Mechanical — Ethylene Oxide Gas	Sterilize — Mechanical — Dry Heat Hot Air	Packaging — Wrap (15)	Packaging — Wrap Optional (16)	Packaging — Include With Other Articles (17)	Packaging — No Wrap — Does Not Apply (18)	Packaging — Protect (19)	Sterilize — Mechanical — Steam Autoclave	Sterilize — Mechanical — Ethylene Oxide Gas	Sterilize — Mechanical — Dry Heat Hot Air
3. Instruments used in operative procedures, delivery room procedures, treatment and diagnostic trays, emergency procedures or come in contact with any kind of wound:																
heat resistant — metal, nylon or plastic: e.g., fiber optic light carrier, general operating instruments, razors (3)					X				X					X		
heat sensitive — plastic, nylon: lensed instruments, resectoscopes, fiber optic light carriers (3)				X			X		X						X	
steam sensitive: knife blades, cataract knives, keratomes, iris scissors (3)				X			X	or — X	X						X	or — X
metal instruments with sliding parts which cannot be separated					X			X	X							X
4. Instruments used for post-mortem procedures. (10)					X	X			X					X		
5. Hollow needles to be used for any purpose throughout the hospital:																
subcutaneous, intravenous, spinal (11), and other needles with obturators (biopsy)					X				X	or	X			X	or — X	
diagnostic and therapeutic needles with nylon or plastic lead (3)				X			X		X	or	X				X	or — X

MATERIEL PROCESS CHART

To Render Safe for Employee Handling (Terminal Treatment or Decontamination to Prevent Cross Contamination)
to Render Safe for Next Patient (Pre-Use and Preoperative Treatment to Prevent Contamination)

Order of Processing is from Left to Right — ARTICLE	Wash & Sanitize — Manual — Hot Water & Detergent	Wash & Sanitize — Manual — Water & Detergent Germicide	Wash & Sanitize — Mechanical — Hot Water & Detergent	Disinfection — Manual — Chemical Solution	Wash & Sterilize — Mechanical — Water & Detergent & Steam @ 270°	Sterilize — Mechanical — Steam Autoclave	Sterilize — Mechanical — Ethylene Oxide Gas	Sterilize — Mechanical — Dry Heat Hot Air	Packaging — Wrap (15)	Packaging — Optional (16)	Packaging — Include With Other Articles (17)	Packaging — No Wrap / Does Not Apply (18)	Packaging — Protect (19)	Sterilize — Mechanical — Steam Autoclave	Sterilize — Mechanical — Ethylene Oxide Gas	Sterilize — Mechanical — Dry Heat Hot Air
6. Suture needles.					X				X	or	X			X _ or		X
7. Utensils used for general and special procedures: operating rooms, delivery rooms, emergency room, patient care units or other clinical areas.																
metal			X		X				X					X		
reusable plastic (3)							X		X						X	
8. Utensils used for diagnostic and therapeutic procedures, newborn and premature care, preparation of infant formulas: e.g., foot soak kettle, paracentesis bucket, nursery bath basin, suction irrigating container, pitcher for mixing formulas.					X				X					X		
9. Glass syringes used for any purpose in the hospital.				X	X				X	or	X			X _ or		X
10. Glass and rubber syringes: e.g., asepto, Ellik Evacuator.					X	X			X					X		
11. Special syringes:																
glass with metal piston				X	X		X _ or	X	X					X _ or	X	
glass with fiber piston					X				X	or				X		X

MATERIEL PROCESS CHART

To Render Safe for Employee Handling (Terminal Treatment or Decontamination to Prevent Cross Contamination) to Render Safe for Next Patient (Pre-Use and Preoperative Treatment to Prevent Contamination)

Order of Processing is from Left to Right

ARTICLE	Wash & Sanitize — Manual: Hot Water & Detergent	Wash & Sanitize — Manual: Water & Detergent Germicide	Wash & Sanitize — Mechanical: Hot Water & Detergent	Disinfection — Manual: Chemical Solution	Wash & Sterilize — Mechanical: Water & Detergent & Steam @ 270°	Sterilize: Steam Autoclave	Sterilize: Ethylene Oxide Gas	Sterilize: Dry Heat Hot Air	Packaging: Wrap (15)	Packaging: Wrap Optional (16)	Packaging: Include With (17) Other Articles	Packaging: No Wrap — Does Not Apply (18)	Packaging: Protect (19)	Sterilize: Steam Autoclave	Sterilize: Ethylene Oxide Gas	Sterilize: Dry Heat Hot Air
12. Syringe (autoclavable plastic). (3)					X				X	or	X			X		
13. Formula bottles.					X					X				X.		
14. Bottle carriers.					X											
15. Nipples.			X			X							X	X		
16. Nipple guards (paper).								destroy	**X**					**X**		
17. Infant formula. (12)						X destroy		destroy						X		
18. Catheters, drains, flask collars, flask caps, tubing, ear bulbs, ureteral catheters, filiform catheters and followers, cardiac catheters and the like: (3) — heat resistant: plastic, rubber, nylon				X	X or	X			X or		X			X		
18. — heat sensitive: plastic, woven fiber				X			X		X or		X				X	
19. Rubber sheeting, drapes, bed protectors.			X		X or	X			X					X		
20. Gloves (re-usable).			X	X or	X	X			X					X or	X	
21. Ampoules — spinal drugs (outside surface). (3)	X														X	
22. Anesthesia induction equipment and accessories:																

MATERIEL PROCESS CHART

To Render Safe for Employee Handling (Terminal Treatment or Decontamination to Prevent Cross Contamination)
to Render Safe for Next Patient (Pre-Use and Preoperative Treatment to Prevent Contamination)

ARTICLE (Order of Processing is from Left to Right)	Wash & Sanitize — Manual: Hot Water & Detergent	Wash & Sanitize — Manual: Water & Detergent Germicide	Wash & Sanitize — Mechanical: Hot Water & Detergent	Disinfection — Manual: Chemical Solution	Wash & Sterilize — Mechanical: Water & Detergent & Steam@270°	Sterilize — Mechanical: Steam Autoclave	Sterilize — Mechanical: Ethylene Oxide Gas	Sterilize — Mechanical: Dry Heat Hot Air	Packaging: Wrap (15)	Packaging: Optional Wrap (16)	Packaging: Include With Other Articles (17)	Packaging: No Wrap — Does Not Apply (18)	Packaging: Protect (19)	Sterilize — Mechanical: Steam Autoclave	Sterilize — Mechanical: Ethylene Oxide Gas	Sterilize — Mechanical: Dry Heat Hot Air
endotracheal tubes, breathing bags, airways, nasal catheters, laryngoscopes, suction tips, ether masks, spirometer reservoir, and the like — heat resistant					X				X					X		
heat sensitive				X			X		X						X	
23. Bottles, jars, flasks.					X				X		X	or X		X		
24. Glass connectors.				or	X				X		or X			X		
25. Manual breast pump.					X		X		X					X		
26. Electric hair clippers.					X				X					X		
27. Dishes, glass drinking tubes, medicine glasses. (3)					X								X			
28. Carafes: (2) — metal					X				X		or		X			
glass					X				X		or		X			
plastic (3)			X	or					X		or		X			
29. Hand scrub brushes.					X				X					X		
30. Nail files.					X				X					X		
31. Bath tubs, Sitz baths: — fixed or portable (3)		X											X			
32. Tops of suction bottles with floating cutoff valves. (3)					X								X			

MATERIEL PROCESS CHART

To Render Safe for Employee Handling (Terminal Treatment or Decontamination to Prevent Cross Contamination)
to Render Safe for Next Patient (Pre-Use and Preoperative Treatment to Prevent Contamination)

Order of Processing is from Left to Right — ARTICLE	Wash & Sanitize · Manual · Hot Water & Detergent	Wash & Sanitize · Manual · Water & Detergent Germicide	Wash & Sanitize · Mechanical · Hot Water & Detergent	Disinfection · Manual · Chemical Solution	Wash & Sterilize · Mechanical · Water & Detergent & Steam@270°	Sterilize · Mechanical · Steam Autoclave	Sterilize · Mechanical · Ethylene Oxide Gas	Sterilize · Mechanical · Dry Heat Hot Air	Packaging · Wrap (15)	Packaging · Optional Wrap (16)	Packaging · Include With Other Articles (17)	Packaging · No Wrap—Does Not Apply (18)	Packaging · Protect (19)	Sterilize · Mechanical · Steam Autoclave	Sterilize · Mechanical · Ethylene Oxide Gas	Sterilize · Mechanical · Dry Heat Hot Air
33. Electric drills, saws used in surgery. (3)		X				X – or	X		X					X – or	X	
34. Decubitus pad (autoclavable Polyester® pile) (5) (13)			X Launder			X			X							
35. Decubitus pad (lambs wool pile). (5) (14)			X Launder						X							
36. Canister (container for dressings). (1)					X									X		
B. Instruments and other articles used for examining purposes or care, which come in contact with body surfaces only:																
Examples:																
1. Diagnostic instruments such as:																
tuning fork, pelvimeter																
stethoscope, percussion hammer.		X								X						
2. Hot water bottles, ice caps, invalid cushions.			X				X			X						
3. Alternating pressure mattress, heating and cooling mattresses, heating pads.		X					X		X		or		X			
4. Anesthesia examining equipment:																
stethoscopes, sphygmomanometer			X				X			X			X			

MATERIEL PROCESS CHART

To Render Safe for Employee Handling (Terminal Treatment or Decontamination to Prevent Cross Contamination)
to Render Safe for Next Patient (Pre-Use and Preoperative Treatment to Prevent Contamination)

Order of Processing is from Left to Right — ARTICLE	Wash & Sanitize — Manual — Hot Water & Detergent	Wash & Sanitize — Manual — Water & Detergent Germicide	Wash & Sanitize — Mechanical — Hot Water & Detergent	Disinfection — Manual — Chemical Solution	Wash & Sterilize — Mechanical — Water & Detergent & Steam@270°	Sterilize — Mechanical — Steam Autoclave	Sterilize — Mechanical — Ethylene Oxide Gas	Sterilize — Mechanical — Dry Heat Hot Air	Packaging — Wrap (15)	Packaging — Optional (16)	Packaging — Include With (17) Other Articles	Packaging — No Wrap — Does Not Apply (18)	Packaging — Protect (19)	Sterilize — Mechanical — Steam Autoclave	Sterilize — Mechanical — Ethylene Oxide Gas	Sterilize — Mechanical — Dry Heat Hot Air
blood pressure cuff (bandage type) (5) (6)			X Launder										X			
5. Plastic arm boards.																
6. Goggles.		X		X			X			X						
C. Utensils and other articles used in routine and daily care of patients; also terminal treatment.																
1. Bedpans, urinals. (2)																
Daily Care:																
metal			X	or	X											
reusable plastic, nylon (3)			X	or	X											
Terminal Care:																
metal					X				X					X		
reusable plastic, nylon (3)					X				X						X	
2. Patient utensils such as wash basins, emesis basins, soap dishes.																
Daily Care:																
metal			X	or	X											
reusable plastic, nylon (3)			X	or	X											
Terminal Care:																
metal					X									X		

MATERIEL PROCESS CHART

To Render Safe for Employee Handling (Terminal Treatment or Decontamination to Prevent Cross Contamination)
to Render Safe for Next Patient (Pre-Use and Preoperative Treatment to Prevent Contamination)

Order of Processing is from Left to Right → ARTICLE	Wash & Sanitize — Manual: Hot Water & Detergent	Wash & Sanitize — Manual: Water & Detergent Germicide	Wash & Sanitize — Mechanical: Hot Water & Detergent	Disinfection — Manual: Chemical Solution	Wash & Sterilize — Mechanical: Water & Detergent & Steam @ 270°	Sterilize — Mechanical: Steam Autoclave	Sterilize — Mechanical: Ethylene Oxide Gas	Sterilize — Mechanical: Dry Heat Hot Air	Packaging: Wrap (15)	Packaging: Wrap Optional (16)	Packaging: Include With Other Articles (17)	Packaging: No Wrap — Does Not Apply (18)	Packaging: Protect (19)	Sterilize — Mechanical: Steam Autoclave	Sterilize — Mechanical: Ethylene Oxide Gas	Sterilize — Mechanical: Dry Heat Hot Air
reusable plastic, nylon (3)					X				X					X		
3. Thermometers. (2)				X			X			X	or		X			
4. Thermometer holders, containers, trays and the like:																
heat sensitive plastic (2) (3)			X		X		X				or	X				
heat resistant metal or nylon		X			X						or	X				
D. Bedding and linen:																
1. Mattresses. (3)		X					X		X		or		X			
2. Mattresses and pillows covered with plastic or rubber. (3)							X		X		or		X		X	
3. Blankets:																
cotton (5)			X Launder						X					X		
wool (3)			X Launder						X						X	
4. Pillows:																
feather (5)			X Launder						X						X	
fiber (acrylic) (5)			X Launder						X							
foam rubber (5)			X Launder				X		X							
5. Linens used for patient care. (5)			X Launder						X		or		X	X		

MATERIEL PROCESS CHART

To Render Safe for Employee Handling (Terminal Treatment or Decontamination to Prevent Cross Contamination) to Render Safe for Next Patient (Pre-Use and Preoperative Treatment to Prevent Contamination)

ARTICLE (Order of Processing is from Left to Right)	Wash & Sanitize — Manual: Hot Water & Detergent	Manual: Water & Detergent Germicide	Mechanical: Hot Water & Detergent	Disinfection — Manual: Chemical Solution	Wash & Sterilize — Mechanical: Water & Detergent & Steam@270°	Sterilize — Mechanical: Steam Autoclave	Mechanical: Ethylene Oxide Gas	Mechanical: Dry Heat Hot Air	Packaging: Wrap (15)	Wrap Optional (16)	Include With Other Articles (17)	No Wrap — Does Not Apply (18)	Protect (19)	Sterilize — Mechanical: Steam Autoclave	Mechanical: Ethylene Oxide Gas	Mechanical: Dry Heat Hot Air
6. Linens used for special procedures in operating room, delivery room, emergency room and patient care units. (5) (6) (9)			X Launder						X					X		
7. Linens used for isolation patients. (5) (6) (9)			X Launder							X	or		X			
8. Linens used in care of infants; for therapeutic procedures; for formula preparation. (5) (9)			X Launder						X					X		
9. Linens used for burn patients and other special situations (kidney transplant, germfree environment). (5) (6) (9)			X Launder						X					X		
E. Infant furniture; therapeutic and diagnostic apparatus; orthopedic and fracture apparatus.																
1. Bassinets: basket metal					X				X					X		
plastic (3)			X				X		X						X	
frame			X													
2. Incubators: heat and moisture sensitive parts:									X		or		X		X	
plastic hoods, nebulizers, gauges, cabinets and the like (3)		X							X		or		X		X	

MATERIEL PROCESS CHART

To Render Safe for Employee Handling (Terminal Treatment or Decontamination to Prevent Cross Contamination)
to Render Safe for Next Patient (Pre-Use and Preoperative Treatment to Prevent Contamination)

Order of Processing is from Left to Right

ARTICLE	Wash & Sanitize · Manual · Hot Water & Detergent	Wash & Sanitize · Manual · Water & Detergent Germicide	Wash & Sanitize · Mechanical · Hot Water & Detergent	Disinfection · Manual · Chemical Solution	Wash & Sterilize · Mechanical · Water & Detergent & Steam@270°	Sterilize · Steam Autoclave	Sterilize · Ethylene Oxide Gas	Sterilize · Dry Heat Hot Air	Packaging · Wrap (15)	Packaging · Wrap Optional (16)	Packaging · Include With Other Articles (17)	Packaging · No Wrap — Does Not Apply (18)	Packaging · Protect (19)	Sterilize · Steam Autoclave	Sterilize · Ethylene Oxide Gas	Sterilize · Dry Heat Hot Air
heat and moisture resistant parts:																
i. e., water jars, mattress trays, filters and the like (3)					X				X					X		
3. Parts of therapeutic and diagnostic apparatus which come in contact with patient or bedding:																
oxygen tent canopy, bed cradle, perineal light (3)		X					X				or		X			
4. Parts of apparatus which do not come in contact with body discharge or patient:																
cabinet for oxygen apparatus, suction pump, resuscitator, blood oxygenator, I.P.P.B., pacemaker, defibrillator (3)		X					X		X				X			
5. Parts of apparatus which come in contact with body discharge:																
suction bottles, tubes, tips and bottles, masks, mouth pieces, nasal catheters																
heat resistant				X	X – or	X			X							
heat sensitive				X			X		X							
6. Fracture equipment:																
metal bars, frames, trapeze, Bucks extension			X			X							X			

MATERIEL PROCESS CHART

To Render Safe for Employee Handling (Terminal Treatment or Decontamination to Prevent Cross Contamination) to Render Safe for Next Patient (Pre-Use and Preoperative Treatment to Prevent Contamination)

ARTICLE (Order of Processing is from Left to Right)	Wash & Sanitize — Manual — Hot Water & Detergent	Wash & Sanitize — Manual — Water & Detergent Germicide	Wash & Sanitize — Mechanical — Hot Water & Detergent	Disinfection — Manual — Chemical Solution	Wash & Sterilize — Mechanical — Water & Detergent & Steam@270°	Sterilize — Mechanical — Steam Autoclave	Sterilize — Mechanical — Ethylene Oxide Gas	Sterilize — Mechanical — Dry Heat Hot Air	Packaging — Wrap (15)	Packaging — Wrap Optional (16)	Packaging — Include With Other Articles (17)	Packaging — No Wrap — Does Not Apply (18)	Packaging — Protect (19)	Sterilize — Mechanical — Steam Autoclave	Sterilize — Mechanical — Ethylene Oxide Gas	Sterilize — Mechanical — Dry Heat Hot Air
7. Orthopedic hammocks, slings, belts.																
canvas (5) (6)			X Launder										X			
leather		X					X	or X	X							
8. Traction bow and splints, Thomas splints (plastic). (3)		X				X	or X						X			
9. Weights and weight holders:																
plastic covered weights			X				X						X			
holders for liquid weights			X				X						X			
metal weights					X — or — X								X			
10. Sandbags:																
canvas cover		X					X		X				X			
rubber cover		X					X		X				X			
plastic cover		X					X						X			
11. Foam cushions.																
12. Cast cutters (electric). (3)		X					X	destroy								
13. Rope (sash cord for traction).		X					X									
14. Anesthesia gas machine; positive pressure machine.																
15. Whirlpool bath.		X											X			

MATERIEL PROCESS CHART

To Render Safe for Employee Handling (Terminal Treatment or Decontamination to Prevent Cross Contamination) to Render Safe for Next Patient (Pre-Use and Preoperative Treatment to Prevent Contamination)

ARTICLE (Order of Processing is from Left to Right)	Wash & Sanitize — Manual — Hot Water & Detergent	Wash & Sanitize — Manual — Water & Detergent Germicide	Wash & Sanitize — Mechanical — Hot Water & Detergent	Disinfection — Manual — Chemical Solution	Wash & Sterilize — Mechanical — Water & Detergent & Steam@270°	Sterilize — Mechanical — Steam Autoclave	Sterilize — Mechanical — Ethylene Oxide Gas	Sterilize — Mechanical — Dry Heat Hot Air	Packaging — Wrap (15)	Packaging — Wrap Optional (16)	Packaging — Include With Other Articles (17)	Packaging — No Wrap — Does Not Apply (18)	Packaging — Protect (19)	Sterilize — Mechanical — Steam Autoclave	Sterilize — Mechanical — Ethylene Oxide Gas	Sterilize — Mechanical — Dry Heat Hot Air
F. General equipment entering into one or more aspects of patient care and which may contribute to environmental sepsis:																
1. Beds, bed rails, bedside stands, dressers, clothing lockers. (7) (8)		X														
2. Wheelchairs, stretchers, walkers, portable utility carts (special attention to treads, wheels, tires).			X										X			
3. Orthopedic frames, traction and the like. (3) (7) (8)		X											X	X		
4. Operating tables, delivery tables and accessories. (7) (8) (10)		X														
5. Food service carts; supply distribution carts. (3)			X													
6. Mayo stands, ring stands, setup tables and other furniture in operating room and delivery room. (7) (8)		X														
7. Lavatories, commodes, clinical sinks.		X														
8. Flashlights.		X							X				X	X	X	
9. Cellulose padding (sheet wadding, combine padding).																

MATERIEL PROCESS CHART

To Render Safe for Employee Handling (Terminal Treatment or Decontamination to Prevent Cross Contamination)
to Render Safe for Next Patient (Pre-Use and Preoperative Treatment to Prevent Contamination)

ARTICLE (Order of Processing is from Left to Right)	Wash & Sanitize — Manual: Hot Water & Detergent	Wash & Sanitize — Manual: Water & Detergent Germicide	Wash & Sanitize — Mechanical: Hot Water & Detergent	Disinfection — Manual: Chemical Solution	Wash & Sterilize — Mechanical: Water & Detergent & Steam @ 270°	Sterilize — Mechanical: Steam Autoclave	Sterilize — Mechanical: Ethylene Oxide Gas	Sterilize — Mechanical: Dry Heat Hot Air	Packaging: Wrap (15)	Packaging: Wrap Optional (16)	Packaging: Include With Other Articles (17)	Packaging: No Wrap — Does Not Apply (18)	Packaging: Protect (19)	Sterilize — Mechanical: Steam Autoclave	Sterilize — Mechanical: Ethylene Oxide Gas	Sterilize — Mechanical: Dry Heat Hot Air
10. Scales:																
nursery		X					X						X			
adult		X														
cart		X														
11. Shades; Venetian blinds.		X														
12. Books.							X									
13. Motors or pumps which do not come in contact with body surfaces. (3)		X					X			X			or X			
14. Toys. (3)		X	or X				X									
15. Lamps. (3)		X					X									
16. Soap dispensers: operating suite, delivery suite and throughout hospital. (3)		X parts	X parts			X parts										
17. Mops. (5) (6)			X launder			X										
18. Wood; cork; wooden bedboards.		X					X	or X		X			or X			
19. Plastic covered bedboards.		X					X			X			or X			
20. Telephone.		X		or X			X									
21. Room radiators.		X					X									
22. Patient's clothing, shoes.							X									

MATERIEL PROCESS CHART

To Render Safe for Employee Handling (Terminal Treatment or Decontamination to Prevent Cross Contamination)
to Render Safe for Next Patient (Pre-Use and Preoperative Treatment to Prevent Contamination)

Order of Processing is from Left to Right

ARTICLE	Wash & Sanitize — Manual: Hot Water & Detergent	Wash & Sanitize — Manual: Water & Detergent Germicide	Wash & Sanitize — Mechanical: Hot Water & Detergent	Disinfection — Manual: Chemical Solution	Wash & Sterilize — Mechanical: Water & Detergent & Steam @ 270°	Sterilize — Mechanical: Steam Autoclave	Sterilize — Mechanical: Ethylene Oxide Gas	Sterilize — Mechanical: Dry Heat Hot Air	Packaging: Wrap (15)	Packaging: Wrap Optional (16)	Packaging: Include With Other Articles (17)	Packaging: No Wrap — Does Not Apply (18)	Packaging: Protect (19)	Sterilize — Mechanical: Steam Autoclave	Sterilize — Mechanical: Ethylene Oxide Gas	Sterilize — Mechanical: Dry Heat Hot Air
23. Intravenous standards.		X														
24. Drapes (window). (5)			X Launder or Dry Clean				X						X			
25. Wet vacuum, other floor cleaning apparatus. (7) (8)		X														
26. Refuse or garbage containers: plastic, metal			X	— or —	X											
27. Floor or kick buckets in operating room and delivery room (waste container). (7) (8)					X											
28. Money (paper).							X									
29. Floors.			X Scrubber													
30. Lights: delivery or operating		X														
31. Laboratory cultures for discard.						X						X				

SUB-NOTE REFERENCES:

1. Use not recommended.
2. Articles used daily by the patient during his hospital stay should be sanitized after each use. This represents minimum treatment in concurrent care.
3. Certain products are heat-sensitive and do not tolerate temperatures as high as 250° - 270° F. The manufacturers recommendations should be checked before processing.
4. These instruments can be autoclaved if treated with an oil-in-water emulsion beforehand.
5. Designates laundry procedure — classified as a sanitization process.
6. Contaminated linen requires special handling in the laundry. Consult the Manual on Laundry Practice, American Hospital Association.
7. Wheels and treads on wheelchairs, stretchers, other vehicles and furniture are commonly neglected. They require special attention.
8. A mechanical washer incorporating a flowing steam facility may be used to wash and sanitize refuse containers, some types of wheeled equipment and furniture.
9. Where the need exists to decontaminate linen prior to laundering, as in isolation or for the control of communicable disease, ethylene oxide gas sterilization is recommended.
10. If used to remove tissue or bone grafts, instruments require sterilization after decontamination.
11. A new spinal needle is recommended for each use.
12. Approved methods for terminal heating of infant formulas employ a time-temperature relationship of either 212° F. for 30 minutes or 230° F. for 10 minutes.
13. Requires exposure in steam autocalve after laundering to complete decontamination.
14. Gas sterilization not generally recommended as procedure shortens life of product.
15. Wrap — Enclose and secure in a protective cover. If article is to be sterilized after wrapping, a wrapper suitable for the sterilizing process should be used.
16. Wrap optional — The operator must determine whether the article requires wrapping.
17. Include with other articles — Usually pertains to articles which may be part of an instrument set, treatment tray or piece of apparatus.
18. No wrap — Specific protection after decontamination not required. Article in most instances is returned to patient unit for storage.
19. Protect — Cover article or apparatus with fabric or plastic sheet or bag; store in clean drawer or closed cupboard.

Defective linen should be marked and placed into a receptacle for transfer to the mending or patching station. Heat-pressure patching for linen repair is rapid and preferable to mending by sewing as the many needle holes created by the sewing machine become portals for contamination.

There are many different articles of linen with varied dimensions to be handled in the pack room. A table having minimum dimensions of 30 × 72 inches will facilitate folding of large drapes used in surgical packs as well as provide work stations for several persons for the wrapping of small items. Three kinds of holding facilities have proven to be satisfactory to receive inspected, folded linen and to make the linen readily accessible for pack assembly: 1) portable cart with approximate dimensions of 52 × 52 × 18 inches, 2) wall-mounted shelves, and 3) pass-through shelves. Folded linens should be located on the shelves in sequence of use for pack assembly.

A portable cart with top surface of 24 × 44 inches can be used efficiently as a work base for pack make up when any of the aforementioned holding facilities are used for inspected linens, and especially helpful when fixed or pass-through shelves are part of the pack room. The worker merely pushes the cart by the shelf units, removes pack contents, and assembles the pack. When a work table is used for pack make up, portable shelf units of folded linen are desirable. The filled portable cart is moved to one corner of the narrow end of the work table, and an empty cart is placed on the opposite corner of the table. The linen is removed from storage shelves, placed on work table, assembled into unit or pack, then placed on the empty receiving cart. Other pack contents and securing material should be available at the work area on either shelves or work table.

Assembled linen packs may be placed directly on portable shelved carts, floating bottom or self-leveling carts, sterilizer loading cars, or sterilizer baskets for transfer to the sterilizers. Space should be available in the pack room for holding carts filled with assembled linen packs. Storage facilities for reserve linen items and other pack contents such as cotton balls, applicators, radiopaque sponges, and 4 × 4 inches and 4 × 8 inches sponges should be provided.

A writing facility should be available in the pack room. Drawer storage should be available beneath the writing surface to hold requisition forms, records, guide cards. A bulletin board for posting of memos, time sheets, and assignments is helpful. Blackboard and chalk should not be used. An intercom unit connected to the laundry supply room or other areas in Central Service will save time communicating needs or events. Sitting stools with height adjustments are recommended for personnel as some wrapping activities can take place while they are seated. A lavatory for hand washing is conducive to good hygiene. A small vacuum cleaner equipped with attachments for shelf, wall, and floor cleaning will help decrease lint buildup and maintain a good standard of cleanliness in the room.

Preparation of Treatment Trays

A good treatment tray must have the following characteristics:

—The proper equipment so that the procedure may be performed according to a predetermined technique.

—Contents arranged so that there will be minimal handling to insure convenience and safety at time of use.

—Correct packaging and handling for sterilization and storage to achieve and maintain sterility.

The preparation of treatment trays follows the same general pattern as the processing of other materials. Collection, cleaning and decontamination, reassembly, wrapping, sterilizing, storage, and redistribution for use takes place. A prescribed routine for handling of trays after use should be made known to personnel in order to prevent dissemination of contamination into the environment and loss of articles to be reprocessed. The routine should describe the manner of handling waste and disposable articles, precleaning, if any, packaging of tray contents to confine soil (this is a commonly neglected practice), and location of tray in the utility room for reclaiming by Central Service. If decontamination will take place at point of use, personnel must be competent to carry out the procedure.

Since treatment trays are comprised of a variety of items, different cleaning methods are required. Therefore, upon return to central processing, sorting of articles according to type takes place. If decontamination will take place in Central Service, procedures necessary to accomplish this for the varied articles must be ahdered to. The Materiel Process Chart, starting on page 388, is recommended for this purpose and it can be adapted to various arrangements of physical facilities. Following cleaning and decontamination, assembling and wrapping of trays of a kind or those having similar contents can be done at one work station. A work place arranged so that assembly of trays takes place with little effort and unnecessary movement on the part of the worker, increases productivity. This means availability of tray contents, wrappers, securing tape, labels, and a place to put assembled trays for sterilization.

In order to provide optimum conditions for sterilization of treatment trays, certain guide lines in the selection of contents and processing need to be observed. A shallow-base tray should be used, as it is lighter to handle and less likely to trap air. Articles should be arranged on the tray so there is minimal need for handling or rearrangement at time of use. Items which can trap air or hold water must be placed on the tray in a manner to avoid such occurrence when the tray is placed on edge in the sterilizer.

Central Service personnel have found through experience that certain economics can be realized if some disposable articles are used in the treatment tray. Unwaxed paper cups, aluminum foil bowls, fiber towels, prepackaged scalpel blades, lubricants, soaps, and disinfectants are a few examples. The presterilized, prepackaged items should be checked for sterilizing temperature tolerance before they are selected for use in this manner.

Whenever possible, the contents of the trays should be cross-indexed and those with similar contents be studied and redesigned so that the variety will be decreased and still meet the needs of the various procedures. Trays must be positioned in the autoclave on edge without interference from other packs or supplies. Tray assembly will take place more efficiently and accurately if a file of guide cards (5 × 8 inches in size) with list of contents, pertinent processing notes, and photograph of arrangement is available. A reference set of such cards assembled by the Hospital Medical Facilities Branch of the United States Public Health Service is available from the Government Printing Office.[21]

Control of Supplies

Standard quantity dispensing

Standard quantity supply dispensing means that a predetermined quantity of supplies are provided for a patient care unit or department. This quantity should be adequate for patient care needs for a specific period of time. After the designated time period has elapsed, the remaining quantity is checked and the used items replaced to bring the supplies available to the original standard. There are several ways standard quota dispensing may be accomplished.

PERSONNEL AND CART. A cart loaded with supplies is moved to each using unit by a worker from Central Service. The person monitoring the distribution cart replaces the used supplies in the respective storage facility and records the quantity left.

EXCHANGE CART. A cart containing a predetermined quantity of material usually sufficient for 24 hours is left on each using unit. Each day at a specified time, this cart is removed from the using unit and replaced by another cart, filled with supplies. The original cart is returned to Central Service for cleanup, rotation of supplies, and restocking. Authorities differ in opinion on two points of technique relative to handling unused supplies returned on an exchange cart: Should the supplies be reissued or go through a complete reprocessing because they have been exposed to a potentially contaminated environment during transit and storage out of Central Service? Should such supplies be taken into the sterile storage area of Central Service to be combined with new supplies?

STANDARD REQUISITION. A specific quantity of supplies is stored in the using unit. Once each day, or oftener if this is the policy, personnel in the using unit check the standard and then request supplies from Central Service to replenish stock. This method is most often used when an automated system which moves supply containers on a vertical conveyor is available or when dumb waiters and self-guided or electromechanically guided carts are in the hospital.

Demand Dispensing

All supplies are requested just prior to the time of use. Very few or no supplies are maintained on the using unit. This method is not used frequently, but, when it is employed, there is usually an automated vertical conveyor system available. If an automated vertical conveyor system is not used, there is considerable delay between request of item and arrival for use. This method causes considerable interruption in Central Service operation to fill the frequent requests and consumes personnel time on the using unit to order supplies.

Frequency of Dispensing

The frequency at which supplies should be dispensed is determined by hospital policy related to distribution of supplies and charge for materials, quantity of materials in circulation, amount of storage space in Central Service and using area, and kinds of materials used most frequently. Distribution schedules for supplies which are frequently used should be consolidated as much as possible and take place only once or twice each day. The dispensing of a great many items in small quantities consumes time and contributes to an unnecessary handling of supplies when taking the inventory. Effort should be made to decrease the time spent filling orders and delivering supplies. Some hospitals have found that it is advantageous to deliver or dispense the basic or standard list of supplies once or twice each week. Special supplies may be requested at time of need. Such practice is worthy of study for possible acceptance by more Central Service Departments.

Return of Supplies for Reprocessing

In situations where automated vertical transportation systems are available, these may be used to return material for reprocessing. Any vehicle or container used to collect or hold soiled supplies should not be used to dispense supplies unless subjected to decontamination first. Supplies may be returned for reprocessing in several ways.

ROUTINE COLLECTION. Person from Central Service is assigned to take a cart and collect soiled articles from using units and return them to Central Service.

RETURN AT WILL. Soiled supplies and apparatus are returned whenever convenient to personnel on the using unit or whenever a load accumulates. This method takes a considerable number of people away from the patient unit and contributes to hospital traffic.

RETURN AFTER USE. Soiled supplies or apparatus are returned to Central Service immediately following discontinuance of use. When this procedure is followed there is less chance for articles to become lost or misplaced, and soiled material is not likely to contribute to contamination of the environment.

EXCHANGE CART. A cart is placed in the utility room (soiled area) or other area specified for holding soiled material in each using unit and left there for a specific period of time (12 to 24 hours). After the predetermined time lapse the cart is transferred to Central Service and another clean cart is left in its place to receive soiled articles during the ensuing 24 hours.

The frequency at which supplies are returned for reprocessing is dependent upon the policy relative to keeping of soiled contaminated material on the using unit, amount of holding space available on the using unit and in receiving area of Central Service, inventory available for use, and whether or not an automated vertical transportation system is available. Generally, soiled articles should be returned two or three times in a 24-hour period following periods of peak use of supplies. Too frequent collection trips contribute to traffic through the hospital, and often times there is not enough material collected to make all the tours worthwhile.

Length of Time Supplies May Be Considered to Remain Sterile

The question of how long after sterilization may wrapped supplies be considered to remain sterile is frequently asked by Central Service supervisors. Answers have been given which range in time from one week to an indefinite period. Most people concerned with this problem do not appreciate that it is of dual significance to the hospital. First, there is the desire on the part of all to preserve the sterile state of processed articles for a maximum period of time. This can be done and within practical working limits of time. Sooner or later, however, a point is reached at which the contamination on the exterior of the package defies opening the wrapper at the risk of contaminating the contents and the immediate environment.

It is known that protection against contamination of sterile wrapped supplies is largely dependent upon the porosity of the wrapper and the method of wrapping. The most serious aspect of contamination is that due to insects and vermin (ants, roaches, silverfish), which may gain access to the interior of a package through the folds of the wrapper. In general, the storage areas for sterile supplies in hospitals can be depended upon to be free of insects and vermin. In the tropics, the problem of insect control may be difficult, and occasionally it has been found necessary to institute rather elaborate methods such as specially designed containers to protect supplies against contamination.

Aside from the problem of insect contamination, there is a possibility, however remote it may seem, of bacteria eventually penetrating the muslin or paper barrier. Just when this will occur or under what conditions is difficult to determine in hospital practice. Changes in atmospheric conditions surrounding the packages, handling the packages so as to force air in and out, are contributing factors to possible contamination. In the author's laboratory, studies have been made to determine how long syringes and needles will remain sterile when wrapped in muslin as compared to packaging in paper bags and then held in clean storage. The results indicated that bacterial contamination does not gain access to syringes or needles packaged in either muslin or paper bags for at least four weeks. Certainly, under normal conditions of clean storage, supplies properly wrapped in double thickness muslin, made up of four layers, can be depended upon to remain sterile for at least four weeks. This also applies to articles placed in plastic coverings without being hermetically sealed. There is no need to resterilize supplies at the end of one or even two weeks storage. Beyond this period, most articles will have been issued for use.

If there are a great number of supplies which have not been dispensed before this length of time, attempts should be made to reduce the need for resterilization. It may be possible to decrease the sterile inventory of the articles which have not been used. Articles which have a low turnover rate and are hermetically sealed in plastic wrappers or bags after sterilization should be marked with an expiration date. Under no conditions should any package be considered sterile in storage for longer than six months.

Why continue the controversy on the maximum period of time that the contents of a sterilized package will remain sterile? Everything has an expiration date, and here the evidence indicates that with each passing day the probability of contamination gaining access to, or invading the wrapping barrier becomes greater, either directly or indirectly. We have a far more serious problem when we face up to the fact that microbial contamination is released from the exterior of every package, when it is opened, to the surrounding area. This should be of vital concern to everyone who opens or unwraps the packages in the operating room or other critical areas.

Rotation of Supplies

A procedure for placing sterile supplies on storage shelves and a procedure for removing them should be established for every Central Service Department. Supply rotation is facilitated by the use of pass-through shelf storage units. It is also necessary that personnel on the patient care unit and in other supply-using departments be taught the patterns for removal and replacement of materials in the storage facilities.

A procedure for rotation of supplies is necessary to eliminate the wasteful practice of reprocessing articles which have become outdated before they are used, as well as to preclude the possibility of the use on a patient of an article which, due to unnecessary rehandling and exposure in the storage facility, may be no longer sterile. If standard quantity distribution is practiced, the rotation of supplies is done by Central Service personnel during the checking and restocking of the supply quota. If supply standards are monitored by a service manager[22] or supply clerk in the patient care unit, the rotation of supplies should be the responsibility of these persons.

There are several methods which can be used to assist in the rotation of supplies.

DATING. The use of an expiration date is recommended because it is easy to follow and personnel can associate the expiration date with the calendar date. This practice coincides with the expiration dates put on some medications by pharmaceutical companies and on some foods available in retail stores. The public is used to looking for expiration dates; therefore, this method can easily be followed by hospital personnel for rotation of supplies. Articles should be dated before sterilization as they are placed on the sterilizer loading car.

COLOR CODING. Another method which permits rapid identification of outdated supplies is color coding. Each package or article is marked with a color after sterilization. The colored mark may be a piece of tape which is commercially available or a mark from a wax pencil. The method works in the following manner: A chart is developed to designate the color coding on each package dispensed from Central Service for a specific period of time. For example, all processed supplies issued from Central Service can be marked with either red, blue, green, or yellow color. Each color is used for a one week period—the calendar dates noted on the color coding guide chart. As supplies marked with color are dispensed and those with the fourth color, yellow, appear, those having a mark with the first color, red, should be moved to the front of the storage shelf for immediate use or returned to Central Service for reprocessing. If packages are serially numbered, and dated with sterilization and expiration dates, the use of color coding is superfluous.

Sterilizer Load Identification

In order to maintain a positive record of the relationship of the sterilizer used and the specific operating cycle to the article sterilized, a means of load identification must be established. The method of load identification as related to the individual article should be similar to the product-lot control numbers used by pharmaceutical manufacturers. Conditions in the sterilizer during each operating cycle should be recorded on a chart which is a standard part of the sterilizing equipment. The number of the cycle should also be recorded on the chart. The charts are replaced and dated daily. They should be retained by the hospital for reference for at least two years. Each package and article subjected to the sterilization cycle should be marked prior to placement on the sterilizer loading car. For the record, essential information includes

sterilizer number, e.g.:	1
load number:	6
date sterilized:	7-13-68
expiration date:	8-13-68

The establishment of a lot control number for *all* packages and articles subjected to a sterilization cycle should become routine procedure in all hospitals. Maintenance of a written record of what transpired during each sterilization cycle is a part of the responsibility of those individuals who are charged with the preparation and sterilization of supplies.

Staffing the Department

Along with changes in the functions being performed by Central Service Departments there has been a change in philosophy about who should manage the department. The nurse supervisor in many hospitals has been replaced by persons of varied backgrounds and titles. Central Service Departments[23] are now being managed by industrial engineers, pharmacists, licensed practical nurses, purchasing agents, nurses, technicians, laundry managers, and personnel with special training received in the armed forces Medical Corps. Administration in each hospital must designate the comprehensiveness of operation desired by their Central Service Department and determine the level of educational preparation and experience required by the person engaged to manage the department. The person selected for the role must be familiar with administrative and supervisory duties, have knowledge related to technical processing procedures, basis for technics in supply use, problem-solving methods, work simplification, communication practices, and an awareness of the importance of continuing in-service education for the employees. Because we live in an era of rapid technological development, the supervisor must be aware of changes as they affect hospitals, must be flexible in accepting these changes, and must have a long-range perspective that harmonizes with the administration's objectives and plans for the overall improvement of the department and the hospital. The supervisor must be a good teacher, as the level of employee performance is largely dependent upon the quality of instruction received. When the Central Service Department is not managed by a nurse, it is beneficial to have a nurse advisor, a liaison person from the department of nursing service or an advisory committee which includes a nurse to promote interdepartmental cooperation. Attendance at institutes, seminars, hospital association meetings, expansive reading of hospital and related literature, along with visits to other Central Service Departments, will enhance the supervisor's knowledge and administrative ability. The role of manager in Central Service does not yet certify professional status to the individual, but there are persons engaged in a movement to make this a reality.[24]

No established guide exists to automatically determine the number of people required to operate a Central Service Department of any size. The number of workers employed in hospitals of various sizes has been reported in a study made by the Public Health Service—Division of Hospital Central Medical and Surgical Supply Services.[25] Each hospital must determine the number of workers necessary to furnish the services outlined. This will depend on several things:

- The degree of centralization for processing of materials and apparatus.
- Collection and distribution methods.
- Work schedules and number of hours the department is open to provide service.
- Number of disposable articles being used.
- Number and kinds of mechanical aides available for processing.
- Inventory of reprocessable material available in circulation in relation to need.

Even though the variables which affect manpower requirements are known, experience in worker utilization reveals that the actual number required can only be stated after a study of the time it takes the workers to carry out their assigned tasks.

In-Service Programs

A planned orientation program should be conducted to stimulate worker interest and enable him to do his tasks correctly and efficiently. An organized continuing in-service education program is necessary for several reasons:

- To provide information for all personnel and give them more insight into their role in the hospital organization.
- To convey pointers on how to improve work habits.
- To instruct the staff in use and care of new equipment.
- To acquaint them with changes in operation of the department.
- To introduce new concepts and trends in patient care which affect the functioning of the department.
- To prevent the "stagnant worker syndrome"—he arrived, was taught, released from supervision, and dismissed to carry on eternally.

The supervisor should present the worker with a clear guide to his individual work responsibilities. A designated time for carrying out each activity will eliminate piecemeal processing. Rotation of activity assignment will keep employees interested as they learn and become proficient in most activities. It is also advantageous to have the workers trained to carry out more than one assignement, as this will insure that someone will be able to perform any task when absences occur. Specific written procedures for carrying out each activity should be available for reference at the respective work stations. Wasteful practices, sloppy techniques, and employees whose productivity is below par will not permit the best designed and equipped department to be utilized effectively and economically.

Personnel Attire

All personnel assigned to Central Service should change into an outer uniform which is clean to the department and hospital, each day before reporting to the work area. Apparel change should take place in a locker room located nearby, preferably having direct access to the department and assigned exclusively for Central Service personnel. An easy to don wraparound dress is suggested for female workers and scrub-type suit for male workers. Head covering should be worn by all personnel and changed daily. A style which is comfortable, confines the hair, and made of a fabric which does not permit hair strands to protrude through it, is desirable. Careful visual inspection of material being processed to prevent the inclusion of foreign matter is a requirement of every worker even though head covering is worn.

When personnel leave the department for "breaks" or meals, a protective coat is worn over their uniform. A control system for receiving clean uniforms daily and replacing covering gowns needs to be established for each hospital. Personnel interchange between clean and contaminated areas should be discouraged.

Maintenance of the Physical Environment

Due to the nature of activities being carried on in the Central Service Department, the standard of cleanliness must be very high. Environmental conditions within the plant have a bearing on the type of housekeeping schedule required for the individual hospital. The cleaning schedule should be developed according to need and some housekeeping activities scheduled more frequently than in other hospital areas. A good housekeeping program is one of shared responsibility between Housekeeping and Central Service which follows a plan developed by both departmental supervisors. A detailed maintenance plan is especially important when housekeeping services are contracted to an outside agency. The plan should include routine daily cleaning, the kind of cleaning to be done at specific intervals and periodic project cleaning. Workers from the housekeeping department may be responsible for cleaning windows; complete and spot washing of walls; vacuuming and scrubbing of floors; maintenance of sterilizer access area; care of ventilation grilles, vents, and air conditioning baffles; exterior cleaning of water stills, light fixtures, and tops of cupboards; emptying linen hampers, and replacement of same.

Major cleaning is best accomplished when there is the least amount of activity in the department, such as during the night or evening hours. A housekeeping plan defining the responsibility of the Central Service Department could include the cleaning of insides of sterile and unsterile storage cupboards, drawers, open shelves, work counters, stations, and tables; the sanitizing of carts used to collect soiled material and distribute clean supplies, and the maintenance of mechanical washing apparatus. Mechanical cleaning units used in the department including floor scrubbers, wall cleaners, pickup vacuum require disassembly and sanitization regularly so that they will not become reservoirs and dispersers of bacteria. Only through the maintenance of high sanitation standards in the Central Service Department will all the efforts for cleaning, processing, and sterilizing of materials be worthwhile.

THE CHALLENGE FOR CENTRAL SERVICE

There is an increasing concern about the need to control microorganisms on objects used for patient care and throughout the hospital physical plant. This concern has directed more attention to potential sources of contamination throughout the hospital environment. Techniques of handling articles used for patient care or treatment, as well as those in the environment, are under constant surveillance. Centralized processing permits better control of work performance, and techniques can be upgraded. If centralized processing for decontamination is not provided for in today's hospital, where will items be decontaminated to make them safe for personnel handling and for use by the next patient? The unveiling of the reservoirs of contamination and their relationship to hospital acquired infections has brought about this change in the concept of materiel handling.

REFERENCES

1. "Preliminary Report of a Survey and Study of Surgical Dressings and Materials," Research and Information Dept. American College Surgeons, Oct. 1928.
2. UNDERWOOD, W. B.: Notes on the planning and organization of the central sterile supply. *Surgical Supervisor, 4,* 1944.
3. UNDERWOOD, W. B.: More about that central sterile supply. *Surgical Supervisor, 5,* 1945.
4. LONDON, J.: The future of central service. *JAHA, 39*:74-75, 1965.
5. DAVIS, E. L.: From central dressing room to central service department. *Hospital Topics, 43*:119, 120-122, 1965.
6. SR. MARIE CLAIRE, Personal Communications, July 1959, June 1965, Mar. 1967.
7. DEITZ, A. F., and JEFFREY, L. P.: Developing a comprehensive transportation service. *Hosp Manage, 101*:108-110, 1966.
8. FIERRELL, J. R., and O'CONNELL, J. A.: An established hospital converts to materials management. *Hosp Progr, 48*:56, 60, 62, 64, 67, 1967.
9. DAVIS, E. L.: Central service: a department in transition. *Hosp Topics, 43*:131-138, 1965.

10. Rosenberger, Donald M.: Changing Concepts of the Central Service Department. Paper presented at Instructional Conference, New England Hospital Assembly, 1965.
11. Central Sterilizing Club of the British Isles: Resume of the Sixth Meeting of the Club held at St. Bartholomews Hospital, London, 1964.
12. Murray, S.: New system for central supplies. *Lancet 1*:1207-1209, 1964.
13. Weymes, C.: Regional central sterile supply serves a group of hospitals. *Hosp Topics, 44*:139-142, 1966.
14. Nuffield Provincial Hospital Trust: *Central Sterile Supply, Principles and Practice.* London, Oxford U. P., 1963.
15. Weymes, C., Black, J. M., and Currie, E. R.: *Planning a Regional Central Sterile Supply Department, Western Regional Hospital Board and Glasgow Victoria Hospitals.* Glasgow, McCorquodale & Co., 1964.
16. Allen, S. M.: Central sterile supply. *Hospital Equipment News, 9*:18-20, 1963.
17. Schafer, M. K.: The nurse's role in architectural planning. *Nurs Outlook, 1*:141-143, 1953.
18. Craft, N. B.: Logistics and central service programming. *Hospitals, 39*:75-78, 80, 1965.
19. Unpublished Report, American Sterilizer Co., 1967.
20. Unpublished Report, American Sterilizer Co., 1966.
21. Superintendent of Documents, U. S. Government Printing Office, Washington, D. C. 20402: Treatment Trays and Sets Prepared in the Hospital Central Medical and Surgical Supply Services. 72 cards. Catalog No. FS 2.74-3: C-13 cards.
22. Brodt, D. E.: The service manager, innovation for nursing and health organization. *Hosp Progr, 47*:69, 70, 74, 1966.
23. Pendleton, R.: A changing role for central service. *Hospitals, 38*:75-78, 1964.
24. Letourneau, C. U.: Professionalism in central service. *Hosp. Progr, 47*:32-39, 1966.
25. U. S. Department of Public Health Service, Division of Hospital and Medical Facilities: *A Study of Hospital Medical and Surgical Supply Services.* PHS. Publication No. 930-C-10. Washington, D. C., U. S. Gov. Print. Office, 1965.

Chapter 16

PREPARATION OF STERILE SOLUTIONS

I N CLINICAL practice, sterile solutions or fluids as they are commonly known are employed for specific purposes. They are administered to the patient through the parenteral route, given orally, applied to the skin, and used to irrigate or bathe body tissues, organs, and deep cavity wounds. It is the purpose here to familiarize the reader with the basic fundamentals of preparing sterile solutions, particularly those solutions which are used for other than parenteral applications, together with the flasking technique and equipment for their preparation. Solutions normally referred to as external are customarily labeled as *irrigating solutions, topical solutions* and *surgical solutions* in hospitals. An external solution may be defined as any aqueous medium in which water serves as the solvent for one or more solutes (chemical compounds) used for applications on the skin in nursing care and for purposes of wound irrigation, including the moistening of sponges during surgical procedures.

OBJECTIVES FOR THE PREPARATION OF EXTERNAL SOLUTIONS

The objective of any planned program for the preparation of external solutions using the sterile-flask technique should be to provide a quality product which, when administered to the patient, is exactly as originally prepared. A philosophy of merely providing a preparation at a lower cost than that available from commercial sources is illogical. The deciding factors should be the upgrading of the present solution-preparation technique to produce at lower cost a solution which has been prepared with accuracy, stability and safety; and the assurance that each finished flask is not only sterile, but also chemically pure. In other words, external solutions should be prepared to the same standards, and be of the same high quality, as parenteral solutions. The premise is that any solution used to irrigate a deep wound or a cavity, or to bathe tissue, has the same physiological absorption characteristics as fluid administered by the parenteral routes.

Originally, solutions were prepared by a physician or the pharmacist. Today, the preparation of solutions has assumed the volume of mass production. The extensive use of sterile fluids suggests that the preparation be concentrated in one place. A hospital Central Service Department, because of its similarity to the production facilities of industry, is a logical place for the production of sterile external solutions. In many instances this activity is supervised by the pharmacist. The operative procedures can be easily and effectively controlled with an appreciable amount of economy, a high rate of efficiency, and maximum safety; and the solutions produced can be of a quality in which one can have complete confidence.

In the past, many sterile solutions were prepared with water obtained from water sterilizers located in specific departments where sterile fluids were necessary. Typical areas were the surgical suite, the obstetrical department, the emergency and outpatient departments, the milk formula room, and utility rooms on the nursing units. Fortunately in most hospitals water sterilizers have been replaced by the flask system. Solutions in flasks are prepared at a central point, under the supervision of a qualified person. A program for the preparation of external solutions, no matter how well conceived and preevaluated, is dependent upon properly trained personnel. This involves not only adequate training in the specialized techniques required in preparation, but also an understanding of, and an obligation to adhere to, the concepts behind these techniques. In addition, such persons involved in the preparation must be meticulous with regard to cleanliness, understanding of the details of the required procedures, and critically observant of each step so that the objective may be uncompromisingly attained.

If persons lacking a professional background are entrusted with certain aspects of the procedure, close supervision is essential. This will keep the personnel vigilant and will avoid instances leading to confusion, difficulty, and opportunities for error and contamination. A procedure detail ignored can make the difference between a satisfactory and an unsatisfactory product.

Personnel of reasonable intelligence, well-trained and well-supervised by either the pharmacist or the Central Service supervisor are quite satisfactory for practically all the tasks involved in the preparation of sterile external solutions. Equipment must, of course, receive its share of consideration in the program. The selection of items should be based on established principles of facility of operation, available space, ease of cleaning, quality and quantity of product required, reliability, and definite safety factors.

WATER STILLS

Modern usage of the term "distilled water" signifies a process involving evaporation of raw water by boiling, followed by immediate condensation of the liberated steam or water vapor. The quality or purity of the condensate produced by this process can vary greatly and still conform to the basic characteristics of distilled water. If the distilled water is to be used in critical applications demanding unusual quality, such as for the preparation of injectables or intravenous infusions, it must be substantially free from impurities of a mineral, metallic, or organic nature and, above all, free from pyrogenic substances. Of the methods currently available for the preparation of low residue water, that of distillation when carried out in a properly designed and correctly operated still stands unequalled as the best method for producing nonpyrogenic water of the highest purity. Evidence confirming the superiority of the distillation process is not always easily obtainable because of the mediocre performance of the average water still.

The principle upon which most water stills operate is essentially the same. The source of heat may be either steam, electricity, or gas, depending upon the type of still. The larger capacity stills ranging from 5 to 150 gallons per hour output are usually heated by steam, while those of small capacity from 1 to 5 gallons per hour are usually heated by electricity. The basic parts of the still consists of an evaporator pan or boiler, a medium of heating, a vapor tower, or stillhead, and a condenser. In operation, the raw water is fed into the evaporating pan where it is heated and converted into steam (see Fig. 16-1). The steam rises in the vapor tower where it contacts a series of baffle plates, the purpose of which is to eliminate entrainment of droplets of spray or foam from the rising steam. After passing the baffle plates, the dry steam continues upward to the condenser where it contacts a cooling coil, is condensed into water, and finally flows by gravity to the collecting vessel or storage bottle.

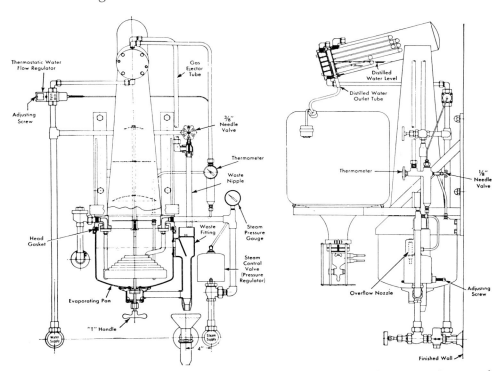

FIGURE 16-1. Sectional view of single effect water still designed for the production of nonpyrogenic distillate. The side view shows a storage carboy mounted in front of still.

Water distillation is a process consisting of three steps:

Evaporation. This means changing the required amount of water to steam. The heat necessary to bring about this change is calculated by first multiplying the number of gallons of distilled water per hour required by 8.3 to convert to pounds per hour. For example, a 10-gallon-per-hour still requires 83 pounds of water to be evaporated per hour. However, the water to be evaporated must first be heated to 212°F. Heat is measured by BTU's (British thermal units). If we assume the temperature of the feedwater to be 50°F, then to raise the temperature of one pound of water to 212°F will require 212°F − 50°F = 162°F or 162 BTU. To convert one pound of water to steam at 212°F requires an additional 970 BTU of heat. This makes 1032 BTU the total heat required per pound of water. For a 10-gallon-per-hour still, the total heat required then becomes 1032 × 83 pounds or 85,656 BTU. This amounts to 88.3 pounds of steam heat.

Vapor conduction. Pure water is obtained from water containing impurities by conducting the steam away from the evaporator to a condenser. As boiling takes place in the evaporator, the steam rises from the water to the vapor tower carrying with it water droplets. These entrained droplets contain dissolved solids and they must be removed before the steam enters the condenser. This feature is usually accomplished by means of a series of baffles in the vapor tower and by maintaining a low vapor velocity.

Condensation. The last step is converting the steam to pure water by condensation. To change one pound of steam to water means that 970 BTU must be removed. This is the purpose of the cooling water in the condenser coil. The normal operating conditions of a still specify that the water leaving the condenser should be at a temperature of about 160°F. Thus, every pound of cooling water has a temperature change of 110°F which means that 110 BTU of heat can be removed. On this basis, it is necessary to supply approximately 9 pounds of cooling water for every pound of distilled water produced. This same ratio holds true whether expressed as pounds or gallons of distillate.

The mechanical-design features of any still will largely determine its efficiency in producing distillate of high purity. The cross-sectional area or diameter of the evaporating pan is an important factor. The larger the water area in the evaporator pan with generous allowance for steam space above the water surface, the less opportunity there is for violent boiling. When the water boils violently there is proportionately more carry-over of nonvolatile substances than when the water is subjected to moderate controlled boiling. In addition, the evaporator pan should be easily removable without the use of tools, within convenient reach of the operator, to facilitate daily cleaning of the pan and heating coil.

The height of the vapor tower is another important factor in the design of the still. This determines the disengaging distance between the water level in the evaporating pan and the condenser. It has a direct bearing on the amount of entrainment or possible carry-over of droplets of raw water into the condenser. The vapor tower should also be of wide cross section so that the velocity of the steam can be maintained at a low level, thereby discouraging entrainment. The 30-inch rise of the vapor tower on the 10-gallons-per-hour still shown in Figure 16-1, including the proper placement of baffles, insures optimum conditions for the prevention or removal of entrained spray or foam from the steam. The entrainment-separation efficiency in a still is controlled not only by the mechanical equipment, the boiling rate, and the water level in the evaporator, but also by the surface tension, dissolved solids, and liquids in the evaporator.

One of the most difficult problems to cope with in any water still is the removal of released gases from the condenser. Unless some positive and efficient means is incorporated on the still to promptly remove liberated gases ascending from the evaporator, such as carbon dioxide, chlorine, and ammonia, it is difficult to prevent their reabsorption into the distillate. When this occurs in the average still the purity of the distilled water is markedly lowered as can be demonstrated by means of the conductivity meter. If these foreign gases are forcefully and continuously ejected from the condenser, a water of higher purity is obtained. Some water stills depend on a slight emission of steam vapor from the condenser to force ejection of the foreign gases and to visibly indicate that the gases are not stratified in the condenser. A more efficient method is the installation of a controlled jet evacuator, which introduces a slight negative pressure on the condenser, thereby assuring automatic removal of the gases as rapidly as they collect in the condenser.

All water stills should be equipped with a deconcentrator or bleeder device on the evaporating pan to permit continuous formation of steam from a flowing stream of water. This prevents concentration of impurities, which in the case of hard water, may produce excessive foaming with resulting entrainment of droplets to the distillate. Stills should also be provided with automatic regulating valves on both water and steam lines to prevent priming or surges in boiling, and to maintain the correct balance between water supply to evaporator and the rate of heating. An automatic diversion device is advantageous, especially when the quality of distillate must be constant and rigidly controlled. It should automatically open the waste line at any moment the quality falls below a specified level of resistance and close it when the water quality returns to standard.

The metals used in the construction of a still also influence the quality of distillate. Tin, stainless steel, Monel, nickel, aluminum, copper, and brass are the commonly used metals. Copper and brass should be plated with pure block tin if it is anticipated that these metals will come in contact with the distillate. A still fabricated of corrosion-resistant Monel metal with nickel condensing coil has proved to be a satisfactory combination. Aluminum is not a suitable material for fabrication of the evaporating pan because of its susceptibility to attack by alkaline water.

Traditionally, pure tin or tin-coated copper have been recommended for water-distilling systems because it was assumed that tin was nonreactive with water below 250°F. The literature reveals that there is no technical basis for the exclusive use or specification of tin in distilled water systems. In fact, current research studies show that both stainless steel (type 304) and tin are acceptable materials for high-purity water systems.[1] Moreover, it has been demonstrated experimentally by spectrographic analysis that the quality of distillate from a still made of Type 304 stainless steel is as good as, or of slightly higher quality than, the distillate from a tin still.

The water still shown in Figures 16-2 and 16-3 represents a significant advance in the design of equipment for the production of high-purity distilled water in hospitals, laboratories, and industry. It is probably the first all-stainless steel water-processing system, including still, piping, storage, and distribution facilities. The still operates under an internal pressure of 2 to 10 psig. The free rise of vapor under pressure substantially increases the operating efficiency. The steam-jacketed, distillate-collecting bowl superheats the distillate and frees it from dissolved gases. By discharging the distillate under low pressure it becomes possible to place the storage tank at a higher elevation than the still. This permits the still and storage tank to be installed in rooms with ceiling heights too low for conventional equipment of the same capacity.

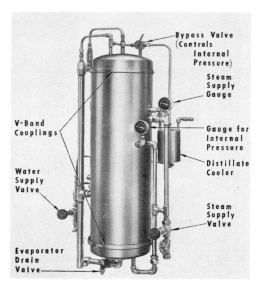

FIGURE 16-2. All-stainless steel water still of new design for operation under an internal pressure of 2-10 psig.

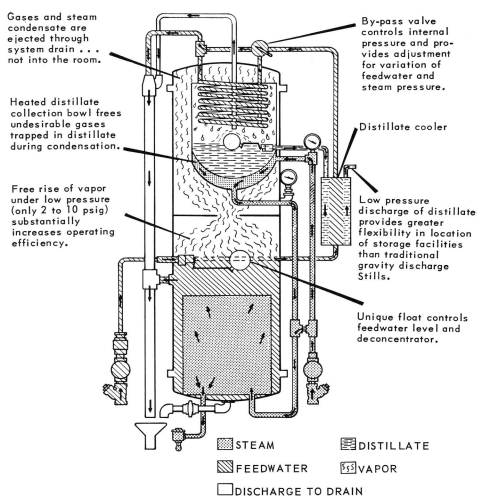

Gases and steam
condensate are
ejected through
system drain . . .
not into the room.

By-pass valve
controls internal
pressure and pro-
vides adjustment
for variation of
feedwater and
steam pressure.

Heated distillate
collection bowl frees
undesirable gases
trapped in distillate
during condensation.

Distillate cooler

Free rise of vapor
under low pressure
(only 2 to 10 psig)
substantially
increases operating
efficiency.

Low pressure
discharge of distillate
provides greater
flexibility in location
of storage facilities
than traditional
gravity discharge
Stills.

Unique float controls
feedwater level and
deconcentrator.

▨ STEAM   ▤ DISTILLATE

▨ FEEDWATER   ⁵ˢˢ VAPOR

☐ DISCHARGE TO DRAIN

FIGURE 16-3. Sectional view of water still shown in Fig. 16-2. The free rise of vapor under pressure substantially increases operating efficiency.

Myers[6] has described a "thermocompressor" still which operates on the principle of vapor compression for evaporation of water. It is designed to overcome the wastage of heat and water involved in condensing steam by conventional methods. By this method it is possible to evaporate several pounds of water per pound of steam supply through the addition of a relatively small amount of energy (input) to the compressor. Vapor-compression stills employ the heat-pump principle of salvaging the latent heat of evaporation, with the heat economy of fifteen or more effects of multiple-effect evaporation. The prime disadvantage of this type of still is that it must be fed with either softened or demineralized water. This means that in hard water areas two processes have to be used in order to supply a distillate suit-

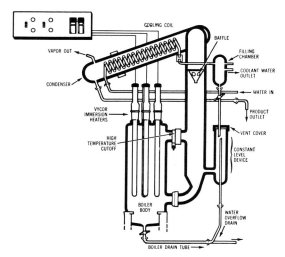

FIGURE 16-4. Glass still designed for production of high purity distillate. The surfaces coming in contact with water or vapor are made of inert Pyrex® and Vycor.®

able for injection. Compression stills may be electric-driven or they may be powered by prime movers.

The glass still shown in Figure 16-4 is a new development in water purification apparatus. All surfaces coming in contact with water or vapor are fabricated of inert Pyrex and Vycor® ware, with Teflon® stopcock plugs. It has a capacity of 10 liters per hour. The water in the boiler body is preheated by the condenser. A high temperature cutoff on the boiler shuts off the power supply if the water falls below the operating level. Four 2000-watt heaters are used to evaporate the water, and the vapors pass through a uniquely designed baffle to the condenser. After condensation, the distilled water drains through the product outlet to a storage vessel. The quality of distillate from this still is of the order of 1.7 megohm/cm with total solids of less than 0.3 ppm. It is particularly well adapted to laboratory requirements for high purity water.

Operation and Maintenance of Water Stills

The water still must be kept clean. This point has been recognized by authorities for years, but too frequently stills are put into service and operated for long periods of time with no cleaning of the interior parts until something goes drastically wrong. Practice has clearly demonstrated that the distillate from a single-effect still of good design is entirely suitable for parenteral solutions when, but only when, the still is clean. Frequent cleaning is a fundamental requirement in the operation of any still. The frequency of cleaning will depend upon the quality of the raw water supply and the design characteristics of the still.

When parenteral solutions first came into extensive use, serious difficulties were experienced with distillate collected from inefficient or foul stills. In an effort to solve the problem, double or triple stills were widely advocated, users forgetting that while double or triple effect distillation might postpone the day, that ultimately these stills would also become foul and their product unfit for use. Cleaning double or triple stills involves twice or three times the labor, expense, and delay needed for cleaning a single-effect still. Any still in continuous service will become increasingly foul until, regardless of all the protective baffles and intricate passageways with mysterious names, the product becomes unfit for use. Ultra refinements in the performance of a clean still are not significant. The intent should be to provide an apparatus, instead, which will produce initially water of satisfactory purity, with the all-important provision of means for maintaining that quality by easy daily cleaning.

The still shown in Figure 16-1 was designed specifically for production of distillate for preparation of external and parenteral solutions. Performance tests over a period of several years in various laboratories have shown the distillate to be nonpyrogenic, with the average purity ranging from 400,000 to 800,000 specific ohms resistance. (The purity of the distillate coming from any still is, of course, dependent upon the quality of the feed water.) Interior parts of the still are easily accessible for inspection and cleaning, without the use of tools. The evaporating pan may be detached from the body of the still by loosening the tee handle and then applying a twisting motion which actuates a bayonet joint. The pan should be removed daily for thorough flushing, to remove sludge and scale.

Hard scale adhering to the steam coil of any still will slow down the performance and cause the still to produce less than its rated capacity. When the coil or heat exchanger becomes badly coated, it should be disconnected and a clean spare coil put in its place. The coated coil can then be treated with a dilute (5%) hydrochloric acid solution to remove the scale, after which it is retained as a spare. The high-purity water still described in Figures 16-2 and 16-3 is designed and constructed in such a manner as to eliminate the need for daily cleaning of the evaporator. At the end of each day it is only necessary to drain out the evaporator by opening the steam supply valve, closing the water supply valve and opening the drain valve. This is sufficient to remove adherent scale from the surfaces of the heat exchanger.

STORAGE OF DISTILLED WATER

The question frequently arises as to the most satisfactory material for construction of distilled-water storage tanks and distribution systems. According to Friend,[2] metals such as stainless steels, nickel alloys, or aluminum are required to handle high-purity water. Others[3] have reported that the most desirable metal is aluminum for temperatures up to 350°F (177°C). Surprisingly few quantitative data are available concerning the corrosion resistance of tin in distilled water. According to Britton[4] there is almost no reaction of tin to distilled water, although some tarnishing occurs under boiling conditions. Lowenheim and associates[5] reported that tin would probably be the principal material for conveying water if it were not for cost and strength limitations. Water containing salts of chlorides, sulfates, and nitrates may cause pitting of tin with the appearance of black spots.

In a recent evaluation of the tank storage and distribution systems for high-purity distillate it was found that metallic-ion pickup, from all storage containers, increases with time and increasing specific resistance of the stored water.[1] Analyses of water sampled after 4- and 24-hour storage in a tin-lined, a tin-coated, a Type 304 stainless steel, and a Pyrex glass tank showed iron (4-11 ppb) was dissolved in the distillate regardless of the construction material. However, no tin or copper was found in samples from the stainless steel or Pyrex tanks. About 7 ppb tin was dissolved from the tin-lined tanks, and copper was definitely dissolved from the tin-coated tanks.

As a current recommendation, it may be said that Type 304 stainless steel and tin are equally satisfactory materials for use in distillation equipment or for the storage and distribution (valving and piping) of high-purity water. If the water distribution system is pressurized from a central source, the pressure pumps must be of stainless steel construction with stainless valving and piping throughout the distribution system. Tin-lined brass is unsuitable for pressure systems because of the galvanic action with the stainless steel pump. In general, plastic materials are not satisfactory for use in storage tanks or water distribution systems. They are porous materials and unreacted chemical components may be leached out by the distilled water.

HARDNESS OF WATER

Pure water is a rare commodity in nature. When formed in the clouds, it is in a relatively pure state, but its composition is soon altered due to the absorption from the air of gases such as oxygen and carbon dioxide during the course of precipitation. Upon reaching the earth, water dissolves mineral substances with which it comes in contact, the amount dependent upon the composition of the soil or rocks in the particular locality. Water also becomes polluted with industrial and sewage wastes from factories and cities.

Total hardness is the accepted basis for classifying industrial waters as good or bad. In this context total hardness means a characteristic of water generally accepted to represent the total concentration of calcium and magnesium ions.[7] Hardness is usually expressed in parts per million (ppm) of the equivalent amount of calcium carbonate. Other dissolved substances, principally iron, manganese, aluminum, and zinc, also contribute to the total hardness. The hardness of natural waters varies considerably in different sections of the country. Surface waters in the Atlantic Coast area and in the

Pacific Northwest are generally softer than waters found elsewhere in the U.S. Waters of average hardness are found in the Great Lakes areas, parts of the Midwest, and in areas of natural impounded waters in the Southwest. Waters are classified as hard when the total hardness exceeds 150 ppm. Table 16-1 gives the descriptive classifications.

TABLE 16-1

CLASSIFICATION OF WATER

Total Hardness, ppm	Classification
<15	Very soft water
15–60	Soft water
61–120	Medium-hard water
121–180	Hard water
>180	Very hard water

The map below shows the hardness as calcium carbonate and the pH in average values per area for waters in the United States. Most natural waters fall within the nearly neutral pH range of 6.0 to 8.0. The exceptions are swamp waters with a pH of 3.0 to 5.0, some mine waters with a pH as low as 2.0, and natural Western brines with a pH of 9.5. The pH of ocean water is in the range of 8.0 to 8.4. *Brackish* waters are those containing extremely high concentrations of chlorides.

The pH value influences greatly the scale-forming and corrosive tendencies of water. A low or acid pH value favors corrosion of metallic equipment in contact with the water. A high or alkaline pH may precipitate calcium car-

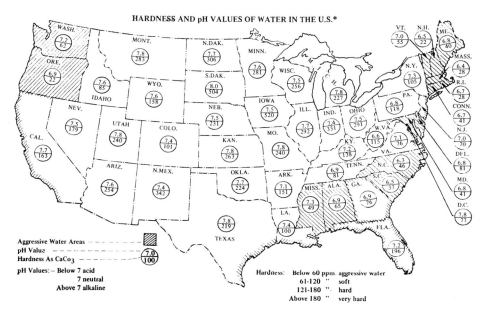

HARDNESS AND pH VALUES OF WATER IN THE U.S.*

Aggressive Water Areas
pH Value
Hardness As CaCo₃

pH Values: – Below 7 acid
7 neutral
Above 7 alkaline

Hardness: Below 60 ppm. aggressive water
61-120 " soft
121-180 " hard
Above 180 " very hard

* Reprinted by permission of the American Iron & Steel Institute

bonate from solution to form scale on the surfaces of boiler tubes, heat exchangers, and condensers.

DEIONIZED WATER

Deionization, oftentimes referred to as demineralization, is a process of purification by which ions are removed from the water. In comparison, purification of water by simple distillation means the removal of water from the impurities; purification by deionization means the removal of the impurities (ionizable) from the water. The process of ion exchange is the "reversible exchange of ions between a solid (synthetic resin) and a liquid in which there is no substantial change in the structure of the solid."[14]

In a deionizer the synthetic resins constitute the ion-exchangers. As the water is passed through a series of resin beds the ionic content is removed by chemical reaction. The result is a chemically pure water from the stand-point of freedom from ionic constituents, but organic compounds or non-electrolytes and microorganisms may not be removed. Deionized water can be used for many laboratory applications, in air-conditioners, and, if sterile, in humidifiers. It is an excellent feedwater to the evaporator pan of a still. By changing an existing still from city-water feed to deionized-water feed the quantity of distillate produced can be increased as much as 50 per cent, and the quality improved proportionately.

The chief disadvantage of deionized water is that it may contain onionic and colloidal impurities that are incompletely removed from the feed water. Also, the resin beds are liable to become heavily contaminated with certain organisms—*Pseudomonas aeruginosa* is a particular hazard. Deionized water should not be used for the preparation of parenteral solutions or external irrigating solutions. In this connection, it should be noted that some solutions such as acriflavine and benzalkonium chloride are incompatible with deionized water.[15] It has been pointed out by Jeffrey and Fish[16] that deionized water may not be safe to use in certain pharmaceutical preparations used in the care of hospitalized patients.

PURITY OF DISTILLED WATER

There are many definitions of high purity water. According to Eckel,[8] the one accepted in the nuclear-power field states that high-purity water is water that has been distilled and/or deionized so that it will have a specific resistance of 500,000 ohm/cm or greater. In terms of freedom from dissolved solids (ionizable impurities) this definition would seem to apply equally well for high-purity water requirements in hospitals. Suggested working standards for degrees of water purity are given in Table 16-2.

Distilled water for injection or water intended for use as a solvent for the preparation of parenteral solutions must be nonpyrogenic and conform to

TABLE 16-2

GRADES OF WATER PURITY
DISTILLED AND/OR DEIONIZED

Grade	Specific Resistance in Ohms (25°C)	Specific Conductance in Micromhos (25°C)	Electrolytes (ppm)
Low purity	<300,000	>3.3	1.4
Average purity	300,000– 1,000,000	1.0–3.3	0.4–1.4
High purity	1,000,000–10,000,000	0.10–1.0	0.02–0.4
Ultrapure	10,000,000–17,000,000	0.060–0.10	0.002–0.02
Theoretically pure	18,000,000	0.055	0.000

the standards of purity as outlined in the Pharmacopeia of the United States. Water of an equivalent purity should be used in the preparation of sterile external solutions. To meet these requirements a continuous and accurate monitoring of the purity of the distillate is a necessity. The simplest overall method for monitoring the quality of distilled water is by measurement of the specific conductance.

Electrolytic or solution conductivity is a measure of the ability of a solution to carry an electric current. Specific conductance is defined as the reciprocal of the resistance in ohms of a 1-centimeter cube of the liquid at a specified temperature. The unit of specific conductance is the reciprocal ohm or *mho*. Since this is a very large value of electrolytic conductivity, the practical unit commonly employed is 1 millionth of a mho or 1 *micromho*. In practice, conductance measurements are usually made in terms of resistance since resistance is the reciprocal of conductance. Resistance is measured in ohms, and the term *specific resistance* is, therefore, ohms per centimeter cube. Resistance is also expressed in terms of millions of ohm/cm or megohm/cm. In the electronic industry, it has become fairly common to speak of "15 megohm water," meaning water with a total dissolved solid content of the order of 0.01 ppm.

Aqueous solutions of acids, alkalies, and salts have high conductivity because these chemicals, when dissolved in water, dissociate into positively and negatively charged ions which carry electrical current as they migrate through the solvent. In the process of distillation or deionization, there is a reduction in the number of both positive and negative ions in the water, resulting in poorer conductivity or, the reverse, higher resistance. The relationship of parts per million of sodium chloride in solution to specific resistance and specific conductance is given in Table 16-3. Even absolutely pure water will conduct electricity to some degree. However, the dissociation of water increases as the temperature rises, and this means that the conductivity of ultimately pure water varies with the temperature.

Theoretically pure water has a specific conductance of about 0.055 micromhos or 18,000,000 specific ohms at 25°C (77°F). Water of this purity cannot be produced by the distillation process but it has been obtained by the deionization process. Actually, the production of 20, 10, or even 5 mil-

TABLE 16-3

RELATIONSHIP OF IONIZABLE IMPURITIES IN WATER TO SPECIFIC RESISTANCE AND
SPECIFIC CONDUCTANCE AT 25°C
(*Data from Michalson[10]*)

ppm as Sodium Chloride	Specific Resistance in Ohms/cm	Specific Conductance in Micromhos/cm
20.8	23,000	44.
10.3	45,000	22.
5.1	90,000	11.
4.1	115,000	8.7
3.0	150,000	6.5
2.0	230,000	4.4
1.0	450,000	2.2
0.5	900,000	1.1
0.4	1,000,000	0.91
0.3	1,500,000	0.69
0.2	2,000,000	0.48
0.10	4,000,000	0.26
0.04	7,000,000	0.15
0.03	9,000,000	0.11
0.01	12,000,000	0.085
0.004	16,000,000	0.063
0.002	17,000,000	0.060
0.000	18,000,000	0.055

lion ohms water is chiefly of academic interest, since water exceeding 1 million ohms is of adequate purity for almost all applications, with the exception of ultrapure requirements for manufacturers of semiconductors, electron tubes, and nuclear power plants.

It is obviously not difficult to meet the requirements of the Pharmacopeia for distilled water with total dissolved solids of not more than 10 ppm. In terms of ionizable solids, this would mean a distillate of approximately 50,000 ohms resistance. Almost any still, even one that is carelessly operated, will produce distillate of this purity. The problem is to provide assurance that the water shall be nonpyrogenic. The measurement of conductance or resistance in terms of specific ohms is a direct function of the quantity of electrolytes or ionizable impurities present in the water. Admittedly this does not constitute a direct measurement of pyrogenic content, but it should be understood that pyrogens are nonvolatile and their presence in freshly distilled water is proportional to the amount of entrainment or carry-over of droplets of raw (feed) water from the evaporating pan of the still. Therefore, continuous measurement of the ionizable impurities by means of the conductivity meter provides a logical method for checking performance of the still and also a reliable indication of the possibility of pyrogen contamination.

A convenient and accurate method for determining the purity of distilled water is shown in Figure 16-5. The recording conductivity meter is attached to the wall, adjacent to the storage tank. The conductivity cell with self-contained thermistor (automatic temperature compensator) is sealed into the drawoff cock of the stainless steel storage tank. This feature assures the op-

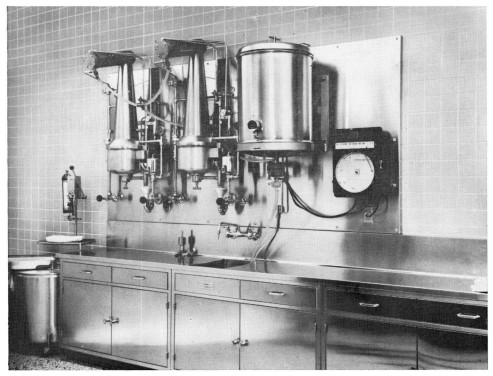

FIGURE 16-5. Sterile fluids room showing an arrangement of two 10 gallons per hour water stills, with stainless steel storage tank and recording conductivity meter.

erator of known purity of the distillate at the point of use. When water is drawn from the tank, or when water is fed into the tank from the condenser on the still, it passes through the conductivity cell, and the specific resistance is indicated on a 10-inch horizontal scale located at the top of the conductivity meter. The resistance is also recorded on the 12-inch circular chart which rotates once each 24 hours.

Distilled water acceptable for use in preparation of parenteral solutions should have a purity equal to or better than the following characteristics:

Resistance (specific ohms) 500,000
Specific conductance (micromhos) 2.0
pH 5.7-6.0
Residue after evaporation (1 hr. @ 105°C) .... 1.0 ppm
Chloride (Cl) .... 0.1 ppm
Ammonia (NH$_3$) .... 0.1 ppm
Heavy metals (as Pb) .... 0.01 ppm

As a general rule, it is advisable to reject all distilled water which gives a reading of 250,000 specific ohms or less on the conductivity instrument. This is equivalent to about 2 ppm of electrolytes. If the conductivity meter is equipped with an automatic diversion device, it will automatically open the waste line at any moment the quality of distillate falls below this level of resistance.

The reaction of ordinary distilled water is always acid because of the absorption of carbon dioxide. Water which has taken up carbon dioxide from the air until equilibrium has been established, will contain about 0.03% carbon dioxide by volume, and the calculated pH should be 5.7. In fact, this is the value usually found in distilled water which has been freely exposed to the air. Water from an efficient still, collected and stored in closed, nonsoluble glass or metal containers, will usually have a pH of 6.0 to 6.4.

DISTILLATE FOR MICROBIOLOGICAL APPLICATIONS

A standard of quality of distilled water for laboratory use apparently does not exist. It is usually accepted, however, that water for microbiological applications should be free of inorganic and organic substances, either toxic or nutritive, that might influence survival or growth of bacteria and viruses. In addition, the distilled-water supply system should be free of organisms that might contribute inhibitory substances to media and the *in vitro* growth of tissue cells such as *Pseudomonas*[9] and algae. Spoehr, *et al.*[11] demonstrated antibacterial activity in material obtained from killed cells of *Chlorella*. Distilled water containing more than 0.1 ppm of chlorine will inactivate biotin.[12]

Price and Gare[12] have reported that traces of volatile short-chain fatty acids may occur in distilled water and they may be a source of inhibitory interference in microbiological assays. These volatile organic contaminants are supposedly derived from dead organisms which have accumulated in the water still. To determine if a particular distillate is satisfactory for microbiological applications, it has been proposed by Geldreich and Clark[13] that a biological suitability test be performed on the water source in question. A good quality water for general use in the laboratory should have a specific resistance of not less than 500,000 ohms. Correct interpretation of this figure is important because specific conductance measurements do not differentiate between toxic or nontoxic metallic ions present in the distilled water and they do not indicate the presence of any organic contaminants.

WATER REQUIREMENTS FOR THE HOSPITAL

Water requirements for hospitals vary in accordance with the services performed. In some departments water of high purity, usually distilled, is considered a necessity in order to prepare or process certain materials.

In Central Service Department it is used for the rinsing of instruments, syringes, needles, tubing, flasks, and closures and for the preparation of sterile solutions.

In the pharmacy it is used for preparing injectables, surgical fluids, and

I.V. solutions and for the preparation of germicides, disinfectants, lotions, emulsions, syrups, detergents, and cleaning agents.

In the laboratory it is used for the preparation of diagnostic and chemical reagents, biological stains, and culture media.

The greatest demand for high-purity water is in the preparation of sterile (external) solutions. As a rule, the requirements for this purpose can be calculated on the basis of 3 liters per bed per week. For example, a 100-bed hospital would use $100 \times 3 \times 52 = 15,600$ liters per year. In estimating requirements it is helpful to consider the following needs:

> 4 liters per surgical operation
> 2 liters per delivery
> 2 liters per cystoscopic procedure
> 16 liters per TUR procedure
> 1 liter per day postnatal care.

CHEMICALS

All chemicals used in the preparation of injectables or external solutions must be of a high degree of chemical purity and free from pyrogenic substances. The standard of purity of each chemical should conform to the requirements of the U.S. Pharmacopoeia, or preferably the American Chemical Society Specifications for Reagent Chemicals. Wherever possible, the chemicals should be purchased on a tested, pyrogen-free and known chemical assay basis in preweighed quantities, protected against contamination in well-closed containers. The acceptance of any particular lot of chemical also depends upon the quantity of foreign matter present. Excessive dust or dirt is evidence of careless handling prior to packaging and sufficient cause for rejection. The presence of foreign particles such as parts of insects indicates serious contamination.

Only the highest purity dextrose should be used for the preparation of solutions. Certain lots of dextrose may contain acid-dehydration products or protein-split products formed by side reactions during the course of manufacture. These impurities may give rise to a yellow color, often mistaken for caramelization, upon sterilization of the dextrose solutions. They may also lead to the formation of white, flocculent precipitates in the final solutions.[17]

PYROGENS

Familiarity with the basic facts concerning pyrogens is essential to the successful preparation, dispensing and administering of parenteral and external solutions. The term "pyrogen" which means "fever producing" was introduced by Burdon-Sanderson in 1876.[18] Although the chemical composition of pyrogens has not been definitely established, the latest evidence suggests that they are complex polysaccharides apparently attached to another radical containing nitrogen and phosphorus.[19,20,21] It is generally accepted that pyrogens are by-products of bacterial growth or metabolism closely related to or identical with bacterial O antigen and commonly called endotoxin.

Landy and his associates [22,23,24] have purified O antigen from a strain of typhoid bacilli and thereby isolated a phosphorylated lipopolysaccharide essentially free of protein which was capable of producing the various biological phenomena attributed to endotoxins including pyrogenicity. It is known that pyrogens occur only in media which have been contaminated with bacteria. Many species of bacteria, including airborne contaminants, yeasts, and molds, produce pyrogens.[25] They have been shown to be of a particulate nature, larger than 50 millimicrons, but smaller than 1 micron.

The concept of a pyrogenic substance produced by bacteria was firmly established by Seibert,[27] who showed that the substances designated "pyrogens" were products of bacilli usually found in river water. Rademaker[28] also found them in varying amounts of tap water in numerous cities, their concentration varying with the seasons. Pyrogens are extremely soluble in water, and they cannot be removed by passage through a Berkefeld filter. They may, however, be removed by adsorption on an activated asbestos filter or on activated charcoal.[26,29,30,31]

Pyrogens cannot be destroyed by autoclaving except at very high temperatures for a prolonged period of time. Banks,[32] for example, found that pyrogenic water was rendered innocous by heating to a temperature of 284°F (140°C) for 30 minutes. Sterilization is of no practical value as a safeguard in removing pyrogen from solutions intended for parenteral administration. According to Wiley and Todd,[33] sterilization through autoclaving at 240°F (116°C) for 30 minutes will destroy about 25 per cent of the pyrogenic activity of a concentrated solution, yet this process will have little effect on a dilute solution such as might arise from accidental contamination of water.

Quantitative information describing the pyrogenic capacity of intact organisms of different species added to parenteral solutions which were then autoclaved has been reported by Marcus, Anselmo, and Perkins.[34] Multiple tests on solutions to which had been added known numbers of various bacterial species showed that 1,000 or more organisms/ml had to be present before the U.S.P. rabbit pyrogen test yielded a positive result. This work led to the description of a culture method employing memebrane filters to test freshly prepared parenteral solutions for pyrogenic capacity.[35] Evidence was presented to show that freshly prepared solutions which immediately prior to autoclaving yielded counts of less than 10,000 bacteria per liter, without regard to species, were nonpyrogenic by the U.S.P. rabbit test. On the basis of extensive laboratory and field trial, it was concluded that the bacteriological assay for this purpose was at least as specific and sensitive as the rabbit assay for pyrogenicity.

One major source of pyrogens is distilled water which has become contaminated with airborne pyrogenic bacteria. A poorly designed water still or one that is operated incorrectly may also produce distillate containing pyrogenic substances. Although pyrogens are nonvolatile, they are still capable of passing through the ordinary distillation process by means of entrainment or carry-over with mineral impurities to the distillate. Tap water is the usual source of contamination, and any glassware or tubing rinsed or washed in tap water will produce pyrogen unless sterilized within an hour. Rademaker[36] found that pyrogen can be developed within 2 hours at room temperature in the drying films of moisture remaining in such tubing and equipment. Similarly, a sufficient amount of pyrogen can be formed within an intravenous needle rinsed in tap water to produce a reaction.

A pyrogenic or febrile reaction may occur any time from 15 minutes to 8 hours following the injection of a solution containing pyrogenic substances. Such reactions from intravenous solutions occur in hospitals even though the means to eliminate them entirely are well known. In the opinion of certain authorities,[17,37] these reactions are inexcusable in the light of present day knowledge. The precautions necessary for the prevention of reactions in routine parenteral therapy are as follows:

· Use only freshly distilled water from an efficient still in the preparation of solutions and for the rinsing of all apparatus.

· Provide for intelligent and reliable operation of the water still. Discard the first fraction of distillate at the beginning of each day's operation. Frequent cleaning of the water still at regular intervals is necessary.

· Prepare solutions and sterilize the final products within a few hours after the water has been distilled.

· Immediately sterilize all tubing, needles, and glassware after rinsing with distilled water to prevent production of pyrogens in residual moisture films.

· If nondisposable intravenous sets are used, permit 50 to 100 ml of nonpyrogenic solution to be run through the set and wasted, before inserting the needle into the vein.

EXTERNAL SOLUTIONS

Sterile external solutions are used in almost every department of the hospital in one form or another. Their therapeutic effect is based upon compatibility with the tissues being irrigated. The most popular and commonly used external solutions are the following:

> sterile distilled water
> sterile isotonic sodium chloride solution
> sterile glycine solution
> sterile boric acid solution
> sterile magnesium sulfate solution

Saline Solution

Saline is probably the oldest and most commonly used solution for both intravenous and irrigating applications. Besides its cleansing properties, it has been proven to act as a stimulant to the tissues, and the red corpuscles are preserved in it, whereas they are destroyed by plain water.

External solutions are usually prepared to be isotonic with the body fluids and with blood. A hypotonic fluid such as distilled water will cause the red cells to swell and burst. Conversely, a hypertonic solution may cause crenation of the red cells. But an isotonic solution is one compatible with blood and body fluid. It exerts the same osmotic pressure as the blood and is easily absorbed by the blood and lymph. The U.S. Pharmacopoeia refers to an isotonic solution as one containing not less than 0.85% and not more than 0.95% of sodium chloride in water.

Isotonic sodium chloride solution of 0.9% is rapidly becoming the preferred solution, not only for replacing deficits of fluids in the body but, also, for irrigating and bathing the tissues and cavities.

Any solution used to irrigate a deep wound or body cavity, or to bathe tissue can enter the blood stream by capillary action. Therefore, the requirements for the preparation of external solutions in the "open system" of administration are first, that the basic fluid be free of impurities, and second, that it be isotonic with the body fluids. In addition, external solutions must receive the same consideration for accuracy, safety, and sterility as parenteral solutions.

This absorption of fluid through irrigation of wounds or other routes may be great, depending on the circumstances, as, for example, in urological cases. During a transurethral resection, 5 or more liters of irrigating fluid can be absorbed through the open capsular venous sinuses, depending on resection time, the irrigating fluid, and the number of open venous sinuses.[38] The use of sterile external solutions to flush out the deep cavities during operative procedures and postoperative treatment may have consequences which have not been fully studied, and are still unknown to us at the present time.

Sterile isotonic sodium chloride solution is used extensively in almost every department of the hospital. Some typical examples are given below.

1. The Operating and Delivery Rooms.
    a. To bathe tissues and irrigate cavities exposed during an operative procedure.
    b. To moisten sponges and dressings of all kinds.
    c. To rinse blood, tissue, and other matter from instruments and the surgeon's hands.
2. The Emergency and Outpatient Departments.
    a. To bathe and irrigate wound sites.
    b. To keep dressings moist, or to remove them.

3. The Nursing Units.
   a. To moisten, or keep wet, dressings of all kinds.
   b. For irrigation of orifices.
   c. For irrigation of cavities postoperatively.

Sterile Boric Acid Solution

In the past, boric acid was used in hospitals for practically every condition—infected wounds, burns, eczema, by mouth for peritonitis, diarrhea, kidney conditions. During recent years the fatalities from the use of boric acid have been largely limited to newborn infants, with most of the cases occurring on the newborn services. The presence of boric acid in hospitals, especially in the newborn nursery and pediatric sections, constitutes a potential health hazard and has been associated with repeated accidental deaths over the years. Boric acid powder is one of the weakest antiseptics in use, and any good qualities it may have are outweighed by its poisonous one.

The literature emphasizes that when a boron product enters the body by swallowing, or through the mucous membrane of mouth, eyes, or through wounds, chafed buttocks or otherwise, once in the body it acts as a poison.

Boric acid solution has no place in today's modern hospital. Although it is not highly toxic, poisonings and deaths may occur after absorption from various types of open lesions or as a result of a human error such as occasions where milk formulas are mistakenly made with sterile boric acid solution instead of sterile distilled water. Despite its weak germicidal property, boric acid is, for some inexplicable reason, still widely used. This usage continues regardless of the fact that concentrations greater than 3% may inhibit phagocytosis, the ability of the body to defend against bacteria, thus negating one of the body's primary defenses against bacterial invasion.

In the past few years, more and more doctors have taken a serious view of this so-called mild antiseptic. The American Academy of Pediatrics[39] states

> Since it is possible to provide satisfactory care for patients without the presence of this substance, it is recommended that rigid controls over hospital use be required, and the elimination of boric acid from the newborn nursery and pediatric ward of all hospitals be required.

Perhaps with the greater awareness of the untoward effects possible with boric acid, the use of this substance in all its forms will be discontinued in hospitals.

Magnesium Sulfate Solution

A saturated solution of magnesium sulfate is generally used to combat inflammatory conditions of the skin, and to reduce swelling, redness, and pain. Its saturation point depends on the hardness or softness of water and the temperature of the solvent. Heat increases the saturation point, and cold decreases it. Crystallization usually occurs at temperatures of 100°F and lower. The most common use for a sterile solution of magnesium sulfate is for wet compresses applied locally to the skin. In a more dilute form, it has been used for medicinal baths and soaks for various parts of the body. The preparation of a magnesium sulfate solution for external use involves the same hazards, and must be regarded with the same precautions as boric acid.

Urological Fluids

It is generally agreed that solutions used for irrigation during urological diagnostic examinations and therapeutic procedures should be sterile. If a water sterilizer is used to provide water for urological procedures, it is located so that the water is either drawn off in a pitcher (for transfer into a Valentine percolator) or piped directly to the point of use. The fittings and piping are difficult to clean and the sterility of the solution doubtful. There is also the possibility of high-temperature water reaching the patient. The water sterilizer, however, can provide large volumes of solution more easily than the flasking technique. The disadvantages, however, far outweigh the advantages. For example, the height above the bladder (7 to 10 feet) causes an undesirably high pressure capable of rupturing a bladder. There also is danger of rapid extravasation of water, which is hypotonic and injurious, into the open tissue spaces and blood stream.[40] Besides, there is no convenient means of adding substances to the water for making an isotonic solutions.

The advantage of the sterile flasking technique is its insured sterility. The sterile solution is used directly from the sealed flask. The sterile flasking technique employs the principle of siphonage, similar to tidal drainage. The solution flows into the bladder by gravity. As many as four interconnected flasks of 2000-milliliter capacity are held in an inverted position, and while one flask is being replaced, the solution is drawn from the second flask, thus insuring a continuous supply of sterile solution. The water used in the preparation is assured to be nonpyrogenic by distillation, and the vacuum sealed flasks maintain sterility. A concentrate of heat sensitive solute may be added directly to the flasks of sterile distilled water at the time of use; or prepared sterile isotonic solutions and flasks of water may be stored, ready for use to meet any emergency need.

In recent years, considerable attention has been focused on irrigating solutions used during surgical procedures of cystoscopy, suprapubic cystostomy, transurethral resection, and others. Recognition of irrigating solutions entering the circulation as being a case of postoperative reactions was due to the clinical observations reported in 1948 by McLaughlin, *et al.*[41] Considerable evidence has accumulated in the literature to support these observations. The absorption of significant quantities of irrigating solution through the opening of capsular venous sinuses early during the course of a resection may lead to the absorption of as much as five or more liters of the fluid. A result of this absorption is the syndrome known as water intoxication. This is a clinical condition resulting from the acute expansion of the volume of body water.[42]

Since the appearance in 1947 of several articles discussing the now well-known syndrome of intravascular hemolysis during transurethral prostatectomy, efforts have been made to prevent hemolysis by the use of isotonic irrigating solutions. The first solution tried was glucose in 5% concentration. This satisfactorily prevented intravascular hemolysis but was found to have undesirable effects on the patient. In addition, the glucose solution interfered with clear vision on the part of the physician. The general opinion now is that other solutions are probably better especially glycine and mannitol. Both have been found satisfactory. There is evidence in the literature that the use of an isotonic solution for irrigation during transurethral resections has resulted in a striking reduction of morbidity and mortality.[43]

Pennisi and associates[44] give the following characteristics for an ideal irrigant:

- Economical and with a refractory index akin to water.
- Easy to prepare, handle, and store.
- Nontoxic.
- Nonhemolytic.
- Bactericidal.
- Easily diffusible in the intracellular as well as the extracellular compartment.
- Osmotic diuretic.
- Of a nature to allow the return flow of sodium from the intracellular to the extracellular compartment.
- Of a physical and/or chemical nature to cause contracture of newly opened vascular orifices.

STERILE FLASK TECHNIQUE

The flasking technique is a method that provides sterile distilled water and isotonic solutions at the operating table or treatment site with certainty that they will be sterile. Today, the amount of sterile solution being used is greater than ever before, and medicine is requiring a more reliable and an ever-increasing variety of solutions.

The flasking technique for the preparation of sterile solutions is usually carried out in the Central Service Department. Briefly, it consists of using borosilicate glass containers which are filled with freshly distilled water, or the desired solution, and sterilized at 250° to 254°F for an appropriate period of time depending upon the size of the container. Special flask closures are used which are designed to allow air and vapor to escape from the solution during sterilization. After sterilization, when the temperature drops below

212°F an hermetic seal automatically forms, insuring sterility of the solution for an indefinite period of time. The closure also provides a sterile lip over which the solution can be poured when the flask is opened for use. Disposable closures are also available which simplify the procedure.

Flasks and closures (except the disposable closures) not only fill immediate needs for sterile, uniform solutions, but they can be safely and economically reused. The preparation of external solutions using the sterile flask technique is not a difficult procedure. The basic facilities required are the following:

· A solution room of adequate space, designed specifically for processing solutions, as shown in Figures 16-6A and 16-6B.
· Equipment especially designed for all phases of processing—cleaning of apparatus, preparation of fluids, and their sterilization.
· Solution flasks and closures which will (except for the disposable closures) withstand repeated exposure to high temperatures, resist chemicals, and can be closed in a manner maintaining sterility of contents.
· Ingredients of high purity.
· Personnel qualified for this particular type of work.

A completely integrated technique furnishes safe procedures for operating a solution room. It relies principally upon equipment produced by specialists who understand the exceptional standards imposed by hospital practices. The technique provides the following essentials for successful operation:

· Close planning cooperation between equipment experts and hospital personnel.
· Proper cleaning facilities which include special counters with built-in sinks and automatic flask washer and rinser.
· Flasks, closures, and accessories designed to withstand rough handling, repeated high temperature sterilization and chemical action.
· Purity of distilled water, rigidly controlled by a conductivity meter.
· Disposable irrigation sets. Their use. is safer than the older method of cleaning rubber tubing, containers, and reservoirs prior to assembly of units and sterilization. Prepackaged and presterilized disposable irrigation sets are now firmly established as the safe, positive way to protect the patient's welfare.
· Proper supervision. The solution room provides for centralized production with competent supervision of all phases of preparation, sterilization, and storage.
· Efficient sterilizers. While any pressure steam sterilizer may be used for the sterilization of flasked solutions, modern techniques suggest the additional requirements of an automatic control and a solution accelerator exhaust valve.
· A method of control to confirm the quality and safety of the finished product.

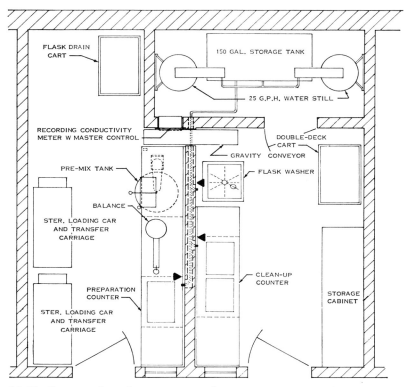

FIGURE 16-6A. Layout of a solution room with equipment and facilities for the production of external and parenteral solutions.

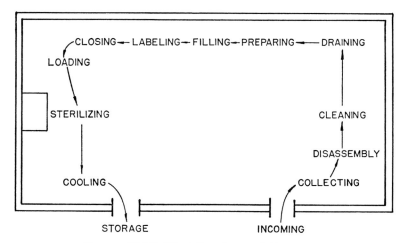

FIGURE 16-6B. Work flow for a solution room.

GLASS CONTAINERS

The solution containers should be made of nonsoluble, borosilicate, heat-resistant glass. Pyrex glass has been found most satisfactory for this purpose. Its low expansion coefficient minimizes breakage due to thermal shock, its physical hardness resists breakage due to careless handling, and its chemical stability resists hydrolysis by the solutions when subjected to repeated use. The containers should be designed for heavy, thick-wall fabrication so as to withstand repeated use, moderately rough handling, and both positive and negative pressures created during the sterilization and cooling process. All surfaces must be smooth and free from depressions or crevices which would hinder thorough cleaning.

Solution flasks of square design, as shown in Figure 16-7 offer several advantages over the round or pear-shaped types. The square shape provides an almost flat contact surface between flasks when placed side by side, thus avoiding pressure cracks or fractures when the flasks are forcibly bumped against each other. The square shape also permits a greater number of flasks to be sterilized per load and requires less storage space in shelf area following sterilization.

The thorough cleaning of flasks and all other items of glassware is essential to the successful preparation of safe solutions. The cleaning process should be conducted as follows:

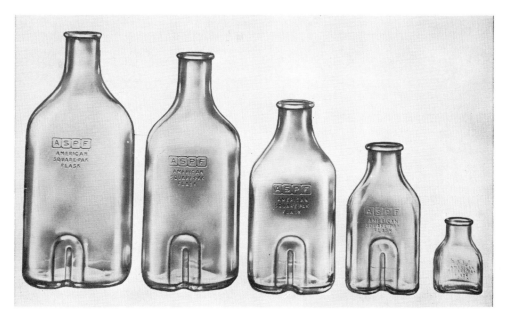

FIGURE 16-7. Solution flasks of square design. For use in preparation of external or parenteral solutions.

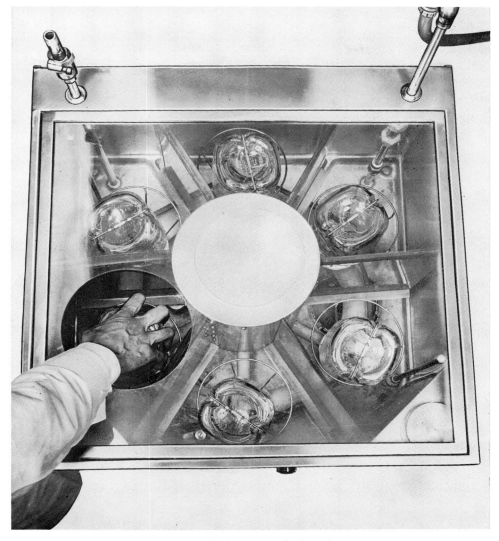

FIGURE 16-8. Automatic flask washer.

· Rinse each flask with tap water to remove any residue of solution.

· Wash in solution of 0.5% Calgonite or other equally effective detergent in distilled water. Rinse three times with freshly distilled water. (The use of an automatic flask washer and rinser as shown in Figure 16-8 provides a more efficient method of cleaning.)

· Inspect each flask for "water breaks." The interior should be crystal clear with no spots in the film of distilled water left on the glass after the final rinsing.

· Invert on portable flask drain cart for draining, as in Figure 16-9.

· The flasks should be filled with solution as promptly as possible after

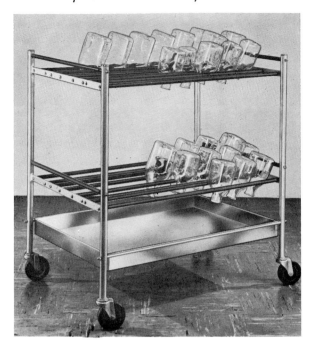

FIGURE 16-9. Portable flask drain carriage.

washing. If they are permitted to stand for several hours before filling, the final rinsing process with freshly distilled water must be repeated.

Reclaimed flasks or bottles such as commercial intravenous solution bottles should never be used for the preparation of solutions. Such containers are made of soft glass, which chips and breaks easily. Investigations show also that the glass itself breaks down after repeated exposure to chemicals and intense heat.

FLASK CLOSURES

An automatic self-sealing closure should be used on all parenteral or external solution flasks. The combination closure consisting of collar and cap when applied to the glass container must provide safe storage of the sterilized solution under hermetically sealed conditions. The collar should be of molded, nontoxic, heat-resistant neoprene or equal which retains its resiliency after repeated sterilization. It should not become tacky nor should it stick to either the container or the cap. The cap should be fabricated from a heat-resistant plastic, with smooth surfaces accurately formed to fit perfectly and securely over the top and flanged edge of the companion collar. All collars and caps must be free from easily detached fragments or particles.

A typical example of one kind of self-sealing closure is shown in Figures

16-10A, 10B, and 10C. The first illustrates the collar in position on the flask with the cap engaged. The cap locks on the collar and it will not fall off when the flask is moved about. The lip of the collar is slightly compressed by the cap when in proper position, thus sealing out possible airborne contamination.

Figure 16-10B shows the position of the cap and collar during sterilization. Due to the rise in temperature and pressure during sterilization, the liquid and air in the flask expand, and when an internal pressure of 1½ pounds is reached, the seal between the lip of the collar and the top of the cap is broken, thus permitting the trapped air to escape. In this manner all excess vapor and air are evacuated from the flask during sterilization.

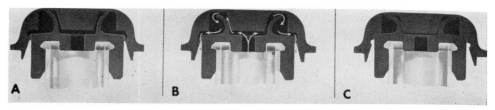

FIGURE 16-10 A. Automatic sealing and venting closure. This shows position of cap on collar before sterilization. B. Position of cab on collar showing pathway for escape of air from flask when 1½ pounds pressure has developed in flask during sterilization. C. Position of cap automatically sealed on collar by vacuum after solution has been sterilized.

Figure 16-10C shows the collar and cap after sterilization. When the internal pressure of the flask drops below 1½ pounds, the seal between the lip of the collar and cap will again be in effect. In the process of cooling, the liquid in the flask will revert to its original volume less the amount lost by vaporization. Since the primary seal between the lip of the collar and the cap will not permit entry of air, a vacuum results which draws the cap down tightly onto the collar forming a triple seal as illustrated. All collars and caps must be thoroughly cleaned and rinsed with freshly distilled water before placing on flasks.

The new disposable closure (Fig. 16-11) is specially designed to free vapors from the flask during the sterilization cycle. When the temperature of the solution falls below 212°F, a positive hermetic seal is formed by the closure. This vacuum seal maintains sterility indefinitely, a condition indicated visually by the depression in the closure created by the vacuum. If the vacuum seal is broken at any time prior to actual use of the solution, the closure pops back to its normally contoured position. The closure can be removed aseptically from the flask by pulling the tab back gently as shown. When closures show signs of softening, cracking, or hardening, they should be discarded. Closures which have deteriorated reduce the reliability of the her-

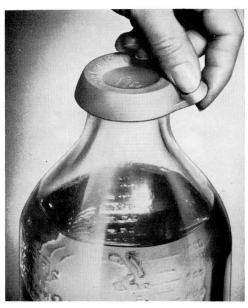

FIGURE 16-11. Disposable closure for solution flasks. It provides a positive hermetic seal, indicated visually—not by hand testing for water hammer.

metic vacuum seal and some leakage may take place. When this occurs, the sterility of the contents of the flask is doubtful. Attempted reuse of disposable closures is hazardous and should not be permitted.

PHYSICAL FACILITIES

The space for the solution room should be adequate to permit selective placement of all equipment, free movement of working personnel, and storage of all materials. Arrangement of the various work stations should be in logical sequence, conducive to efficient workflow and segregation of cleanup activities from preparation and flasking activities. The work flow for a solution room is shown in Figure 16-6B.

The solution room should be completely enclosed to control air-borne contaminants. Air is a source of contamination since it contains dust particles and droplets. A clear understanding of air contamination is very important, not only in the operation of a solution room but also in the planning.

The quality of distilled water is dependent on the type of still, the method of maintenance, and the efficiency of operation. Only distilled water measuring above 250,000 specific ohms resistance should be used. The interval of time between the collection of distilled water and its use for the preparation of solutions is of the utmost importance. Solutions should be prepared as soon as possible after the distilled water is collected—within 4 hours. Equally important is control of the time lapse between preparation of solutions and their sterilization. Sterilization should follow as soon as possible, within one hour, to prevent a substantial increase in microbial populations.

Mechanical equipment is of primary importance in the solution room and it should be used wherever possible as an aid in decreasing the chance of human error. Items such as portable automatically controlled flask washer, a premix tank, a flask filler, portable carts, flask draining carts, borosilicate flasks, and automatic sealing closures are desirable for the efficient operation of the solution room.

The portable automatic flask washer, while designed for rapid and efficient washing of flasks, is flexible in function. It can also be used for other purposes such as washing laboratory bottles and other related glassware. The portable automatic flask washer (Fig. 16-8) operates at the rate of six flasks per minute. During the automatic cycle, each flask is given an initial rinse inside and out with hot tap water. This is followed by two detergent washes and a rinse of hot tap water. A final rinse of distilled water leaves the flask clean. The complete cycle requires 1 minute during which time six soiled flasks are inserted and six clean flasks removed. An automatic cutoff stops the washer if the distilled water supply is exhausted, thus eliminating risk of missing the final rinse. Distilled water consumption averages about 400 ml per flask, so that 20 gallons will rinse approximately two hundred flasks. Manual washing and rinsing is a tedious and monotonous task. When a large number of flasks is involved, it is difficult to insure thorough cleaning unless a mechanical washer is used. Mechanical cleaning not only provides standard cleaning for each flask, but also reduces labor and cost.

The processing of flasks can be further expedited through the use of the portable flask drain cart, shown in Figure 16-9. This cart is designed to allow thorough draining of flasks after washing and rinsing. It will hold flasks in an inverted position, protecting the inside from air contamination. It also provides a means of transporting flasks in volume to the filling area.

Hospitals using sterile saline and other external solutions in large volumes may find it more efficient to use a premix tank for their preparation. The premix unit (Fig. 16-12) is a highly practical device for mixing, filtering, and filling accurately compounded solutions. The capacity and simplicity of the unit make it ideal for the large volume of isotonic solutions required. Accurately determined amounts varying from 40 to 200 liters of solution can be made, mixed, and flasked in an extremely short time. The responsibility for weighing and measuring the solute should be that of the pharmacist. Another external solution preparation facility is shown in Figure 16-13. This mobile unit fills flasks automatically with no overflow and no underfill.

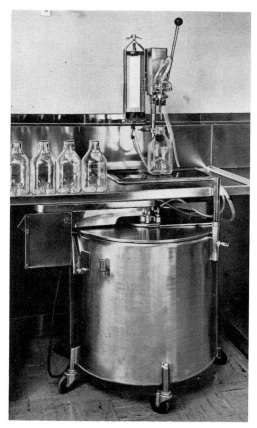

FIGURE 16-12. Portable premix tank of 200 liters capacity. For use with batch method for preparation of solutions.

PREPARATION OF PARENTERAL SOLUTIONS

The subject of parenteral therapy is of the utmost importance to clinicians and hospitals. The word "parenteral" is derived from the Greek, meaning "not through the alimentary canal."[45] In normal usage the term parenteral therapy is applied to the method of administering fluids through veins. The purposes of parenteral therapy are to maintain or replace body stores of water, electrolytes, calories, vitamins, and protein; to restore acid-base balance; and to restore blood volume. Safe intravenous solutions are, therefore, required to achieve these purposes and to meet the individual needs of each patient.

There are a number of courses available to hospitals to meet the increasing demands for safe parenteral solutions. The institution may purchase the commercially prepared products, or may manufacture its own solutions, or engage in both these procedures. Manufacture of solutions in the hospital is particularly attractive because the economics involved results in a marked

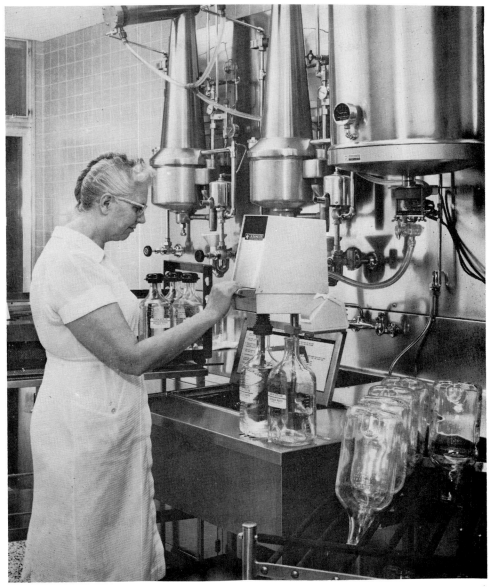

FIGURE 16-13. External solution preparation facility, for the automatic filling of flasks with no overflow and no underfill.

savings for the institution. Many hospitals currently prepare their own solutions, and there is a convincing body of evidence to show that these solutions are safe, economical, and practical.[17,46,47,48] Other hospitals are also desirous of reducing costs of solutions used in parenteral therapy, but they are reluctant to undertake the manufacturing program because of fear of untoward allergic or febrile reactions. This fear complex is founded largely upon unsatisfactory past experiences in certain hospitals where the solutions were prepared under conditions believed to be safe and practical at the time. It is now known that these past failures to produce satisfactory solutions were almost invariably due to inadequate cleaning facilities, lack of control on quality of distilled water, improvised equipment, and lack of skilled supervision.

The preparation of chemically pure, sterile, and nonpyrogenic solutions is not a difficult matter, provided the materials used in manufacturing are of high purity, and if the personnel responsible for cleaning of the apparatus are thoroughly reliable. A dependable system for hospital-made solutions comprises the following major elements:

· *Proper planning of the solution room.* Adequate space should be provided in a room designed specifically for this purpose. It may be located as a part of or adjacent to the pharmacy or in the Central Service Department.

· *Adequate cleaning facilities.* Efficient methods must be used for the cleaning of all apparatus, bottles, and closures entering into the manufacture of solutions.

· *Purity of distilled water.* A source of high purity, nonpyrogenic distillate is essential. Water stills should be equipped with conductivity recorders for a continuous check on the purity of the distillate.

· *Purity of chemicals.* All chemicals used in making the solutions must be of high purity and free from pyrogenic substances.

· *Disposable intravenous administration sets.* It is no longer considered safe or practical for the hospital to employ reusable intravenous sets. The availability of disposable commercial sets which are sterile, nontoxic and nonpyrogenic is an added incentive to the hospital-made-solution program.

· *Needle cleaning facilities.* Chemical cleanliness of needles is essential for safe, reactionless infusions. There is an increasing trend to use disposable needles.

· *Skilled supervision.* Centralized responsibility for the preparation of solutions should be delegated to the hospital pharmacist, microbiologist, or pathologist.

STERILIZATION OF HEAT-SENSITIVE SOLUTIONS

Careless operation of the sterilizer, use of too much heat or an unduly prolonged exposure period will destroy or seriously impair the quality of certain solutions. When difficulty is encountered, the cause is almost invariably oversterilization. The exposure period selected must be adequate for each individual flask or bottle in the sterilizer. The total number of flasks placed in the sterilizer is not important. The time required for the sterilizer to reach 250°F will vary with the size of the load. Exposure at this temperature is dependent upon the largest flask in the load. For example, 1000-milliliter flasks of dextrose solution are normally and properly sterilized in

30 minutes exposure, with the sterilizer operating at maximum controlled temperature of 250° to 254°F. The average small bottle or flask of procaine solution (1 or 2 ounces) will receive the same sterilizing effect in 12 to 15 minutes at this temperature. Obviously the two containers should not be sterilized in the same load, unless the procaine solution is of the correct pH which increases heat stability.

Murphy and Stoklosa[49] have studied the effect of autoclaving on the stability of solutions of alkaloidal salts, including procaine hydrochloride. Their findings indicated that such solutions may be sterilized by autoclaving, under properly controlled conditions, without significantly affecting their potency. The optimum pH range for maximum stability of solutions of alkaloidal salts was found to be from 2.9 to 4.8, before and after sterilization. According to Bullock and Cannell,[50] procaine hydrochloride solutions are most stable at a pH of 3.0 to 3.5. In this range they may be autoclaved at 250°F for as long as 2 hours with only 2.5 per cent decomposition.

The reliability of low heat (marginal) sterilization with the addition of preservatives such as chlorobutanol, thiomerosal, and benzyl alcohol to heat-labile parenteral solutions has been questioned. Studies[51] have shown that preservatives do not enhance the destructive effect of heat. A low pH is more efficacious than an auxiliary agent in promoting sterilization at lower temperatures.

The importance of heat sterilization of spinal anesthetic ampuls should not be overlooked. If ampuls are autoclaved with the spinal anesthetic tray or setup, they are subjected to sterilization for a prolonged time which may cause deterioration of the anesthetic agents. This subject has been investigated by Golden[52] and Gerlich *et al.*[53] Their findings indicated that spinal anesthetic drugs could be reautoclaved (15 to 20 minutes at 248°F) up to five times without serious loss of potency. However, it has been mentioned by others[54] that excessive autoclaving of Pontocaine® and Novocain® solutions may result in a hydrolytic breakdown of the anesthetics. The indications are that most spinal anesthetic drugs may be autoclaved *once* at a temperature of 250°F for 15 minutes. The vasoconstrictor compounds such as epinephrine are more heat labile and the exposure time should be reduced to 10 minutes at 250°F. They should not be reautoclaved.

After sterilization, pressure in the sterilizer must be exhausted slowly. Otherwise, violent ebullition will take place which will result in blown stoppers and an undue loss of fluid. At best, under the most careful regulation of exhaust, there will be a loss of 3 to 5 per cent of the fluid by vaporization. This establishes a general rule for making up solutions which should be observed. Add an extra 5 per cent of distilled water to each flask so that the sterilized product will have the concentration intended.

The practice of permitting the entire sterilizer to cool down slowly after solution sterilization prolongs exposure to excessive heat. In the case of heat-sensitive solutions, this may be detrimental, as evidenced by discoloration. The most satisfactory method calls for some skill and care in regulation of the exhaust, as follows:

> At the close of the exposure period, turn off all heat to the sterilizer. Close the valve admitting steam to the chamber, and then adjust the chamber exhaust valve slightly open to a degree that will permit exhaust of pressure to zero in not less than 10 to 15 minutes. With this method, the heat of the solution will be dissipated without violent ebullition, and at about the same rate at which the pressure is reduced.

INFANT FORMULAS

The preparation of infant formulas is not directly associated with the preparation and sterilization of solutions. Three principal methods for providing formulas to nursery infants are currently recognized in the United States. They are 1) preparation of the formula entirely in the hospital formula room, 2) final preparation of formula in the hospital from components, presterilized, packaged, and delivered from an outside source, and 3) use of individually packaged presterilized formula delivered by an outside source.

Wherever formulas are prepared, it is necessary to subject them to a terminal heating process. This is the only practical method which gives assurance of bacteriologically safe milk mixtures for infants. The time-temperature relationship of the process must be adequate to destroy pathogens, including the inactivation of viruses. Whereas sterility of the formula is desirable, it is not always attainable. The amount of heat that can be applied is limited by the fragile character of milk which, if heating is too severe, will undergo both physical and nutritional damage.

At the present time authorities recognize two methods for terminal heating of formulas: the nonpressure (flowing steam) process at 212°F for 30 minutes and the pressure steam method conducted at 230°F for 10 minutes. Both methods have their advantages and disadvantages. The pressure method may give a higher percentage of sterile formulas; but it also presents several opportunities for chemical or physical changes such as carmelization of the sugar in formulas, coagulation of milk proteins, boiling of formulas resulting in clogged nipples, and the plugging of the chamber drain line of the sterilizer which occurs when formulas boil over and coagulated milk gains access to the outlet valve. The nonpressure method is regarded by many as the superior technic for the terminal heating of formulas. When the pressure method is followed in an automatically controlled sterilizer with careful attention given to all phases of the sterilizing cycle, the results are satisfactory.

Upon completion of the terminal heating process, the formulas are removed from the sterilizer, cooled at room temperature for one hour, and then placed in a refrigerator of adequate (cooling) capacity with a holding temperature of 40°F (5°C). Cooling of formulas in tap water is not recommended because of the possibility of contamination being transferred to the exterior of the bottles, then carried into the refrigerator and, finally, to the nursery.

COOLING SOLUTIONS BY EXTERNAL ABSORPTION OF HEAT

Various systems are available for cooling solutions in either flint or borosilicate glass bottles. All depend upon the external absorption of heat by applying a cooling medium to the outside of the containers of solution. This is accomplished as follows:

> Upon completion of the sterilizing period, compressed air is admitted to the chamber to raise the pressure about 3 psig above the sterilizing range. This seals the self-venting flask closures and prevents the cooling water, introduced subsequently, from entering the flasks. Finally, when the compressed air has reduced the load to approximately 240°F (115°C), cold tap water is sprayed over the bottles, after which the water flows to the waste.

The kind of spray cooling system selected is determined by the type of solution containers used. Borosilicate glass bottles withstand the thermal shock caused by direct spraying with cold tap water. Flint glass bottles require the temperature of the spray water to be reduced gradually during the cooling period. The system is best applied when made a part of the automatic controls on the sterilizer. Spray cooling systems make it possible to process a load of solutions in about one-half the time required with a standard solution exhaust accelerator valve.

STORAGE OF SOLUTIONS

The amount of space and the location required for storage depend upon the volume of solutions consumed in the hospital. The type of storage at the point of use depends upon the temperature preferences of the medical staff. Although the fear of causing shock by application of cold has largely disappeared, the tendency to employ hot compresses in hemostasis is still present to some degree.[55] Many authorities concur that the sterile solution used to moisten sponges during an operation should be kept at approximately body temperature. In urological procedures, the trend is to introduce the solution into the patient at body temperature. However, solutions at room temperature are still generally used.

In view of the change in philosophy concerning the applications of hot solutions, storage facilities should no longer present a problem. The external solutions may be stored in Central Service at room temperature and distributed daily as needed. Critical areas requiring higher temperature solutions can be serviced by keeping reserve flasks in thermostatically heated cabinets as shown in Figure 16-14.

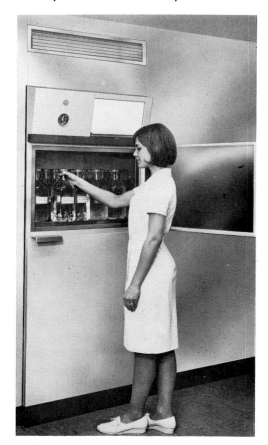

FIGURE 16-14. Flask warming cabinet.

SIGNIFICANCE OF TESTS TO DETERMINE QUALITY
OF PARENTERAL SOLUTIONS

Can hospitals make satisfactory solutions without an elaborate testing program? This question is frequently asked by administrators, medical and surgical staffs, and other professional workers who concern themselves with the problems of parenteral therapy. Many of these people labor under the impression that it is essential to maintain a biologics testing laboratory, including an animal colony, in order to make pyrogen and sterility tests on each batch of solutions prepared in the hospital. Such an understanding is not entirely correct. To be sure, if pyrogen tests are to be performed routinely on solutions, it is necessary to have available a sufficient number of test animals. The availability of a simple bacteriological test for pyrogens has been mentioned.[35] Although this test is not official in the U.S. Pharmacopoeia, it is apparently as valid as the rabbit test and would yield the same information as is given by the rabbit test. This procedure, as well as sterility tests, can be performed in the bacteriology section of the clinical laboratory of any hospital. The basic reasons for concern about the element of testing stem from unsatisfactory experiences in certain hospitals in the past when solutions were made under adverse conditions with makeshift equipment, and more recently from "scare selling" on the part of biased individuals trying to prevent hospitals from making their own intravenous solutions.

The significance of tests to determine the quality of solutions should be thoroughly understood. Certainly it is not the author's intent to discourage the testing of solutions in any hospital providing that suitable facilities are available. Rather, it is the intent to point out that the hospital need not institute an elaborate testing program to safeguard the production of intravenous solutions. It is acknowledged, however, that in the beginning and for the first few months' operation of a new solution room, the quality of the solutions produced should be firmly established, in order to convince doubtful persons as to the safety and quality of product. This factor of safety and assurance is as much a responsibility of the manufacturer of the equipment as it is of the hospital. When a new solution room is opened, it should be the responsibility of the equipment supplier to thoroughly instruct the hospital personnel in the preparation of solutions, as well as to periodically collect samples of the solutions for pyrogen test, sterility test, and chemical assay. These tests should be made by some responsible laboratory and a report issued in writing to the hospital as substantial proof of the safety of the system and to show that the quality of the solutions meets the requirements of the U.S. Pharmacopoeia in every respect.

When parenteral solutions are properly prepared from freshly distilled water and high-purity chemicals, it is not necessary to routinely test each lot for pyrogenic reactions. Of the many hospitals now making their own solutions, very few routinely perform pyrogen tests. There are a few authorities, however, who insist upon a biologic test as an additional safeguard in establishing the quality of the product or as an occasional check on a lot of material which may be under suspicion. Even then it must be admitted that the biologic test for pyrogens is not conducted routinely but rather on a periodic basis, either monthly or semi-monthly, on random samples taken from the stock of freshly prepared (sterile) solutions made the day of the test. If an occasional pyrogen test is required it should be conducted as follows:

> Use rabbits (1500 gm or more) maintained at least 1 week on an unrestricted diet and which are not losing weight. Animals which have been previously used for pyrogen tests must have a rest period of at least 2 days. Use clinical thermometers previously tested to determine time required to record a maximum temperature. Two days before test, take 4 temperature readings every 2 hours and reject animals with temperatures above 39.8° C. House test animals in individual cages and keep them at

uniform environmental temperature ± 5° for at least 48 hours before the test day.

Performance of Test

· Perform test at the same temperature as the animal quarters.

· Use three animals for each test.

· Withhold food 1 hour before test is started and for the duration of the test. Water may be allowed.

· Take a control test 15 minutes before injection of test material. Animals may be used if the control temperature is above 38.9°C and below 39.8°C.

· Warm product to be tested to about 37°C and inject through ear vein 10 ml/kg. (Use only syringes and needles known to be pyrogen-free by heating in a muffle furnace at 250°C for 30 minutes.)

· Record temperature every hour for 3 hours.

· A positive test for pyrogens is demonstrated if two of the three rabbits show a temperature rise of 0.6°C or greater. If only one animal shows such a rise, or if the sum of the temperature rises of the three animals exceeds 1.4°C, the test must be repeated, using five rabbits. The test shall be considered positive if two or more of the group of five rabbits show an individual rise in temperature of 0.6°C or more above the normal established for these animals.

SUMMARY

Procedure for Processing External Solutions

The objective of any program for the preparation of external solutions should be to produce solutions of high quality—solutions in which the user can have complete confidence. To accomplish this, a procedure must be followed that is both technically sound and functionally practical. In addition, it must be carried out by well trained and reliable personnel. The following outlined procedure at the end of this chapter is offered as a guide for implementation into a variety of situations.

REFERENCES

1. IRWIN, J. R., BECK, W. D.; FOLK, R. M.; HEFFELFINGER, R. E., and MILLER, P. D.: An Evaluation of the Effect of Materials of Still Construction on Quality of Distillate. Report from Battelle Memorial Institute, Columbus, Ohio, Dec. 30, 1965.

2. FRIEND, W. Z.: The importance of high purity water data to industrial applications. *Corrosion, 13*:81-85, 1957.

3. STRUBLE, R. W.: Materials for Handling Deionized Water. Technical Memorandum No. 51, (Battelle Institute), NYO, Sept. 6, 1957.

4. BRITTON, S. C.: The Corrosion Resistance of Tin and Tin Alloys. Tin Research Institute, April, 1952.

5. LOWENHEIM, F. A.; WOOFTER, R. A., and HARTWELL, R. R.: Tin and tin plate. In *Corrosion Resistance of Metals and Alloys*. Laque, F. L., and Copsen, H. R. (Eds.) ACS Monograph No. 158, Chap. II, New York, Reinhold, 1963.

6. MYERS, J. A.: The thermocompressor still. *Pharm J*, Aug. 4, 1962, p. 109-111.

7. *Manual on Industrial Water*. ASTM Publication No. 148-B, Am. Soc. Test. Materials, Philadelphia, 1956, p. 422.

8. ECKEL, J. F.: Introduction to symposium on corrosion by high purity water. *Corrosion,* 13:70, 1957.

9. REITLER, R., and SELIGMANN, R.: *Pseudomonas aeruginosa* in drinking water. *J Appl Bact,* 20:145-150, 1957.

10. MICHALSON, A. W.: Monitoring water quality with the Solu Bridge. *The Analyzer,* 8:18-20, 1967.

11. SPOEHR, H. A., SMITH, J. H. C.; STRAIN, H. H.; MILNER, H. W., and HARDIN, G. J.: *Fatty Acid Antibacterials from Plants.* Carnegie Institution of Washington, Publication No. 586, Washington, D.C., 1949.

12. PRICE, S. A., and GARE, L.: A source of error in microbiological assays attributable to a bacterial inhibitor. *Nature, 183*:838-840, 1959.

13. GELDREICH, E. E., and CLARK, H. F.: Distilled water suitability for microbiological applications. *J Milk Food Tech,* 28:351-355, 1965.

14. HIESTER, N. K., and PHILLIPS, R. C.: Ion exchange. *Chem Eng, 61*:161, 1954.

15. MOON, B. H.: A report on deionized water in hospital pharmacy use. *Hosp Manage,* 97:78-84, 1964.

16. JEFFREY, L. P., and FISH, K. H., JR.: Deionized water—an evaluation. *Amer J Hosp Pharm,* 21:497-500, 1964.

17. WALTER, C. W.: The relation of proper preparation of solutions for intravenous therapy to febrile reactions. *Ann Surg, 112*:603-617, 1940.

18. WHITTET, T. D.: The occurrence and importance of pyrogens. *J Pharm Pharmacol, 6*:304-309, 1954.

19. NESSET, N. M.; MCLALLEN, J.; ANTHONY, P. Z., and GINGER, L. G.: Bacterial pyrogens. I. Pyrogenic preparation from a *Pseudomonas* species. *J Amer Pharm Ass, 39*:456-459, 1950.

20. WALKER, J.: A method for isolation of toxic and immunizing fractions from bacteria of the *Salmonella* group. *Biochem J, 34*:325, 1940.

21. NOWOTNY, A.: Molecular biology of gram-negative bacterial lipopolysaccharides. *Ann N Y Acad Sci, 133*:277-786, 1966.

22. WEBSTER, M. E.; SAGIN, J. F.; LANDY, M., and JOHNSON, A. G.: Studies on the O antigen of *Salmonella typhosa.* I. Purification of antigen. *J Immunol, 74*:455-465, 1955.

23. LANDY, M., and JOHNSON, A. G.: Studies on the O antigen of *Salmonella typhosa.* IV. Endotoxic properties of the purified antigen. *Proc Soc Exp Biol Med, 90*:57-62, 1955.

24. LANDY, M.; JOHNSON, A. G.; WEBSTER, M. E., and SAGIN, J. F.: Studies on the O antigen of *Salmonella typhosa.* II. Immunologic properties of the purified antigen. *J Immunol,* 74:466-478, 1955.

25. CO TUI, F. W., and SCHRIFT, M. H.: Production of pyrogen by some bacteria. *J Lab Clin Med,* 27:569-575, 1942.

26. LEES, J. C., and LEVVY, G. A.: Emergency preparation of pyrogen-free water. *Brit Med J,* 1:430-432, 1940.

27. SEIBERT, F. B.: Fever producing substance found in some distilled waters. *Amer J Physiol,* 67:90-104, 1923, and The case of many febrile reactions following intravenous infusions. *Amer J Physiol,* 71:621-651, 1924.

28. RADEMAKER, L. A.: The cause of elimination of reactions after intravenous infusions. *Ann Surg,* 92:195-201, 1930.

29. CO TUI, F. W.; MCCLOSKEY, K. L.; SCHRIFT, M., and YATES, A. L.: New method of preparing infusion fluids based on removal of pyrogens by filtration. *JAMA,* 109:250, 1937.

30. CO TUI, F. W., and WRIGHT, A. M.: The preparation of nonpyrogenic infusion and other intravenous fluids by adsorptive filtration. *Ann. Surg, 116*:412-425, 1942.

31. BRINDLE and RIGBY: Preparation of nonpyrogenic water and infusion fluids. *Quart J Pharm Pharmacol, 19*:302, 1946.

32. BANKS, H. M.: Study of hyperpyrexia reaction following intravenous therapy. *Amer J Clin Path, 4*:260, 1934.

33. WYLIE, D. W., and TODD, J. P.: An examination of the sources and the quantitative methods of testing pyrogen. *Quart J Pharm Pharmacol,* 21:240-252, 1948.

34. MARCUS, S., ANSELMO, C., and PERKINS, J. J.: Studies on bacterial pyrogenicity. I. Quantitative basis. *Proc Soc Exp Biol Med, 99*:359-362, 1958.

35. MARCUS, S.; ANSELMO, C., and LUKE, J.: Studies on bacterial pyrogenicity. II. A bacterial test for pyrogens in parenteral solutions. *J Amer Pharm Assn,* (Sci ed), *49*:616-619, 1960.

36. RADEMAKER, L.: Intravenous solutions: Facts and fancies. *J Int Coll Surg, 11*:194-199, 1948.

37. RADEMAKER, L.: Reactions to intravenous administration of solutions. *JAMA, 135*:1140-1141, 1947.

38. PIERCE, J. M., JR.: The treatment of water intoxication following transurethral prostatectomy. *J Urol, 87*:181, 1962.

39. NOTES and COMMENTS: Hazards of boric acid. Hospitals. *JAHA, 35*:66, 1961.

40. FOLEY, F. E. B.: Fluid supply apparatus for cystoscopy and transurethral operations. *J Urol, 79*:896, 1958.

41. HOYT, S.; GOEBEL, J. L.; LEE, H., and SCHOENBROD, J.: Types of shock-like reaction during transurethral resection and relation to acute renal failure. *J Urol, 79*:500-506, 1958.

42. PIERCE, J. M., JR.: The treatment of water intoxication following transurethral prostatectomy. *J Urol, 87*:181-183, 1962.

43. HAGSTROM, R. S.: Studies on fluid absorption during transurethral prostatic resection. *J Urol, 73*:852, 1955.

44. PENNISI, S. A.; ROWLAND, H. S., JR.; VINSON, C. E., and BUNTS, R. C.: Hyponatremia as affected by various irrigants used during transurethral electroresection of the prostate. *J Urol, 86*:249-258, 1961.

45. DORLAND, W. A. N.: *Dorland's Illustrated Medical Dictionary,* 24th ed. Philadelphia, Saunders, 1965, p. 1102.

46. LARSEN, F. L.: Considerations in the preparation of parenteral solutions—a case study. *Bull Amer Soc Hosp Pharm, 10*:210-219, 1953.

47. LISWOOD, S., and FINER, N. S.: The best "buy" in parenteral solutions? *Mod Hosp,* pp. 90-94, May, 1955.

48. ZUGICH, J. J.: Parenteral fluids in the hospital. *Pharm Internat, 4*:9-48-54, 1950.

49. MURPHY, J. T., and STOKLOSA, M. J.: Effect of autoclaving on the stability of solutions of certain thermolabile substances. *Bull Amer Soc Hosp Pharm, 9*:94-97, 1952.

50. BULLOCK, K., and CANNELL, J. S.: The preparation of solutions of procaine and adrenaline hydrochlorides for surgical use. *Quart J Pharm Pharmacol, 14*:241-251, 1941.

51. KRAMER, N.: The influence of preservatives on low heat sterilization. *Bull Parenteral Drug Ass, 12*:10, 1958.

52. GOLDEN, A. A.: Sterilization of ampuls for spinal anesthesia. *J Amer Osteopath Ass, 57*:261, 1957.

53. GERLICH, N. A., NICHOLES, P. S., and BALLINGER, C. M.: Heat sterilization of spinal anesthetic ampuls. *Anesthesiology, 19*:394-399, 1958.

54. SLEVIN, D.: Personal Communication. Dec. 2, 1965.

55. WILLMANN, V. L., and HANLON, R. C.: The influence of temperature on surface bleeding, favorable effects of local hypothermia. *Ann Surg, 143*:660, 1956.

Procedure	Directives to Be Incorporated in Technique	Explanation of Directives
I. PRE-PREPARATION Care of used flasks—point of use.	Empty any remaining solution from flask; replace cap.	Assembled units simplify handling and cleaning. Less loss of caps. Protects inside of flasks from soil.
	Place flask in designated holding area.	
Transfer to solution room.	Hold flasks in collection area and transfer at predetermined intervals.	
	Place in cleanup area of solution room.	Used flasks should be confined to soiled area. Places them in proper location for cleaning.
II. CLEANING OPERATIONS Start water stills.	First, open water valve. When water overflows, open steam valve.	Only freshly distilled water should be used for rinsing. One gallon of distilled water is required for rinsing approximately ten (10) flasks.
	Turn on conductivity meter; discard initial distillate; begin collecting distillate when conductivity meter indicates a resistance exceeding 250,000 specific ohms.	Only distilled water with a reading above 250,000 specific ohms resistance is suitable.
Disassemble flasks.	Remove and discard date sticker from cap; remove cap; place in washing sink.	Flask closures must be disassembled for thorough cleansing of all surfaces.
	Remove collar, using collar remover; place collars in sink with caps.	Collar remover simplifies and speeds removal.
	Remove identification label.	
	Place flasks as near cleaning facilities as possible.	Cart facilitates handling and transfer.
Wash and rinse flask units.		Thorough cleaning of flask closures is essential.
Reusable flask closures.	Use hot water (110°–120°F) containing a low-sudsing detergent.	Free rinsing detergent should be used.
	Scrub each cap and collar with brush; be sure to reach all surfaces.	Nylon bristle brush is preferred.

Procedure	Directives to Be Incorporated in Technique	Explanation of Directives
	Place in rinsing sink; rinse thoroughly with tap water.	Rinsing should include copious use of water. There should be no trace of residual detergent.
	Rinse thoroughly with distilled water.	
	Inspect caps and collars for quality; discard chipped or cracked caps; discard collars that are worn, cracked, or distorted.	Damaged closures will not maintain seal.
	Reassemble caps and collars.	Caps and collars should be assembled before they are applied to flasks. If the collar is applied to the flask separately, the lip may be crimped when the cap is applied.
	Place in plastic bag; fill with distilled water; agitate; drain water from bag; twist top to form closed package with caps and collars inside.	Provides protection until time when closures are needed.
	or	
	Place in stainless steel container (bucket); fill with distilled water; cover container with plastic canopy.	Protects closures until needed. Cover should be lint-free.
	Transfer to filling area.	Ready for use.
Treatment of new reusable flask closures before initial use.	Immerse collars and caps in a container of low-sudsing detergent.	This process conditions the caps and collars, and also removes dust and particles acquired during manufacturing and storage.
	Place container in the autoclave and process for 30 minutes at 250°F.	
	Remove from detergent solution and rinse thoroughly with tap water.	All residual detergent must be removed.
	Rinse thoroughly with distilled water.	
	Place in circulation.	

Procedure	*Directives to Be Incorporated in Technique*	*Explanation of Directives*
Disposable closures.	Place in distilled water prior to use.	This permits final rinse; also simplifies applying to flask.
Identification labels.	Disposable—Pregummed.	Apply and date.
	Transfer to filling area.	Ready for use.
Flasks.		Thorough cleansing of flasks is essential for preparation of safe solutions.
	Mechanical Cleaning (preferred method)	Provides a standard cleaning method which is efficient and rapid.
	Use mechanical flask washer whenever one is available.	
	Follow manufacturer's operating instructions. The cycle includes: Initial rinse inside and outside with hot tap water Two jet washes inside and outside with hot water containing low-sudsing detergent Hot tap water rinse Final rinse with distilled water.	Removes residue of solution. Free rinsing detergent is necessary.
	Remove from washer.	
	Inspect each flask for "water breaks" and damage. Return unclean flasks for rewash; discard damaged flasks.	Interior should be crystal clear with no breaks (spots) in distilled water film left on glass after final rinse. Chipped or cracked flasks should not be used.
	Place on drain cart in the inverted position.	Inverted position allows final rinse water to drain; less chance of dust or other foreign particles settling on mouth or inside of flask.
	Transfer drainage cart to filling area.	Flasks are ready for use.
	Repeat distilled water rinse if not filled within four hours.	Removes any foreign particles which might have collected during holding period.
	Manual Cleaning (alternate method)	Standard cleaning of each flask is difficult to insure.

Procedure	Directives to Be Incorporated in Technique	Explanation of Directives
	Rinse each flask with hot (110°–120°F) tap water.	Removes any residue of solution.
	Wash each flask in hot water (110°–120°F) containing a low-sudsing detergent.	Detergent should be free rinsing.
	Use long handled brush to scrub inside of flask.	Nylon bristle brush is preferred.
	Rinse thoroughly with tap water.	Rinsing should include copious use of water.
	Rinse thoroughly with distilled water.	
	Inspect each flask for "water breaks" and for damage; re-wash unclean flasks; discard damaged flasks.	Chipped or cracked flasks should not be used.
	Place on drain cart in the inverted position.	Inverted position allows final rinse water to drain; less chance of dust or other foreign particles settling on the mouth or inside flask.
	Transfer drainage cart to filling area.	Flasks are ready for use.
	Repeat distilled water rinse if not filled within four hours.	Removes any foreign particles which might have collected during holding period.
III. PREPARATION OF EXTERNAL SOLUTIONS Distilled water	Use only freshly distilled water from an efficient water still equipped with conductivity meter. Reading must be above 250,000 specific ohms resistance.	Purity of water used for external solutions should equal that for parenteral solutions.
	Fill flasks by use of hand dispenser attached to Tygon tubing leading from reservoir of still.	Facilitates filling of flasks.
	Insert dispenser in mouth of flask and fill to required level.	
	Apply identification label for distilled water.	Labels applied to flasks as filled reduce the risk of errors.
	Apply preassembled reusable cap and collar or disposable closure to flask.	Assembled unit is easier to apply; less chance of faulty closure.
		Disposable closures are more dependable.
	Place finished flasks on sterilizer loading car.	Minimizes handling of flasks.

Procedure	Directives to Be Incorporated in Technique	Explanation of Directives
Normal saline.	Use only chemically pure sodium chloride.	Conforms to requirements of U. S. Pharmacopoeia.
	Use only freshly distilled water of above 250,000 specific ohms resistance.	Purity of water used for external solutions should equal that for parenteral solutions.
	Bulk (Batch) *Method*	
	Use large mixing tank equipped with facilities for bulk dilution, filtration, and semiautomatic dispensing of finished solution.	Facilitates production of normal saline when volume is required.
	Follow mixing and dispensing instructions provided by the manufacturer.	
	Use sodium chloride weighed by pharmacist to the prescribed grams per 100 m distilled water (weight to volume).	Pharmacist should be responsible for weighing of all chemicals used in preparing external solutions. Assures accuracy of finished product.
	Apply identification label for Normal Saline.	Labels applied to flasks as filled reduce the risk of errors.
	Apply preassembled reusable cap and collar or disposable closure to flask.	Assembled unit is easier to apply; less chance of faulty closure.
		Disposable closures are more dependable.
	Place finished flasks on sterilizer loading car.	Minimizes handling of flasks.
	Single Unit Method	Used when pre-mix tank is not available or whenever small number of flasks are prepared.
	Use premeasured (weight or volume) concentrate of sodium chloride supplied by pharmacist.	Pharmacist should prepare and dispense concentrate.
	Use distilled-water hand dispenser attached to Tygon tubing leading from reservoir of still.	
	Insert dispenser into mouth of flask and fill to required level.	The required level is indicated by the mark above the 250 ml, 500 ml, 1000 ml, 1500 ml or 2000 ml graduation; it allows for evaporation during sterilization process, leaving solutions of proper concentration.

Procedure	Directives to Be Incorporated in Technique	Explanation of Directives
Boric acid solution.	Follow labeling and closure instructions for Bulk (Batch) Method.	Quantity is usually limited
	Follow instructions for preparation of solutions (filling, labeling, and closing), using single unit method, as described under Normal Saline.	Eliminates chance for error by operator.
	Never combine the preparation of boric acid solution with preparation of other solutions.	Pharmacist must prepare concentrate used in making external solutions.
	Use preweighed boric acid crystals (weighed by pharmacist) for desired concentration.	
Magnesium sulfate solution.	Follow instructions for preparation of solutions (filling, labeling, and closing), using single unit method, as described under Normal Saline.	Eliminates chance for error by operator.
	Never combine the preparation of magnesium sulfate solution with the preparation of other solutions.	Pharmacist must prepare concentrate used in making external solutions.
	Use preweighed magnesium sulfate crystals (weighed by pharmacist) for desired concentration.	
Glycine solution.	Follow instructions for preparing solutions, using single unit method, as described under Normal Saline.	For suspension of flasks at time of use when continuous irrigation is involved.
	Place bails on flasks.	For use with irrigation sets.
	Use collar or closure which fits the urology set to be used.	Available commercially.
	Use glycine concentrate—15% in water.	Makes a 1.5% glycine solution.
	Pour 200 ml of glycine concentrate in 2000 ml flask; add distilled water to required level.	Single-use labels (paper) are available.
	Apply identification label.	Provides a sterile hermetically sealed unit with indefinite shelf life.
	Sterilize with other solutions in routine manner.	

Note: It is recommended that other urological solutions be diluted to the desired concentration by injection of the concentrate into the sterile solvent at time solution is needed.

Procedure	Directives to Be Incorporated in Technique	Explanation of Directives
IV. Sterilization of Solutions	Sterilize solutions as soon as preparation and flasking have been completed.	Prepared solutions should never stand longer than 1 hour before sterilization.
	Sterilize by steam under pressure Gravity Discharge Type Sterilizer Set the Selector to "slow exhaust" Use temperature of 250°–254°F	To avoid violent boiling during exhaust period.
	Exposure periods: 75 ml–250 ml flask—20 minutes 500 ml–1000 ml flask—30 minutes 1500 ml–2000 ml flask—40 minutes	Only flasks requiring the same exposure time may be combined in load.
	Prevacuum Type Sterilizer Set Selector to: Liquids—1 liter for flasks of 1000 ml or less Liquids—2 liter for 1500 ml–2000 ml flasks	The Selector automatically determines the correct temperature and exposure period.
	Remove load from sterilizer after completion of cycle, or when chamber pressure gauge shows zero.	To avoid overexposure.
	Cool to room temperature in nondrafty location.	
	Date each flask; place date directly on single-use label.	Insures effective rotation of flasks during storage.
	After cooling to room temperature, check each flask for vacuum seal by lightly striking the top or bottom of flask with heel of hand; should hear a distinctive click, known as water hammer.	Water hammer click indicates flask is hermetically sealed.
	or	
	Visible indentation of disposable closure.	Assures hermetic seal.
	Discard any flask without water hammer.	Flask is not sealed.
	Transfer flasks of sterile solutions to storage shelves.	Solutions are safe for use immediately or indefinitely.

DISCARD DISPOSABLE CLOSURES AFTER USE
(Contamination of solution may occur if closure is reused)

Procedure	Directives to Be Incorporated in Technique	Explanation of Directives
V. CARE OF SPECIAL EQUIPMENT		
Water stills	Drain distilled water reservoir (tanks or carboys) at end of working day.	Distilled water should not be held over from one day to the next.
	Turn off conductivity meter; replace recording chart, date the used chart; keep used charts for 6 months.	Each chart covers 24-hour period; used charts serve as reference records.
	Remove evaporating pan from still; clean pan and steam coil with tap water, using a cellulose sponge to loosen soil.	A clean pan and coil insure high grade distillate.
	Replace pan.	
Mechanical flask washer	Turn toggle switch and thermostat to OFF.	
	Turn off distilled water supply; turn off hot tap water supply.	
	Drain reservoir of washer.	Discard washing solution.
	Clean strainers in tub as necessary.	Strainers can be removed for cleaning.
	Clean plastic cover inside and outside.	
	Clean outside of tub with water containing a detergent. Use cellulose sponge to wipe tub.	No need to clean inside of tub.
Mixing tank	Follow detailed cleaning instructions supplied by manufacturer.	
General cleaning of solution room	Clean thoroughly all work counters, sinks, drain carts, portable carts.	Solution rooms should be kept scrupulously clean.
		Use cellulose sponges for cleaning.
	Clean storage areas as necessary to maintain cleanliness.	
	Wet-mop floor.	Use clean lint-free mop.
	Keep door (or doors) to solution room closed at all times.	Helps in maintaining a clean solution room.

Chapter 17

LABORATORY AND INDUSTRIAL STERILIZERS

ATTEMPTS to confine bacteriological sterilization to the use of a single type of laboratory sterilizer are no longer justified. The unusual requirements of sterile techniques and processes evolving from research in infectious diseases and allied fields demand highly specialized sterilizing equipment. Many of these sterilizers are a combination type for use with either saturated steam under pressure or ethylene oxide gas mixed with suitable diluent gases. The latter method is a substitute for steam in sterilizing heat-sensitive or moisture-sensitive materials. Also deserving of mention are the many double-door laboratory sterilizers which operate under automatic controls for applications where the transfer of material from an unsterile environment to a sterile room is required. It is not intended to explain in detail the form and functions of these different types of laboratory sterilizers employed in microbiological research and industrial process control; only basic principles can be covered in this book.

It is regrettable that in many laboratories which are otherwise equipped with highly efficient apparatus there are hopelessly and, indeed, hazardously obsolete autoclaves in use. Some are twenty to thirty years old—relics of a period when the fundamentals of steam sterilization as we now recognize them were not understood thoroughly. Dependable operation and uniform results certainly cannot be expected from such equipment. Specific reference is made to those sterilizers from which air is discharged, if at all, by some type of hand regulation and in which the thermometer, if one is provided, is located at the top of the chamber. It is true that these sterilizers can be operated so that air will be eliminated adequately from the chamber. However, it usually is impractical to apply the expert knowledge of the control and the close supervision required to assure accurate, dependable performance. Another deficiency of old sterilizers, especially those heated by gas or electricity, is the slow rate of heating which makes it almost impossible to sterilize heat-sensitive fluids and media without destructive effect. Such sterilizers have been largely responsible for the erroneous assumption that lower pressures and temperatures or fractional sterilization must be resorted to for all heat-sensitive fluids.

MODERN LABORATORY STERILIZERS

About 1933, the fundamental principles upon which modern steam sterilizers function were first applied in this country. This development resulted in radical design and manufacturing changes which led, initially, to the establishment of the single shell pressure chamber as the most popular type. Such equipment functions satisfactorily in sterilizing bacteriological culture media and solutions. However, it is not well adapted to the sterilization of wrapped supplies or for any load that requires drying after sterilization. Because of the single shell construction, the chamber retains an excessive quantity of moisture following sterilization. Lacking the heat radiated from the steam jacket of a double shell sterilizer, the residual moisture cannot be evaporated readily in a single shell unit. Also, this type of sterilizer cools down after each load is withdrawn, thus decreasing the output volume made possible by a double shell sterilizer.

Thus, quite logically, the most widely accepted laboratory sterilizer now is the double shell, jacketed type shown in Figure 17-1. This sterilizer matches all the performance capabilities of the single shell unit and provides for some which are not possible in that outmoded equipment. The double shell sterilizer provides a controlled temperature range of 212°F (110°C) to 273°F (134°C) for processing laboratory supplies, culture media, and other heat-stable and moisture-stable materials. Nonpressure (streaming steam) conditions are employed for processing substances requiring a temperature of 212°F (100°C). Coagulation ("trapped air") processing of heat-coagulable media is accomplished by manual operation of the control system. The sterilizer has a steam jacket surrounding the side walls of the chamber, the same as provided on all surgical supply sterilizers. Pressure is first generated in the jacket and maintained constant at 15 to 17 pounds throughout the operating cycle or the entire working day. The hot side walls prevent condensate formation, and the load absorbs only that amount of moisture from the steam that is required to heat the load. Thus, this laboratory sterilizer functions as efficiently as any surgical supply sterilizer in sterilizing and drying wrapped or porous materials. Drying is achieved either by the vacuum dryer device or by the "cracked door" method (see page 215 describing "cracked door" method). Since pressure is maintained in the steam jacket continuously throughout working hours, the sterilizer is ready for immediate and more rapid use than is possible with a single shell chamber.

The discharge of air and movement of steam through the laboratory sterilizer is the same as in any modern pressure steam sterilizer. When the steam enters the air-filled chamber, it immediately rises to the top, compressing the air at the bottom. As the pressure increases in the chamber, the air is gradually forced out through a screened outlet leading to the chamber

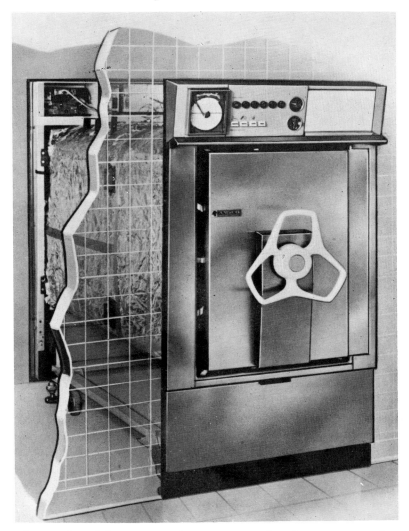

FIGURE 17-1. Modern laboratory sterilizer; steam jacketed type; recessed; equipped with automatic controls.

discharge line, past the temperature-sensing element or thermometer, through the thermostatic trap, and finally to the atmospheric vent. When the air has been evacuated from the chamber, saturated steam contacts the thermostatic element of the trap. The trap gradually closes, controlling the flow of steam. Air pockets and condensate accumulating thereafter in the lower areas of the chamber are eliminated by intermittent opening and closing of the thermostatic trap. All laboratory sterilizers should have the indicating thermometer or temperature-sensing element located in the chamber discharge line. The primary purpose is to detect any interruption in the normal flow of air and condensate from the chamber. If the chamber discharge line becomes clogged with sediment or residue from spillage of media in the chamber, the temperature rise will be retarded markedly, although the pressure may rise to the normal operating range. When this occurs, the air and steam stratify in the chamber, with the steam concentrating in the upper area. A thermometer at the top of the chamber will indicate the temperature of relatively pure steam, while the lower or bottom areas will be filled with air or an air-steam mixture at a much lower temperature. A thermometer located correctly in the chamber discharge line will promptly indicate faulty operation, the need for cleaning or maintenance, and the quality of the steam contacting the load. An additional safeguard in the laboratory sterilizer is an automatic time-temperature control. The thermostat which actuates the timer should also be located in the chamber discharge line, adjacent to the thermometer. Unless the chamber is filled with saturated steam at the right temperature, the control will fail to function.

THE ISOTHERMAL CONTROLLED STERILIZER

Laboratories have an established need for sterilizers with a much wider range of temperature control than is available in standard design units. The requirements cover not only sterilization by steam under pressure, but also fractional sterilization, inspissation, pasteurization, and low-temperature moist heat. To perform all of these functions, a sterilizer must provide a controlled range of operating temperatures from 140°F (60°C) to 273°F (134°C). This broad range of temperature is useful to the microbiologist because it permits him to evaluate the properties of solutions and media sterilized at progressively higher temperatures and shorter periods of time. It also permits fractional sterilization and processing of heat-coagulable culture media, including egg and blood serum slants. Moreover, the broad temperature range provides a convenient means of investigating marginal methods of sterilization of solutions or biologics where a moderate degree of heat plus chemical action, or the synergistic activity of combined energies, produces the required sterilizing effect.

The requirements for such a versatile unit have been fulfilled by the widely accepted laboratory-isothermal steam sterilizer, the latest development in laboratory sterilizer design. The chamber is steam-jacketed and constructed for a maximum operating pressure of 36 pounds. The automatic master control allows the operator to select the desired programming cycle by pressing the appropriate button on the main control panel. Steam pressure is thus maintained to yield temperatures anywhere in the range of 221°F (105°C) to 273°F (134°C). The timing instrument of the automatic control is adjustable for any exposure period between 3 and 90 minutes. The timer resets automatically when the sterilizing cycle has been completed, if the electric power fails, or if the temperature drops 2°F

(1.1°C) below the set sterilizing value. For low-temperature operation an isothermal control system is employed to prevent air-steam stratification in the chamber. This system converts the sterilizer to a fully automatic, non-pressure, low-temperature machine for processing heat-coagulable and heat-sensitive materials between 158°F (70°C) and 219°F (104°C). When operating under isothermal control, the atmospheric conditions in the chamber approximate saturation with water vapor through the cycle.

Figure 17-2 is a diagram showing the principle of operation of the isothermal control.* Steam from the supply line enters the chamber through a nozzle. It immediately contacts the cooling coil, through which water circulates. The steam is reduced in temperature before it reaches the chamber

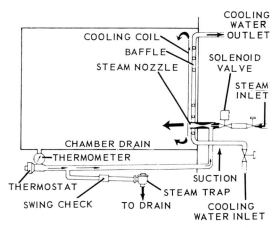

FIGURE 17-2. Components of isothermal control system.

proper. As steam passes through the nozzle and into the chamber, a negative pressure is created at the nozzle and is transmitted to the chamber drain opening through the system of piping. This suction draws incoming steam from the nozzle toward the front end of the chamber and circulates it back to the nozzle via the discharge line and into the chamber again. This action assures an isothermal condition throughout the chamber and prevents air-steam stratification. This circulatory process permits the thermometer to indicate the actual temperature conditions within the chamber. The supply of steam to the chamber is governed by a solenoid valve actuated by the thermostat. The following test data indicate the typical accuracy of temperature control in the isothermal sterilizer:

Sterilizer: 20 x 20 x 36″ Laboratory Sterilizer, steam heat, equipped with Cyclomatic control and Isothermal control.
Load: 235 test tubes (18 x 150 mm) in baskets, each ⅓ filled with media and stoppered with cotton plugs.

* U. S. Patent No. 2713702.

Location of thermocouples: In tubes located at 1) front bottom, 2) center, and 3) top rear of chamber. Temperature readings recorded by potentiometer.

Series of tests:

5 at 140°F (60°C)
3 at 160°F (71°C)
3 at 180°F (82°C)
3 at 200°F (93°C)
3 at 210°F (98.5°C)

Conditions of test: Each test was preceded by a chamber warm-up period of 15 minutes at the operating temperature. Observations were continued for a 30-minute period after the load had reached thermostat setting temperature. Water flow through cooling coil was regulated at 20 gallons per hour for all tests below 200°F (93°C). No water was used above this temperature.

Results:

Thermostat Setting °F °C	Thermometer Reading During 30-Min. Period °F °C	Time to Heat Load to Processing Temperature Minutes- Average	Deviation of Load Temp. from Thermometer Temp. at Thermocouple Positions F° °C
140	141.5±1.5	36	−5.5 to +4.5
60	61.0±1.0		−3.0 to +2.5
160	163.0±1.0	20	−6.5 to +4.0
71	73.0±0.5		−3.5 to +2.5
180	181.5±1.0	16	−3.5 to +3.5
82	83.0±0.5		−2.0 to +2.0
200	200.0±1.0	9	−1.0 to +3.0
93	93.0±0.5		−0.5 to +1.5
210	210.0±0.5	10	−1.5 to +0.
99	99.0±0.3		−0.8 to +0.

INDUSTRIAL STERILIZERS

Pressure steam sterilizers are widely used by manufacturers of sterile products and commodities. The sterilizers vary in their accessory and installation characteristics to meet the requirements of the user. Proper installation is influenced by the need for ease of operation, throughput capacity, access for maintenance, cleanliness, and other factors. Industrial sterilizers may have doors at one or both ends of the chamber. The single-door sterilizer is the most commonly used. The double-door sterilizer provides for loading of nonsterile material at one end and removal of the sterilized material at the other. Supplemental instrumentation provides necessary monitoring and gives assurance of safe operation.

Although doors of the smaller sterilizers are light enough to be operated manually without difficulty, doors on the larger sterilizers are heavy and may be difficult to close. Power assists are commonly employed for the opening and closing of heavy doors. Doors that swing either to the left or the right can be obtained in manually or power-operated types.

Industrial sterilizers are usually mounted without panel enclosures, or they may be recessed into a wall or mounted into a pit. Cabinet enclosures are especially suitable for individual units at different locations. Such enclosures eliminate costly recessing rooms, enhance cleanliness, and permit slow, even dissipation of heat from the chamber.

Recessing is most desirable in a multiple-unit installation. Recessed units have a neat appearance and permit maintenance work to be done in the recessing room, thus excluding maintenance personnel from clean, or restricted, areas. Moreover, recessing of larger units is an effective way to handle their radiant heat loss. Where work flow is from a contaminated area (through a double-door sterilizer) to a clean area, a cross-contamination seal is required.

Cross-contamination Seal and Door Interlocks

This arrangement is for double-door (pass-through) sterilizers. It affords positive cross-contamination control by preventing airborne microorganisms or other particulate matter from passing from one work area to the other via the space around the sterilizer body at the wall opening. The work areas should be so planned that the cross-contamination seal will be opposite the control end of the sterilizer. The cross-contamination seal is always employed in conjunction with a door interlock system which permits only one sterilizer door at a time to be opened. Once the door on the unclean end is closed, the door to the clean or noncontaminated end cannot be opened until the sterilization cycle is completed. The system includes a signal light at each end of the sterilizer to show whether the door at the opposite end is open or closed. The automatic lock may be bypassed by using a tumbler-type lock, with removable key (see Figs. 17-3, 17-4, and 17-5).

STERILIZERS FOR ATTACHMENT TO BIOLOGICAL HOODS

Hoods for containing contaminate-free material are essential in many research and production activities by government, university, and commercial enterprises. Accordingly, specialized equipment must be used to meet such critical requirements as, for example, double-door sterilizers for attachment to biological hoods. Such facilities make practicable the passing of sterilized materials and supplies into the hood and the subsequent return of materials from the enclosure. A sealing flange prevents the entry of contaminants from the exterior environment. Where double-door sterilizers are installed, it is essential to provide electric interlocking doors to prevent either door from

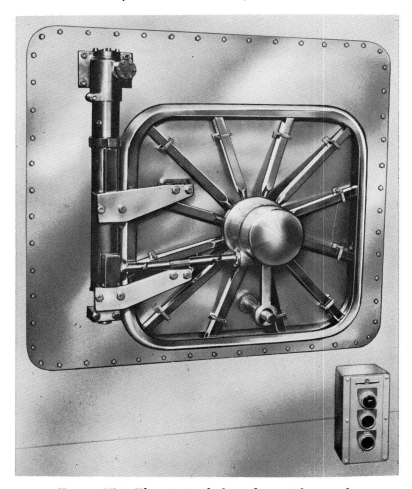

FIGURE 17-3. Electric interlocking door, with controls.

being opened before completion of the sterilizing cycle. Only the door on the hood side can be opened following the cycle (see Fig. 17-6). The experience gained in developing and manufacturing biological hood combinations makes it possible to meet many highly critical and specialized processing needs. The variety of combinations may include special construction materials, various power-door arrangements, automatic process controls and instrumentation, and special mounting arrangements.

DECONTAMINATION

The daily routine in an infectious disease laboratory may result in widespread contamination of the atmosphere, work materials, and the operator.[1] Even when an operation is performed under the most careful precautions, the equipment must be cleaned up after the operation. In case of an acci-

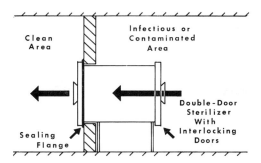

FIGURE 17-4. Diagram of double-door sterilizer between contaminated and clean areas, with sealing flange located on clean side.

dent or spill, decontamination of an entire room or a building and its contents may be required. In either event, more than one method of decontamination may be needed. Heating is the simplest and most widely used method of sterilization; it also is the most effective. This method should be used whenever possible. Also a wide variety of liquid decontaminants are available. These substances have been evaluated for many applications.[2]

The selection of decontaminants and procedures for their use for the broad spectrum of microorganisms and situations cannot be detailed here. However, it is strongly suggested that the efficacy of every liquid disinfectant proposed for use in the laboratory be evaluated for each specific application. Optimal organism recovery techniques should be employed; consideration should be given to the amount of solid organic matter present, the temperature, the acidity (pH), and other variables which may make published data inapplicable. Liquid germicides are suitable for decontaminating glassware and small apparatus pending sterilization in an autoclave.

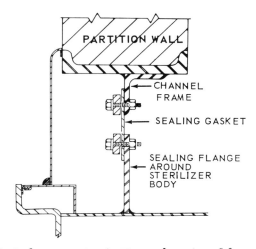

FIGURE 17-5. Typical cross-contamination seal as viewed from side of sterilizer

The germicide selected should be one which will not etch the glass or leave a residue. Hypochlorite solutions should be inactivated with thiosulfate before terminal sterilization in the autoclave. This is necessary to avoid release of gaseous chlorine in the chamber. Liquid germicides for personnel decontamination should be selected not only for specific action against the agents involved but, additionally, for minimal effect on the skin and mucous membranes.

DISPOSAL OF CULTURES

It is the practice in many microbiological laboratories to terminally heat discarded cultures for 30 minutes at 250°F (121°C); others employ the old "rule of thumb" procedure of 15 pounds for 15 minutes. These exposure times may or may not be adequate for sterilization, depending upon the rate of heat-up of the chamber, the depth of the culture container, and the presence of water in the container. Slow heating autoclaves may be almost self-compensating in that when the chamber has attained sterilizing temperature the load is approximately at that temperature. In comparison, many of the modern laboratory sterilizers utilize thermostatic temperature control instead of the conventional pressure regulator control. This feature enables the sterilizer to reach the selected operating temperature rapidly. In certain instances the chamber heat-up time may be less than 5 minutes to 250°F (121°C). Consequently, this factor must be taken into consideration when attempting to carry out safe disposal of cultures and other kinds of contaminated material.

STERILIZERS FOR TISSUE CULTURE PROCESSING

The need for special sterilizing systems to permit tissue culture processing and similar critical applications has advanced in the past decade because steam from a conventional boiler system usually has boiler contaminants and other toxic impurities. In a tissue culture sterilizer, steam from the building supply line heats only the jacket. This facilitates poststerilization drying, if desired; it also preheats the chamber before high-purity steam is

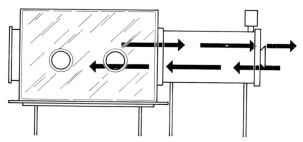

FIGURE 17-6. Diagram of double-door sterilizer attached to biological hood. Arrows indicate passage of sterilized materials into the hood and subsequent return of materials from the enclosure.

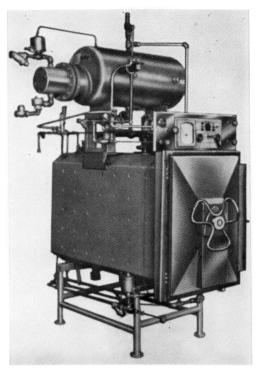

FIGURE 17-7. Rectangular steam sterilizer with high-purity indirect steam generating system.

admitted directly to the chamber. The high-purity-steam generating system produces the required amount of chamber steam from either distilled or deionized water. The steam generator is mounted either on top of, or adjacent to, the sterilizer, as shown in Figure 17-7. The heavy-duty stainless steel coil of the generator utilizes steam from the building supply line to heat water in the generator. Water may be fed automatically to the generator, or the generator may be filled manually. All tissue culture sterilizing systems should be equipped with programing controls and instrumentation that will provide an automatic cycle which includes charging the chamber with high-purity steam (generated from distilled or deionized water) to the selected sterilizing temperature and maintaining it for the selected time, timing the exposure period, and exhausting the chamber, either slowly or quickly, in conformance with the selected exhaust phase of the processing cycle.

STERILIZATION OF LIQUIDS

The sterilization of liquids in flasks, bottles, or test tubes involves a different use of steam than is required for sterilization of dry goods. In the latter case it is necessary to permeate the porous materials with steam in order that both heat and moisture shall be absorbed by the fibers. In solution sterilization, the problem is simply a matter of absorbing heat from the steam. The solution, if aqueous, contains the necessary moisture. When steam contacts the cold flasks or bottles it condenses, and the condensate drains to the bottom of the sterilizer and then out to the waste by means of the chamber discharge line. This process will continue until the solution has been heated to the temperature of the surrounding steam. The time required for heating governs the exposure period. This will vary with the size and shape of the container, the volume of liquid, the thickness of the container walls and the heat conductivity of the container. Measurements to determine the time required for a given container of solution to attain a temperature of 250°F (121°C) are usually made by means of a thermocouple and potentiometer. The graphic data given in Figure 17-8 are illustrative of the different rates of heat transfer through commonly used flasks and bottles.

Common errors in solution sterilization can often be avoided through a clear understanding of the operating cycle. During the period of heating the solution and as long as the exposure continues, there will be no visible indication of boiling of the liquid, even though the temperature may be far above the normal boiling point of water at atmospheric pressure. This is due to steam pressure maintained in the sterilizer, at all times equal to or in excess of the pressure possible to develop from the heat in the liquid. Until this condition reverses there can be no ebullition. When the chamber pressure is reduced, after sterilization, the pressure corresponding to the temperature of the liquid will then be greater than the steam pressure and the liquid will begin to boil. If chamber pressure is exhausted rapidly, boiling will be so violent that stoppers will be blown out of the flasks and some of the solution will escape into the chamber. Experience has shown that when pressure is exhausted at a uniform rate through a period of not less than 10 to 15 minutes, the solution will lose its heat at about the same rate as the pressure reduction, and violent boiling will not occur. With heavy loads of solutions in flasks or bottles it may be necessary to extend the exhaust period to 20 or 30 minutes, depending upon the characteristics of the sterilizer exhaust valve and the type of closure on the flasks or bottles.

Even when the cooling down process is conducted with the greatest of care there will be an evaporation loss of fluid of 3 to 5 per cent, unless the containers are hermetically sealed. This has established the general practice in preparing solutions of adding about 5 per cent more distilled water to the container so that after sterilization the product will have the intended concentration. On the other hand, too slow cooling is objectionable. If the period is overextended, the effect is the same as overexposure. If the heat is turned off at the end of the exposure time and the sterilizer allowed to cool down without opening the exhaust, one hour or longer may elapse before the pressure in the chamber is reduced to zero gauge. During this period, the liquid will be maintained between the maximum temperature of 250°

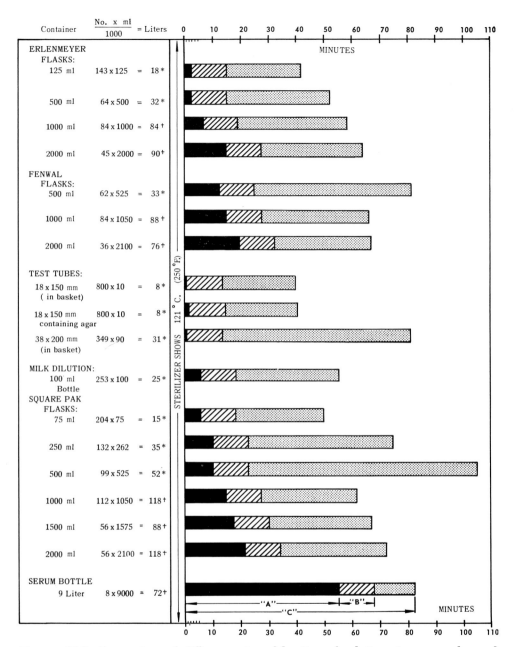

FIGURE 17-8. Comparison of different rates of heating of solutions in commonly used containers. Section "A" of each bar represents additional (heat-up) time required for solution to reach 250°F after sterilizer shows this temperature. Section "B" is the holding time (minimum standard of 12 minutes) after solution has reached 250°F. "A" plus "B" equals required exposure period. Entire bar length "C" is total time solution remains above 212°F during sterilizing cycle, including slow exhaust.

The symbol * designates a 20″ × 20″ × 38″ gravity-discharge-type sterilizer with fully loaded chamber. The † designates a 24″ × 36″ × 36″ sterilizer, gravity type, equipped with solution accelerator exhaust valve. Steam pressure (psig): supply 60-75; jacket 19-20; chamber 18-19.

to 254°F (121° to 123°C) and 212°F (100°C). For many solutions this prolonged exposure to temperatures above 212°F (100°C) is not harmful, but for bacteriological media containing carbohydrates or agar, the destructive influence is marked.

Assuming that a modern sterilizer is in use, destructive effects usually follow the incorrect practice of sterilizing all loads of solutions for the same period, the old "15 pounds for 20 minutes" rule or something equally unscientific. It takes much longer to sterilize a 1000-ml flask of liquid than a test tube containing 10 ml, yet it is not uncommon to find laboratory sterilizers filled with large flasks and small tubes, all in the same load. The size and type of flask used, not the number of flasks in the sterilizer, establishes the exposure period. If the flasks are all alike, the exposure period will be the same for one or any number placed in the sterilizer. The time required to heat the containers to the sterilizing temperature will, of course, vary with the size of load, but exposure period should not vary. Containers should not be filled to more than 75 per cent of their capacity, to allow for fluid expansion and to prevent overflow.

Exposure Periods for Solutions

The following exposure periods for aqueous solutions or liquids in various types of containers will afford a reasonable factor of safety in sterilization:

Container	Capacity	Minutes Exposure 250°–254° F (121°–123° C)
Test tubes	18×150 mm	12–14
Test tubes	32×200 mm	13–17
Test tubes	38×200 mm	15–20
Erlenmeyer (Pyrex) flask	50 ml	12–14
Erlenmeyer (Pyrex) flask	125 ml	15–20
Erlenmeyer (Pyrex) flask	200 ml	15–20
Erlenmeyer (Pyrex) flask	500 ml	17–22
Erlenmeyer (Pyrex) flask	1000 ml	20–25
Erlenmeyer (Pyrex) flask	2000 ml	30–35
Fenwal (Pyrex) flask	500 ml	25–30
Fenwal (Pyrex) flask	1000 ml	25–30
Fenwal (Pyrex) flask	2000 ml	35–40
Square-Pak (Pyrex) flask	75 ml	20–25
Square-Pak (Pyrex) flask	250 ml	25–30
Square-Pak (Pyrex) flask	500 ml	25–30
Square-Pak (Pyrex) flask	1000 ml	30–35
Square-Pak (Pyrex) flask	1500 ml	30–35
Square-Pak (Pyrex) flask	2000 ml	35–40
Milk dilution bottle	100 ml	20–25
Serum bottle (Pyrex)	9000 ml	70–75

Minimum exposures as given above represent the least periods under which sterilization should be attempted and the maximum periods should not normally be exceeded.

BACTERIOLOGICAL MEDIA

Some bacteriological media are known to be heat-sensitive. Prolonged sterilization or excessive heating of media containing sugars (glucose, lactose, and saccharose) frequently causes hydrolysis, with the production of acid. Phenol red lactose broth, for example, sterilized at 250°F (121°C) for 15 minutes, or sterilized by filtration, produces no demonstrable amount of acid when inoculated with S. *typhosa,* but when sterilized for 30 to 45 minutes at this temperature, an appreciable amount of acid is produced. Excessive heating may also cause formation of a precipitate in agar media. Overexposure may cause an increase in acidity, break down the peptones, and diminish the ability of agar to produce a firm gel. Oversterilization of media such as wort agar, with a normal pH of 4.8, will destroy the agar. Peroxide formation may occur in certain types of media such as papaic digest broth, or when citrate is autoclaved with manganese in a synthetic medium.[9]

Nutrient agar should be sterilized immediately after it is made—while still fluid—because of the destructive influence of each additional heating. Most sugars contained in media can be sterilized by autoclaving if overheating is avoided. In fact, it has been shown[3] that maltose and lactose undergo less destruction by rapid autoclaving than by fractional or intermittent sterilization in the Arnold apparatus. If the medium is contained in test tubes, the tubes placed in wire baskets (not overloaded) so steam can circulate freely around each tube, an exposure period of 12 minutes at 250°F (121°C) will usually be satisfactory.

Heat-labile compounds like glutamine and thiamine should be sterilized by filtration. The autoclaving of glucose-containing media may result in caramelization, but this reaction is not necessarily responsible for inhibition of growth. The critical factor appears to be associated with the heating of the glucose media at an alkaline pH and in the presence of phosphate. A solution of glucose, phosphate, and peptone at a pH of 7.2 becomes inhibitory after autoclaving at 250°F (121°C) for 15 minutes, but at a pH of 5.4 it is not inhibitory.[4] At a pH of 6.8, it is believed that pressure steam sterilization of glucose-salts solutions results in a partial conversion of glucose to other sugars, including gentiobiose.[5] Smith[6] reported that autoclaving at 250°F (121°C) for 20 minutes, at a pH of 7.5, destroys 20% glucose and 50% maltose; the degree of destruction is accelerated by the presence of phosphate.

FRACTIONAL STERILIZATION

Occasionally it is necessary to sterilize bacteriological media at temperatures no higher than that of atmospheric steam. Also, solutions of certain chemicals, such as cocaine and epinephrine, which are unstable at autoclaving temperatures, may be sterilized with flowing steam. For this purpose a special type of nonpressure sterilizer (Arnold) is commonly used in which the material is subjected to the free-flowing steam from boiling water for periods of time varying from 20 to 60 minutes on each of 3 consecutive days. The modern laboratory sterilizer should permit operation with nonpressure or flowing steam.

Between exposures to steam the material is kept at incubation temperature or room temperature. The principle of this method is that the first exposure to flowing steam destroys the vegetative forms of bacteria but not the spores. Then when the material is incubated overnight, or for 24 hours, most of the spores will develop into the vegetative stage and will be killed by the second period of heating. Again the material is incubated, allowing the remainder of the spores to germinate so they may be killed on the third heating. Although sterilization usually results after the third period of heating, failures may also occur. Optimum conditions must prevail in the media in order for the spores to develop into vegetative forms during the incubation period. The presence of proper nutrients, correct pH, and the absence of bacteriostatic substances influence the effectiveness of the process. *Fractional sterilization has application only for those materials which will support microbial growth.* It is useless to attempt to sterilize dry goods by this process.

INSPISSATION

The process of inspissation is a combination of pasteurization with intermittent or discontinuous heating for a period of 4 to 7 days. It consists of heating the solution or material in a water bath or an inspissator once daily for 30 to 60 minutes at 140°F (60°C) to 176°F (80°C), or at the highest temperature below 212°F (100°C) which the substance can tolerate without change, for 4 to 7 days. It is not regarded as a reliable method of sterilization, but frequently must be used for heat-sensitive pharmaceuticals or chemicals which are injured by higher temperatures. A bacteriostatic agent is usually added to the medicinal preparations sterilized by this process.

One of the most useful applications of the inspissation process is the preparation of heat-coagulable media for use in diagnostic bacteriology. Loewenstein's, Jensen's, Petroff's, Locke's, blood serum, and other heat-coagulable media call for special treatment in order to prepare culture slants with the proper degree of hardness and to avoid formation of broken bubbles on the surface caused by engendered pressure. Many laboratories process such media in the Arnold sterilizer or in the autoclave with air trapped in the chamber so that the partial pressure of steam in the air-steam mixture produces a temperature of 176°F (80°C) to 200°F (93°C). Neither of these methods is satisfactory because of the difficulty in maintaining accurate temperature control, the nonuniformity of temperature throughout the chamber and the load, and the long time required for inspissation. Even with a specially designed electrically heated inspissator, the time required to produce a satisfactory medium is 2 hours.[7] The isothermal controlled sterilizer (Fig. 17-2) functions ideally for the processing of heat-coagulable media. Slants coagulate satisfactorily at 176°F (80°C) for 30 minutes or 200°F (93°C) for 20 minutes. The degree of hardness may be altered as desired by increasing temperature or lengthening exposure period, or both.

STERILIZATION OF EMPTY FLASKS OR BOTTLES

Empty flasks or bottles can be sterilized in the autoclave if they are placed on their sides in the chamber so as to provide a horizontal path for the escape of air. If the container has no stopper or cover air will be displaced quickly in this position and sterilization will occur in 15 minutes at 250°F (121°C). If the container is tightly sealed or stoppered, sterilization will not occur, regardless of the position of the container, because steam will be excluded. Even when flasks are lightly stoppered with cotton and placed bottom side up in the sterilizer, air evacuation will be somewhat retarded and exposure should be not less than 30 minutes. This method of sterilizing lightly stoppered containers can only be recommended with reservation because of the uncertainty of air elimination. It is preferable to sterilize stoppered flasks by the hot air method.

HOT AIR STERILIZATION OF GLASSWARE

Exposure to hot air is the method of choice for the routine sterilization of glassware common to the bacteriological laboratory. This includes such items as Petri dishes and pipettes (wrapped in paper or placed in special metallic holders), empty test tubes (plugged), centrifuge tubes, fermentation tubes, bottles, flasks, and any other empty glass, porcelain, or metallic containers required as sterile stock laboratory supplies.

Prior to sterilization, all glassware must be thoroughly cleaned and free from traces of organic matter; otherwise during the heating process the residue may char and leave stains on the containers after sterilization. Glassware containing cultures or infectious material should first be sterilized by means of steam under pressure, then emptied, and thoroughly cleaned in hot detergent solution. A temperature of 338°F (170°C) for at least one hour is recommended for the hot air sterilization of glassware. Although a prolonged exposure to this temperature is not deleterious to the glassware, excessive heating will definitely char the paper wrappers or cotton plugs. Test tubes plugged with cotton wool and sterilized by dry heat at 320° to 356°F (160° to 180°C) may show a greasy film on their inner surfaces which contains sufficient acid to inhibit microbial growth.[8]

REFERENCES

1. UMBREIT, WAYNE W. (Ed.): *Advances in Applied Microbiology.* New York and London Academic Press, 1961, vol. 3, p. 173.

2. REDDISH, G. F. (Ed.): *Antiseptics, Disinfectants, Fungicides, and Chemical and Physical Sterilization.* Philadelphia, Lea & F. 1957.

3. BENTON, A., and LEIGHTON, A.: Actual temperatures attained by mediums in autoclave sterilization. *J Infect Dis, 37:*353-358, 1925.

4. LEWIS, I. M.: The inhibition of *Phytomonas malvacearea* in culture media containing sugars. *J Bact, 19:*423, 1930.

5. KHAN, A. W., and WALKER, T. K.: The formation of gentiobiose and other saccharides during pressure-steam sterilization of a glucose-salts solution of pH 6.8. *J Appl Bact, 21:*278, 1958.

6. SMITH, M. L.: The effect of heat on sugar solutions used for culture media. *Biochem J, 26:*1467, 1932.

7. LEVIN, W.; BRANDON, G. R., and McMILLEN, S.: The culture method of laboratory diagnosis of tuberculosis. *Amer J Public Health, 40:*1305-1310, 1950.

8. POLLOCK, M. R.: Unsaturated fatty acids in cotton wool plugs. *Nature* (London), *161:*853, 1948.

9. BARRY, V. C.; CONALTY, M. L.; DENNENY, J. M., and WINDER, F.: Peroxide formation in bacteriological media. *Nature, (London), 178:*596, 1956.

Chapter 18

STERILIZER CONTROLS, STERILIZATION INDICATORS, AND CULTURE TESTS

STERILIZATION failures occur in hospitals even though personnel charged with this responsibility have instructions to correctly prepare and expose the surgical supplies to saturated steam under pressure at 250°F for 30 minutes. As a rule, surgeons recognize that all instruments and supplies used in the performance of an operation constitute a potentially major source of contamination for operative wounds. Dandy,[1] for example, has attributed the majority of postoperative infections to inadequate sterilization of the towels, gowns, gauze, and other supplies that pass through the sterilizers.

It has been reported that there is a special hazard of gas gangrene attendant with the intramuscular injection of adrenaline in oil.[2] Patel[3] and others reported thirty-two cases of tetanus following injection of a drug. The availability of the most modern sterilizing equipment, as well as published methods for safe sterilization of supplies, still does not entirely prevent the occurrence of fatal postoperative infections resulting from inadequate sterilization.[4] Faulty and improperly operated sterilizers, even those of modern design, may allow spores to survive on instruments, gloves, and other articles.[5] Far too few workers recognize that the organisms carried into a wound by the hands and instruments of a surgeon are apt to be more harmful and virulent than those occurring there by accident.

For the most part, sterilization failures are the result of a series of factors, either singly or combined, which make up the human equation in sterilizer operation. Those of primary importance are the following:

· Unfamiliarity with the characteristics of the individual sterilizer, such as method of air removal, rate of heating, penetration time, safety factor, method of drying load.

· Incorrect methods of packaging and wrapping of supplies with little or no regard for the size and density of the individual packs.

· Carelessness in loading the sterilizer, with disregard for the necessity of providing for complete air removal and for free circulation of steam throughout the load.

· Failure to time correctly the proper period of exposure—usually due to ignorance or negligence on the part of the operator.

· Failure to carry out the correct sequence of operations in the sterilizing cycle, as the result of carelessness, fatigue, or distraction.

· Attempts to sterilize materials which are impervious to steam, such as talcum powder, anhydrous oils, and petrolatum.

· Attempts to short-cut established methods of sterilization on the basis of limited bacteriological tests with organisms of unknown heat resistance and unknown populations.

· Faulty equipment resulting from lack of maintenance and lack of basic knowledge concerning the principle of operation and care of sterilizers.

RECORDING THERMOMETERS

When properly installed and used, the recording thermometer is a practical detector of faulty sterilization. This instrument contains a standard clock mechanism, electrically driven, which revolves a 6-inch diameter chart once in 24 hours. The thermometer system consists of a helical pressure element connected to the sensing bulb by a flexible capillary tube. It indicates and records the same temperature as that shown by the indicating thermometer located in the discharge system of the sterilizer chamber. It also records the duration of each exposure and the absolute pressure. Lacking the recorder, the operator can, and frequently does, forget to time the exposure when the temperature has advanced to the prescribed sterilizing range. Without the recorder, it is difficult to maintain the required uniformity where several individuals have access to the sterilizers or to prove what has or has not been done in routine practice. If the exposure periods are greater or less than prescribed, or if the temperature has not been maintained within the proper limitations, there is a positive record of the errors, thus providing evidence needed upon which to act in correcting discrepancies.

Recording thermometers are subject to some distortion of the highly flexible pen arms, but means for easy readjustment are provided on the instrument. Accuracy of the recorder should be checked at weekly intervals or oftener as follows: Operate the sterilizer in the routine manner until the temperature becomes stable at the maximum range which should not be less than 250°F, nor more than 254°F, as shown by the indicating thermometer on the sterilizer. If there is any deviation, adjust the screw on the pen arm until the temperature of the recorder is the same as that shown by the indicating thermometer. Recorders are delicate instruments and only minor adjustments should be undertaken. If there is any reason to question the accuracy of the instrument or in the event of malfunction, a qualified serviceman should be consulted.

In the author's opinion, the recording thermometer should be considered a necessary part of every surgical supply sterilizer because its proper use most certainly promotes safer performance. It should be regarded as standard equipment, not a luxury. The ability to prove with daily chart records that definite standards of time and temperature are being maintained for each cycle of sterilization should appeal to those who must shoulder the responsibility for sterilization. Without the recorder, the supervisor is helpless in detecting discrepancies.

INDICATING AND RECORDING POTENTIOMETERS

The most dependable physical method for testing the functional efficiency of sterilizers, the penetration of steam through a porous load, or the rate of heat transfer through solution containers involves use of a potentiometer, an instrument for measuring temperature in the most inaccessible portion of the load during sterilization. When using this instrument, access to the load is gained through a thermocouple, two small wires of dissimilar metals (usually copper-constantan) soldered together at the ends and inserted in the load. The terminal ends of the thermocouple are usually brought out under the door of the sterilizer, impinging against the door gasket, and connected to the potentiometer, as in Figure 18-1. (An alternate method for instrumentation is to install a thermocouple gland directly through the sterilizer shell or backhead.) Any change in temperature at the joined ends of the couple develops a thermoelectric current which is immediately indicated on the dial of the instrument.

A reliable potentiometer normally has an accuracy of adjustment of the order of $\pm 0.5°$F. In this manner, the penetration of steam through a load can be followed, readings being taken at frequent intervals and the results then plotted on graph paper. With such data one can easily determine if a given sterilizing cycle provides a reasonable factor of safety. When using the potentiometer, the chamber of the sterilizer should be filled to the maximum contemplated for routine loading.

The test pack selected for observation should be the largest and most densely arranged one, and it should be located near the front bottom of the chamber to which point the steam will travel with the greatest lag. The thermocouple should be buried in the most compact part of the pack, usually in the center, to which steam will gain access most slowly. If the method of preparing the packs follows the standardized procedure and if the loading of the packs in the chamber is typical of routine practice, such tests are highly significant. Care should be used, however, to guard against superheating by using only freshly laundered fabrics for the test pack.

For bulk loads of surgical packs, both large and small, 30 minutes' exposure at 250° to 254°F should show a reasonable margin of safety in time beyond that required to meet the minimum standard. For example, if the test pack with thermocouple showed that a time of 12 minutes was required to reach 250°F, measured from the time the discharge line thermometer on the sterilizer reached this temperature, it would require an exposure of 24 minutes to meet the minimum standard. To this should then be added an

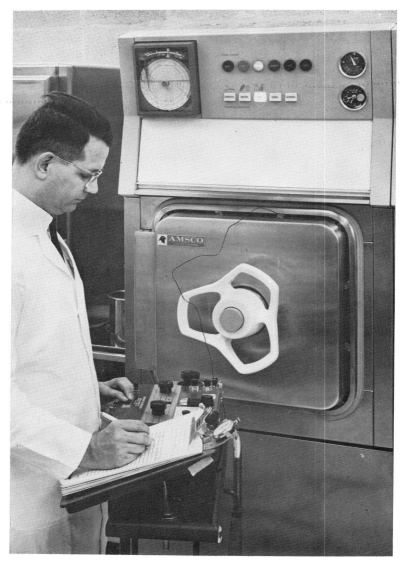

FIGURE 18-1. The potentiometer is a useful instrument for testing the efficiency of sterilizers or in determining rate of heating of a given load. Thermocouple may be inserted under edge of door or through gland in shell. Point of thermocouple is located in center of a test pack.

additional 6 minutes for a fair margin of safety, making a total of 30 minutes exposure. If the test data show that the pack is so dense that the minimum standard of 12 minutes at 250°F cannot be maintained in 30 minutes' exposure, the correct procedure would be to revamp the package, perhaps remove some of the more compact articles and wrap those separately. Sterilization should not continue for much longer than 30 minutes, because added exposure becomes increasingly harmful, especially to certain materials.

AUTOMATIC TIME-TEMPERATURE CONTROLS

The human element must be reckoned with in order to safeguard the hospital against failures in sterilization of supplies. Sterilizer manufacturers have recognized this problem and accepted the responsibility of doing their part in bringing about better control and more effective methods for sterilization in hospitals. The development of automatic control mechanisms designed to minimize the human element and to increase the mechanical reliability in sterilizer operation is a good example of industry's attack on the problem. Typical of the class of automatic controls with program selectors is the instrument shown in Figure 8-9. The function of any such control should not be limited to automatic timing of the selected exposure period, but rather it should extend to all phases of the sterilizing process, to the end that all steps in the cycle normally carried out manually by the operator are conducted automatically according to a predetermined pattern established by the supervisor. This means that when the control is set for operation, it will automatically eliminate air from the chamber and the load, time the established exposure period at the correct temperature, exhaust the steam from the chamber, govern the process of drying, and, finally, sound an alarm announcing completion of the cycle.

Since all exposure periods are based upon maintenance of a minimum standard temperature, for the specific kind of sterilizer, the control should be of the type that will insure automatic recycling in the event that the temperature in the sterilizer falls below the standard at any time during the exposure period. The speed of response of the temperature sensing and measuring instrument is also important, especially in the high speed autoclaves. For the exact measurement of temperatures developed during the steam phase of the cycle, only control instruments rapid in response should be used, preferably those with an intermediate time value of less than 6 seconds. The intermediate time value means the time in which half of the temperature change has been reached.

In discussing the functional efficiency of automatic controls in pressure steam or ethylene oxide gas sterilization, it should be understood that any such control instrument must, of necessity, have certain limitations because it cannot indicate or compensate for faulty methods used in the preparation, packaging, and loading of supplies in the sterilizer. Regardless of the degree of mechanical perfection exhibited by the sterilizer and the controls which guarantee so-called unvarying uniformity of operation, sterilization of the load is still dependent upon correct methods of packaging and strict adherence to established rules for loading the sterilizer. This statement applies to all types of sterilizers—gravity displacement, high speed, prevacuum high temperature, or otherwise. Do not be misled by rhetorical claims with emphasis upon speed of operation.

The prime purpose of any automatic control is to effect economy and uniformity of results and to guard against the inaccuracies of human behavior in sterilizer operation. To this end, it is essential that the instrument eliminate the mental burden of remembering the time at which the exposure period began and when it should end. Likewise, it should eliminate errors in the reading of the thermometer, insure the proper sequence of each step in the sterilizing cycle, and protect the load against under-exposure or over-exposure. The reliability of the control should merit complete confidence on the part of the operator to the extent that once it is set in operation, the exact period of continuous exposure at the correct temperature, as well as the entire cycle of performance, will be carried out with accuracy and precision not obtainable through manual operation. The use of automatic program controls on sterilizers naturally presupposes the need for frequent inspection and servicing to insure peak efficiency of operation. A properly trained mechanic or serviceman familiar with the equipment should always be engaged for this work. If these requirements are met, sterilizers equipped with automatic controls can be depended upon to afford a greater factor of safety in routine sterilization with a substantial savings in personnel time, materials and supplies.

TELLTALE INDICATORS

Authoritative opinion is seemingly divided on the actual worth of all sterilization indicators or controls of the "telltale" type. For long this subject has been a controversial one, and not infrequently the utilitarian value of such indicators is questioned. Ecker,[6] for example, in evaluating the efficiency of these devices found that their turning points, based on melting of the indicator substance or on color changes, had not been standardized and they varied in the time-temperature ratios required for complete change. In contrast to these findings, Hoyt[7] reported that one type of indicator, when properly used and interpreted, was found to be an adequate check on the efficacy of sterilization of rubber gloves. On the basis of hundreds of tests under widely varying conditions of application in hospitals, Underwood[8] reported that the hermetically sealed, pellet in glass tube control reacted (fused) uniformly when subjected to temperatures of 248° to 252°F for 5 to 8 minutes. At slightly lower temperature (245°F) the time required to fuse the control ranged from 20 to 30 minutes. These results encouraged Underwood to make the recommendation that approved sterilization indicators can be used to advantage as an occasional check against faulty packaging, loading and performance of sterilizers. An evaluation of a group of telltale indicators by Walter[9] revealed marked discrepancies in individual controls

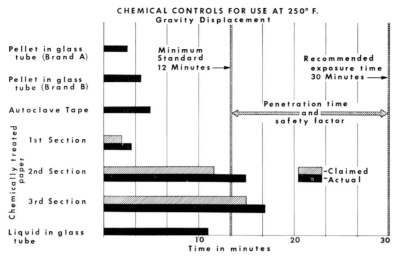

FIGURE 18-2. Evaluation of commonly used sterilization indicators under hospital conditions of operation in a gravity displacement sterilizer.

with a sufficient number showing delayed changes in end points so as to confuse operators and to cause unnecessary resterilization of supplies.

The results of a recent evaluation of a group of sterilization indicators by Smith and Perkins[10] are given in Figure 18-2. As can be seen the fusible pellet-type controls (Brands A and B) fall far short of meeting the minimum standard of 12 minutes at 250°F for sterilization. Of 300 controls tested (Brand A) all were fused in 2½ minutes at 250°F; of 100 samples tested all were fused in 4 minutes at 245°F (118°C)—a hazardous condition. Brand B control gave slightly better results in which no fusion or melting occurred in 170 samples tested for 3 minutes at 250°F. However, all samples were fused in 4 minutes at 250°F.

The liquid in glass tube control was found to have a precise, uniform endpoint. Out of 200 tubes tested at 250°F, for 10 minutes or less, not one changed color to green, but when exposed to 250°F for 11 minutes all tubes were changed to green. It is interesting to note, but of little practical value, that this liquid in glass tube control when suspended in boiling water vapor changed color to green in 6½ hours.

The chemically treated paper indicators were found to respond uniformly to physical conditions of time-temperature-moisture in the autoclave and they gave the most reliable response of all controls tested. Specifically, the paper indicators exceed somewhat the minimum standard of 12 minutes at 250°F saturated steam as well as the manufacturer's claims—an unexpected result.

In the case of autoclave tape the findings would seem to indicate that this product should not be placed in the same category as the other time-temperature controls. Under actual hospital conditions of sterilization, tape which was exposed to temperatures ranging from 230°F for 10 minutes through 250°F for 14 minutes could easily be interpreted as a safe color change. Nevertheless, it is important to note that autoclave tape is useful for identifying packages and articles which have been exposed to the physical conditions of an autoclave cycle. In addition, it is valuable as a test for adequacy of removal of air from chamber and load in a prevacuum type sterilizer.

It is the author's belief, based upon observations over a period of twenty-five years, that all sterilization indicators possess the same general disadvantage, to a greater or lesser degree, in that a percentage will be found to react to a time-temperature ratio inadequate for sterilization or that the end points are not sufficiently clear so as to permit accurate interpretation of the results. These controls do not indicate the actual buildup of temperature in the test pack nor do they indicate how much overexposure may have been applied. It is unfortunate for the user that the manufacturers of such controls have not attempted to bring about uniformity or standardization of end points to conform to a safe time-temperature relationship required for sterilization of supplies. Consequently, one type of indicator used in one hospital may react to a different time-temperature relationship than another type employed in another hospital.

The majority of glass tube indicators contain essentially the same material, namely, a pellet of sulfur which in the pure state has a melting point of about 248°F (120°C). In the process of manufacture certain changes may be introduced in the material which alter the melting point. Also, variations in the thickness or composition of the hermetically sealed glass tube affect the rate of heat transfer and the time-temperature conditions to which the control will react. It is doubtful if there is any control commercially available that can be depended upon to react exactly the same every time without failure. Studies have shown that rarely will any of the glass tube indicators melt at a temperature as low as 240°F (116°C) for 30 minutes. A fair percentage will, however, undergo partial or complete melting at 245°F (118°C) for 10 minutes. Certain of the paper indicators which undergo color change when exposed to moist heat at 250°F for 5, 12½ and 20 minutes are fairly reliable. However, they occasionally pose a problem for the untrained operator because the color change or end point is not sharp and correct interpretation is difficult.

If sterilization indicators are to be used, the indicator of whatever form it may be should be placed in the center of the largest and most densely wrapped package in the load. *This package should then be placed on the perforated tray or shelf in the front bottom of the sterilizer chamber.* The correct method for placing indicators in packs is shown in Figure 18-3. When indicators are used for setting up standards for sterilizing systematically pre-

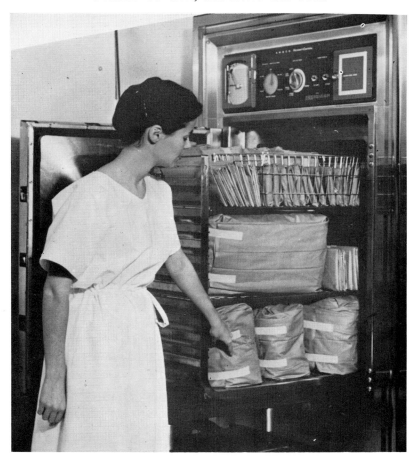

Figure 18-3. Correct method for using sterilization indicators or culture tests. Indicators should be located in center of largest packs—near bottom and in coolest area of chamber. Coolest portion of chamber is at front bottom, near outlet to discharge pipe.

pared loads, a heavy load of supplies as large and dense as any that will be encountered in routine practice should be assembled. Then select six of the heaviest and most densely wrapped packages. Place one indicator or control in the center of each of these packs, then place the packs on edge in the bottom of the sterilizer. Add the remainder of the load as it will normally be placed. Sterilize for 30 minutes, timing the exposure when the thermometer shows 250°F, with the sterilizer regulated to produce a maximum of 250° to 254°F. Upon completion of the cycle, remove the load and examine the controls. For greater reliability this method should be supplemented with culture tests, using bacterial spores of standardized heat resistance.

Sterilization indicators, culture tests and other detectors are often placed at the extreme top of the chamber, tied to the end frames of loading cars, or located just under the covers of packages. Tests made under such careless conditions mean nothing, and may develop a false sense of security in a highly inefficient sterilizer.

THE BOWIE-DICK TEST

This test derives its name from J. H. Bowie and J. Dick, Department of Microbiology, Royal Infirmary, Edinburgh, Scotland.[11] It was developed originally to expose the pattern of residual air within a challenge load consisting of a single pack in a high-vacuum sterilizer. In utilizing the test, autoclave (indicating) tape* is placed on the surface of a fabric in a crisscross manner, usually consisting of 3 pieces of tape about 8 inches long. This layer of fabric is then arranged in the test pack so that strips of tape extend from the outer edge to the center of the pack at a given layer depth. Usually 3-layer depths are tested in the pack. Following exposure in a prevacuum sterilizer, the pack is opened, the tape examined, and conclusions drawn as to the pattern of residual air, if any, that remained in the pack during the sterilizing cycle. Figures 18-4 and 18-5 show the influence of residual air on the autoclave tape exposed in a test pack.

The principle and the significance of the Bowie-Dick test is not clearly understood by all those who should use it in monitoring prevacuum sterilizers. This is apparent both in the United States and the United Kingdom as evidenced by Kelsey.[12] The following quotation lists several points that must be observed.

1. The Bowie-Dick test was designed for high-vacuum sterilisers for porous loads. It is quite irrelevant to downward-displacement sterilisers,

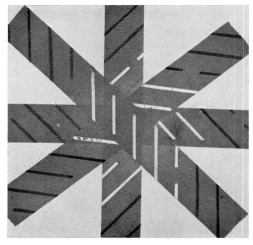

FIGURE 18-4. Typical pattern of changes in autoclave tape suggesting presence of residual air in pack and a faulty high-vacuum sterilizer.

* Type 1222 Tape. Minnesota Mining & Mfg. Co.

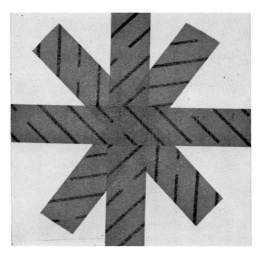

FIGURE 18-5. Pattern of changes in autoclave tape suggesting complete elimination of air from test pack.

whether used for fabrics, instruments, or bottled fluids.

2. The test-pack must be used by itself in an otherwise empty chamber [see p. 215 for contents of test pack].

3. The test is for adequacy of removal of air from chamber and load during the pre-vacuum stage, so that when steam is subsequently admitted its penetration of the load may be virtually instantaneous. It is not a test for adequate exposure to heat in terms of time-at-temperature.

4. The significant finding is not the intensity of the colour-change undergone by the heat-sensitive tape but its uniformity.

5. Any contrast in colour between the centre and the edge of the tape cross will be reduced and become unreadable if extended holding-times are used. The holding-time at 134°C must not exceed 3½ minutes.

6. High-vacuum sterilisers which cannot be made to pass the Bowie-Dick test must be relegated to the category of assisted downward-displacement sterilisers and treated accordingly. They cannot be reinstated merely by extending the holding-time until a uniform colour change is obtained.

7. Heat-sensitive tape, as used in this test, shows a colour-change which is only qualitative. Strips of tape may be useful on individual packages as indicators of exposures to heat, to prevent the issue of unsterilised items as sterile—they must not be used as indicators of successful sterilisation.

BIOLOGICAL TESTS FOR DETERMINING EFFICIENCY OF STERILIZATION

The best means at our disposal to confirm the sterility of an article or to determine the efficiency of a sterilizing process are strictly of a biological nature. Bacteriological culture tests designed to confirm the presence or absence of living microorganisms constitute the most commonly employed methods. Mechanical controls or sterilization indicators of the "telltale" type which supposedly react to some minimum of time and temperature do not constitute a direct approach to the lethality of the sterilizing process. When properly conducted, culture tests are more reassuring to bacteriologists and surgeons in general. Unfortunately, the delay entailed in determining the results of culture tests makes them somewhat impractical except for the periodic check on the maintenance of minimum standards. If they are not properly planned they may be distinctly misleading. The usual culture test is meaningless unless dry spores of established heat resistance in known populations are used.

The use of culture tests for regularly determining the efficiency of sterilizing processes in hospitals should be established as a standard control procedure. If the hospital has a properly equipped laboratory and a qualified bacteriologist or trained technician to do this work, then the culture test becomes a reliable means for the periodic testing of sterility of supplies. The bacterial spore strip technic described below is a safe and practical procedure. It can be used as an effective method of control in both large and small hospitals.

Spore-bearing Organisms

1) *Bacillus subtilis var. globigii,*
   U.S.D.A. Strain 1221a,
   A.T.C.C. No. 9372.
2) *Bacillus stearothermophilus,*
   N.C.A. Strain 1518,
   A.T.C.C. No. 7953.

Preparation of Spore Strips*

Inoculate a Kolle flask, containing nutrient agar, with a suspension of cells from a 24-hour nutrient agar slant culture of desired organism. The addition of 0.01% manganese sulphate to the nutrient agar will stimulate sporulation. Incubate the flask at 32°C for *B. subtilis* or 55°C for *B. stearothermophilus.* After 5 to 7 days incubation, prepare a smear of the growth and stain with malachite green spore stain. If microscopic examination shows heavy spore production, the growth is washed from the agar with a small quantity of sterile water and aseptically filtered through several layers of gauze. The suspension is then ready for standardization.

Prepare a 1:100 dilution of the suspension in sterile water, heat in water at 84°C for 5 minutes, and cool immediately. This will destroy the vegetative cells and the less resistant spores. From the boiled suspension prepare serial dilutions, plate on nutrient agar, incubate for 48 hours, and then make spore counts. Standardize suspension.

* A product of American Sterilizer Co., Erie, Pa.

Small strips of filter paper, 1½″ × ¼″, are then inoculated with a measured amount of the suspension so as to give a spore count of 100,000 or more per strip. The strips are dried at room temperature for several hours, inserted in small *sterilizable glassine* paper envelopes, sealed, and placed in clean storage.

Heat Resistance of Spore Strips

Contrary to popular belief, the spores of *B. subtilis* are not highly resistant to moist heat. Spores from most strains of this organism will show a uniform resistance to moist heat equal to or greater than the pathogenic organisms, including dry spores of *Cl. tetani* and *Cl. welchii*. Strips with populations of 1,000,000 spores each will uniformly survive exposure to saturated steam at 215°F (102°C) for 5 minutes, but will be killed in 15 minutes at 220°F (104°C). *This organism should not be used for checking the efficiency of pressure steam sterilizers.* It is satisfactory for dry heat and ethylene oxide gas.

B. stearothermophilus is one of the most resistant organisms known. Spore strips with populations of about 10,000 to 100,000 will survive exposure to saturated steam at 250°F (121°C) for at least 5 minutes, but will be killed in 12 minutes. This is the organism of choice for determining the efficiency of steam sterilizers.

Use of Spore Strips

When using bacterial spore strips for determining the efficiency of sterilizing processes, care must be taken to insure proper placement of each strip in the most inaccessible to steam portion of the test package. The correct procedure is to select two or more of the largest and most dense packs which comprise a part of the routine load of bulk supplies. Open the packs and insert two envelopes containing the bacterial spore strips in the center of each pack, as shown in Figure 18-6. Rewrap the packs and identify by marking with a Venus 6B pencil or other means. Place the packs on edge on the bottom shelf of the sterilizer chamber, near the front, as in Figure 18-3. Add the remainder of the load in the usual manner and operate the sterilizer according to standard procedure. If the test is being performed in a prevacuum-type sterilizer the load should consist of a single test pack. This constitutes the greatest challenge. Upon completion of the sterilizing cycle, including the drying period, remove the envelopes containing the spore strips from the test pack(s) and deliver them to the laboratory for sterility testing.

Spore strips may also be used for determining the efficiency of sterilization of rubber gloves. In this application it is necessary to insert the envelope containing the strip in one of the glove fingers, and then wrap in the usual manner. Do not attempt to sterilize gloves for less than 15 minutes at 250°F. The supervisor should record and file the following sterilization test

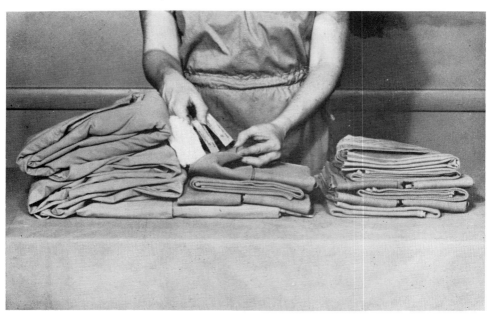

FIGURE 18-6. Bacterial spore strips or other culture tests should be placed in most dense portion of test pack.

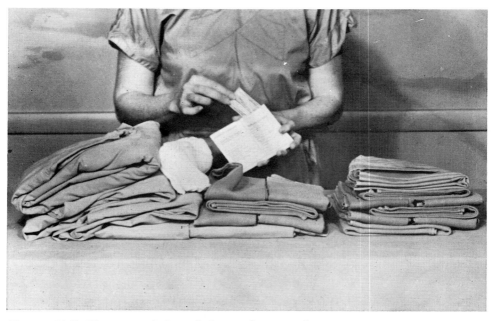

FIGURE 18-7. Upon completion of the sterilizing cycle, remove test strips from pack, place in protective envelope and deliver to laboratory.

data each time spore strips or other culture tests are made:

Date of test ....
Sterilizer ....
Type of load ....
Number test strips used ....
Location of test strips in load ....
Sterilizing conditions:
    Temperature (Indicating thermometer) ....°F
    Temperature (Recording thermometer) ....°F
    Exposure period ....minutes
Test conducted by ....
Department ....

STERILITY TEST PROCEDURE

All tests for sterility should be conducted in a clean and dust-free area of the laboratory, with as nearly static air circulation as is possible. Do not work in front of open windows or in drafty areas. A more reliable arrangement is to use a laminar flow hood or a completely enclosed cabinet such as are employed in control laboratories for the testing of disposable medical devices. The bacteriologist or technician should observe rigid bacteriologic technic throughout the procedure.

Cut open one end of the spore strip envelope with sterile scissors. Carefully withdraw the spore strip with sterile forceps (Fig. 18-8) and immerse it in the culture tube (18 × 150mm) containing 10 ml of sterile trypticase soy broth.

Incubate the tubes for 7 days at 32°C for *B. subtilis* strips and 55°C for *B. stearothermophilus* strips. Observe the tubes daily during the incubation period. If turbidity develops in the medium at any time during incubation it is indicative of bacterial growth—presumably due to spores which have survived the sterilizing process.

Controls: One or more *positive* controls should be included in each test series, performed on a monthly or semimonthly basis. This requires the transfer of an unexposed spore strip from the envelope to the tube of freshly prepared trypticase soy broth, followed by incubation at the correct temperature. A positive result indicates that the medium possesses suitable growth-promoting properties and that the spore strips contained viable spores prior to the sterilizing process. A *negative* control should also be included in each test series consisting of one or two tubes of the trypticase soy broth only. The absence of growth, following incubation, shows that the medium was effectively sterilized before use in the sterility test procedure.

Upon completion of the sterility test, the bacteriology laboratory should send a report to the supervisor giving the following information:

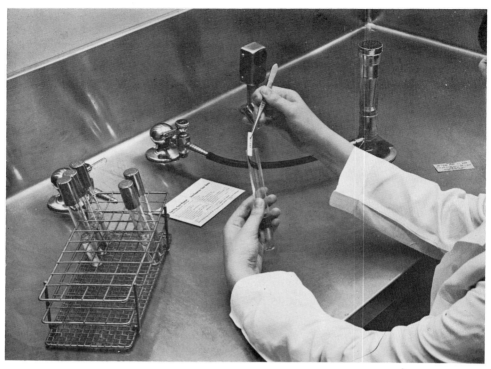

FIGURE 18-8. Carefully withdraw spore strip from envelope with sterile forceps and immerse in tube of culture medium. Sterility tests can be performed with a higher degree of reliability by using a laminar flow hood or a completely closed cabinet.

To .... (Supervisor)

Dept. ....

Date Test Strips were Cultured ....

Results of Culture Tests (Check One):

    One Strip Negative; Other Positive ☐

    Both Strips Positive ☐

    Should test be repeated? Yes ☐ No ☐

    Was Control Strip Cultured? Yes ☐ No ☐

    Control Strip Test Result:

                Positive ☐   Negative ☐

Signature ....

Date ....

HEAT RESISTANT SPORE SOIL AS TEST MATERIAL

In 1937, Ecker[6] recommended a culture test procedure involving the use of air dried and powdered garden soil (1 gram) samples in paper packages inserted in the center of test packs or drums. Since that time many workers,[13,14,15] particularly in European countries, have utilized this procedure or a modification thereof for determining and approving the functional capability of sterilizers. The argument advanced in favor of using native spore soil as a test material rather than spore cultures is that the former closely resembles the practical conditions under which medical and surgical supplies become contaminated with dust or dirt particles containing resistant spores. It is further contended that the spore soil represents a combination of numerous soil spore species of variable thermal stabilities which permits one to use a single test material rather than a multitude of tests with many different species for evaluation of autoclaves.

The views expressed on the advantages of a spore test soil as opposed to use of one organism, such as spores of *B. stearothermophilus* of known heat resistance are not enthusiastically endorsed by all microbiologists. It is known that samples of garden soil or compost vary in heat resistance, species and numbers of organisms, depending upon the area from which the soil is collected. Moreover, it is believed by some that spore soil is an unrealistic test because of the protection afforded organisms encased in mineral or organic matter. The heat resistance of spore soil is determined initially by exposing 50-mg samples of the finely pulverized soil, previously dried at 220°F (105°C), to streaming steam at 212°F (100°C) for 12 hours.

FREQUENCY OF CULTURE TESTS

A standard procedure should be set up for the routine evaluation of each sterilizer in the hospital on a semimonthly basis by means of culture tests. The procedure should also include ethylene oxide gas and dry heat or hot air sterilizers. If practical, the frequent checking of commercially prepared "sterile" supplies should be instituted as a quality control function on outside purchased supplies. Wherever possible, all bulk supplies should be sterilized with saturated steam at 250°F for 30 minutes or under equivalent conditions in high vacuum sterilizers. The operating room supervisor and the central service supervisor should put forth every possible effort toward the standardization of sterilizing and disinfecting technics. Frequent checking of the sterilizing process by means of culture tests, the maintenance of exact standards for the preparation, packaging, and loading of supplies in the sterilizer, plus intelligent and painstaking supervision are factors recognized as essential to the effective sterilization of hospital supplies.

REFERENCES

1. DANDY, W. E.: Importance of more adequate sterilization processes in hospitals. *Bull Amer Coll Surg,* 16:11-12, 1932.
2. MARSHALL, V., and SIMS, P.: Gas gangrene after injection of adrenaline in oil. *Med J Aust, ii:*653, 1960.
3. PATEL, J. C.; DHIRAWANI, M. K.; MEHTA, B. C., and AGARWAL, K. K.: Tetanus following intramuscular injection. *J Indian Med Ass,* 35:505, 1960.
4. SEVITT, S.: Source of two hospital-infected cases of tetanus. *Lancet,* 2:1075, 1949.
5. SCHMIDT, B.: Gasbrand als Hospitalinfektion und seine Verhütung. *Chirurgie,* 28:497, 1957.

6. ECKER, E. E.: Sterilization based on temperature attained and time ratio. *Mod Hosp*, 48:86-90, 1937.

7. HOYT, A.: Rubber glove sterilization and use of sterility indicators. *J Lab Clin Med*, 19:382-390, 1934.

8. UNDERWOOD, W. B.: *Textbook of Sterilization*. Chicago, Lakeside, Donnelley, 1941, p. 100.

9. WALTER, C. W.: Evaluation of sterility indicators. *Surgery*, 2:585-589, 1937. Also in *Aseptic Treatment of Wounds*, New York, Macmillan, 1948, p. 93.

10. SMITH, G., and PERKINS, J. J.: Unpublished data, Research Labs, American Sterilizer Co., 1967.

11. BOWIE, J. H.; KELSEY, J. C., and THOMPSON, G. R.: The Bowie and Dick autoclave tape test. *Lancet*, 1:586-587, 1963.

12. KELSEY, J. C.: The Bowie-Dick test. *Lancet*, II:911-912, 1966.

13. STUTZ, L., VON: Die Bedeutung der höchstresistenten thermophilen Sporenbildner bei der Sterilisation. *Med Klin*, 39:1722-1723, 1960.

14. FLURY, F.: Thesis. Beitrag zur Sterilisationstechnik und Sterilisationskontrolle in einer Spitalapotheke. Swiss Federal Institute of Technology, Zurich, 1962. (No. 3202).

15. KURZWEIL, H.: Neue Methoden der bakteriologischen Testung von Dampfsterilisationsapparaten. *Schweiz Z Path Bakt*, 20:505-510, 1957.

Chapter 19

STERILIZATION OF MEDICAL AND SURGICAL SUPPLIES WITH ETHYLENE OXIDE

T HE USE OF volatile or gaseous agents for purposes of disinfection and disinfestation has been a common procedure for a long time in many institutions. However, their use as sterilizing agents has been very limited primarily because of their inability to destroy bacterial spores and because of their adverse physicochemical effects on certain materials as well as for other important reasons. In a search for a more effective agent of this type, a chemical compound, ethylene oxide, was found which showed definite microbial and sporocidal properties in both its liquid and vapor phases. It was further found that heat-labile and moisture-sensitive materials could be sterilized with this agent without the detrimental or deteriorative effects resulting from steam or dry heat sterilization processes. Because of these capabilities, ethylene oxide has become widely used as a sterilant in hospitals and industry during the past decade.

Ethylene oxide was first discovered and described by Wurtz[1] in 1859. The value of this compound as a fumigant and pesticide was recognized in the early 1900's, and in 1929, Schrader and Bossert[2] found that it possessed bactericidal properties. This discovery led to an investigation resulting in a U. S. patent on a "Method of Sterilization" by Gross and Dixon[3] in 1937. During the next few years, interest in ethylene oxide as a sterilizing agent increased and in 1949, a series of four papers by Phillips and Kaye[4,5,6,7] was published in which the parameters for achieving sterility of bacterial spores by ethylene oxide were described. As a result of these reports, and many others [8,9,10,11,12,13] which followed, the practical usage and application of this agent as a sterilant has been established in a wide variety of fields ranging from food processing to interplanetary space vehicles and probes.

PROPERTIES OF ETHYLENE OXIDE

Ethylene oxide is an epoxy compound commonly designated as the simplest cyclic ether. It has a molecular weight of 44.05, a boiling point of 51.3°F (10.7°C), a freezing point of —168.3°F (—111.3°C) at atmospheric pressure and a vapor pressure of 7.3 psig at 70°F (21.1°C). The structural formula of ethylene oxide is as follows:

501

$$\begin{array}{ccc} H & H & \\ | & | & \\ H-C-C-H & \\ \diagdown\diagup & \\ O & \end{array}$$

In the liquid form ethylene oxide is colorless, completely soluble in water at 50°F (10°C) and, in the presence of a basic or acidic catalyst, will react with water to form a number of complex glycols. Ethylene oxide is flammable in both the liquid and gaseous states with the vapors forming flammable or explosive mixtures with air in all proportions from 0.4 to 100 per cent by volume[14] depending upon the type of ignition source. Mixtures of ethylene oxide and air can be ignited by an electric spark, static electricity, excessive heat, open flame, or by other similar means.

Liquid ethylene oxide in a concentrated or dilute form will cause severe burns on the human skin. It acts as a vesicant on exposed skin surfaces resulting in bleb formation of varying sizes and possible sensitization. Gaseous ethylene oxide is moderately toxic if inhaled. It will cause irritation of the skin, eyes, and mucous membranes as well as dizziness and nausea. A maximum tolerance of 100 ppm of vaporized ethylene oxide in air during an 8-hour exposure is recommended by the Manufacturing Chemists Association.[15] However, Hollingsworth, Rowen, Oyen, McCollister, and Spencer[16] have suggested 50 ppm ethylene oxide as a maximum industrial limit, and Thomas[17] feels that a maximum limit of 10 ppm of ethylene oxide in air should be required because of its toxic effects.

MICROBICIDAL ACTION OF ETHYLENE OXIDE

The destruction of microorganisms by liquid and gaseous ethylene oxide has been definitely established by a large number of investigators. Since the classical studies of Phillips and Kaye[5,6,7] in which the sporicidal action of ethylene oxide was determined under laboratory-controlled conditions of temperature, concentration, time, and humidity, the destruction of viruses,[18,19] molds,[20] and pathogenic fungi[21] have also been reported. Pappas and Hall[22] demonstrated the ability of ethylene oxide to kill highly resistant thermophilic bacteria found in food materials.

The virucidal properties of ethylene oxide are of prime interest to those in the medical-surgical fields who are concerned with such virus diseases as serum hepatitis (SH) and infectious hepatitis (IH). It is generally considered by authorities in the field of gaseous sterilization that, since a large variety of infectious animal viruses can be readily destroyed by ethylene oxide, there is no reason to believe that the SH and IH viruses are anymore resistant to ethylene oxide than the animal viruses. It is unfortunate that the inability to isolate and grow the hepatitis viruses on normal tissue culture media or by other means precludes actual experimentation on determining the resistance and virucidal effects of ethylene oxide on these particular viruses.

Studies to determine the specific reactions by which ethylene oxide destroys microorganisms have been neglected to a large degree. Of the several theories which have been proposed, the more commonly accepted hypothesis concerns the alkylating effects which ethylene oxide and other alkylating agents have on microbial cells. Alkylation is a chemical term usually defined as the replacement of an available hydrogen atom within a chemical group such as the amino, carboxyl, or hydroxyl groups with a hydroxy ethyl radical.

Some investigators[23,24] have demonstrated that ethylene oxide and similar compounds react with the nucleic acids of enzymic systems within the cells and that the cellular synthesis of these nucleic acids is disrupted by the alkylating agents resulting in the inability of the cell to normally metabolize and/or reproduce. Others[4] also suggest a similar reaction in which ethylene oxide reacts with certain chemical groups within the cell such as the sulfhydryl, amino, carboxyl, or hydroxyl groups and that because of this reaction the normal metabolic and/or reproductive processes of the microbial cell are seriously altered resulting in the inactivation or death of the cell. It is not definitely known which of these groups is actually attacked first by ethylene oxide; however, it is believed that the sulfhydryl group is the most reactive or susceptible to the agent. A simple illustration of alkylation as related to this discussion is shown in Figure 19-1. Shown are some of the chemical constituents of a living bacterial cell which may react chemically with ethylene oxide. When in contact with this agent, a chemical reaction occurs resulting in the death or inactivation of the cell. The rate at which destruction of organisms occurs would appear related to the rate of diffusion of the gas through the cell wall and the availability or accessibility

ALKYLATION

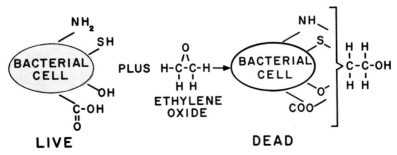

FIGURE 19-1. Theoretical chemical reactions of ethylene oxide on a bacterial cell by alkylation.

of one of the chemical groups to react with ethylene oxide. The rate of destruction also may depend upon whether the cell is in a vegetative or spore state. Phillips[25] and Bisset[26] have reported that in the formation of a bacterial spore, the sulfhydryl group may be protected by changes in the protein molecule, and the sterilizing action of ethylene oxide would then be restricted to one of the other chemical groups which are not as reactive. If the process of alkylation is accepted as the mode of action, the killing of microorganisms by ethylene oxide is a chemical interference and, probably, it is closely related to the inactivation of the cell reproductive process.

ETHYLENE OXIDE MIXTURES

Ethylene oxide in the pure form is not recommended for routine hospital sterilization in either the liquid or vapor state because of its flammability and toxic hazards. For practical usage, mixtures of ethylene oxide and inert gases such as carbon dioxide or fluorinated hydrocarbons are suggested. Coward and Jones[27] reported that all possible mixtures of ethylene oxide and air can be made nonflammable at ordinary temperatures and pressures by mixing 7.15 volumes of carbon dioxide with each volume of ethylene oxide. Haenni, Affens, Lento, Yeomens, and Fulton[28] described studies on the flammability characteristics of various ethylene oxide-halogenated hydrocarbon (Freon®, Ucon®, Genetron®* mixtures. These studies were significant, as they related to the flammability limits of mixtures of ethylene oxide and chlorofluorohydrocarbon at temperatures of 132.8° to 161.6°F (56° to 72°C) in various-size chambers. They found marked differences in the flammability limits of ethylene oxide-inert gaseous mixtures when determined in large-size chambers as opposed to smaller conventional apparatus. They further showed that the following two gaseous mixtures were nonflammable in any proportion of air at temperatures up to 130°F (54.4°C):

> Mixtures containing dichlorodifluoromethane (Freon-12 or Genetron-12) and ethylene oxide in concentrations up to 12 per cent by weight.
> Mixtures containing equal parts of Freon-12 and trichloromonofluoromethane (Freon-11 or Genetron-11) and ethylene oxide up to 11 per cent by weight.

At the present time, there are several ethylene oxide mixtures which can be safely employed as sterilizing agents under normal conditions. These mixtures and the types of containers in which they are sold are shown in Table 19-1. The ethylene oxide-carbon dioxide mixtures (Carboxide® and Oxyfume Sterilant-20®) are the least expensive and are both reasonably safe to use in properly constructed sterilizing equipment. The Oxyfume Sterilant-20 mixture is sometimes preferred over the Carboxide mixture because of its higher ethylene oxide concentration.

---

* Products of E. I. DuPont Co., Linde Products Co., and Allied Chemical Co., respectively.

TABLE 19-1

ETHYLENE OXIDE MIXTURES USED IN GASEOUS STERILIZATION PROCEDURES

Mixtures	Manufacturer	Type of Container Cylinders		
		Gross Wt.	Net Wt.	Tare Wt.
Ethylene oxide and carbon dioxide:				
Carboxide				
10% Ethylene oxide	Union Carbide Corp.	155	40	115
90% Carbon dioxide	Linde Division, N.Y., N.Y.	193	60	133
Oxyfume Sterilant-20				
20% Ethylene oxide	Union Carbide Corp.	145	30	115
80% Carbon dioxide	Linde Division, N.Y., N.Y.	193	60	133
Steroxide-20				
20% Ethylene oxide	Castle-Ritter-Pfaudler Co.	193	60	133
80% Carbon dioxide	Rochester, N.Y.			
Ethylene oxide and fluorinated hydrocarbons:				
Cry-Oxide				
11% Ethylene oxide	Ben Venue Laboratories	21 oz disposable cans		
79% Trichlorofluoremethane	Bedford, Ohio			
10% Dichlorodifluoromethane				
Benvicide				
11% Ethylene oxide	The Matheson Co.	43	16	27
54% Trichlorofluoremethane	East Rutherford, N.J.	235	100	135
35% Dichlorodifluoromethane		381	270	111
Pennoxide				
12% Ethylene oxide	Pennsylvania Engineering Co.	39	25	14
88% Dichlorodifluoromethane	Philadelphia, Pa.	180	140	40
Steroxide-12				
12% Ethylene oxide	Castle-Ritter-Pfaudler Co.	20 and 36 oz disposable cans		
88% Dichlorodifluoromethane	Rochester, N.Y.			
Anprolene				
84% Ethylene oxide	C. R. Bard Inc.	½ oz disposable glass vials		
16% Inert gases	Murray Hill, N.J.			

The ethylene oxide-halogenated hydrocarbon mixtures (Cry-Oxide,® Benvicide,® and Pennoxide®) differ from the other mixtures in that they have much lower container vapor pressures at ambient or room temperature and contain more ethylene oxide per unit volume than the mixtures of ethylene oxide and carbon dioxide at the same pressure. These mixtures are as safe to handle as the carbon dioxide mixtures and can also be stored at room temperature.

MEASUREMENT OF ETHYLENE OXIDE

The concentration of ethylene oxide in a closed vessel is usually measured in terms of milligrams per liter of chamber space. There are several ways by which the concentration of ethylene oxide can be determined. A simple method is by determining the weight of a gas cylinder before and after the chamber has been charged. The weight difference is equal to the quantity of gas required to fill the chamber to a predetermined pressure. From this weight, the concentration of ethylene oxide can be determined.

Another method for determining concentration is by actual chemical analysis of samples of the gaseous atmosphere taken from the chamber. The more popularly used chemical methods are those devised by Lubatti[29] and Swan[30] or, in some cases, modifications of these methods. Direct measurement by such instruments as the gas chromatograph or the infrared analyzer can also be employed.

There is actually no method by which hospitals can quickly and accurately determine ethylene oxide concentrations because gas sterilizers are usually not equipped with required analytical instrumentation or devices. In most, if not all cases, however, a pressure gauge is installed on the sterilizer which indicates the chamber pressure when the chamber is charged. If the pressure gauge is operating correctly, an estimate of the ethylene oxide concentration can be made from the pressure reading after the chamber has been charged. This is usually achieved by mathematically applying the ideal gas laws since the partial pressures created by the ethylene oxide and its diluent(s) within the chamber constitutes a function of the quantity or volume of gas introduced into the chamber at a given temperature. Figure 19-2 shows the ethylene oxide concentrations at different chamber pressures when the chamber temperature was held at 130°F $\pm$ 5°. The curve was

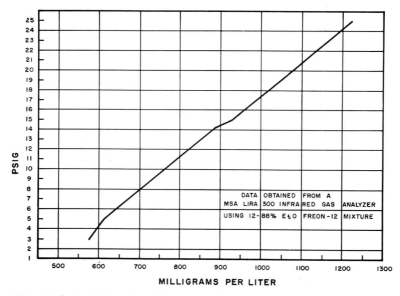

FIGURE 19-2. Relationship of ethylene oxide concentrations (mg/liter) to varying chamber pressures at 130° ±5° F.

drawn from the ethylene oxide concentration readings as they occurred on an infrared gas analyzer.

FACTORS INFLUENCING ETHYLENE OXIDE STERILIZATION

Sterilization by ethylene oxide is a much more complex process than that of steam or dry heat. This complexity lies in the fact that in addition to time and temperature, which are the major factors in steam and dry heat sterilization, ethylene oxide concentration and moisture are equally as important in gaseous sterilization. The relationship of these factors to ethylene oxide sterilization and their influence on the achievement of sterility by this agent are discussed below.

Temperature

Temperature has a marked influence on the sterilizing efficiency of ethylene oxide as it enhances penetration and affords a reduction in the exposure period. This was demonstrated by Phillips,[5] whose studies indicated that the activity of ethylene oxide increases approximately 2.74 times for each 18°F (10°C) rise in a temperature range of 41° to 98.6°F (5° to 37°C). It was assumed that this temperature coefficient was constant for other temperature ranges and ethylene oxide concentrations.

In a later report, Ernst and Shull[31] stated there were at least two temperature coefficient values for the lower and higher temperature ranges. These consisted of a value of 1.8 for ethylene oxide concentrations of 440 mg/liter and 880 mg/liter at the respective temperatures of above 105.1°F (40.6°C) and 92.1°F (33.4°C), and values of 3.2 and 2.3 for the same respective ethylene oxide concentrations but at lower temperatures.

In routine sterilization with ethylene oxide, temperatures of 120° to 140°F (49° to 60°C) are used; however, there are some instances, e.g. the sterilization of heat-labile plastics, where these temperatures may be too high. Gaseous sterilization at room temperature is also conducted in some applications but longer exposure periods are required and there may be difficulty in maintaining in the vapor state the mixtures of ethylene oxide and inert gas at the chamber pressures employed. Temperature is also important from a physical standpoint. It influences the pressure produced by a given volume of gas in a closed vessel. This is important when charging a chamber with gas to provide a predetermined concentration of ethylene oxide. If the chamber has been heated, the volume of gas required to provide the desired concentration will remain in the gaseous state. However, if the temperature is decreased, after the chamber has been charged, some of the gas may condense to a liquid, as the temperature will not support the gas in the vapor state. Conversely, if a chamber has been charged to a given pressure, or has been charged with a given volume of gas at a certain temperature, and more gas is introduced for such purposes as doubling the ethylene oxide concentration, the temperature should also be raised to prevent possible condensation of the gas. As the extent to which the temperature should be raised is not directly proportional to the quantity of gas admitted, precautions should be taken in this situation. Normally, it is more desirable to employ a gaseous mixture containing a higher ethylene oxide concentration than it is to elevate the temperature, particularly if heat-sensitive materials are to be processed.

Concentration

Essential in gaseous sterilization is the concentration or the partial pressure of the sterilizing agent within the chamber. For practical applications, an ethylene oxide concentration of 450 mg/liter is usually recommended as the minimum concentration which will provide sterilization within a reasonable time. Higher concentrations of ethylene oxide ranging up to 1000 mg/liter are more desirable, as exposure periods can be reduced almost one half. Concentrations greater than 1,000 mg/liter do not appreciably affect exposure times. Moreover, one must also consider the fact that the use of higher ethylene oxide pressures to provide higher concentrations is predicated on the temperature of the chamber and the ability of that temperature to maintain the ethylene oxide in a vaporized state.

Moisture

It has been established that moisture is an important adjunct to the sterilizing efficiency of ethylene oxide. Kaye[7] has shown that moisture levels of 20 to 40% relative humidity were required to sterilize aerosolized spores by ethylene oxide and that the rate of kill was ten times as fast at 28% relative humidity as it was at 97%. Mathews and Hofstad[19] showed that of 15 animal viruses studied, all were destroyed by ethylene oxide when in the moist state, but nine, which had been dried by lyophilization, remained viable following exposure. Newman, Colwell, and Jameson[8] reported that tubercle bacilli were readily killed in moist sputum by ethylene oxide but survived when suspended in dried sputum. Merriam and Wiles[32] indicated that the moisture content of an organic product prior to gaseous sterilization was essential. They stated that "the introduction of water vapor, steam, or water may, of course, be controlled so as to adjust the moisture content of the products concerned to the desired point." It was further stated that prehumidification of the products before exposure to ethylene oxide may be desirable.

Kaye and Phillips[7] established the well-known relative humidity levels of 20 to 40 per cent as optimum for the sterilization of aerosolized spores by ethylene oxide and indicated that relative humidites lower than 20 per cent and higher than 65 per cent reduced the sterilizing properties of ethylene oxide. Ernst and Shull[33] reported that prehumidification of a sterilizing chamber containing materials prior to the introduction of ethylene oxide gas was more effective in attaining sterility than the simultaneous injection of water vapor and ethylene oxide. Perkins and Lloyd[34] concluded that the optimum levels of humidity depended to a large degree upon the nature of the materials being sterilized and the porosity of the material surfaces. They showed that highly porous surfaces could be sterilized at relatively low humidities, however, solid surfaces required chamber humidities of 50% relative humidity or more. The relationship of the effects of humidity on the sterilization of porous and solid-surface items by ethylene oxide was also demonstrated in an earlier paper by Opfell, Hohmann, and Latham,[35] who indicated that the absorption and release of moisture by porous surfaces is a contributing factor to the reason porous-surfaced materials are easier to sterilize than solid-surfaced items.

The moisture content of the microbial cell is another important factor in gaseous sterilization. It has been known for some time that dry or desiccated cells are much more resistant to sterilization processes than moist or wet cells. In a recent article, Gilbert, Gambill, Spiner, Hoffman, and Phillips[36] demonstrated that excessive drying of bacterial cells will result in a nonuniform reaction of ethylene oxide, and in order to regain rapid uniformity of reaction, the cells must be rehydrated by direct wetting with water. In view of the above and other available information, it can be concluded that the moisture content of the microbial cell at the time of exposure to ethylene oxide is an important factor, that excessive drying or desiccation of materials to be gas sterilized should be avoided, and that the moisture content of the atmosphere in those areas where material packaging is conducted should be controlled at approximately 50% relative humidity or more so as to avoid unintentional dehydration of contaminating organisms.

Moisture concentration in gaseous sterilization has usually been expressed in terms of per cent relative humidity and measured as such with indicating and/or recording devices calibrated directly in per cent relative humidity. Because of certain disadvantages in using this system in gas sterilizing chambers, a modified method was recently incorporated in the author's laboratory in which moisture is measured in terms of milligrams water per liter. This is accomplished by the use of an infrared analyzer which is connected to a gas sterilizer and measures the water content contained in the gaseous atmosphere directly in milligrams per liter of water. Comparative tests using the infrared analyzer with a per cent relative humidity indicating system revealed comparable results when the relative humidity readings were mathematically corrected to milligrams of water at the test temperature. On the basis of these results, it is our recommendation that moisture concentration in gaseous sterilization would be more meaningful if measured and reported on a weight basis such as milligrams per liter of gaseous atmosphere. To facilitate this recommendation, the theoretical relationship of per cent relative humidity to milligrams of water per liter is illustrated in Figure 19-3.

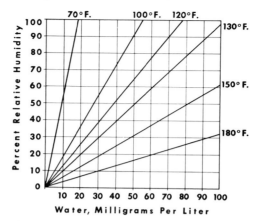

FIGURE 19-3. Relationship of per cent relative humidity to moisture content (mg/liter) at varying chamber temperatures.

Time

Sterilization by vaporized ethylene oxide is not an instantaneous process since it is governed by specific factors—for example, temperature affects the rate of diffusion and permeation of ethylene oxide through packaging materials, thus, low chamber temperatures require longer exposure times than do higher temperatures; packaging materials have differing permeability characteristics to ethylene oxide and moisture; heavily contaminated or soiled materials require longer exposure periods than do clean items; low ethylene oxide concentrations also require longer exposure periods; and the degree of dryness or desiccation of contaminated materials affects sterilization times. Consequently, a given exposure period for one situation may not be adequate for another. In certain instances, exposure periods have to be determined experimentally or on a trial and error basis utilizing acceptable microbiological sterility controls as a basis for determining the required exposure time. It is fundamental to effective ethylene oxide sterilization that all articles are thoroughly cleaned beforehand and properly packaged in approved wrapping materials.

STERILIZATION CONCEPTS

A sterilization process has been traditionally defined as a method by which all forms of life are destroyed. Sterility is normally demonstrated by proving, through the use of accepted microbiological procedures, that no viable or living organism can be recovered from the processed item or material. Sterility is usually confirmed by either the procedure described in the United States Pharmacopoeia, XVIII Edition, in which a qualitative analysis is conducted on exposed materials for the presence of bacteria and molds or by the use of exposed biological sterility controls which are qualitatively analyzed for the presence of bacteria. In both procedures, the results are recorded as growth or no growth with the latter indicative of sterility. These procedures for sterility testing of exposed items are widely accepted at this time. Recently, there has been a trend in certain industries and, particularly, in the spacecraft sterilization field to employ another method for establishing sterility. This method is based on the concept that bacteria, subjected to a lethal process, die at a uniform rate or exponentially with time (see Chapter 4). The importance of this concept resides in the fact that it provides a means for quantitatively evaluating a sterilization process by permitting the computation of bacterial death rates and by determining the resistance of microorganisms to a particular method of sterilization. It also permits the evaluation of the effects of such factors as time and temperature on the destruction of microorganisms in steam and hot air sterilization as well as those of concentration and moisture in gaseous sterilization.

DECIMAL REDUCTION TIME

In practice, the decimal reduction (D value) time, previously explained in Chapter 4, and now applied to ethylene oxide sterilization, is based on determining the thermochemical death-time rates of microorganisms exposed to the gas under controlled conditions of temperature, time, moisture, and gas concentration. Normally, the test organisms are bacterial spores, although bacterial vegetative cells, molds, yeasts, and viruses can also be used. Following exposure, quantitative assays are made to determine the number of organisms surviving the process. Survivor curves are then prepared in which the logarithm of the number of survivors is plotted against time. This results in a straight-line graph which is commonly referred to as a logarithmic order of death. From this curve, D values, or the time required to destroy 90 per cent of the total cell or spore population at a given temperature, or concentration of ethylene oxide can be determined. Studies on the resistance of bacterial spores to ethylene oxide utilizing the D value concept have been conducted by El-Bisi,[37] Vondell,[38] and by Liu, Howard, and Stumbo[39]. Similar studies in the author's laboratories have provided significant data on the resistance of several spore-forming organisms to ethylene oxide under laboratory controlled conditions [500 mg ethylene oxide/liter, 130°F (54°C) and 30 to 50% relative humidity]. Figure 19-4 shows the results of some of these studies. The data illustrate the resistance of spores of the Fort Detrick, Maryland, red strain of *B. subtilis* var. niger, *Clostridium sporogenes* (ATCC 7955), *Clostridium sporogenes* (ATCC 3584), and *Bacillus stearothermophilus* (ATCC 7953) to ethylene oxide when dried on porous surfaces (paper strips) and nonporous surfaces (ceramic tile squares). D values, obtained from these data and D values from similar curves prepared for the nonspore-forming organism, *Micrococcus radiodurans,* are shown in Table 19-2.

Another advantage in establishing thermochemical death-time curves

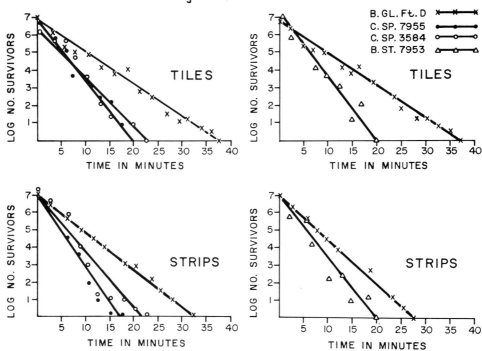

FIGURE 19-4. Resistance of bacterial spores to ethylene oxide under laboratory-controlled conditions and on porous and nonporous surfaces.

concerns the ability of the investigator to plot probability curves of bacterial survival and the minimum exposure periods required to attain sterility under a given set of conditions. Figure 19-5 illustrates this concept.

RESISTANCE AND PROTECTION OF MICROORGANISMS

Failure to attain sterility in gaseous sterilization can be attributed to a number of factors other than irregularities in the basic requirements of temperature, time, moisture, and gas concentration of this process. Among these factors are the natural microbial and viral resistance, barriers to effective gas permeation such as the type and nature of soil on an article, the preparation and packaging of materials, and to variations in the composition of mate-

TABLE 19-2

D VALUE—MINUTES

ORGANISM	NONPOROUS SURFACE	POROUS SURFACE
B. subtilis var. *globigii*	6.0	4.55
C. sporogenes ATCC 7955	3.4	2.6
C. sporogenes ATCC 3584	3.8	2.8
B. stearothermophilus ATCC 7953	2.8	2.8
M. radiodurans	5.4	3.75

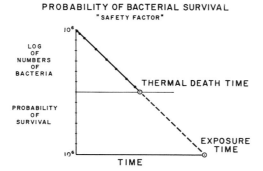

FIGURE 19-5. Use of a bacterial survival curve for determining minimum sterilization times under specified conditions.

rials. The resistance of microorganisms to chemical disinfectants has been the subject of intensive studies by many investigators.

It has been found that bacterial spores can be as much as 100,000 times more resistant to chemical agents than the bacterial vegetative cells. Phillips[25] has shown that there is a comparatively narrow range of resistance between spores and vegetative cells when exposed to ethylene oxide. From studies made with the spores of *B. subtilis* var. *globigii* and the organisms *Micrococcus pyogenes* and *Escherichia coli,* he reported a resistance ratio of between 2 and 6. Among the various factors which influence cell resistance is the presence of lipids (fats and fat-like materials) within the cells, which have been shown to increase their resistance to ethylene oxide. Church, Halvorson, Ramsey, and Hartman[40] reported that aerobic bacterial spores of certain species containing these materials were more resistant to ethylene oxide than those from which lipids had been chemically extracted. This relationship is of importance when selecting culture media for the growth and harvesting of microorganisms for investigating the sterilizing action of ethylene oxide. For example, studies[41] in the author's laboratories have shown that spores of *Clostridium sporogenes,* grown in a meat infusion medium and dried on porous and solid surface materials, are much more resistant to ethylene oxide than similar spores grown in a synthetic medium containing trypticase and peptone and exposed to ethylene oxide under the same conditions. Recent evidence has shown that some nonsporeforming bacteria can be as resistant to ethylene oxide as the most resistant bacterial spores known at this time. To illustrate, Opfell, Shannon, and Chan[42] reported the dry *Staphylococcus epidermidis* cells were more resistant to ethylene oxide vapor than were *B. subtilis* spores and they were capable of surviving in liquid ethylene oxide as well as in a solid propellant mixed with ethylene oxide. The authors indicated that the occurrence of *S. epidermidis* cells on exposed surfaces during the assembly of spacecraft vehicles could interfere with the gaseous sterilization of component parts because of the resistance of these organisms to ethylene oxide. Another example concerns the organism *Micrococcus radiodurans*. Anderson[43] and Hawiger and Jeljaszewicz[44] have reported that this organism, isolated from irradiated ground pork and beef, exhibits a high degree of resistance to gamma radiation and ultraviolet light. It was reported that the organism survived a radiation dose of 4×10^6 roentgen equivalents physical (rep) in meat and up to 6×10^6 rep on tryptone-glucose-yeast-extract agar slants. Interest in the resistance of this organism to radiation led to a series of studies in the writer's laboratory to determine whether the organism was resistant to ethylene oxide. Results of these studies[45] indicated that *Micrococcuss radiodurans* has a resistance to ethylene oxide almost equalling that of *B. subtilis* var. *globigii.*

The state of hydration and the preparation of bacterial suspensions for test purposes also contribute to the resistance of organisms to this agent. The effects of dehydration on the resistance of microbial cells to ethylene oxide and the difficulties in rehydrating such organisms after drying were recently reported by Phillips.[46] His findings showed a definite increase in the resistance of bacteria to ethylene oxide on dehydration and further indicated that rehydration of dried cells is a slow process even at high humidities. Gilbert, *et al.*[36] also reported on the resistance of dehydrated cells to ethylene oxide. The preparation of bacterial suspensions for exposure to ethylene oxide is equally important in determining microbial resistance to this agent. Harvested cells or spores in suspension should be cleaned by proper microbiological procedures to remove all constituents of the growth medium and other debris prior to exposure as these substances will provide a protective barrier around the cell.

Barriers to effective gas permeation or diffusion also create problems in attaining sterility by ethylene oxide. Heavily soiled items or materials inhibit gas permeation. Because of the inhibiting and protective effects of dense soils, heavily contaminated materials should be cleaned prior to sterilization. In hospital practice there are many instances where articles are contaminated with infectious agents which present a hazard to employees if manual cleaning procedures are performed before the articles are sterilized. For these cases it is recommended that such items be decontaminated as soon after use as possible by subjecting them to ethylene oxide for a period of time sufficient to render the materials safe for handling. *This means extending the exposure time to ethylene oxide to at least double the normally recommended exposure time for the specific article or material.* The preparation and packaging of materials to be sterilized by ethylene oxide may also create problems in achieving sterility if not conducted according to approved procedures. Large, dense loads of tightly packed items and improper chamber loading techniques retard the permeation and diffusion of moisture and the gaseous agent as well as heat penetration. Bacteria suspended in physiological saline and dried on solid surfaces show a much greater resistance to ethylene oxide than those suspended and dried in distilled water or blood serum. This was shown by Znamirowski, McDonald, and Roy,[47] who reported that saline suspensions of *B. cereus* spores were very resistant to ethylene oxide when dried on glass surfaces and that sterilization was not achieved in an 18-hour exposure period at 130°F (54.4°C), 850 mg/liter ethylene oxide and approximately 40 to 50% relative humidity. On the basis of these results, it was proposed that a protective cover of salt crystals is developed during the drying of the saline solution, which surrounds the bacteria either collectively or singly, and this crystalline structure is practically impermeable to ethylene oxide.

A final factor in this series which may cause some difficulty in gaseous sterilization is the material composition or the consistency of the commodity being sterilized. For example, powders having a low moisture content are very difficult to sterilize and should be equilibrated to humidities of 50 to 60% relative humidity prior to exposure. Crystalline materials are also difficult or impossible to sterilize if they contain embedded organisms. Doyle and Ernst[48] reported that bacterial spores entrapped in insoluble crystalline materials were very difficult to detect and extremely resistant to ethylene oxide and moist and dry heat. They indicated that crystals, by the nature of their structure, create thermal conductivity barriers. Attempted sterilization of liquids, ointments, lotions, creams, or jellies by ethylene oxide in the vapor state is not practical because of the long exposure periods required and the possibility of chemical reactions in the materials.

MATERIALS COMPATIBLE WITH ETHYLENE OXIDE

The great advantage attached to ethylene oxide processing is the ability to sterilize, without destructive effects, a wide variety of medical equipment articles and materials necessary for patient care. The more commonly used articles are listed in Table 19-3.

TABLE 19-3

Hospital Equipment and Materials Sterilizable by Ethylene Oxide

Telescopic Instruments	Plastic Goods	Rubber Goods	Instruments and Equipment	Miscellaneous
Bronchoscopes	Catheters	Tubing	Cautery sets	Dilators
Cystoscopes	Nebulizers	Surgical gloves	Eye knives	Electric cords
Electrotomes	Vials	Catheters	Lamps	Hair clippers
Endoscopes	Syringes	Drain and feed	Needles	Miller-Abbott tubes
Esophagoscopes	Test tubes	sets	Neurosurgical	Pumps
Ophthalmoscopes	Petri dishes	Sheeting	instruments	Motors
Otoscopes	I. V. sets		Scalpel blades	Books
Pharyngoscopes	Infant incubators		Speculae	Toys
Proctoscopes	Heart lung machines		Syringes	Pottery
Resectoscopes	Heart pacemakers		Dental	Blankets
Sigmoidoscopes	Artificial kidney		instruments	Sheets
Thoracoscopes	machines		Oxygen tents	Furniture
Urethroscopes				Sealed ampules
				Sutures
				Medicine droppers

LIMITATIONS IN ETHYLENE OXIDE STERILIZATION

Although ethylene oxide appears to be an ideal sterilant for most heat-sensitive materials, there are some disadvantages or limitations which require caution in its application. Some acrylic plastic materials and polystyrene are attacked by the mixtures of ethylene oxide and fluorinated hydrocarbon, particularly those containing trichloromonofluoromethane (Freon-11). Bosomworth and Hamelberg[49] reported the occurrence of blebs in certain parts of endotracheal tubes and cuffs following exposure to ethylene oxide and steam cycles.

Certain medicaments and pharmaceuticals are affected by gaseous sterilization. Kaye[9] reported that while penicillin was unaffected, streptomycin calcium sulphate suffered 35 per cent loss in activity when exposed to ethylene oxide. Sutaria and Williams[50] have reported an increase in pH occurring in a number of solutions exposed to ethylene oxide and that sodium iodide crystals are discolored to varying degrees. In respect to solutions contained in plastic or glass vials, it should be emphasized that the exposure of these vials to ethylene oxide vapors will not result in sterile solutions as the gas does not permeate through glass, but it is absorbed to some degree by the plastic. However, gaseous sterilization can be used to sterilize the outer surfaces of the vials when required. A large variety of urological, ophthalmic, surgical, and dental instruments can be gas sterilized. All protein matter and other kinds of soil must, however, be removed by thorough washing and cleaning prior to exposure. All instruments must be dry prior to packaging because wet instruments packaged in plastic wrappers will remain wet during exposure to ethylene oxide and this may induce the formation of a film of ethylene glycol. Gaseous ethylene oxide in water solution will hemolyze red blood cells and inactivate complement and prothrombin. Certain culture media, sterilized by ethylene oxide, were reported by Sykes[51] to be unsuitable for growing certain fastidious bacteria following exposure due to the reaction of the sterilant with the organic components of the media. In addition to these, such materials as dried food powders and other food items, animal diets, and animal bedding are definitely altered by gaseous sterilization. Adverse chemical reactions occur in garden soil when exposed to ethylene oxide which interfere with studies on soil fumigants and herbicides.

Certain component parts of spacecraft assemblies such as electronic circuitries embedded in epoxy resin cannot be sterilized by this process. Difficulties have occurred in the gaseous sterilization of certain types of lensed instruments because of the solvent action of the hydrocarbon diluents on the lens cement and the crazing effects of these diluents on the lenses. It is important, therefore, that those concerned with the practical applications of gaseous sterilization be cognizant of the fact that ethylene oxide is not a satisfactory sterilant for all materials. In general, one should not use ethylene oxide for sterilization purposes if the material is heat-stabile and will withstand sterilization by means of saturated steam under pressure.

RESIDUAL ETHYLENE OXIDE

One serious disadvantage of ethylene oxide sterilization is the time required for dissipation of the residual contained in exposed porous (absorptive) materials. This condition must be understood by hospital professional personnel and allowance made for an adequate aeration period of articles sterilized by this process so as to avoid untoward patient reactions in the clinical use of the articles.

The fact that materials which are porous will sorb such gases as ethylene oxide can be amply demonstrated by the detection of this agent in plastics, rubber, and leather by chemical analysis following exposure. Sorption would not ordinarily be a serious disadvantage of ethylene oxide sterilization if the residual gas were nontoxic and could be readily dissipated or removed from these materials in a short time. Unfortunately, studies have shown that ethylene oxide will persist in exposed products of this nature for several hours and, in some instances, for several days. Phillips[52] reported that he found up to 4% ethylene oxide in rubber immediately following exposure and quantitative amounts still present after 5 hours' aeration, but none after 24 hours. Beard and Dunmire[53] revealed that old and spongy soft leather absorbs and retains ethylene oxide gas much longer than new and smooth-finished leathers. They found that after exposing leather samples to 100 mg ethylene oxide per liter for 16 hours at room temperature, 10 to 18 per cent of the absorbed gas was retained in the samples after approximately 128 hours of aeration under normal conditions of air circulation. Royce and Moore[54] reported that they found as much as 15.4 mg of ethylene oxide per gram of rubber in rubber gloves following exposure; 6.7 mg after 30 minutes and 0.4 mg after 4 hours' exposure. They demonstrated that, on human volunteers, vesicular lesions occurred on the fingers, hands, and forearms when the ethylene oxide concentration was greater than 2 milligrams per gram of rubber. Freeman and Barwell[55] demonstrated that polyvinyl chloride tubing will sorb ethylene oxide and dichlorodifluoromethane (Freon-12 or Genetron-12), and they pointed out that if the tubing is used with a heart-lung machine immediately following exposure, the dissipating gases may form gas bubbles in the blood as it circulates through the tubing. Hirose, Goldstein, and Bailey,[56] in describing the effects of ethylene oxide-exposed plastic tubing on the hemolysis of blood contained in the tubing, indicated that changes are produced which cause extensive hemolysis. They also found marked differences in the quantity of hemolysis produced by different brands of plastic tubing. The greatest extent of hemolytic activity was found to occur in tubing used immediately after exposure to ethylene oxide.

AERATION OF ARTICLES EXPOSED TO ETHYLENE OXIDE STERILIZATION

Most, if not all, materials retain varying amounts of ethylene oxide gas following their removal from a gas sterilizer. It is essential that this residual gas be allowed to dissipate from the materials, to an acceptable tolerance level, prior to their usage. The tolerance level is dependent upon a great number of factors spanning from the individual patient to a variety of materials, implements, and procedures. It is impossible to establish a single criterion for tolerance of residual ethylene oxide which will be acceptable and clinically safe for all situations. This judgment must rest with the particular individual who is responsible for the patient's care.

Methods for rapidly removing sorbed ethylene oxide and its diluent gases from exposed materials have been sought for some time. Such procedures as multiterminal chamber vacuums, in which the exposed load is subjected to repeated air washings, or exposing the load to forced air circulation in a closed chamber have been suggested, as well as placing exposed materials in well-ventilated areas for indefinite periods of time. Freeman and Barwell[55] reported that dissolved ethylene oxide in polyvinyl chloride tubing could be completely removed by holding the tubing under a vacuum greater than 29 inches of mercury for 1 to 2 hours. Hirose, Goldstein, and Bailey[56] recommended that at least three and preferably five days should elapse before using gas-sterilized tubing for clinical extracorporeal bypass. Clarke, Davidson, and Johnston[57] have stated that if ethylene oxide gas sterilization is used for plastic tubing, it should be held for three days' aeration before use. There was little advantage in keeping it aerated for longer periods.

Tests in the author's laboratories indicate that the removal of total residual gases in certain exposed materials can be accelerated by incubating these materials at 120°F (49°C). The data in Table 19-4 illustrate the effects of elevated temperatures on removal of residual gas. Whereas, these studies were limited to the materials indicated and polyethylene film, further observations showed that other materials would react in a similar pattern. For rapid removal of ethylene oxide, exposed materials can be placed

TABLE 19-4

EFFECTS OF ELEVATED TEMPERATURES ON THE REMOVAL OF SORBED
ETHYLENE OXIDE MIXTURES IN EXPOSED MATERIALS

Ethylene Oxide Mixture	Complete Removal of Total Mixture (Hours)		Complete Removal of the EtO Fraction (Hours)	
	Gum Rubber	Vinyl*	Gum Rubber	Vinyl*
Carboxide				
Room temperature	ca. 100	ca. 100	24	ca. 100
49°C (120°F)	4	7	4	7
Cry-Oxide				
Room temperature	150	150	10	50
49°C (120°F)	25	30	5	5
Pennoxide				
Room temperature	150	150	25	ca. 100
49°C (120°F)	12	18	4	6

* Tygon tubing.

in an area or chamber capable of maintaining 120°F (49°C) with a full load and having a good air circulation or transfer system, for approximately 8 hours. Otherwise the exposed materials should be aerated in a well-ventilated area at room temperature for a longer period.

Based on the literature and the experience of many medical institutions and professional personnel over the past ten years, aeration for not less than 24 hours at room temperature has been found satisfactory for a wide variety of articles. On the other hand, aeration quarantines extending to as much as 7 days are employed by some practitioners for certain cases. Such cases include, but are not limited to, implantation devices such as pacemakers and artificial heart valves. *It is imperative that all personnel who use such sterilizers be properly and thoroughly instructed as to the need for aeration of exposed articles.*

STORAGE OF STERILIZED ARTICLES

The length of time during which a gas-sterilized article will remain sterile depends upon the type and condition of the packaging material, the extent of handling during storage, the storage conditions, and the thickness of the wrapping material. When packaging items in heavy wrapping paper or muslin cloth for gaseous sterilization, 2 to 3 layers of these materials are preferred. It is not known exactly how long articles packaged in this manner will remain sterile under normal storage conditions. However, there is no evidence to indicate that correctly packaged articles need to be resterilized at intervals of less than 30 days.

Plastic films of 1 to 3 mils (0.001 to 0.003 inches) in thickness are preferred packaging materials in gaseous sterilization. They are convenient to handle and are sufficiently flexible for wrapping ordinary supplies and materials. Evans[58] reported that articles sterilized in plastic-wrapped packages remain sterile much longer than those packaged in paper or muslin. He stated that items sterilized in a polyester film, such as Mylar®, will remain sterile indefinitely, although it is very difficult to permeate with ethylene oxide and moisture. He stated further that whereas polyethylene or polyvinyl chloride may keep an item sterile for as long as twenty years, evidence was available that products sterilized in polyethylene were still sterile after ten years' storage. Cellophane, if used at all, has poor storage characteristics because it becomes dry and brittle and cracks under normal storage conditions. Plastic films greater than 3-mil thickness have been used in gaseous decontamination procedures in which clothing and bedding materials are placed in large, heavy plastic bags. Ethylene oxide is then introduced into the bag; the bag is sealed and held at room temperature for as long as 16 hours or more. The gas will permeate through the bag but, because of the thickness, permeation is slow and the items are decontaminated by the time the gas has disappeared. This process of delayed or latent permeation of ethylene oxide is advantageous if packaged articles are not going to be used in relatively short periods of time.

PACKAGING MATERIALS

To maintain sterility in an item, some type of packaging and a protective wrapping material must be employed. Requirements of packaging materials comprise permeability to ethylene oxide and moisture, flexibility for wrapping and sealing irregular size articles, capacity to withstand normal handling, low cost, and capacity to withstand normal storage conditions without deterioration. In general, such materials as paper, cloth (muslin), and certain plastic films meet these requirements. Transparent plastic films are preferred in many cases because they allow easy identification and inspection of the wrapped article.

Because of the wide variety of plastic films available on the market today which are being used for packaging, relatively few have been tested and found compatible with ethylene oxide sterilizing processes. Dick and Faezel[59] and Lebovits[60] have reported on the premeabilities of a large number of these plastic films to ethylene oxide and other gases including water vapor. Of the plastic films which have been tested to date as packaging materials and found satisfactory for the ethylene oxide sterilization process, low density polyethylene film of 3.0 mils thickness has met most of, it not all, of the requirements for a packaging material.

ETHYLENE OXIDE STERILIZING CYCLES

Sterilization by ethylene oxide is normally accomplished in a pressure vessel or sterilizing chamber of some type either at atmospheric pressure or at elevated pressures. For reasonable short exposure periods, temperatures of 120° to 140°F (49° to 60°C) and ethylene oxide concentrations of 600 to 800 mg/liter are employed.

In a continuing search for more effective and faster methods of gaseous sterilization, a process was recently developed in which sterility can be achieved in a much shorter exposure time than that normally required. This process* comprises a method of introducing steam into a sterilizing chamber at a preselected absolute pressure. A mixture (12% ethylene oxide and 88% halogenated hydrocarbon gas) is then introduced to provide an ethylene oxide concentration of approximately 720 mg/liter. An exposure period of 1¾ hours is allowed for sterilization, followed by chamber exhaust and evacuation to approximately 26 in. Hg. Freshly filtered air is then admitted to the chamber to atmospheric pressure and the chamber is reevacuated. Filtered air is again admitted to atmospheric pressure and the load removed for aeration. The total cycle time is approximately 2½ hours. The primary advantage of this process lies in the rapid heating of materials

---

* Patent Pending.

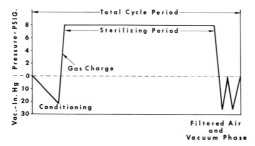

FIGURE 19-6. Flow diagram of cycle phases which occur during an ethylene oxide sterilizing process.

to the desired sterilizing temperature of 130°F ±5° (54°C ±3°). The moisture content of the chamber and load is also raised during the cycle resulting in a chamber relative humidity of 80 to 90% and a load humidity of 60 to 75%. Although these relative humidity ranges are somewhat higher than those normally accepted (30 to 50% relative humidity) for gaseous sterilization, the sterilizing action of ethylene oxide has been found to be essentially unaffected by these conditions. Wrapping or packaging materials such as polyethylene film (3 to 4 mil), paper, and muslin cloth may be employed with this process, however, the latter two packaging materials are preferred. The reason for this lies in the fact that residual moisture in the paper- or muslin-wrapped items dissipates much more rapidly than from the plastic-wrapped items. The use of this process in hospitals has indicated that the exposure of certain moisture-sensitive instruments may be affected by the high moisture content within the chamber. This possibility is noted because of the limitations which are inherent in all sterilizing processes.

A schematic diagram illustrating the various phases of this cycle is shown in Figure 19-6. Figure 19-7 is a schematic drawing of a sterilizing chamber

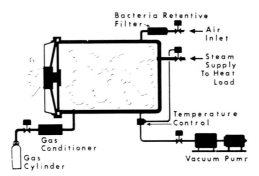

FIGURE 19-7. A schematic drawing of an ethylene oxide sterilizer and the various systems used in its operation.

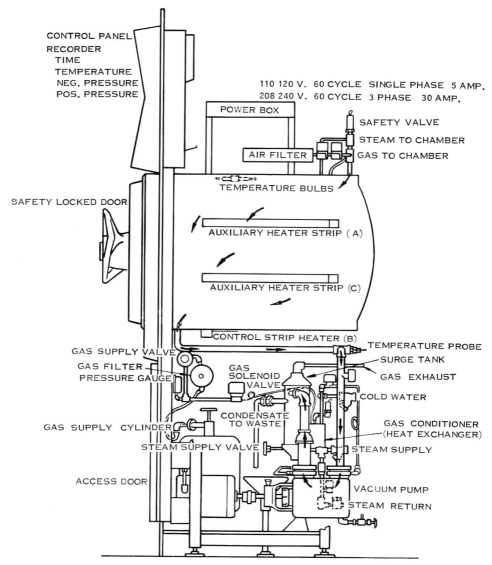

FIGURE 19-8. A schematic drawing of the various mechanical and electrical components of an ethylene oxide sterilizer.

and the various systems (heating, temperature control, and gas charge) which are employed in this sterilizing process, and Figure 19-8 illustrates the various mechanical components of a sterilizer designed to operate under this method.

GAS STERILIZING EQUIPMENT

In hospital applications, gaseous sterilization is usually conducted in commercially produced ethylene oxide sterilizers. These are fabricated steel chambers of various sizes with fully automatic, semiautomatic, or manual control systems. One of the smaller-size chambers, shown in Figure 19-9, is a cylindrical sterilizer with dimensions of 10 $\times$ 16 inches. This table or bench unit is designed for the sterilization of relatively small loads of materials. Larger units are capable of accommodating longer articles such as broncho-scopes, esophagoscopes, catheters, and similar items. The chambers are eas-ily operated and utilize a small cylinder of Pennoxide gas. A source of vac-uum is required for drawing a 26 to 27 in. Hg vacuum on the chamber to facilitate the introduction of the gas into the chamber during the charging phase and for chamber evacuation following the exposure period. Figure 19-10 illustrates a similar chamber installed in a wall dividing two rooms or a room and corridor, separating the clean from the unclean side. This unit is approximately the same size as that described above and can be operated from either a gas cylinder or a 21 ounce disposable can of Cry-Oxide. The open mounted or bench-type chamber is normally preheated to 130°F $\pm$ 5° and approximately 15 ml of water is placed on the chamber floor. The load is inserted and an initial vacuum drawn after the door is closed. When the desired vacuum is reached, the hand valve on the vacuum line is closed and the vacuum source terminated. The hand valve on the gas charge line is opened and the small needle valve on the gas cylinder hose line is turned on slowly to allow the liquid gas to bleed into the chamber, where it vaporizes and raises the chamber pressure. When the desired pressure is reached, the needle valve and hand valve are closed. The timer is then set for the desired exposure period. At the end of the exposure period, the chamber is evacu-ated as before, and the filtered air line then opened to relieve the vacuum to

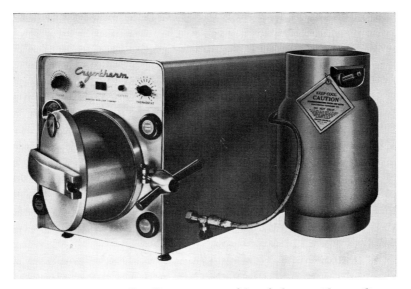

FIGURE 19-9. A small, office-type, portable ethylene oxide sterilizer.

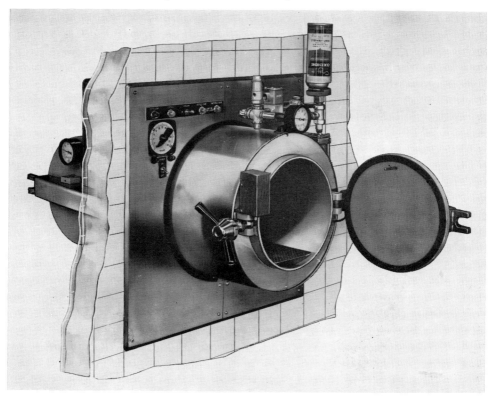

FIGURE 19-10. A small-size, wall, pass-through ethylene oxide sterilizer.

atmospheric pressure. The "pass clave" or through-the-wall unit is operated in a similar fashion if a gas cylinder is utilized. However, for the disposable Cry-Oxide can operation, a calibrated sight-glass, holding the disposable can in an inverted position and connected to the gas charge line on the chamber, must be filled to the desired level with the liquid gas from the can before the chamber can be charged. In operation, the stepwise procedure is identical to that described above. The only exception is the detail for charging the chamber with gas. This is accomplished by opening the hand valve on the gas charge line and allowing the liquid in the sight-glass to enter the chamber. When the sight-glass is empty, the hand valve is closed. The timer is then set for the desired exposure period and the cycle continues as before.

Larger-size ethylene oxide sterilizers representing the medium rectangular or the bulk-size units are illustrated in Figure 19-11. The larger-size gas sterilizers find applications in hospitals for the sterilization and decontamination of bulk equipment and supplies. They are operated in the same manner as the smaller-size sterilizers. For industrial purposes, these units are designed for greater versatility in operational cycles in that chamber temperature, pressures, and other cyclic phases can be varied or changed as desired to permit special processing of products. Different gas mixtures can also be

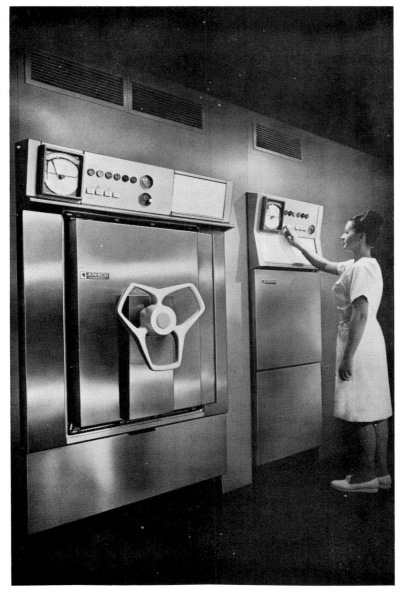

FIGURE 19-11. Medium-size, recessed, combination steam and ethylene oxide sterilizer with gas control console.

employed as well as modified gas cycles programmed on either an automatic or manual operation.

STERILITY CONTROLS

The sterility of processed materials is predicated upon the inability to demonstrate the presence of living organisms on or in the material sterilized when using approved bacteriological techniques. The officially accepted method of determining sterility is described in the United States Pharmacopoeia, XVIII Edition. This is a direct method in which a certain percentage of a number of like articles are cultured in fluid thioglycollate broth and fluid Sabouraud's medium and incubated at 85° to 89.6°F (30° to 32°C) and 71.6° to 77°F (22° to 25°C) for 7 days and 14 days, respectively. The absence of microbial growth, following these incubation periods, signifies that the materials in that particular load are sterile. Whereas this method is employed routinely in many pharmaceutical houses, it is unsuitable for hospitals where the objects to be sterilized by ethylene oxide may be irregular in size and shape and inconvenient to handle, and may include the only one of its kind available at the time. In this case a biological control may be used. The usual method of preparing a biological control is to impregnate a paper strip, swatch of cloth, or some other equally porous material with a culture of bacterial vegetative cells or, as in most cases, spores, in known populations. This control is usually packaged in an envelope, which is permeable to ethylene oxide and moisture. It is placed in the load of materials in various areas, as well as inside the packaged items prior to exposure. Following exposure, the control is aseptically removed from the envelope, transferred to suitable culture medium, and incubated at the optimum temperature of the test organism. If growth has not occurred within a seven-day incubation period, it is inferred that the articles in the load were sterilized.

The preparation of biological controls requires careful consideration in the selection of the test organism, the culture media in which they are grown, and the population employed. Carelessly prepared controls may give misleading results or a false assurance that the exposed items were sterilized. The most commonly used test organism is *B. subtilis* var. *globigii*, although *B. cereus*, *B. pumilus*, and *B. stearothermophilus* have been employed in addition to *M. pyogenes* var. *aureus* and *E. coli*. For routine sterility control work, *B. subtilis* var. *globigii* is recommended, as it is convenient to handle, grows readily on ordinary culture media, and can be easily identified by its orange pigment when grown on solid agar surfaces.

The growth medium should be simple and as free from fats or lipids as possible. If a sporogenic bacterium is used, sporulation should be allowed to continue until the spore population is at least 95 per cent of the total spores and vegetative cells. It is also important that the bacterial spores are properly cleaned prior to inoculation onto the desired substrate. Beeby and Whitehouse[51] reported that spores suspended in methyl alcohol were stable on storage and, when dried on aluminum foil strips, gave the most reproducible results of the spore suspensions tested. Brewer and Arnsberger[62] recommend the use of spores from a thermophilic organism because of the unlikelihood that this organism would be found as a laboratory contaminant in sterility testing. They suggested the use of *B. stearothermophilus* spores suspended in 1% sorbitol solution. Chen, Ortenzio, and Stuart[63] recently reported on the preparation of a biological control using the spores of *B. subtilis* and *Cl. sporogenes* obtained from a soil extract-egg-meat medium. Although the spores are unwashed, the authors claim that the controls provide highly reproducible results and are a practical guide for use in testing the efficiency of ethylene oxide and other sterilizing systems.

It is important that the selection of the use population of cells or spores bear a close relationship to the probable level of contamination on the articles to be sterilized, and that this selection be considered with a liberal margin of safety in mind. It has been proposed that the normal contamination on clean and room-dried articles ranges from a few hundred up to 25,000 bacteria of various species. On this basis, a biological control should contain a substantially higher population of organisms to provide a factor of safety. It is recommended that the biological control to be used for routine gas sterilization should comprise a suitable material which contains a population of 10^5 clean, dry, and viable spores of *B. subtilis* var. *globigii*.

Chemical indicators adaptable to gaseous sterilization are available in several types. These include special tapes which change color in the presence of ethylene oxide, chemically impregnated paper discs, enclosed in plastic envelopes, which change color when exposed to ethylene oxide and chemically treated paper strips which not only change color in the presense of ethylene oxide but also contain bacterial spores, thus, combining a biological control with a chemical indicator. Royce's sachets[64] represent another type of chemical indicator consisting of small plastic envelopes containing a chemical solution which undergoes a color change in an ethylene oxide atmosphere.

FUTURE NEEDS IN GAS STERILIZATION

There is still much to be learned about ethylene oxide gas sterilization and in its applications in the medical and surgical fields. The relationship of moisture to the sterilizing action of ethylene oxide and to the rehydration of dried or desiccated organisms to a point where they exhibit optimum sensitivity to ethylene oxide needs more investigative work. More accurate and sensitive instruments are needed for indicating and measuring moisture levels in gas sterilizing chambers under various temperatures and pressures. Increased knowledge of the kinetics of gaseous sterilization and the manner in which gases permeate the bacterial cell wall and various materials is another important area for research. The search for and development of new gaseous agents or combinations of gases which are less toxic to humans and more rapid in their sterilizing action should be continued. Further development is needed on the standardization of procedures for gaseous sterilization and for equipment which will expand the use of this process to many other areas where sterilization is required.

REFERENCES

1. WURTZ, C. A.: Sur l'oxyde d'ethylene. *C R Acad Sci (Paris)* 48:101, 1859.
2. SCHRADER, H., and BOSSERT, E.: Fumigant Composition. U. S. Pat. No. 2,037,439, 1936.
3. GROSS, P. M., and DIXON, L. F.: Method of Sterilizing. U. S. Pat. No. 2,075,845, 1937.
4. PHILLIPS, C. R., and KAYE, S.: The sterilizing action of gaseous ethylene oxide. I. Review. *Amer J Hyg,* 50:270-279, 1949.
5. PHILLIPS, C. R.: The sterilizing action of gaseous ethylene oxide. II. Sterilization of contaminated objects with ethylene oxide and related compounds: time, concentration, and temperature relationships. *Am J Hyg,* 50:280-288, 1949.
6. KAYE, S.: The sterilizing action of gaseous ethylene oxide. III. The effect of ethylene oxide and related compounds upon bacterial aerosols. *Am J Hyg,* 50:289-295, 1949.
7. KAYE, S., and PHILLIPS, C. R.: The sterilizing action of gaseous ethylene oxide. IV. The effect of moisture. *Am J Hyg,* 50:296-306, 1949.
8. NEWMAN, L. B.; COLWELL, C. A., and JAMESON, E. L.: Decontamination of articles made by tuberculosis patients in physical medicine and rehabilitation (a study using "Carboxide gas"). *Am Rev Tuberc Pulmonary Dis,* 71:272-279, 1955.
9. KAYE, S.: IRMINGER, H. F., and PHILLIPS, C. R.: The sterilization of penicillin and streptomycin by ethylene oxide. *J Lab Clin Med,* 40:67-73, 1952.
10. SKEEHAN, R. A.; KING, J. H., and KAYE, S.: Ethylene oxide sterilization in ophthalmology. *Am J Ophthal,* 42:420-430, 1956.
11. BRUCH, C. W.: Gaseous sterilization. *Ann Rev Microbiol,* 15:245-262, 1961.
12. GILLETTE, W. B.: Ethylene oxide sterilization in dentistry. *J Oral Ther,* 2 (6):440-444, 1966.
13. MEEKS, C. H.; PEMBLETON, W. E., and HENCH, M. E.: Sterilization of anesthesia equipment. *JAMA* 199 (4):276-278, 1967.
14. HESS, L. C., and TILTON, V. V.: Ethylene oxide-hazards and methods of handling. *Ind Eng Chem,* 42:1251-1258, 1950.
15. MANUFACTURING CHEMISTS' ASSOCIATION, INC.: Properties and Essential Information for Safe Handling and Use of Ethylene Oxide, Chemical Safety Data Sheet SD-38., New York, N.Y., 1951.
16. HOLLINGSWORTH, R. L.; ROWE, V. K.; OYEN F.; McCOLLISTER, D. D., and SPENCER, H. C.: Toxicity of ethylene oxide determined on experimental animals. *Arch Ind Health,* 13:217-227, 1956.
17. THOMAS, C. G. A.: Sterilization by ethylene oxide. *Guy Hosp Rep,* 109:57-74, 1960.
18. KLARENBEEK, A., and TONGEREN, H. A.: Virucidal action of ethylene oxide gas. *J Hyg (Camb),* 52:525-528, 1954.
19. MATHEWS, J., and HOFSTAD, M. S.: The inactivation of certain animal viruses by ethylene oxide. *Cornell Vet,* 53:452-461, 1953.
20. KIRBY, G. W.; ATKIN, L., and FREY, C. N.: Recent progress in "rope" and mold control. *Food Indust,* 8:450-451, 1936.
21. FULTON, J. D., and MITCHELL, R. B.: Sterilization of footwear. *U S Armed Forces Med J,* 3:425-439, 1952.
22. PAPPAS, H. J., and HALL, L. A.: The control of thermophilic bacteria. *Food Technol,* 6:456-458, 1952.
23. ROSS, W. C. J.: *Biological Alkylating Agents.* London, Butterworths, 1962.
24. WHEELER, C. P.: Studies related to the mechanisms of action of cytotoxic alkylating agents: a review. *Cancer Res,* 22:651-688, 1962.
25. PHILLIPS, C. R.: Relative resistance of bacterial spores and vegetative bacteria to disinfectants. *Bacteriol Rev,* 16:135-138, 1952.
26. BISSET, K. A.: Evolution in bacteria and the significance of the bacterial spore. *Nature,* 166:431-432, 1950.
27. COWARD, H. F., and JONES, G. W.: Limits of Flammability of Gases and Vapors. U S Bureau of Mines Bull. No. 503, 1952.
28. HAENNI, E. O.; AFFENS, W. A.; LENTO, H. G. YEOMANS, A. H. and FULTON, R. A.: New nonflammable formulations for sterilizing sensitive materials. *Ind Eng Chem,* 51:685-688, 1959.

29. LUBATTI, O. F.: Determination of ethylene oxide. *J Soc Chem Ind* (London), *51*:361-367T, 1932.
30. SWAN, J. D.: Determination of epoxides with sodium sulfite. *Anal Chem, 26*:878, 1954.
31. ERNST, R. R., and SHULL, J. J.: Ethylene oxide gaseous sterilization: I. Concentration and temperature effects. *Appl Microbiol, 10* (4):337-341, 1962.
32. MERRIAM, C. J., and WILES, R.: Treatment of Organic Products. U. S. Pat No. 2,080,179, 1937.
33. ERNST, R. R., and SHULL, J. J.: Ethylene oxide gaseous sterilization: II. Influence of method of humidification. *Appl Microbiol, 10*:342-344, 1962.
34. PERKINS, J. J., and LLOYD, R. S.: *Applications and Equipment for Ethylene Oxide Sterilization.* London, Pharmaceutical Press, 1961.
35. OPFELL, J. B.; HOHMANN, J. P., and LATHAM, A. B.: Ethylene oxide sterilization of spores of hygroscopic environments. *J Am Pharm Ass, Sci Ed, 48*:617-619, 1959.
36. GILBERT, G. L.; GAMBILL, V. M.; SPINER, D. R.; HOFFMAN, R. K., and PHILLIPS, C. R.: Effect of moisture in ethylene oxide sterilization. *Appl Microbiol, 12* (6):496-504, 1964.
37. EL-BISI, H. M.; VONDELL, R. M., and ESSELEN, W. B.: Kinetics of Bactericidal Activity of Ethylene Oxide In the Vapor-Phase: I. Effect of Cellular Water Activity. Bacteriol. Proc. 63rd General Meeting, S.A.B., p. 13, 1963.
38. VONDELL, R. M.: Studies on The Kinetics of The Bactericidal Action of Ethylene Oxide In The Vapor Phase. Dissertation, U. Massachusetts, Amherst, Mass., 1962.
39. LIU, T. S., HOWARD, G. A., and STUMBO, C. R.: The Efficacy of Dichlorodifluoromethane—Ethylene Oxide Mixture As A Sterilant At Elevated Temperatures. Dissertation, U. Massachusetts, Amherst, Mass., 1964.
40. CHURCH, B. D., HALVORSON, H.; RAMSEY, D. S., and HARTMAN, R. S.: Population heterogeneity in the resistance of aerobic spores to ethylene oxide. *J. Bacteriol, 72*:242-247, 1956.
41. Unpublished Data, Amsco Research Laboratories, American Sterilizer Co., Erie, Pa., 1966.
42. OPFELL, J. B.; SHANNON, J. L., and CHAN, H.: Comparison of Methyl Bromide and Ethylene Oxide Resistances of *Staphylococcus epidermidis* and *Bacillus subtilis* Spore Populations. Bacteriol. Proc. 67th General Meeting ASM, 1967.
43. ANDERSON, A. W.; NORDAN, H. C.; CAIN, R. F.; PARRISH, G., and DUGGAN, D.: Studies on a radio-resistant *Micrococcus*. I. Isolation, morphology, cultural characteristics, and resistance to gamma radiation. *Food Technol, 10*:575-577, 1956.
44. HAWIGER, J., and JELJASZEWICZ, J.: Antibiotic sensitivity of *Micrococcus radiodurans*. *Appl Microbiol, 15* (2):304-306, 1967.
45. *Technical Report No. 1967-6 Ethylene Oxide Thermal Chemical Death Studies With The Radiation Resistant Microorganism,* Micrococcus radiodurans. Erie, Pa., American Sterilizer Co., 1967.
46. PHILLIPS, C. R.: *The Sterilizing Properties of Ethylene Oxide.* London, Pharmaceutical Press, 1961.
47. ZNAMIROWSKI, R.; McDONALD, S., and ROY, T. E.: The efficiency of an ethylene oxide sterilizer in hospital practice. *Canad Med Ass J, 83*:1004-1006, 1960.
48. DOYLE, J. E., and ERNST, R. R.: Resistance of Spores Occluded in Crystals to Sterilization. Bacteriol. Proc. 67 General Meeting ASM, 1967.
49. BOSOMWORTH, P. P., and HAMELBERG, W.: Effect of sterilization technics on safety and durability of endotracheal tubes and cuffs. *Anesth Analg (Cleveland) 44* (5):576-586, 1965.
50. SUTARIA, R. H., and WILLIAMS, F. H.: Ethylene oxide sterilization in a hospital pharmacy. *Pharm J, 186*:311-314, 1961.
51. SYKES, G.: *Disinfection and Sterilization.* Bath, England, Pitman Press. 1958, p. 177.
52. PHILLIPS, C. R.: Gaseous sterilization. In G. F. Reddish (Ed.): *Antiseptics, Disinfectants, Fungicides, and Chemical and Physical Sterilization.* Philadelphia, Lea & F., 1954.
53. BEARD, H. C., and DUNMIRE, R. B.: Retention of ethylene oxide fumigant by shoes. *Arch Ind Health, 15*:167-169, 1957.
54. ROYCE, A., and MOORE, W. K. S.: Occupational dermatitis caused by ethylene oxide. *Brit J Industra Med, 12*:169-171, 1955.

55. FREEMAN, M. A. R., and BARWELL, C. F.: Ethylene oxide sterilization in hospital practice. *J Hyg (Camb)*, 58:337-345, 1960.

56. HIROSE, T.; GOLDSTEIN, R., and BAILEY, C. P.: Hemolysis of blood due to exposure to different types of plastic tubing and the influence of ethylene oxide sterilization. *J Thorac Cardi. Surg, 45 (2)*:245-251, 1961.

57. CLARKE, C. P.; DAVIDSON, W. L., and JOHNSTON, J. B.: Hemolysis of blood following exposure to an Australian-manufactured plastic tubing sterilized by means of ethylene oxide gas. *Aust New Zeal J Surg, 36*:53, 1966.

58. EVANS, R. P.: Practical aspects of ethylene oxide sterilization. *Bull Parenteral Drug Ass,* 15:9-15, 1961.

59. DICK, M., and FEAZEL, C. E.: Resistance of plastics to ethylene oxide. *Mod Plastics,* 38:148-150, 1960.

60. LEBOVITS, A.: Permeability of polymers to gases, vapors and liquids. *Mod Plastics, 43*:139-146, 1966.

61. BEEBY, M. M., and WHITEHOUSE, C. E.: A bacterial spore test piece for the control of ethylene oxide sterilization. *J Appl Bact, 28 (3)*:349-360, 1965.

62. BREWER, J. H., and ARNSBERGER, R. J.: Biological-chemical indicator for ethylene oxide sterilization. *J Pharm Sci, 55 (1)*:57-59, 1966.

63. CHEN, J. H. S.; ORTENZIO, L. F., and STUART, L. S.: Application of A.O.A.C. Sporicidal Test to Evaluating Efficiency of Sterilizing Devices and Sporicidal Chemicals. Bacteriol. Proc. 67th General Meeting ASM, 1967.

64. ROYCE, A., and BOWLER, C.: An indicator control device for ethylene oxide sterilization. *Pharm Pharmacol, 11* (Suppl.):294, 1959.

Chapter 20

BRIEF ON HOSPITAL INFECTIONS

THE PROBLEM

THE PHYSICAL environment of the hospital is similar in many respects to that of the industrial community and the potential environmental health problems are largely the same. Also, it may be said that the hospital is a community of ill people, many of whom harbor virulent bacterial or viral pathogens. It follows then that the risk of infection in hospitals is greater than in ordinary life because some patients are admitted to the institution for the treatment of infections and these same patients contribute their resistant microorganisms or etiological agents to the environment. In addition, certain members of the professional staff and other employees of the hospital, not omitting visitors, may be healthy carriers of a variety of pathogens, each person contributing a share to the reservoir of infectious agents. Every person is potentially a carrier of pathogenic organisms, and knowledge of this condition is essential to the first-line defense against the spread of infectious agents from one person to another. Moreover, it must be recognized that all of the common modes of transmission of infectious agents are present in the average hospital, without exception, and including the water supply, food, air, liquid and solid wastes, insects, rodents, and a large number of fomites ("tinder used to carry fire") such as contaminated dressings, laundry, bedding, surgical and diagnostic instruments.

Hospital infections, acquired or developed in the institutional environment, are not new. The staphylococcal disease, for example, is as old as the osteomyelitis lesions observed in Egyptian mummies of 4000 years ago.[1] In terms of a hospital problem this disease is as old as medicine and surgery and certainly as old as hospitals themselves. To say that many hospitals throughout the medically advanced countries of the world do not have a problem with acquired infections would be a gross misstatement. On the other hand, it is most alarming and seemingly unfair to hospital management in general to have to face periodically the dramatic and sensational charges of the problem as has occurred through the medium of newspapers, popular magazines, and other publications. This kind of notoriety carries the inference that many of our better-managed hospitals operate under low standards of adequacy in an insanitary environment leading to propagation of disease, and where prime concern is not for the welfare of the patient but rather for the convenience of the staff—a most disturbing situation if true.

It is not difficult to understand that possibly a large number of our present-day hospitals may be deficient in their capability of conforming to the precept of Florence Nightingale that the hospital "shall do the sick no harm." This deficiency does not, however, provide justification for a priori general condemnation of the quality of patient care in our hospitals, or expressed in other words "no stronger condemnation of any hospital or ward could be pronounced than the simple fact that any zymotic disease has originated in it, or that such diseases have attacked other patients than those brought in with them." The evolution of the modern hospital has been a slow and laborious process, and today it bears little resemblance to those of a century or more ago when almost unbelievable mortality rates resulted from cholera, typhoid, diphtheria, smallpox, and staphylococcal infections; when 2944 of 7650 infants born in one hospital died from neonatal tetanus during the first two weeks; and when puerperal sepsis was the scourge of the lying-in hospitals.[2]

In order that we may be reminded of man's progress in hospital care a brief look into the past in the year of 1788 at the Hotel Dieu in Paris should suffice to renew our confidence in the present and furnish hope for the future:

> There were some 1200 beds, most of which contained from four to six patients, and also 486 beds for single patients. The larger halls contained over 800 patients crowded on pallets, or heaps of straw, which were in vile condition. Acute contagious diseases were often in close relation to mild cases, vermin and filth abounded, and . . . the attendants . . . would not enter in the morning without a sponge dipped in vinegar held to their faces. Septic fevers and other contagia were the rule; the average mortality was about 20 per cent, and recovery from surgical operations was a rarity.[3]

If the modern hospital is to fulfill its basic purpose, it must of necessity bring together both the infected and susceptible individuals. This very act of concentration of patients is not without risk as was so ably expressed by Simpson in 1869[4] when he stated that "in the treatment of the sick, there is ever danger in their aggregation, and safety only in their segregation." Other factors undoubtedly have contributed to the problem, such as the demands for more complicated and longer-duration surgical operations, the use of total body irradiation or cytotoxic agents which destroy the patient's defense mechanism against infection, the overcrowding of hospitals, the shortage of nursing staff, and ineffective measures of contamination control.

The literature discloses that major shifts have occurred in the nature of life-threatening infections in the past 20 years. It seems highly probable that the use of potent antibacterial drugs has been in some measure responsible for these changes, as well as a relaxation in the traditional principles and practice of aseptic and antiseptic techniques. From the several thousand publications and reports on the subject of hospital-acquired infections, dating from 1950 through 1967, it is clear that agreement exists on at least one major aspect of the problem—*the mandatory need for cleanliness and effective decontamination in the most sophisticated and microscopic sense.*

Surveys of a statistically significant nature[5,6,7] do not indicate that staphylococcal and other serious infections are on the increase, nor are they spreading uncontrolled in our hospitals. They do, however, show that some patients in medical wards contract infections and suffer consequences more serious than the conditions for which they entered the hospital. Also, a significant number of hospitalized patients on medical and surgical services continue to die of microbial infections each year. Table 20-1 shows examples of the incidence of wound sepsis as reported in the literature. Does this mean that microbial disease is an integral part of human life and death?[8]

DYNAMICS OF INFECTION
Host-Parasite Relations

For the sake of clarity and to assist in uniformity of understanding, it may be helpful to define certain terms that will be used frequently in this discussion on hospital-acquired infections. Of chief importance is the term *infection*. This is strictly a microbiological term, meaning the introduction of microbes into tissues. It is an expression of parasitism—a normal biological phe-

TABLE 20-1

INCIDENCE OF WOUND SEPSIS REPORTED IN LITERATURE

Type of Surgery	No. Cases Reviewed	Sepsis Rate	Isolated Organism(s)	Source and Mode of Transmission	References
Plastic	1248	0.08	———	———	Dykes and Anderson,[9] 1960–61
Clean Wounds	817	0.7	*Staph., Strep., E. coli*	Direct contact carriers and environment	Culbertson et al.,[10] 1960–61
Clean Wounds	3780	1.2	*Staph.*	Endogenous infection or seeded in O.R. by people. Air contamination unimportant	Howe and Marston,[11] 1959–61
Abdominal, Neuro.	8952	1.6	*Staph.*	Introduced into wound during operation	Cohen, Fekety, and[12] Cluff, 1961–62
Thoracic	2480	2.2	*Staph.*	Cross-infection and glove punctures	Bassett et al.,[13] 1953–56
Orthopaedic	1287	4.3	*Staph.*	Magnitude of dissection	Stevens,[14] 1960
Urologic	100	8.0	*Alcaligenes and Coli*	Urethral instrumentation	Last and Harbison,[15] 1965
General	133	12.7	*Pseudomonas*	Cross-contamination	Sandusky,[16] 1955–60
Intraocular	44	37.0	*Pseudomonas*	Contaminated saline solution	Ayliffe, Barry,[17] et al. 1964
Burn Cases	38	64.0	*Pseudomonas*	Cross-contamination in hospital	Sutter and Hurst,[18] 1964
Thoracic	4	100.0	*Pseudomonas*	Contaminated lignocaine jelly	Phillips,[19] 1966

nomenon in which one living species derives its food requirements in the tissues of another. When this relation causes signs and symptoms of disease in man, or when it destroys a plant or an animal useful to him, the process is abnormal and it becomes an *infectious disease*. When the interaction between the host and the infectious agent results in overt disease and pathology to the host, *progressive infection* is said to have taken place. In contrast, *attenuated infection* may occur, which, in brief, represents a state of truce or peaceful coexistence between the host and the infecting agent.

At the risk of oversimplification, the dynamics of infection may be explained as a delicate balance in which the forces of the host on the one side oppose the forces of the parasite on the other. Generally speaking the side outweighing the other becomes the survivor, but if a condition of equilibrium is reached, the phenomenon then simulates a state of *commensalism*. This means that the host and parasite live in constant and close association, without evidence of injury or of benefit to each other. The normal microbial flora of the respiratory tract and of the skin of man are examples of this condition. In the modern interpretation, an infectious disease is looked upon as a development rather than as an event because of the complex of interactions among the host, the parasite, and the therapeutic (antimicrobial) countermeasures. The selective suppression of bacteria due to antibiotic therapy may upset the delicate host-parasite equilibrium and thereby permit a bacterium of lesser importance to multiply and gain a predominant position.

Pathogenic microorganisms possess certain attributes or inherent characteristics which influence their disease-producing potential and, in turn, the extent of the damage inflicted on the host. These attributes exist in varying degrees, and they are usually designated as pathogenicity, infectivity, invasiveness, toxigenicity, and communicability. In order for a parasite to establish itself and multiply within the host, it becomes necessary that a portal of entry be available so as to permit spread directly through the tissues or through the lymphatic channels to the blood stream. In addition, a portal of exit or method of escape of the parasite from the host is a necessary requirement for perpetuation of the species, including an effective mode of transmission to the next prospective host.

Order of Events in Transmission of Infection

The Etiologic Agent (The causative organism, pathogen, or infectious agent)

PATHOGENICITY. The capacity of the infectious agent to cause disease or to produce progressive lesions in a susceptible host.

VIRULENCE. The degree of pathogenicity.

INVASIVENESS. The ability to enter tissues of the host, multiply, and spread.

TOXIGENICITY. The ability to produce toxic substances. Also, the manifestation of some host-parasite biochemical activity.

PLUS

A Reservoir of Natural Habitat That Permits Survival of the Etiologic Agent

RESERVOIR. A suitable substrate in which an infectious agent lives and multiplies in such a manner that it can be transmitted to a susceptible host. Man himself is the most frequent reservoir of infectious agents pathogenic for man.

SOURCES OF INFECTION. A thing, person, object, or substance from which an infectious agent passes immediately to a host. *Source* is usually applied only to sites of human or animal carriage and to septic lesions in which organisms are actively multiplying.

PLUS

A Method of Escape of the Etiologic Agent from the Reservoir

FOCI OF INFECTION. Open wounds and the respiratory, alimentary, and urinary tracts are potential sources from which infectious disease may be transmitted. Infections in communication with body surfaces, or its natural portals, have convenient pathways through which organisms may be shed.

PLUS

A Mode of Transmission from the Reservoir to the Next Prospective Host

DIRECT CONTACT. Actual touching of the infected person or animal or other reservoir of infection. Hands are especially important in the transmission of pathogenic organisms from septic lesions, portals of the body, or other foci of infection in the host which communicates with the environment.

INDIRECT CONTACT. Touching of contaminated objects such as clothing, bedding, toys, handkerchiefs, surgical instruments, and dressings, with subsequent hand-to-mouth transfer of infective material; less commonly, transfer to abraded skin or mucous membrane.

DROPLET SPREAD. The projection onto the conjunctivae and the face or into the nose or mouth of the spray emanating from an infected person during sneezing, coughing, singing, or talking (see Fig. 20-1). Such droplets usually travel no more than 3 feet from the source. Transmission by droplets is considered a form of contact infection because it involves reasonably close association between two or more persons.

VEHICLE. Water, food, milk, or biological products, including serum and plasma, by which an infectious agent is transported from a reservoir and introduced into a susceptible host through ingestion, inoculation, or by deposit on skin or mucous membrane. Food may serve as a culture medium for pathogens and often is the causal factor in intestinal infections such as food poisoning. Soil may also serve as a source of gas gangrene or tetanus in an open wound.

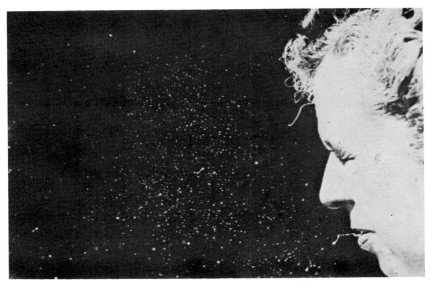

FIGURE 20-1. Late stage of a stifled sneeze. The formation of droplets from the filament of saliva issuing from the mouth can be seen. The diameter of many of the dropets is about 10 microns. (Courtesy American Association for the Advancement of Science.)

AIRBORNE ROUTE. Dissemination and inhalation of microbial aerosols and their deposition on skin, mucous surfaces, or wounds. Microbial aerosols consisting of particles with diameters of 100 microns to less than 1 micron may remain suspended in air for long periods of time. Aerosols arise from droplet nuclei (residue remaining from evaporation of droplets) and from dust particles emanating from contaminated floors, bedding, cotton materials, or soil.

PLUS

A Mode of Entry into the Prospective Host

PORTALS OF ENTRY. These are generally associated with the respiratory tract (mouth and nose), the gastrointestinal tract, and breaks in the superficial mucous membranes and skin. Survival of the infectious agent is dependent upon the size of inoculum and competition afforded between the invading and resident microorganisms.

PLUS

A Susceptible Host

A person not possessing resistance against a particular pathogenic agent and for that reason liable to contract a disease when exposed to an infectious agent is a susceptible host. There are several attributes of host resistance to microorganisms.

SKIN. Sweat and sebaceous secretions have antimicrobial properties which tend to reduce the number of organisms.

MUCOUS MEMBRANES. Microorganisms adhere to the mucous film and are directed by ciliated cells toward the natural orifices. Also, mucous membranes carry a relatively normal microbial flora which militates against the establishment of pathogenic organisms.

PHAGOCYTOSIS. Microorganisms which enter the blood stream, lymphatics, or tissue spaces are engulfed by polymorphonuclear leukocytes and mononuclear phagocytes. The organisms may then be digested by cellular enzymes and thus destroyed.

INFLAMMATORY RESPONSE. When microbial invasion of tissues takes place an inflammatory response occurs.

IMMUNITY. This attribute covers all those properties of the host which confer resistance to a specific infectious agent. The resistance may range from almost complete susceptibility to complete insusceptibility.

The Causes of Wound Sepsis

The fundamental cause of wound sepsis is infection with virulent pyogenic microorganisms. The conditions that support or prevent microbial multiplication in tissues are not clearly understood, but it is well established that frequently organisms in gaining access to wounds fail to initiate a state of sepsis. This indicates that host factors as well as the nature and number of the invading organisms play an important role in the pathogenesis of sepsis. To express this statement in another way, it may be said that *microorganisms are a necessary but not a sufficient condition for the development of a septic complication.* As early as 1890 Cheyne[20] expressed this view as follows:

> If the organisms enter in large numbers sufficient to overcome the resistance of the body, they alone may cause the disease; usually, however, they enter in small numbers, and then other conditions become necessary in order to enable them to act. Of these conditions, the chief are . . . depressed vitality, either local or general, combined with the possibility of their remaining in the weakened tissue. This depression of vitality may be brought about by conditions acting on the body generally, such as acute fevers; or by local conditions, more especially those which induce the early stage of inflammation, such as cold, injury, chemical substances, the products of bacteria themselves, or the products of other kinds of bacteria which may happen to be growing along with them.

At present, there appears to be an increasing awareness among surgeons of the importance of those determinants of postoperative infection which reside within patients themselves, as compared to those concerned with the species or density of the microbial populations in the hospital environment.[5,6] Today, it must be realized that advances in medicine and surgery have resulted in more extensive operations upon more patients with degenerative and metabolic diseases who, as a class, are infection-susceptible. Also, the point must not be overlooked that microorganisms of low virulence, including the so-called saprophytes, can cause sepsis in the presence of devitalized avascular tissues. But there is little information on levels of contamination considered hazardous to patients or personnel.

There is ample evidence in the literature to show that all wounds receive microbial contamination in a random distribution during the operative procedure.[9,10,21] Moreover, most wounds contain viable organisms at the time of closure with levels ranging from tens to hundreds or even greater numbers of microorganisms. In recent years there has evolved the "primary lodgment" concept of Miles and his associates[22,23] which deals with the establishment of microorganisms in tissues and the subsequent development of sepsis. This concept has led to the appreciation clinically that a multitude of independent host factors are at work in the development of a septic complication following clean surgery. Among the more obvious of these factors are the following:

· The kind of tissue.
· Local trauma to the tissue.
· Capillary circulation.
· Blood coagulation mechanism.
· Associated disease in the patient.
· Native resistance of the patient.
  Tissue ischemia during and after operation.
- Effects of anaesthesia on the mobilization of the body's defenses.
· Atraumatic surgical technic.
· Use and type of suture material.
· Meticulous hemostasis.
· Application of skin towels, and previous microbial environment of the
  patient.

Undoubtedly, some wound infections occur as a result of contamination of the wounds with microorganisms carried by operating room personnel, but there is little evidence that staphylococci, for example, in the air of the operating room are commonly responsible for wound infection.[11,24] However, it has been suggested that airborne wound infections occur in proportion to the number of disseminating carriers present during operation.[25] Also, some wound infections are probably related to errors in surgical technic or to unsterile conditions encountered during the operation. Floors, vacuum cleaners, blankets, mattresses, dust particles, air, instruments, dressings, septic fingers, and punctured gloves have been implicated as sources of staphylococci responsible for infection in surgical patients.[26,27,28] On the whole, some authorities[12] believe that these factors probably account for only a small percentage of postoperative wound sepsis under ordinary endemic conditions in hospitals. It seems highly probable, therefore, that many surgical wound infections are caused by staphylococci or other organisms harbored not by the environment but by persons and introduced into the wound at the time of operation. This does not mean that the inanimate environment in the hospital is unimportant. Many inanimate articles have been implicated in hospital infections. Examples are given in Table 20-2. The application of a health rationale based upon cleanliness, sound aseptic techniques, and disinfection of the hospital environment will do much to prevent epidemics and the occurrence of sporadic infections under endemic conditions.

COST OF INFECTIONS

It is difficult to obtain accurate information on the incidence of hospital-acquired infections, and figures to show the increased cost of treatment are even more difficult to obtain. Some years ago, Meleney[47] reported that the length of the hospital stay in infected cases was nearly double that in uninfected cases. A recent five-year study by Ljungqvist[48] in Sweden showed that

TABLE 20-2

INANIMATE ARTICLES IMPLICATED IN HOSPITAL INFECTIONS

Article	Contaminating Organism	Method of Spread	Number of Infections	Reference
Faucet aerator	*Pseudomonas*	Scrub sink	4	Cross, Benchimol, and Diamond[29]
Oxygenator	*Pseudomonas*	Open heart surgery	5	Keown *et al.*[30]
Needles and catheters	*Pseudomonas*	Detergent solutions	40	Plotkin and Austrian[31]
Glassware	Viral Hepatitis	Accidental self-inoculation	2	Byrne[32]
Facial tissues	Variety Pathogens	Direct contact	—	MacPherson[33]
Urethral catheter	*E. coli, Pseudo.*	Catheterization	8	Turck *et al.*[34]
Whirlpool bath	*Staph., Pseudo.*	Open wounds	—	Koepke and Christopher[35]
Suction catheters	*Pseudomonas*	Tracheal suctioning	20	Sutter *et al.*[36]
Endotracheal tube	*Pseudomonas*	Lignocaine jelly	4	Phillips[19]
Cellulose wadding	*Pseudomonas*	Plaster casts	8	Sussman and Stevens[37]
Silk sutures	*Staph.*	During operation	5	Bahnson and Spencer[38]
Urethral instrument	"Water Organism"	Bladder irrigation	11	Last, Harbison, and Marsh[15]
Saline solution	*Pseudomonas*	Contaminated saline solution	44	Ayliffe *et al.*[17]
Needles and syringes	Viral Hepatitis	Inadequate sterilization	8	Dull[39]
Disposable infusion tubes	Viral Hepatitis	Reuse of tubes	41	Dougherty and Altman[40]
Water bath	*E. coli, Pseudo., Proteus*	Formula bottles	32	King and Murphy[41]
Resuscitators	*Salmonella*	Air from resuscitator	51	Rubenstein and Fowler[42]
Catheters	*S. marcescens*	Catheters, towels, and hands	15	Clayton and Graevenitz[43]
Catheters	*Pseudomonas*	Tracheal suctioning	20	Rogers[44]
Saline solution	Flavobacterium	Contaminated saline solution	2	Plotkin and McKitrick[45]
Evacuator and resectoscopes	*Pseudomonas*	Evacuator in operating room	37	Moore and Forman[46]

wound sepsis lengthened the hospital stay by an average of one week. Despite the low infection rate of 1.9 per cent, some 3000 nursing days went into the care of patients with infected wounds during this observation period.

In the 1960 British Public Health Service report on surgical infection, it was estimated hospitalization was prolonged at least ten days solely because of postoperative infection.[49] Cohen[12] and his associates at The Johns Hopkins Hospital showed that the duration of hospitalization prior to operation was similar for infected and control patients, but the total period of hospitalization for infected patients was twice that of the noninfected controls. The increased hospitalization (17.6 days mean) represented a considerable economic expense, but it was often the result of underlying disease rather than of infection. In a study a staphylococcic infections on a surgical service Koch and his co-workers[50] reported that cross infections of postoperative wounds in 18 patients resulted in a total increase in hospital stay of 432 days beyond the usual time required for hospitalization, or a mean of 24 days per patient. The financial impact of such a situation is apparent.

It has been estimated that every major infection costs someone $3000 to $5000. An orthopedic infection may run as high as $12,000 to $15,000. An infection rate of 5 per cent, or 50 per 1000, which equals $150,000 per 1000 cases has been reported in some series.[51] Certainly the collateral effects of a realistic and an attainable infection-control program represent substantial savings to the hospital. Moreover, the financial savings to public and private agencies and organizations providing or paying for medical care, and to those compensating for disability or loss of income should not be disregarded.

THE ASEPTIC BARRIER

The aseptic barrier constitutes the first line of defense against operative surgical infections. This barrier is comprised of a complicated series of procedures designed to prevent the entrance of microorganisms into operative wounds. It has been progressively extended during the past seventy years. Microbial invasion of the aseptic barrier can occur through many pathways, as shown in Figure 20-2. Of chief importance are the following:

- Dust and dirt on the operating room floor.
- Shedding of epidermal scales by staff.
- Discharge from respiratory passages of members of the operating team.
- The "carrier state" of patient and staff.
- Skin of the patient (carelessness in preparation of operative site).
- Conveyance of organisms on hands of staff.
- Wet surgical drapes and gowns.
- Clothing and bedding.
- Airborne contamination resulting from inefficient ventilating system.

In broader terms it may be said that it is generally accepted, but not al-

HOSPITAL SEPSIS

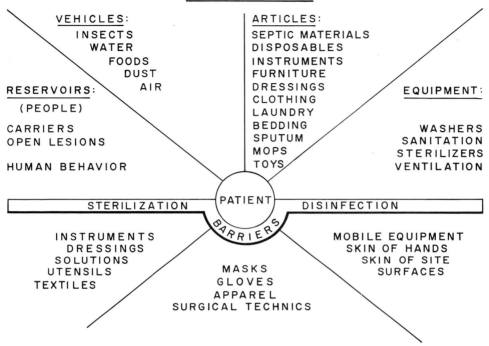

FIGURE 20-2. Basic elements that contribute to hospital sepsis and recognized barriers for protecting the patient against wound contamination.

ways respected, that the leading potential sources of operative-wound contamination are 1) the patient, 2) the operating team, including wound management, 3) visitors in the operating suite, 4) particulate matter in the air, 5) neglect in good housekeeping, and 6) instruments and supplies used in the operation.

The success of any program for the control of infections in a hospital appears to be dependent upon creating a continued awareness of the problem in the minds and actions of all those who care for patients. In summary then, it seems clear that hospitals should never be satisfied with the current rate of progress in reducing the incidence of infections. We must ever work to do more, to institute additional proven methods of control, to upgrade the level of environmental hygiene and sanitation, and with a resoluteness of purpose set forth on a program aimed at the eradication of disease.

REFERENCES

1. BURNEY, L. E.: Staphylococcal disease: National problem. In *Proc. Natl. Conf. on Hospital-Acquired Staphylococcal Disease, Sept. 1958.* Atlanta, Ga., U.S. Public Health Service, Communicable Disease Center, Oct. 1958.

2. RAVENHOLT, R. T., and RAVENHOLT, O. H.: Staphylococcal infections in the hospital and community. *Amer J Public Health, 48*:277-287, 1958.
3. GARRISON, F. H.: *History of Medicine,* 2nd ed. Philadelphia, Saunders, 1917, p. 406.
4. SIMPSON, J. Y.: Our existing system of hospitalism and its effects: Part I. *Edinburgh Med J, 14*:816-830, 1869.
5. BARNES, B. A.; BEHRINGER, G. E.; WHEELOCK, F. C., and WILKINS, E. W.: Postoperative sepsis: Trends and factors influencing sepsis over a 20-year period reviewed in 20,000 cases. *Ann Surg, 154*:585-598, 1961.
6. HOWE, C. H., and MOZDEN, P. J.: Postoperative infections: Current concepts. *Surg Clin N Amer,* June 1963, p. 859-882.
7. REPORT FROM PUBLIC HEALTH LAB. SERVICE. Infections acquired in medical wards. *J Hyg (Camb), 63*:457-477, 1965.
8. DUBOS, R. J.: *Mirage of Health: Utopias, Progress, and Biological Change.* New York, Harper, 1959.
9. DYKES, E. R., and ANDERSON, R.: Atraumatic technic—The sine qua non of operative wound infection prophylaxis. *Cleveland Clin Quart, 28*:157-165, 1961.
10. CULBERTSON, W. R.; ALTEMEIER, W. A.; GONZALEZ, L. L., and HILL, E. O.: Studies on the epidemiology of postoperative infection of clean operative wounds. *Ann Surg, 154*:599-610, 1961.
11. HOWE, C. W., and MARSTON, A. T.: Qualitative and quantitative bacteriologic studies on hospital air as related to postoperative wound sepsis. *J Lab Clin Med, 61*:808-819, 1963.
12. COHEN, L. S.; FEKETY, F. R., JR., and CLUFF, L. E.: Studies of the epidemiology of staphylococcal infection: VI. Infections in the surgical patient. *Ann Surg, 159*:321-334, 1964.
13. BASSETT, H. F. M.; FERGUSON, W. G.; HOFFMAN, E.; WALTON, M.; BLOWERS, R., and CONN, C. A.: Sources of staphylococcal infection in surgical wound sepsis. *J Hyg (Camb), 61*:83-94, 1963.
14. STEVENS, D. B.: Postoperative orthopaedic infections. *J Bone Joint Surg, 46-A*:96-102, 1964.
15. LAST, P. M.; HARBISON, P. A., and MARSH, J. A.: Bacteraemia after urological instrumentation. *Lancet, 1*:74-76, Jan. 8, 1966.
16. SANDUSKY, W. R.: Pseudomonas infections: Sources and cultural data in a general hospital with particular reference to surgical infections. *Ann Surg, 153*:996-1005, 1961.
17. AYLIFFE, G. A. J.; BARRY, D. R.; LOWBURY, E. J. L.; ROPER-HALL, M. J., and WALKER, W. M.: Postoperative infection with *Pseudomonas aeruginosa* in an eye hospital. *Lancet, 1*:1113-1117, May 21, 1966.
18. SUTTER, V. L., and HURST, V.: Sources of *Pseudomonas aeruginosa* infection in burns: Study of wound and rectal cultures with phage typing. *Ann Surg, 163*:597-602, 1966.
19. PHILLIPS, I.: Postoperative respiratory-tract infection with *Pseudomonas aeruginosa. Lancet, 1*:903-904, Apr. 23, 1966.
20. CHEYNE, W. W.: Suppuration and septic diseases. From *Wood's Medical and Surgical Monographs.* New York, W. Wood, 1890, vol. 8, p. 94.
21. WILLIAMS, R. E. O.; BLOWERS, R.; GARROD, L. P., and SHOOTER, R. A.: *Hospital Infection.* London, Lloyd-Luke, 1960, p. 79.
22. MILES, A. A.; MILES, E. M., and BURKE, J.: Value and duration of defense reactions of the skin to primary lodgement of bacteria. *Brit J Exp Path, 38*:79-96, 1957.
23. ELEK, S. D., and CONEN, P. E.: Virulence of *Staphylococcus pyogenes* for man. A study of the problems of wound infections. *Brit J Exp Path, 38*:573-586, 1957.
24. BLOWERS, R.: Postoperative sepsis. *Trans Ass Industr Med Officers, 13*:118-121, 1964.
25. WALTER, C. W.; KUNDSIN, R. B., and BRUBAKER, M. M.: The incidence of airborne wound infection during operation. *JAMA, 186*:908-913, 1963.
26. NAHMIAS, A. J., and EICKHOFF, T. C.: Medical progress. Staphylococcal infections in hospitals. *New Eng, J Med, 265*:77-177, 1961.
27. WALTER, C. W., and KUNDSIN, R.: The floor as a reservoir of hospital infections. *Surg Gynec Obstet, 111*:412, 1960.

28. WESLEY-JAMES, O., and ALDER, V.: Staphylococci in septic fingers. *J Clin Path, 14*:96, 1961.

29. CROSS, D. F.; BENCHIMOL, A., and DIMOND, E. G.: The faucet aerator—A source of pseudomonas infection. *New Eng J Med, 274*:1430-1431, 1966.

30. KEOWN, K. K.; GILMAN, R. A., and BAILEY, C. P.: Open heart surgery: Anaesthesia and surgical experience. *JAMA, 165*:781-787, 1957.

31. PLOTKIN, S. A., and AUSTRIAN, R.: Bacteremia caused by *Pseudomonas Sp.* following the use of materials stored in solutions of a cationic surface-active agent. *Amer J Med Sci, 235*:621-627, 1958.

32. BYRNE, E. B.: Viral hepatitis: An occupational hazard of medical personnel. *JAMA, 195*:118-120, 1966.

33. MACPHERSON, C. R.: Facial tissues: another source of hospital infections? *Ohio Med J, 59*:266-267, 1963.

34. TURCK, M.; GOFFE, B., and PETERSDORF, R. G.: The urethral catheter and urinary tract infection. *J Urol, 88*:834-837, 1962.

35. KOEPKE, G. H., and CHRISTOPHER, R. P.: Contamination of whirlpool baths during treatment of infected wounds. *Arch Phys Med, 46*:261-263, 1965.

36. SUTTER, V. L.; HURST, V.; GROSSMAN, M., and CALONJE, R.: Source of significance of *Pseudomonas aeruginosa* in sputum. *JAMA, 197*:854-858, 1966.

37. SUSSMAN, M., and STEVENS, J.: Pseudomonas pyocyanea wound infection—an outbreak in an orthopaedic unit. *Lancet, II*:734-736, 1960.

38. BAHNSON, H. T.; SPENCER, F. C., and BENNETT, I. L., JR.: Staphylococcal infections of the heart and great vessels due to silk sutures. *Ann Surg, 146*:399-406, 1957.

39. DULL, H. B.: Syringe-transmitted hepatitis: A recent epidemic in historical perspective. *JAMA, 176*:413-418, 1961.

40. DOUGHERTY, W. J., and ALTMAN, R.: A physician-related outbreak of hepatitis. *Amer J Public Health, 53*:1618-1622, 1963.

41. KING, B., and MURPHY, O. M.: Water bath was culprit in nursery infection. *Mod Hosp, 102*:117, 1964.

42. RUBENSTEIN, A. D., and FOWLER, R. N.: Salmonellosis of the newborn with transmission by delivery room resuscitators. *Amer J Public Health, 45*:1109-1114, 1955.

43. CLAYTON, E., and GRAEVENITZ, A. VON: Nonpigmented *Serratia marcescens. JAMA, 197*:1059-1064, 1966.

44. ROGERS, K. B.: Pseudomonas infections in a children's hospital. *J Appl Bact, 23*:533, 1960.

45. PLOTKIN, S. A., and MCKITRICK, J. C.: Nosocomial meningitis of the newborn caused by a flavobacterium. *JAMA, 198*:662-664, 1966.

46. MOORE, B., and FORMAN, A.: An outbreak of urinary *Pseudomonas aeruginosa* infection acquired during urological operations. *Lancet, 11*:929-931, 1966.

47. MELENEY, F. M.: Infection in clean operative wounds: A nine-year study. *Surg Gynec Obstet, 60*:264, 1935.

48. LJUNGQVIST, U.: Wound sepsis after clean operations. *Lancet, 1*:1095-1097, 1964.

49. PUBLIC HEALTH LAB. SERVICE: Incidence of surgical wound infection in England and Wales. *Lancet, 2*:659, 1960.

50. KOCH, M. L.; LEPLEY, D., JR.; SCHROEDER, M., and SMITH, M. B.: Study of staphylococcic infections occurring on a surgical service. *JAMA, 169*:83, 99, 89, 105, 1959.

51. ADAMS, R., and FAHLMAN, B.: Sterility in operating rooms. *Surg Gynec Obstet, 110*:367-376, 1960.

APPENDIX

TEMPERATURE CONVERSION CHART

1°F = 0.56°C
1°C = 1.8°F

Degrees C	Temp. in °C or °F To Be Converted	Degrees F	Degrees C	Temp. in °C or °F To Be Converted	Degrees F	Degrees C	Temp. in °C or °F To Be Converted	Degrees F	Degrees C	Temp. in °C or °F To Be Converted	Degrees F
−17.8	0	32	7.2	45	113.0	48.9	120	248.0	98.9	210	410.0
−17.2	1	33.8	7.8	46	114.8	50.0	122	251.6	100.0	212	413.6
−16.7	2	35.6	8.3	47	116.6	51.1	124	255.2	101.1	214	417.2
−16.1	3	37.4	8.9	48	118.4	52.2	126	258.8	102.2	216	420.8
−15.6	4	39.2	9.4	49	120.2	53.3	128	262.4	103.3	218	424.4
−15.0	5	41.0	10.0	50	122.0	54.4	130	266.0	104.4	220	428.0
−14.4	6	42.8	10.6	51	123.8	55.6	132	269.6	105.6	222	431.6
−13.9	7	44.6	11.1	52	125.6	56.7	134	273.2	106.7	224	435.2
−13.3	8	46.4	11.7	53	127.4	57.8	136	276.8	107.8	226	438.8
−12.8	9	48.2	12.2	54	129.6	58.9	138	280.4	108.9	228	442.4
−12.2	10	50.0	12.8	55	131.0	60.0	140	284.0	110.0	230	446.0
−11.7	11	51.8	13.3	56	132.8	61.1	142	287.6	111.1	232	449.6
−11.1	12	53.6	13.9	57	134.6	62.2	144	291.2	112.2	234	453.2
−10.6	13	55.4	14.4	58	136.4	63.3	146	294.8	113.3	236	456.8
−10.0	14	57.2	15.0	59	138.2	64.4	148	298.4	114.4	238	460.4
−9.4	15	59.0	15.6	60	140.0	65.6	150	302.0	115.6	240	464.0
−8.9	16	60.8	16.7	62	143.6	66.7	152	305.6	116.7	242	467.6
−8.3	17	62.6	17.8	64	147.2	67.8	154	309.2	117.8	244	471.2
−7.8	18	64.4	18.9	66	150.8	68.9	156	312.8	118.9	246	474.8
−7.2	19	66.2	20.0	68	154.4	70.0	158	316.4	120.0	248	478.4
−6.7	20	68.0	21.1	70	158.0	71.1	160	320.0	121.1	250	482.0
−6.1	21	69.8	22.2	72	161.6	72.2	162	323.6	123.9	255	491.0
−5.6	22	71.6	23.3	74	165.2	73.3	164	327.2	126.7	260	500.0
−5.0	23	73.4	24.4	76	168.8	74.4	166	330.8	129.4	265	509.0
−4.4	24	75.2	25.6	78	172.4	75.6	168	334.4	132.2	270	518.0
−3.9	25	77.0	26.7	80	176.0	76.7	170	338.0	135.0	275	527.0
−3.3	26	78.8	27.8	82	179.6	77.8	172	341.6	137.8	280	536.0
−2.8	27	80.6	28.9	84	183.2	78.9	174	345.2	140.6	285	545.0
−2.2	28	82.4	30.0	86	186.8	80.0	176	348.8	143.3	290	554.0
−1.7	29	84.2	31.1	88	190.4	81.1	178	352.2	146.1	295	563.0
−1.1	30	86.0	32.2	90	194.0	82.8	180	356.0	148.9	300	572.0
−0.6	31	87.8	33.3	92	197.6	83.3	182	359.6	154.4	310	590.0
0	32	89.6	34.4	94	201.2	84.4	184	363.2	160.0	320	608.0
0.6	33	91.4	35.6	96	204.8	85.6	186	366.8	165.6	330	626.0
1.1	34	93.2	36.7	98	208.4	86.7	188	370.4	171.1	340	644.0
1.7	35	95.0	37.8	100	212.0	87.8	190	374.0	176.7	350	662.0
2.2	36	96.8	38.9	102	215.6	88.9	192	377.6	182.2	360	680.0
2.8	37	98.6	40.0	104	219.2	90.0	194	381.2	187.8	370	698.0
3.3	38	100.4	41.1	106	222.8	91.1	196	384.8	193.3	380	716.0
3.9	39	102.2	42.2	108	226.4	92.2	198	388.4	198.9	390	734.0
4.4	40	104.0	43.3	110	230.0	93.3	200	392.0	204.4	400	752.0
5.0	41	105.8	44.4	112	233.6	94.4	202	395.6	210.0	410	770.0
5.6	42	107.6	45.6	114	237.2	95.6	204	399.2	215.6	420	788.0
6.1	43	109.4	46.7	116	240.8	96.7	206	402.8	221.1	430	806.0
6.7	44	111.2	47.8	118	244.4	97.8	208	406.4	226.7	440	824.0

VAPOR PRESSURE OF WATER

°F	°C	Pounds per Square Inch	Inches of Mercury	Millimeters of Mercury	°F	°C	Pounds per Square Inch	Inches of Mercury	Millimeters of Mercury
32	0.00	0.08858	0.18035	4.5809	250	121.11	29.823	60.720	1542.3
35	1.67	0.09991	0.20342	5.1668	260	126.67	35.424	72.124	1832.0
40	4.44	0.12164	0.24766	6.2906	270	132.22	41.853	85.213	2164.4
45	7.22	0.14745	0.30021	7.6254	280	137.78	49.196	100.16	2544.2
50	10.00	0.17798	0.36237	9.2040	290	143.33	57.547	117.17	2976.0
55	12.78	0.21394	0.43558	11.064	300	148.89	67.002	136.42	3465.0
60	15.56	0.25614	0.52150	13.246	310	154.44	77.663	158.12	4016.3
65	18.33	0.30549	0.62198	15.798	320	160.00	89.640	182.51	4635.7
70	21.11	0.36297	0.73901	18.771	330	165.56	103.05	209.81	5329.1
75	23.89	0.42969	0.87485	22.221	340	171.11	117.99	240.22	6101.8
80	26.67	0.50689	1.0320	26.214	350	176.67	134.61	274.06	6961.2
85	29.44	0.59588	1.2132	30.816	360	182.22	153.02	311.55	7913.3
90	32.22	0.69816	1.4215	36.105	370	187.78	173.36	352.95	8965.1
95	35.00	0.81537	1.6601	42.167	380	193.33	195.76	398.56	10124
100	37.78	0.94926	1.9327	49.091	390	198.89	220.35	448.62	11395
105	40.56	1.1018	2.2432	56.979	400	204.44	247.29	503.48	12789
110	43.33	1.2750	2.5959	65.936	410	210.00	276.73	563.42	14311
115	46.11	1.4711	2.9952	76.079	420	215.56	308.82	628.77	15971
120	48.89	1.6927	3.4463	87.537	430	221.11	343.72	699.82	17776
125	51.67	1.9423	3.9544	100.44	440	226.67	381.59	776.93	19734
130	54.44	2.2227	4.5255	114.95	450	232.22	422.69	860.60	21860
135	57.22	2.5373	5.1659	131.22	460	237.78	466.90	950.60	24145
140	60.00	2.8890	5.8821	149.41	470	243.33	514.68	1047.9	26617
145	62.78	3.2814	6.6809	169.70	480	248.89	566.15	1152.7	29278
150	65.56	3.7182	7.7503	192.29	490	254.44	621.45	1265.3	32138
155	68.33	4.2034	8.5581	217.38	500	260.00	680.81	1386.1	35208
160	71.11	4.7412	9.6531	245.19	510	265.56	744.38	1515.6	38496
165	73.89	5.3358	10.864	275.94	520	271.11	812.42	1654.1	42014
170	76.67	5.9923	12.200	309.89	530	276.67	855.09	1802.0	45772
175	79.44	6.7156	13.673	347.30	540	282.22	962.63	1959.9	49782
180	82.22	7.5109	15.292	388.42	550	287.78	1045.3	2128.2	54056
185	85.00	8.3886	17.069	433.56	560	293.33	1133.2	2307.3	58605
190	87.76	9.3392	19.015	482.98	570	298.89	1226.7	2497.6	63439
195	90.56	10.385	21.143	537.03	580	304.44	1326.0	2699.8	68576
200	93.33	11.526	23.466	596.05	590	310.00	1431.4	2914.4	74026
205	96.11	12.769	25.998	660.36	600	315.56	1543.2	3143.0	79805
210	98.89	14.122	28.753	730.34	610	321.11	1661.6	3383.1	85932
212	100.00	14.696	29.921	760.00	620	326.67	1787.1	3638.5	92419
215	101.67	15.592	31.745	806.34	630	332.22	1919.8	3908.8	99283
220	104.44	17.186	34.990	888.76	640	337.78	2060.3	4194.8	106549
225	107.22	18.912	38.504	978.02	650	343.33	2208.8	4497.2	114229
230	110.00	20.779	42.306	1074.6	660	348.89	2366.0	4817.2	122357
235	112.78	22.794	46.409	1178.8	670	354.44	2532.3	5155.7	130955
240	115.56	24.968	50.834	1291.2	680	360.00	2708.4	5514.3	140065
245	118.33	27.308	55.598	1412.2	690	365.56	2895.3	5894.8	149730
					700	371.11	3094.3	6299.9	160019
					705.47	374.15	3209.5	6534.5	165977

STEAM CONSUMPTION AND RECOMMENDED BOILER CAPACITY

STEAM STERILIZERS AND WASHER-STERILIZER FOR HOSPITALS

| CHAMBER SIZE (INCHES) | AIR REMOVAL SYSTEM | JACKET | | CHAMBER | RECOMMENDED BOILER CAPACITY (HP) |
| | | STEAM CONSUMPTION AT 50-80 psig FOR STERILIZERS WHICH ARE INSULATED EXCEPT FOR CHAMBER DOOR(S) | | | |
		HEAT-UP WITHIN 30 MINUTES (LBS./HR.)	STANDBY (LBS./HR.)	CONTINUOUS PROCESSING REQUIREMENT (LBS./HR.)	
16x26		20	4	25	1.5
17½x26				21	1.5
20x38		40	8	45	2.0
21½x38	Gravity			28	2.0
16x16x26		35	7	35(50)*	1.5
16x16x26 Washer-Sterilizer				242	7.0
20x20x38		50	9	60(70)*	2.0
24x36x36	Gravity	85	17	80(140)*	4.0
	Mechanical	85	17	190	6.0
24x36x48	Gravity	100	19	105(165)*	6.0
	Mechanical	100	19	255	8.0
24x36x60	Gravity	120	21	140(200)*	6.0
	Mechanical	120	21	335	10.0

* Values in parentheses are for general purpose high speed sterilizers.

1. Steam pressure (50–80 psig) must be dynamic at the sterilizer.
2. The equipment will accommodate line pressure of 50–80 psig. If supply pressure exceeds this, provide a reducing valve. This valve is not included with the sterilizing equipment.
3. Steam consumption values shown above are realistic guide lines for proper sterilizer operation. However, poor steam quality, lack of proper sterilizer insulation, or special loading conditions can drastically increase steam requirements.

STEAM CONSUMPTION AND RECOMMENDED BOILER CAPACITY

STEAM STERILIZERS FOR BIOMEDICAL AND INDUSTRIAL LABORATORIES

CHAMBER SIZE (INCHES)	AIR REMOVAL SYSTEM	JACKET		CHAMBER	RECOMMENDED BOILER CAPACITY (HP)
		STEAM CONSUMPTION AT 50-80 psig SEE NOTE BELOW REGARDING INSULATION			
		HEAT-UP WITHIN 30 MINUTES (LBS./HR.)	STANDBY (LBS./HR.)	CONTINUOUS PROCESSING REQUIREMENT (LBS./HR.)	
24x36x36	Gravity	85	17	80	4
	Mechanical			190	6
24x36x48	Gravity	100	19	105	6
	Mechanical			255	8
24x36x60	Gravity	120	21	140	6
	Mechanical			335	10
36x42x84	Gravity	260	37	250	8
	Mechanical			400	14
42x48x84	Gravity	380	44	350	11
	Mechanical			560	19
48x54x84	Gravity	400	56	400	14
	Mechanical			700	23
48x84x84	Gravity	500	82	600	20
	Mechanical			1000	33
62x66x84	Gravity	500	82	600	20
	Mechanical			1000	33
62x84x84	Gravity	550	97	700	23
	Mechanical			1200	40

1. Steam pressure (50 to 80 psig) must be dynamic at the sterilizer.
2. The equipment will accommodate line pressure of 50 to 80 psig. If supply pressure exceeds this, provide a reducing valve. This valve is not included with the sterilizing equipment.
3. Steam consumption values shown above are realistic guide lines for proper sterilizer operation. However, poor steam quality, lack of proper sterilizer insulation, or special loading conditions can drastically increase steam requirements.

HEAT LOSSES

Steam Sterilizers

CHAMBER SIZE (INCHES)	HEAT RELEASED (BTU PER HOUR–IN THOUSANDS) TO ROOM AT 70 F (CONTINUOUS OPERATION)[1]							UPON REMOVAL AND COOLING OF LOAD (MAXIMUM)
	LOSSES FROM STERILIZER ONLY[2]							
	RECESSED MOUNTED				WITH CABINET ENCLOSURE	WITHOUT ENCLOSURE		
	FRONT OF WALL	BACK OF WALL		BETWEEN WALLS				
	Single or Double Door	Single Door	Double Door	Double Door	Single Door	Single Door	Double Door	
16x26	1.2	1.1			2.3			5.2
17½x26	1.2	1.1			2.3			5.2
20x38	2.6	4.5			7.0			11.7
21½x38	2.6	4.5			7.0			11.0
16x16x26	1.6	2.7	3.5		4.3			6.9
16x16x26 Washer-Sterilizer	1.6	2.7	3.5		4.3			2.4
20x20x38	2.5	4.5	5.3	1.7	7.0			15.2
24x36x36	5.0	7.5	11.3	6.3	12.55			20.2
24x36x48	5.0	9.6	13.8	8.8	14.65			27.6
24x36x60	5.0	11.8	16.5	10.5	16.8			34.5
36x42x84	15.0	19.5	34.0	19.0		34.5	49.0	81.0
42x48x84	19.0	22.5	41.0	22.0		41.5	60.0	110.0
48x54x84	27.0	26.0	52.0	25.0		53.0	79.0	147.0
48x84x84	40.0	37.0	71.0	36.0		77.0	114.0	232.0
62x66x84	38.0	38.0	70.0	33.0		76.0	108.0	236.0
62x84x84	49.0	43.0	84.0	36.5		92.0	133.0	285.0

[1] Cylindrical, small and medium rectangular sterilizers as insulated at the factory with 1-inch thick aluminum-covered glass fiber over exterior chamber walls. Data shown for large rectangular sterilizers are based on sterilizers being insulated.

[2] Total heat loss = sterilizer loss + load cooling loss.

PRODUCTIVITY OF BIOMEDICAL AND INDUSTRIAL LABORATORY STERILIZERS

Chamber Size (Inches)	Type Load	Productive Capacity see note 1	Laboratory/ Isothermal 250 F	Laboratory/ Isothermal 270 F	Cyclomatic/ Thermostatic 250 F	Cyclomatic/ Thermostatic 270 F	Industrial Cyclomatic/ Thermostatic 250 F	Industrial Cyclomatic/ Thermostatic 270 F	Vacamatic "S" see note 3	Vacamatic "RSP" see note 3
24x36x36"	Hard goods	14 Units		8-14		8-14		8-14	21-14	23-26
	Fabrics	6 Units			49-55		49-55		18-22	20-24
	Liquids	120 Units	68-76		68-76		68-76		75-85	75-85
24x36x48"	Hard goods	16 Units		9-15		9-15		9-15	22-26	24-28
	Fabrics	8 Units			53-59		53-59		21-26	23-29
	Liquids	165 Units	78-87		78-87		78-87		83-93	83-93
24x36x60"	Hard goods	20 Units		9-15		9-15		9-15	24-27	26-29
	Fabrics	10 Units			56-62		56-62		25-27	27-29
	Liquids	210 Units	87-98		87-98		87-98		92-100	92-100
36x42x84"	Hard goods	48 Cu Ft			16-20		16-20		32-36	36-40
	Fabrics				76-82		76-82			
42x48x84"	Hard goods	68 Cu Ft					18-22		34-38	38-42
	Fabrics							81-87		
48x54x84"	Hard goods	92 Cu Ft					20-24		42-46	46-50
	Fabrics							86-92		
48x84x84"	Hard goods	153 Cu Ft					21-25		44-48	48-52
	Fabrics							89-95		
62x66x84"	Hard goods	155 Cu Ft					21-25		44-48	48-52
	Fabrics							89-95		
62x84x84"	Hard goods	204 Cu Ft					29-34		52-56	56-60
	Fabrics							97-104		

Notes:

1. Includes allowances for shelves or other loading equipment, space for steam circulation and correct loading; figures shown are based on test loads as follows:

   For Medium Sterilizers
   (Through 24×36×60")

   Hard goods—unwrapped stainless steel adult bedpans.
   Fabrics—packages (each 12×12×20") of muslin wrappers, surgical gowns, sheets or similar linens.
   Liquids—one liter capped and collared borosilicate glass flasks each containing 1050 ml water.

   For Large Sterilizers
   (36×42×84" and Larger)

   animal cages and racks.

   absorbent cotton, gauze bandages.

   (Note: Productive chamber capacities and cycle times for liquid loads in large sterilizers will vary widely according to product and processing requirements. (1)

2. Cycle time is based on starting cycle with sterilizer load at 70° to 76°F, atmospheric pressure about 14.7 psia, and steam supply of 50 to 80 psig at the sterilizer. Does not include time for loading and unloading the sterilizer, opening and closing door or achieving proper jacket pressure. Time to achieve jacket pressure would be considered only at the beginning of each work day as it is normal practice to reduce processing time to a minimum by maintaining constant jacket pressure throughout the work day.

3. Liquids processed with sterilizer operating on the gravity air removal principle at 250°F.

INDEX